CW00456447

Lecture Notes in Electrical Engineering

Volume 545

The book series *Lecture Notes in Electrical Engineering* (LNEE) publishes the latest developments in Electrical Engineering - quickly, informally and in high quality. While original research reported in proceedings and monographs has traditionally formed the core of LNEE, we also encourage authors to submit books devoted to supporting student education and professional training in the various fields and applications areas of electrical engineering. The series cover classical and emerging topics concerning:

- Communication Engineering, Information Theory and Networks
- Electronics Engineering and Microelectronics
- Signal, Image and Speech Processing
- Wireless and Mobile Communication
- Circuits and Systems
- Energy Systems, Power Electronics and Electrical Machines
- Electro-optical Engineering
- Instrumentation Engineering
- Avionics Engineering
- Control Systems
- Internet-of-Things and Cybersecurity
- Biomedical Devices, MEMS and NEMS

For general information about this book series, comments or suggestions, please contact leontina. dicecco@springer.com.

To submit a proposal or request further information, please contact the Publishing Editor in your country:

China

Jasmine Dou, Associate Editor (jasmine.dou@springer.com)

India

Swati Meherishi, Executive Editor (swati.meherishi@springer.com)
Aninda Bose, Senior Editor (aninda.bose@springer.com)

Japan

Takeyuki Yonezawa, Editorial Director (takeyuki.yonezawa@springer.com)

South Korea

Smith (Ahram) Chae, Editor (smith.chae@springer.com)

Southeast Asia

Ramesh Nath Premnath, Editor (ramesh.premnath@springer.com)

USA, Canada:

Michael Luby, Senior Editor (michael.luby@springer.com)

All other Countries:

Leontina Di Cecco, Senior Editor (leontina.dicecco@springer.com)
Christoph Baumann, Executive Editor (christoph.baumann@springer.com)

** Indexing: The books of this series are submitted to ISI Proceedings, EI-Compendex, SCOPUS, MetaPress, Web of Science and Springerlink **

More information about this series at http://www.springer.com/series/7818

V. Sridhar · M. C. Padma ·
K. A. Radhakrishna Rao
Editors

Emerging Research in Electronics, Computer Science and Technology

Proceedings of International Conference, ICERECT 2018

Volume 2

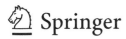 Springer

Editors
V. Sridhar
Department of Electronics and
Communication Engineering
PES College of Engineering
Mandya, Karnataka, India

M. C. Padma
Department of Computer Science
and Engineering
PES College of Engineering
Mandya, Karnataka, India

K. A. Radhakrishna Rao
Department of Electronics and
Communication Engineering
PES College of Engineering
Mandya, Karnataka, India

ISSN 1876-1100   ISSN 1876-1119 (electronic)
Lecture Notes in Electrical Engineering
ISBN 978-981-13-5801-2   ISBN 978-981-13-5802-9 (eBook)
https://doi.org/10.1007/978-981-13-5802-9

Library of Congress Control Number: 2018965440

This Springer imprint is published by the registered company Springer Nature Singapore Pte Ltd.
The registered company address is: 152 Beach Road, #21-01/04 Gateway East, Singapore 189721, Singapore

Preface

This conference proceedings volume contains the written versions of most of the contributions presented during the Third International Conference on Emerging Research in Electronics, Computer science and Technology—ICERECT 18, held during 23 and 24 August 2018, at PES College of Engineering (PESCE), Mandya, Karnataka, India. The conference was held in association with Binghamton University, State University of New York, USA. The vast experience of PESCE in organizing international conference has come to use in bringing out this proceedings. PESCE is a pioneering technical school decimating engineering knowledge for 56 years. The accreditation from NBA and NAAC is testimonials to its credit. Being the beneficiary of World Bank's Technical Quality Improvement Programme (TEQIP) component 1.3, this conference and publication of this proceedings are funded by TEQIP-III.

The motivation for this international conference is due to the fact that the present trends in computers and communications have received attention recently and noticeable progress towards useful applications to mankind is reported. The conference aims to provide an excellent international forum for sharing knowledge and results in theory, methodology and applications in electronics, electrical and computer science. The theme of the conference has been kept generic intentionally with an aim to provide a wide exposure to delegates of this conference. This proceedings while it is exhaustive meets the quality specifications. Articles from wide areas of electronics, communication, computer science and electrical engineering are included.

This proceedings has 121 research articles from different areas of research of both theoretical nature and application nature. We are very sure it will be of great use to budding researchers to kick start and to progress their research as well.

The research papers are organized into three main streams of electronics, electrical and computer technology for the ease of readers. The presentation sessions were also held in the same manner. The areas of electronics cover signal processing and its applications, wireless technology, solid-state devices, VLSI, radar and antennas. The field of computer technology has a focus on algorithms for image and video processing, parallel algorithms, IoT, data mining, machine learning, cloud computing and big data analytics. The papers in the electrical engineering category cover power systems, power converts, drives, machines and control.

The experience of three ICERECT has been very pleasant and made us look forward to the fourth ICERECT. PESCE has the potential and willingness to conduct many other international conferences, and researchers can look forward to many in the days ahead.

Mandya, India   Dr. V. Sridhar
                                                         Dr. K. A. Radhakrishna Rao
                                                                Dr. M. C. Padma

Acknowledgements

This special issue is a result of collective endeavours from several research scholars and scientists from electronics and communication, computer science and engineering, electrical and electronics and information science and engineering from various parts of India and abroad. The authors are indebted to their efforts and their outstanding technical contributions. We would like to express our appreciations to Springer publishers for helping us to create this special issue on the proceedings of the Third International Conference on Emerging Research in Electronics, Computer science and Technology—ICERECT 18, held during 23 and 24 August 2018, in association with Binghamton University, State University of New York, USA, at PESCE campus.

We would like to thank NPIU, TEQIP, Department of Technical Education and Government of Karnataka for extending their financial support to this conference. We would also like to thank TEQIP mentor and coordinator of our institute. We also express our thanks to the editorial board of Springer LNEE. Our thanks are due to President and Trustees of PET® for their constant support and encouragement in organizing this conference successfully.

We thank all our patrons and especially Dr. V. Sridhar profusely for his encouragement to research activities in our institute.

Thanks are also due to the conference committee chair, Dr. H. V. Ravindra, and other committee members, heads of various departments, specifically the organizing departments, CSE, ECE, EE and ISE, the reviewers of the research papers, chairpersons and coordinators of various sessions, staff and student volunteers who made this conference a grand success.

Contents

Editors and Contributors

About the Editors

Dr. V. Sridhar obtained his B.E. from University of Mysore in electronics and communication engineering, M.E. from Jadavpur University, Calcutta, in electronics and telecommunication engineering and Ph.D. from Institute of Technology, New Delhi. He carried out postdoctoral research in the Department of Electrical and Electronics, Universiti Tenaga Nasional, 43009 Kajang, Malaysia. He is serving this institution since 1982, and presently, he is Principal of this institution. His fields of interest are VLSI design, digital signal processing, biomedical engineering and instrumentation and cognitive studies, computer and mobile communications. He was also Registrar (Evaluation) at Visvesvaraya Technological University, Belgaum, from 2004 to 2006 and Acting Vice Chancellor for 6 months. He has more than 100 research publications to his credit in conferences and journals. He has guided ten students for the doctoral degree, and many are pursuing it under his supervision. He is instrumental in establishing a CAD Centre for VLSI design as Center of Excellence at the institution. He is Member of IEEE (M), IETE (F), ISTE (M) and BMSI (M) and has participated in various national and international conferences and seminars in India and abroad.

Dr. M. C. Padma obtained her B.E. from University of Mysore in computer science and engineering, M.Sc. Tech. by research from University of Mysore and Ph.D. from VTU, Belgaum. She is serving this institution since 1990 and presently heading the Department of Computer Science and Engineering. Her fields of interest are image processing, pattern recognition, natural language processing, machine translation, artificial intelligence and expert systems, document image analysis and recognition. She has published about 65 papers in national and international journals. She is also guiding research candidates for Ph.D. programme. She is Life Member of ISTE, IEI, AKECTA, IVPR and CSI and has participated in various national and international conferences and seminars in India and abroad.

Dr. K. A. Radhakrishna Rao obtained his B.E. from University of Mysore in electronics and communication engineering, M.Tech. from IIT Madras and Ph.D. from IISc Bangalore. He is serving this institution since 1985, and presently, he is Professor and heads the Department of Electronics and Communication Engineering. His fields of interest are signal processing, biometrics, medical image processing and embedded systems. He has published about 50 papers in conferences and journals. He is involved in guiding research candidates for Ph.D. programme. He is Senior Member of IEEE and resumed charge of student branch counsellor right from its inception. Apart from this, he is Life Member of BMSI, IETE and ISTE and has participated in various national and international conferences and seminars in India and abroad.

Contributors

Mohammed Ahmed Ali Abdualrhman Department of Computer Science and Engineering, PES College of Engineering, Mandya, Karnataka, India;
Department of Computer Science, College of Engineering and Information Technology, Al-Saeed University, Taiz, Yemen

John M. Acken Department of Electrical & Computer Engineering, Portland State University, Portland, USA

A. Adarsh Department of Electronics and Communication Engineering, Dayananda Sagar Academy of Technology & Management (DSATM), Bangalore, India

H. J. Adarsha Centre for Research in Medical Devices, National University of Ireland (NUI), Galway, Ireland

Rudreshi Addamani PES College of Engineering, Mandya, Karnataka, India

Vinayak Adimule Department of Chemistry, Jain College of Engineering and Technology, Hubli, Karnataka, India

Animikh Aich RNS Institute of Technology, Bangalore, India

Maganalli S. Akhil Global Academy of Technology, Bangalore, India

V. Akhilesh RNS Institute of Technology, Bangalore, India

Basavaraj S. Anami KLE Institute of Technology, Hubballi, India

M. Anand Kumar Center for Computational Engineering and Networking (CEN), Amrita School of Engineering, Coimbatore, Amrita Vishwa Vidyapeetham, Coimbatore, India

Harsha Anantwar Dayananda Sagar College of Engineering, Bangalore, India

K. M. Anil Kumar Department of CS & E, Sri Jayachamarajendra College of Engineering, Mysuru, India

H. Anusha Department of Electrical and Electronics Engineering, Siddaganga Institute of Technology, Tumakuru, India

U. Arjun Department of IS & E, PESITM, Shivamogga, India

M. R. Arulalan Department of ECE, NITK, Surathkal, India

Vanishri Arun SJCE, JSS Science and Technology University, Mysuru, India

B. V. Arunkumar Apollo BGS Hospital, Mysuru, India

Rahul Manjunath Ashlesh Tandon School of Engineering, New York University, New York City, USA

Gangadhar Bagihalli Department of Chemistry, KLE Institute of Technology, Hubballi, Karnataka, India

M. K. Banga Department of Computer Science, Dayananda Sagar University, Bangalore, Karnataka, India

S. S. Behera Indian Institute of Technology Bhubaneswar, Bhubaneswar, India

R. Bhagya Department of Telecommunication Engineering, R.V. College of Engineering, Bangalore, India

S. R. Bhagyashree Department of ECE, ATME College of Engineering, Mysuru, India

C. Bhanuprakash Department of Master of Computer Applications, Siddaganga Institute of Technology, Tumakuru, India

R. K. Bharathi Department of Master of Computer Application, Sri Jayachamarajendra College of Engineering, JSS Science & Technology University, Mysuru, Karnataka, India

N. S. Bhargavi R.V. College of Engineering, Bangalore, India

Mahabaleshwar Bhat Department of Electronics & Communication Engineering, PES University, Bangalore, India

G. Bhavya Department of ISE, BMSIT&M, Bangalore, India

S. N. Bhavya Siddaganga Institute of Technology, Tumakuru, Karnataka, India

S. P. Bhavyashree Department of Computer Science and Engineering, University Visvesvaraya College of Engineering, Bangalore University, Bangalore, India

R. C. Biradar REVA University, Bangalore, India

Debdas Bowmik High Energy Materials Research Laboratory, Defence Research and Development Organization, Ministry of Defence, Government of India, Pune, India

S. M. Bramesh Department of IS & E, PES College of Engineering, Mandya, India

Buddesab Department of Computer Science and Engineering, University Visvesvaraya College of Engineering, Bangalore University, Bangalore, India

J. Chaithra BMS Institute of Technology and Management, Bangalore, India

D. G. Chandani Department of Electronics & Communication, B.V. Bhoomaraddi College of Engineering & Technology, Hubli, Karnataka, India

K. T. Chandrashekhara Department of ISE, BMSIT&M, Bangalore, India

S. Chandrika Department of Electronics and Communication Engineering, Dayananda Sagar Academy of Technology & Management (DSATM), Bangalore, India

Channegowda Department of Animal Husbandry & Veterinary Services, Mysuru, India

Mohamed Rafiq A. Chapparband Department of Electrical Engineering, UVCE, Bangalore, India

Ruhul Amin Chaudhary Lovely Professional University, Phagwara, Punjab, India

G. Chayashree Department of Information Science and Engineering, GSSS Institute of Technology, Mysuru, India

G. S. Chethan Department of Information Science & Engineering, JNNCE, Shivamogga, India

Y. D. Chethan Maharaja Institute of Technology, Srirangapatna Tq, Mandya, Karnataka, India

Ruhul Amin Choudhury Lovely Professional University, Phagwara, Punjab, India

G. Deborah BMS Institute of Technology and Management, Bangalore, India

Deepika Department of CS & E, PES College of Engineering, Mandya, India

Vijayasenan Deepu Department of ECE, NITK, Surathkal, India

T. M. Devegowda Department of Mechanical Engineering, PES College of Engineering, Mandya, Karnataka, India

Kunj Dhonde Department of Electronics and Communication Engineering, Amrita School of Engineering, Amrita Vishwa Vidyapeetham, Bangalore, India

Praveen M. Dhulavvagol School of Computer Science & Engineering, KLE Technological University, Hubli, Karnataka, India

M. G. Ganavi Department of Telecommunication Engineering, R.V. College of Engineering, Bangalore, India

J. Gayathri BMS Institute of Technology and Management, Bangalore, India

Bhat Geetalaxmi Jayaram Department of ISE, The National Institute of Engineering Mysuru, Mysuru, India

T. M. Geethanjali ISE Department, PES College of Engineering, Mandya, Karnataka, India

Siripurapu Geethika Computer Science and Engineering, National Institute of Technology, Andhra Pradesh, Tadepalligudam, Andhra Pradesh, India

C. N. Gireesh Babu Department of ISE, BMSIT&M, Bangalore, India

Anitha Girish JSS Academy of Higher Education and Research, Mysuru, India

Athira Gopalakrishnan Center for Computational Engineering and Networking (CEN), Amrita School of Engineering Coimbatore, Amrita Vishwa Vidyapeetham, Coimbatore, India

E. A. Gopalakrishnan Center for Computational Engineering and Networking (CEN), Amrita School of Engineering, Coimbatore, Amrita Vishwa Vidyapeetham, Coimbatore, India

P. S. Gotekar Priyadarshini College of Engineering, RTMN University, Nagpur, India

M. R. Harshith Gowda Department of Electrical and Electronics Engineering, Siddaganga Institute of Technology, Tumakuru, India

Mukunda Byre Gowda REVA University, Bangalore, India

Sanju P. Gowda Department of Information Science and Engineering, JSS Science and Technology University, Mysuru, Karnataka, India

M. Gowtham Department of Computer Science, Rajeev Institute of Technology, Hassan, Karnataka, India

Shankru Guggari Department of Computer Science and Engineering, BMS College of Engineering, Bangalore, India

Deepa Gupta Department of Mathematics, Amrita School of Engineering, Amrita Vishwa Vidyapeetham, Bangalore, India

D. S. Guru Department of Studies in Computer Science, University of Mysore, Mysuru, India

H. R. Gurupavan Department of Mechanical Engineering, PES College of Engineering, Mandya, Karnataka, India

C. D. GuruPrakash CS&E, SSIT, SAHE, Tumakuru, India

N. Guruprasad Department of Information Science and Engineering, New Horizon College of Engineering, Bangalore, India

Ravindra S. Hegadi School of Computational Sciences, Solapur University, Solapur, Maharashtra, India

Chetana Hegde Manipal Global Education Services, Bangalore, India

Ganga Holi Department of ISE, Global Academy of Technology, VTU Belagavi, Bangalore, India

B. Honnaraju Maharaja Institute of Technology Mysore, Mysuru, Karnataka, India

Amruta Hosur VLSI Design and Embedded Systems, Rashtreeya Vidyalaya College of Engineering, Bangalore, India

Manjunath Jadhav Department of Electronics and Communication, BMS College of Engineering, Basavanagudi, Bangalore, Karnataka, India

G. Jagadamba Department of Information Science and Engineering, Siddaganga Institute of Technology, Tumakuru, India

Divya K. Jain Department of ISE, Global Academy of Technology, VTU Belagavi, Bangalore, India

M. A. Jayaram Department of Master of Computer Applications, Siddaganga Institute of Technology, Tumakuru, India

K. Jeeva Priya Department of Electronics and Communication Engineering, Amrita School of Engineering, Amrita Vishwa Vidyapeetham, Bangalore, India

P. Jhansi Rani CMRIT, Bangalore, India

Vijayakumar Kadappa Department of Computer Applications, BMS College of Engineering, Bangalore, India

Abdullah Mohammed Kaleem Department of Electronics and Telecommunication, MPGI School of Engineering, Nanded, Maharashtra, India

Pattar Gayatri Kallappa Department of Electrical and Electronics Engineering, Siddaganga Institute of Technology, Tumakuru, India

G. M. Kamalakannan CSMST, CSIR-NAL, Bangalore, India

S. Kanthimathi PES University, Bangalore, India

B. S. Kariyappa Department of ECE, R.V. College of Engineering, Bangalore, India

M. L. Kavya Priya Department of CSE, Maharaja Institute of Technology, Mysuru, India

Shivaraj Kengond School of Computer Science & Engineering, KLE Technological University, Hubli, Karnataka, India

Asif Khan University of Electronic Science and Technology of China, Chengdu, Sichuan, People's Republic of China

Akshay Khot Department of Electronics & Communication, B.V. Bhoomaraddi College of Engineering & Technology, Hubli, Karnataka, India

J. Kiran Department of ECE, ATME College of Engineering, Mysuru, India

N. Kishor Department of Electronics and Communication Engineering, Dayananda Sagar Academy of Technology & Management (DSATM), Bangalore, India

Rajendra D. Kokate Department of Instrumentation Engineering, Government College of Engineering, Jalgaon, Jalgaon, Maharashtra, India

Mohan Kumar Kotgire Hochschule Darmstadt, Darmstadt, Germany

D. P. Kothari IIT Delhi, New Delhi, India;
VIT Vellore, Vellore, India;
VRCE, Nagpur, India

Mahesh Koti PES College of Engineering, Mandya, India

A. Vamsi Krishna Department of Electrical and Electronics Engineering, Amrita School of Engineering, Bangalore, Amrita Vishwa Vidyapeetham, Bangalore, India

Akshay Krishna RNS Institute of Technology, Bangalore, India

Namboodiri Akhil M. M. Krishnan Department of Electronics and Communication, BMS College of Engineering, Basavanagudi, Bangalore, Karnataka, India

Y. T. Krishne Gowda Maharaja Institute of Technology Mysuru, Mandya, Karnataka, India

K. ShankarJois Krupa Global Academy of Technology, Bangalore, India

Deepak Kumar Department of Electronics and Communication Engineering, Dayananda Sagar Academy of Technology & Management (DSATM), Bangalore, India

G. Hemantha Kumar University of Mysore, Mysuru, India

N. Kumar Department of EEE, NIE Mysuru, Mysuru, India

Rakesh Kumar Department of Computer Science and Engineering, National Institute of Technical Teachers Training & Research, Chandigarh, India

Sumit Kumar IIIT Manipur, Imphal, India

Y. H. Sharath Kumar Maharaja Institute of Technology, Mysuru, India

Akanksha Kumari BNMIT, Bangalore, India

B. K. S. P. Kumar Raju Alluri Computer Science and Engineering, National Institute of Technology, Andhra Pradesh, Tadepalligudam, Andhra Pradesh, India

Vaishnavi Kumbargeri Department of ECE, R.V. College of Engineering, Bangalore, Karnataka, India

Beenu Kunjumon Department of Computer Science & Engineering, New Horizon College of Engineering, Bangalore, India

D. Lakshmi Department of Electrical and Electronics Engineering, Amrita School of Engineering, Bangalore, Amrita Vishwa Vidyapeetham, Bangalore, India

B. R. Lakshmikantha Dayananda Sagar Academy of Technology and Management, Bangalore, India

C. LakshmiNarayana Department of Electrical Engineering Science, BMSCE, Bangalore, India

Qingsong Li Chengdu Neusoft University, Chengdu, Sichuan, People's Republic of China

Chuanlin Liu Chengdu Neusoft University, Chengdu, Sichuan, People's Republic of China

R. K. Madhu School of Computer Science & Engineering, KLE Technological University, Hubli, Karnataka, India

J. Madhusudhana Department of Electrical Engineering, UVCE, Bangalore, India

Anusha Mahale Department of ECE, R.V. College of Engineering, Bangalore, Karnataka, India

P. K. Mahesh Department of ECE, ATME College of Engineering, Mysuru, India

R. Mala Department of Electronics and Communication Engineering, Dayananda Sagar Academy of Technology & Management (DSATM), Bangalore, India

Mala Power Systems, NIE Mysuru, Mysuru, India

K. N. Manasa PES College of Engineering (Affiliated to University of Mysore, Mysuru), Mandya, Karnataka, India

Bappaditya Mandal Keele University, Staffordshire, UK

A. V. Manjula Department of Electronics, PET Research Foundation, PES College of Engineering, Mandya, India

T. N. Manjunath Department of ISE, BMSIT&M, Bangalore, India

R. Manjunatha PES College of Engineering, Mandya, India

N. Manohar Amrita School of Arts and Sciences, Amrita Vishwa Vidyapeetham, Mysuru, India

S. B. Manojkumar PET Research Foundation, Mandya, India

Bharat Manvi SJCE, Mysuru, India

Rudrayya Math NIE Mysuru, Mysuru, India

M. K. Meghana School of Computer Science & Engineering, KLE Technological University, Hubli, Karnataka, India

Vijay Krishna Menon Center for Computational Engineering and Networking (CEN), Amrita School of Engineering, Coimbatore, Amrita Vishwa Vidyapeetham, Coimbatore, India

Minavathi Department of Information Science and Engineering, PES College of Engineering, Mandya, Karnataka, India

Shakti Mishra Department of ISE, NMIT, VTU, Bangalore, India

S. D. Mohana Department of Master of Computer Application, Sri Jayachamarajendra College of Engineering, JSS Science & Technology University, Mysuru, Karnataka, India

Laveena Monis Department of Computer Science & Engineering, New Horizon College of Engineering, Bangalore, India

Peter Joseph Basil Morris SO-D, FRD Division, Radar-V, LRDE, DRDO, Bangalore, India

S. P. Muley Priyadarshini College of Engineering, RTMN University, Nagpur, India

Mohammed Moin Mulla School of Computer Science & Engineering, KLE Technological University, Hubli, Karnataka, India

S. Murali Maharaja Institute of Technology Mysore, Mysuru, Karnataka, India

K. N. Muralidhara Department of Electronics and Communication, PES College of Engineering, Mandya, India

K. Murugesh Department of ECE, ATME College of Engineering, Mysuru, India

Nagarathna Department of CS & E, PES College of Engineering, Mandya, India

C. H. Nagesh IIIT Manipur, Imphal, India

R. Nagesh Centre for PG Studies Muddenahalli, VTU, Muddenahalli, India

Ravindran Nambiar Jyothi Department of Computer Science & Engineering, Amrita School of Engineering, Bangalore, Amrita Vishwa Vidyapeetham, Bangalore, India

Jayalaxmi G. Naragund School of Computer Science & Engineering, KLE Technological University, Hubballi, Karnataka, India

D. G. Narayan School of Computer Science & Engineering, KLE Technological University, Hubli, Karnataka, India

V. Nattarasu Department of ECE, JSS Science & Technology University, Mysuru, India

S. B. Naveen Kumar Department of Electrical and Electronics Engineering, Siddaganga Institute of Technology, Tumakuru, India

Y. S. Nijagunarya Department of Computer Science and Engineering, Siddaganga Institute of Technology, Tumakuru, India

L. Nikitha R.V. College of Engineering, Bangalore, India

M. G. Ninad SJCE, Mysuru, India

S. Niranjan SJCE, Mysuru, India

S. Nithin Department of Computer Science and Engineering, New Horizon College of Engineering, Bangalore, India

Lu Niu Chengdu Ncusoft University, Chengdu, Sichuan, People's Republic of China

M. C. Padma Department of Computer Science and Engineering, PES College of Engineering (Affiliated to University of Mysore, Mysuru), Mandya, Karnataka, India

S. K. Padma SJCE, JSS Science and Technology University, Mysuru, India

Likhitha S. Padmini Department of ECE, ATME College of Engineering, Mysuru, India

Paramesha Department of Electronics and Communication Engineering, Government Engineering College, Hassan, Karnataka, India

S. S. Parthasarathy Department of Electrical and Electronics, PES College of Engineering, Mandya, India

Honey Pasricha Department of CSE, National Institute of Technical Teachers Training & Research, Chandigarh, India

Anusha Patil Department of Electronics & Communication, B.V. Bhoomaraddi College of Engineering & Technology, Hubli, Karnataka, India

Mallanagouda Patil Department of Computer Science, Dayananda Sagar University, Bangalore, Karnataka, India

Rajashekhargouda C. Patil Department of ECE, DBIT, Bangalore, India

Sushmitha Pattanashetty Department of Electronics and Communication Engineering, Dayananda Sagar Academy of Technology & Management (DSATM), Bangalore, India

K. M. Poornima Department of CS&E, JNNCE Shivamogga, Shimoga, Karnataka, India

Rakshitha R. Prabhu Department of Electrical Engineering, UVCE, Bangalore, India

M. R. Prajwal Sri Jayachamarajendra College of Engineering, Mysuru, India

V. Prajwal SJCE, JSS Science and Technology University, Mysuru, India

Gopalakrishnan Prakash Department of Computer Science & Engineering, Amrita School of Engineering, Bangalore, Amrita Vishwa Vidyapeetham, Bangalore, India

Prajwal Prakash Department of Electronics & Communication Engineering, PES University, Bangalore, India

M. Pranav Department of Computer Science and Engineering, New Horizon College of Engineering, Bangalore, India

Chandrakala Prasad Discipline of Orthodontics, Faculty of Dentistry, University of Toronto, Toronto, ON, Canada

Karthik Prasad University of Waterloo, Waterloo, ON, Canada

S. J. Prashantha Department of CS&E, AIT Chikmagalur, Chikmagalur, Karnataka, India

R. J. Prathibha Department of Information Science and Engineering, SJ College of Engineering, Mysuru, Karnataka, India

J. Prathima Mabel Department of Information Science and Engineering, Dayananda Sagar College of Engineering, Bangalore, India

D. T. Pratish Department of Computer Science, Rajeev Institute of Technology, Hassan, Karnataka, India

N. Praveena Department of ECE, Rashtreeya Vidyalaya College of Engineering, Bangalore, India

N. S. Prema Department of Information Science and Engineering, Vidyavardhaka College of Engineering, Mysuru, India

B. S. Premananda Department of Telecommunication Engineering, R.V. College of Engineering, Bangalore, India

B. Premjith Center for Computational Engineering and Networking (CEN), Amrita School of Engineering Coimbatore, Amrita Vishwa Vidyapeetham, Coimbatore, India

B. K. Priya Department of Electronics and Communication Engineering, Amrita School of Engineering, Amrita Vishwa Vidyapeetham, Bangalore, India

N. Pruthvi BMS Institute of Technology and Management, Bangalore, India

N. B. Puhan Indian Institute of Technology Bhubaneswar, Bhubaneswar, India

M. B. Punith Kumar PES College of Engineering, Mandya, India

Shrinivasacharya Purohit Department of Information Science and Engineering, Siddaganga Institute of Technology, Tumakuru, India

S. K. Pushpa Department of ISE, BMSIT&M, Bangalore, India

M. P. Pushpalatha Department of Computer Science and Engineering, Sri Jayachamarajendra College of Engineering, Mysuru, India

P. S. Puttaswamy Department of Electrical Engineering, PES College of Engineering, Mandya, Karnataka, India;
Department of Electrical and Electronics Engineering, PES College of Engineering, Mandya, Karnataka, India

Gopalapillai Radhakrishnan Department of Computer Science & Engineering, Amrita School of Engineering, Amrita Vishwa Vidyapeetham, Bangalore, India

Sarika Raga Department of DECS, VTU, CPGS, Muddenahalli, Chikkaballapur, India

M. M. Raikar School of Computer Science & Engineering, KLE Technological University, Hubli, Karnataka, India

C. Vidya Raj Department of CS&E, NIE Mysuru, Mysuru, India

B. R. Rajeev Department of Electrical and Electronics Engineering, Siddaganga Institute of Technology, Tumakuru, India

Uppara Rajesh Siddaganga Institute of Technology, Tumakuru, Karnataka, India

B. G. Rakesh SJCE, Mysuru, India

N. Rakshith PES College of Engineering, Mandya, Karnataka, India

C. Rama Krishna Department of Computer Science & Engineering, National Institute of Technical Teachers Training & Research, Chandigarh, India

K. N. Rama Mohan Babu Department of Information Science and Engineering, Dayananda Sagar College of Engineering, Bangalore, India

Radhika Rani SBRR Mahajana First Grade College, Mysuru, India

Pooja R. Rao Department of Information Science and Engineering, JSS Science and Technology University, Mysuru, Karnataka, India

M. R. Rashmi Department of Electrical and Electronics Engineering, Amrita School of Engineering, Bangalore, Amrita Vishwa Vidyapeetham, Bangalore, India;
Department of CS&E, NIE Mysuru, Mysuru, India

H. K. Ravikiran Department of Electronics and Communication Engineering, Rajeev Institute of Technology, Hassan, Karnataka, India

K. M. Ravikumar Department of ECE, S J C Institute of Technology, Chikkaballapur, Karnataka, India

H. V. Ravindra Department of Mechanical Engineering, PES College of Engineering, Mandya, Karnataka, India

H. V. Ravish Aradhya Department of ECE, R.V. College of Engineering, Bangalore, Karnataka, India

M. Revanesh Department of E&CE, PES College of Engineering, Mandya, Karnataka, India

K. Rithesh Department of Computer Science and Engineering, National Institute of Technology Karnataka, Surathkal, Mangalore, India

K. C. Rupesh Department of Electrical and Electronics Engineering, Siddaganga Institute of Technology, Tumakuru, India

B. Sagar East West Institute of Technology, Bangalore, India

Inavalli Sai Sree Computer Science and Engineering, National Institute of Technology, Andhra Pradesh, Tadepalligudam, Andhra Pradesh, India

H. V. Saikumar Department of EEE, NIE Mysuru, Mysuru, India

P. Saleena Department of Computer Science & Engineering, Amrita School of Engineering, Amrita Vishwa Vidyapeetham, Bangalore, India

Ananth Saligram Department of ECE, JSS Science & Technology University, Mysuru, India

Vimuktha E. Salis BNMIT, Bangalore, India

S. Sandhya Department of Electronics and Communication Engineering, Dayananda Sagar Academy of Technology & Management (DSATM), Bangalore, India

H. M. Sanjay CS&E, PESCE, Mandya, India

H. Sathishkumar Department of Electronics, PET Research Foundation, PES College of Engineering, Mandya, India

K. Shalini Center for Computational Engineering and Networking (CEN), Amrita School of Engineering, Coimbatore, Amrita Vishwa Vidyapeetham, Coimbatore, India

U. Shama Firdose Department of ECE, BGSIT, Mandya, India

B. R. Shambhavi Department of ISE, BMS College of Engineering, Bangalore, India

Aadarsh Sharma Department of Computer Science & Engineering, National Institute of Technical Teachers Training & Research, Chandigarh, India

Shivam Sharma Lovely Professional University, Phagwara, Punjab, India

N. S. Shashank Sri Jayachamarajendra College of Engineering, Mysuru, India

D. Shashidhara PES College of Engineering, Mandya, Karnataka, India

B. M. Shashikala Sri Jayachamarajendra College of Engineering, Mysuru, India

H. S. Sheshadri Department of ECE, PES College of Engineering, Mandya, India

Nagashree S. Shetti School of Computer Science & Engineering, KLE Technological University, Hubli, Karnataka, India

K. C. Shilpa Dr. Ambedkar Institute of Technology, Bangalore, India

R. Shilpa Department of Electrical and Electronics Engineering, PES College of Engineering, Mandya, Karnataka, India

K. B. Shiva Kumar Department of TCE, SSAHE, Tumakuru, India

C. S. Shivaraj Department of Electrical and Electronics Engineering, The National Institute of Engineering, Mysuru, Mysuru, India

G. P. Shivshankar Department of Civil Engineering, PES College of Engineering, Mandya, India

T. Shreekanth Sri Jayachamarajendra College of Engineering, Mysuru, India

H. U. Shruthi Department of Electrical and Electronics Engineering, Siddaganga Institute of Technology, Tumakuru, India

P. S. Shruthi Department of CS&E, PES College of Engineering, Chennai, India

V. Shyam Forus Health Private Ltd., Bangalore, India

M. K. Shyla SSAHE, Tumakuru, India

N. Shylashree Department of ECE, Rashtreeya Vidyalaya College of Engineering, Bangalore, India

K. L. Sindhudhar Department of Telecommunication Engineering, R.V. College of Engineering, Bangalore, India

Animesh Singh BNMIT, Bangalore, India

Jaiteg Singh Department of Computer Science and Engineering, Chitkara University Institute of Engineering and Technology, Chandigarh, India

Kamalpreet Singh Lovely Professional University, Phagwara, Punjab, India

Manoj Kumar Singh Manuro Tech Research, Bangalore, India

Suraj Pal Singh National Institute of Technical Teachers Training & Research, Chandigarh, India

Pratiksha Ramesh Sisodia Department of Computer Science, CHRIST (Deemed to be University), Bangalore, India

Shano Solanki Department of Computer Science and Engineering, National Institute of Technical Teachers Training & Research, Chandigarh, India

K. Soman Center for Computational Engineering and Networking (CEN), Amrita School of Engineering, Coimbatore, Amrita Vishwa Vidyapeetham, Coimbatore, India

K. P. Soman Center for Computational Engineering and Networking (CEN), Amrita School of Engineering Coimbatore, Amrita Vishwa Vidyapeetham, Coimbatore, India

T. Sonal Singh Department of ECE, ATME College of Engineering, Mysuru, India

Shubham Sourabh School of Computer Science & Engineering, KLE Technological University, Hubli, Karnataka, India

B. S. Sowmya Lakshmi Department of ISE, BMS College of Engineering, Bangalore, India

R. Sreehari Department of ECE, NITK, Surathkal, India

G. Sridevi Department of ECE, JSS Science & Technology University, Mysuru, India

V. Sridhar Department of E&CE, PES College of Engineering, Mandya, Karnataka, India

Mahamad Suhil Department of Computer Science, GFGC, Paavagada, Tumukuru, India

Shanmukha Sundar Dayananda Sagar College of Engineering, Bangalore, India

K. Sundar Karthikeyan Department of Electronics and Communication Engineering, Amrita School of Engineering, Amrita Vishwa Vidyapeetham, Bangalore, India

Sunjay Suri Graduate Orthodontics, Faculty of Dentistry, Burlington Growth Centre, Toronto, ON, Canada

K. Swarnalatha Department of Information Science & Engineering, Maharaja Institute of Technology Thandavapura, Mysuru, India

Tanya Lovely Professional University, Phagwara, Punjab, India

K. K. Thashrifa Department of Telecommunication Engineering, R.V. College of Engineering, Bangalore, India

J. Thriveni Department of Computer Science and Engineering, University Visvesvaraya College of Engineering, Bangalore University, Bangalore, India

M. Thungamani University of Horticultural Sciences, Bagalkot, India

A. Thyagarajmurthy Electronics and Communications, SJCE, Mysuru, India

N. Tilakraj Department of ECE, S J C Institute of Technology, Chikkaballapur, Karnataka, India;
VTU-RRC, Belgaum, India

S. G. Totad School of Computer Science & Engineering, KLE Technological University, Hubli, Karnataka, India

V. Umadevi Department of Computer Science and Engineering, BMS College of Engineering, Bangalore, India

D. R. Umesh Department of CS&E, PES College of Engineering, Chennai, India

Suma Umesh BMS Institute of Technology and Management, Bangalore, India

Nidhin A. Unnithan Center for Computational Engineering and Networking (CEN), Amrita School of Engineering, Coimbatore, Amrita Vishwa Vidyapeetham, Coimbatore, India

P. Vageesha VTU Recognized Research Centre for Engineering Chemistry, Department of Chemistry, KLE Institute of Technology, Hubballi, Karnataka, India

Vaishali Department of Computer Science and Engineering, National Institute of Technical Teachers Training & Research, Chandigarh, India

K. A. Vani Department of Information Science and Engineering, Dayananda Sagar College of Engineering, Bangalore, India

Prakruthi Vasanth Department of Electrical and Electronics Engineering, The National Institute of Engineering, Mysuru, Mysuru, India

K. S. Vasundhara Patel Department of Electronics and Communication, BMS College of Engineering, Basavanagudi, Bangalore, Karnataka, India

K. Vatsala Department of Electronics and Communication Engineering, Dayananda Sagar Academy of Technology & Management (DSATM), Bangalore, India

M. Veena Department of CS & E, PES College of Engineering, Mandya, Karnataka, India

K. R. Venugopal Department of Computer Science and Engineering, University Visvesvaraya College of Engineering, Bangalore University, Bangalore, India

Aman Ranjan Verma IIIT Manipur, Imphal, India

Vidhyotma Department of Computer Science and Engineering, Chitkara University Institute of Engineering and Technology, Chandigarh, India

B. Vijaya JSS Medical College, Mysuru, India

A. Vijayalakshmi Department of Computer Science, CHRIST (Deemed to be University), Bangalore, India

K. U. Vinayaka Department of Electrical and Electronics Engineering, Siddaganga Institute of Technology, Tumakuru, India

S. Vinay Department of Computer Science & Engineering, PESCE, Mandya, India

Vivek Vinayan Center for Computational Engineering and Networking (CEN), Amrita School of Engineering Coimbatore, Amrita Vishwa Vidyapeetham, Coimbatore, India

B. R. Vishwanath P.E.T. Research Center, PES College of Engineering, Mandya, Karnataka, India

Sujith Viswanathan Center for Computational Engineering and Networking (CEN), Amrita School of Engineering, Coimbatore, Amrita Vishwa Vidyapeetham, Coimbatore, India

Shashidhara B. Vyakaranal School of Computer Science & Engineering, KLE Technological University, Hubballi, Karnataka, India

Deyin Wan Chengdu Neusoft University, Chengdu, Sichuan, People's Republic of China

Amit Yadav Chengdu Neusoft University, Chengdu, Sichuan, People's Republic of China

Design of Low-Power Square Root Carry Select Adder and Wallace Tree Multiplier Using Adiabatic Logic

M. G. Ganavi and B. S. Premananda

Abstract Power dissipation is a significant issue in many digital and VLSI systems. Adiabatic logic is a promising technique in minimizing the power dissipation, and positive feedback adiabatic logic (PFAL) proves to be efficient. The arithmetic operations in the digital systems are incomplete without the use of adders and multipliers. In this paper, a 16-bit square root carry select adder (SQRT CSLA) is implemented using ripple carry adder (RCA). The limitation of power and area in SQRT CSLA using RCA is overcome by incorporating Binary to Excess-1 Converter (BEC) in place of RCA. An 8 × 8 Wallace tree multiplier (WTM) is implemented using the concept of carry-save addition. The limitation of area in WTM is overcome by implementing reduced complexity WTM (RCWTM). The adders and multipliers are realized in both static CMOS and PFAL in Cadence Virtuoso 180 nm technology and simulated in Spectre. The static CMOS-based SQRT CSLA using BEC dissipates 50.25% less power as compared to SQRT CSLA using RCA which makes SQRT CSLA using BEC a better choice w.r.t. power dissipation and area. The PFAL-based SQRT CSLA using RCA and SQRT CSLA using BEC dissipates 54.5 and 83.5% less power as compared to static CMOS designs. PFAL-based RCWTM dissipates 81.8% less power than the static CMOS design. Circuits designed using PFAL dissipates less power as compared to those designed using static CMOS logic with a tradeoff in area.

Keywords CMOS · PFAL · SQRT CSLA · Wallace tree multiplier

M. G. Ganavi (✉) · B. S. Premananda
Department of Telecommunication Engineering, R.V. College of Engineering, Bangalore, India
e-mail: ganavimg6@gmail.com

B. S. Premananda
e-mail: premanandabs@gmail.com

© Springer Nature Singapore Pte Ltd. 2019
V. Sridhar et al. (eds.), *Emerging Research in Electronics, Computer Science and Technology*, Lecture Notes in Electrical Engineering 545,
https://doi.org/10.1007/978-981-13-5802-9_67

1 Introduction

Power is the crucial criterion in the systems such as processors, filters, and VLSI systems. The use of portable devices such as mobile phones and laptops is rapidly increasing with time, which has increased the demand for low-power devices. With the increase in the architecture and operations of the computational systems, the power dissipation also increases which makes it necessary to implement low-power techniques in the design of circuits. Adders and multipliers are the vital building blocks in performing arithmetic computations in the circuits ranging from communication systems, digital signal processors, and VLSI systems to high-end multimedia systems. Carry is generated by the adder such as RCA which reduces the speed and increases the delay. This can be overcome by using adders such as carry-lookahead adder, carry-save adder (CSA), and CSLA [1]. Parallel prefix adders have less delay but consume larger area. Different adders are preferred for different application. The delay in the circuit can be minimized by implementing SQRT CSLA when compared to RCA. The SQRT CSLA using RCA is not efficient w.r.t. area because of number of RCAs [2]; limitation is overcome by using BEC in the second stage of SQRT CSLA in place of RCAs which reduces the area, thereby reducing the power dissipation of the circuit. Multiplication is also an imperative arithmetic operation which is implemented using addition of partial products. Many adders are implicated in the multiplication process.

Various types of multipliers such as Array, Booth, Wallace tree, Dadda, Sequential, and Vedic multiplier exist [3]. The WTM occupies minimum area and also reduces the number of computations as compared to the conventional multiplication by grouping three rows of partial products into one group. The WTM is implemented using CSAs in which addition of three bits is possible at once, by storing carry in the present stage and adding it in the next stage [4]. Different approaches such as reversible logic [5], sleepy stack, and adiabatic logic are the emerging low-power techniques. Adiabatic logic demonstrates to be an efficient technique in minimizing the power dissipation. Adiabatic refers to a thermodynamic process where the heat is not dissipated to the environment [6]. The energy in the adiabatic systems is supplied back to the power clock [7]. There are two types of adiabatic logic circuits, namely fully and quasi/partially adiabatic.

The complete charge in the capacitance is recovered and provided back to the power clock in case of fully adiabatic logic, and in quasi-adiabatic circuits, only a part of energy is recovered back to the circuit [8]. The quasi-adiabatic logic family includes efficient charge recovery logic (ECRL), 2 N-2N2P adiabatic logic, PFAL, NMOS energy recovery logic (NERL), clocked adiabatic logic (CAL), true single phase adiabatic logic (TSEL), and source coupled adiabatic logic (SCAL), and the fully adiabatic logic family includes pass transistor adiabatic logic (PAL), split rail charge recovery logic (SCRL), and so on [9]. The complexity in the circuit implementation is larger in case of fully adiabatic logic circuits than the quasi-adiabatic circuits though the power dissipation is minimized in the former case. PFAL is an efficient quasi-adiabatic technique in which the power dissipation is minimum compared to other quasi-adiabatic techniques.

Power is the critical parameter in portable devices. Design of low-power circuits is a very important concern in ICs. Adiabatic is one of the promising approaches to minimize power dissipation of the devices. The static CMOS- and PFAL-based adders and multipliers are implemented in Cadence Virtuoso 180 nm technology and simulated using Spectre. The circuits implemented using PFAL dissipate less power as compared to those implemented using static CMOS logic.

Organization of the paper is as follows: An insight into the literature is presented in Sect. 2. Section 3 provides an overview of design and implementation of SQRT CSLA using RCA, SQRT CSLA using BEC, WTM, and RCWTM using static CMOS logic and description of adiabatic logic. Section 4 includes the simulation results and comparative analysis of both adders and multipliers implemented using CMOS and PFAL w.r.t. power and area. Section 5 provides the conclusions and the future scope of the work.

2 Literature Review

A decision-based CSLA is proposed where BEC is activated only when required. A comparison is made between decision-based CSLA and modified CSLA using BEC w.r.t. speed, area, and power dissipation by synthesizing the design using Cadence RTL compiler [1]. The power and area of the decision-based CSLA are optimized by 17 and 11.57% compared to CSLA using BEC. Abhiram et al. [2] have proposed 32-bit, 64-bit, and 128-bit SQRT CSLA based on the gate level modification for the regular CSLA which are among one of the fastest adders. Synopsys 90 nm technology is used to design the circuits. The modified CSLA is analyzed and compared with conventional CSLA w.r.t. power, area, and delay. The area and power are minimized in the modified CSLA with an increase in delay.

Biradar et al. [3] have proposed a signed and unsigned Baugh-Wooley and Braun multipliers, and the speed and power of the multipliers are analyzed. Multipliers are designed using CMOS, split-path data-driven dynamic logic (SPD3L), and domino logic. SPD3L increases the power dissipation and provides best performance when speed is considered. Multipliers designed using domino logic provide better results w.r.t. both area and speed. WTM is implemented using compressors to reduce the number of adders [4]. The 5:3 and 7:3 compressors are implemented using the property of both binary counters and compressor. The use of compressors has reduced the number of stages and the delay in the circuit. 7:3 compressor increases the speed by reducing the delay. The use of compressors also reduces the number of stages and the critical path. The WTM reduces the area, the number of stages, and computations.

Alam et al. [6] have designed a 4-bit comparator using PFAL and ECRL using Cadence Virtuoso in gpdk 180 nm technologies and compared it with the static CMOS logic w.r.t. power and area. ECRL comparator provides 13.64%, and PFAL comparator provides 54.54% efficiency compared to static CMOS design. The number of transistors is least in case of ECRL as compared to PFAL and CMOS. Conventional CSLA and CSLA using BEC were designed and analyzed using Cadence

Virtuoso 180 nm technology [7]. The power dissipation of the CSLA using BEC is less compared to conventional CSLA. The delay in the CSLA using BEC is also reduced. ECRL is used to design the adders which prove to be an efficient technique in minimizing the power dissipation.

PFAL dissipates less power as compared to other adiabatic techniques. SQRT CSLA using RCA overcomes the delay in RCA, and the modified SQRT CSLA using BEC minimizes the power dissipation and area occupied by the circuit by replacing RCA by BEC. The SQRT CSLA using BEC proves to be efficient w.r.t. area, power, and delay. WTM reduces the number of stages as compared to conventional multiplication. RCWTM reduces the area as compared to WTM by reducing the number of adders. SQRT CSLA and RCWTM are implemented using PFAL where the power dissipation is minimized as compared to CMOS logic design. The adders and multipliers designed using PFAL can be implemented in several applications where minimizing the power is a foremost concern.

3   Design and Implementation of Adders and Multipliers

3.1   Square Root Carry Select Adder

A 16-bit SQRT CSLA is designed using RCAs and multiplexers of varying bit size as shown in Fig. 1. Full adders (FA) are cascaded to form RCA [10], where the carry out (COUT) of one FA is fed as carry in (CIN) to the succeeding FA. In the first

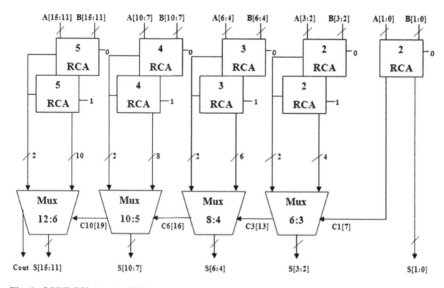

Fig. 1 SQRT CSLA using RCA

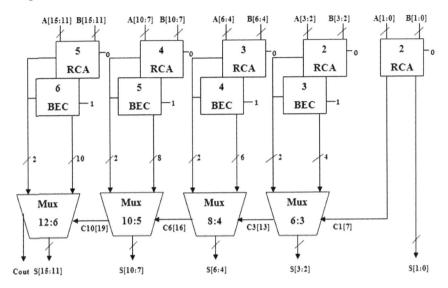

Fig. 2 SQRT CSLA using BEC

stage of the SQRT CSLA using RCA, the inputs are fed into RCAs by considering CIN = '0'; the second stage computes the sum by considering CIN = '1.' The sum of the first and second stages is fed as input to the multiplexers such that it selects the output of first stage when the select line S = '0' and the output of second stage when S = '1' thereby selecting the appropriate output. SQRT CSLA using BEC is as shown in Fig. 2.

SQRT CSLA using RCA is not efficient w.r.t. area as multiple RCAs are used which in turn increases the power dissipation. RCAs in the second stage of SQRT CSLA are replaced by BECs. The input to the first stage RCAs in SQRT CSLA using BEC is the same 16-bit inputs as in SQRT CSLA using RCA, but the input to the second stage BECs is the output of first stage RCAs. The outputs of both first and second stages are fed to the multiplexer to select the appropriate output.

3.2 Wallace Tree Multiplier

Multiplier is a vital arithmetic block in the digital system. WTM is area efficient as compared to the other multipliers, and it is also power efficient. The complete multiplication process involves three steps, namely partial product generation, grouping and reduction of the partial products, and finally addition. In an 8 × 8 multiplication, the three rows of the partial products are considered as a single group, thereby forming two groups of three rows and one group of two rows.

Full adders are used where there are three inputs, half adders are used where there are two inputs, and the sum and carry are generated for each group as shown in

Fig. 3. The same procedure is repeated till the final product is obtained. The dotted representation of modified RCWTM is as shown in Fig. 4. WTM uses FAs and HAs in the addition of partial products with the concept of carry-save addition. The FAs reduce three rows into two rows by considering an input of three bits and producing an output of two bits, i.e., the carry and sum. Unlike FA, HA does not reduce the number of rows; it considers two-bit input and produces two-bit output which proves that using HA is a waste of area. So, it is evident that reduction in the count of HAs reduces the complexity of the circuit.

In the RCWTM, the partial products form a pyramidal shape and the three rows of partial products are considered as a single group. Three bits in a column are added using FA, and the remaining single bits are carried to the next row for addition. The procedure is repeated until the last step is reached, and at the last step, carry propagate adder is used. RCWTM uses less number of HAs with an insignificant

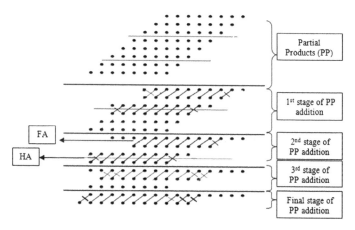

Fig. 3 8 × 8 Wallace tree multiplier [12]

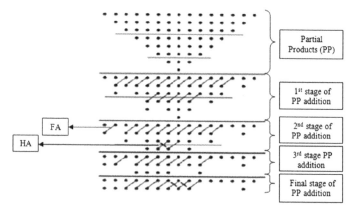

Fig. 4 8 × 8 RCWTM [13]

increase in the number of FAs. The circuit's area is reduced by implementing the RCWTM compared to WTM.

3.3 Adiabatic Logic

Adiabatic logic is a low-power technique which is efficient in minimizing the power dissipation of the circuit. PFAL is an efficient adiabatic technique as compared to other adiabatic techniques in minimizing the power dissipation. The switching power dissipation in static CMOS circuits with capacitive load has a lower limit of $CV_{dd}^2/2$ where V_{dd} and C are the supply voltage and capacitive load, respectively. This power dissipation can be minimized by using adiabatic logic. The charge stored in the capacitor is recycled back to the power clock in the adiabatic logic which minimizes the power dissipation. There are four phases of power clock, and each phase has four intervals. Each phase of the power clock leads the preceding power clock by 90° as shown in Fig. 5 implemented and simulated in Cadence Virtuoso and Spectre.

The energy dissipated is supplied through a constant current source in an adiabatic logic when considering the charge is provided by,

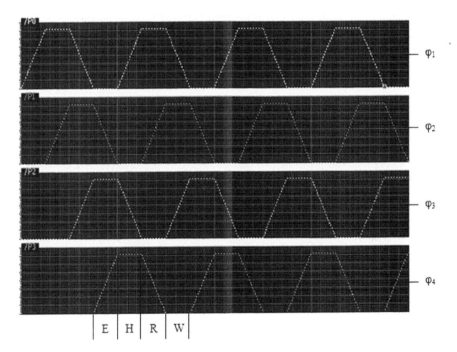

Fig. 5 Power clock

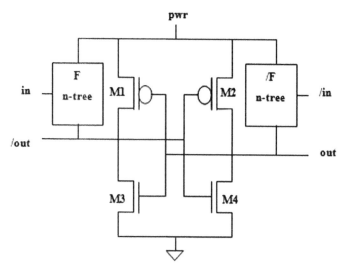

Fig. 6 Basic PFAL structure

$$E = \frac{RC}{T} V^2 \qquad (1)$$

where load capacitance is represented as C, voltage of the power clock or power supply by $V_{dd,}$ and the charging/discharging time by T.

The energy dissipation is less in the adiabatic circuit than the static CMOS circuit if $T \gg 2RC$ [11]. The PFAL circuit consists of a latch made by two PMOS and NMOS that avoids degradation in the logic level on the output nodes out and /out as shown in Fig. 6. The F n-tree and /F n-tree indicates the functional blocks which are placed in parallel with PMOS transistors. The 'pwr' indicates the power clock which minimizes the power dissipation in the circuit. Another advantage of adiabatic logic is that a single circuit provides two outputs; PFAL-based inverter circuit provides the output of inverter at out and output of buffer at /out implemented in Cadence Virtuoso.

The power clock is responsible for the charge recovery in adiabatic circuits. The four intervals of the power clock are evaluate (E), hold (H), recovery (R), and wait (W). The stable input signal is used to evaluate the output in the E interval. The output is provided to the next stage as input by keeping it stable in the H interval. R interval provides the recovery of energy, and symmetry is provided in the W interval [9]. Different phases of power clocks are used at different stages. If the power clock at the first stage is φ_1, then the power clock at the second stage is φ_2, which leads φ_1 by 90°. The four phases of the power clock are applied to four stages of the circuit, and then the same power clocks are repeated in the succeeding stages. The design of adiabatic circuit is such that output of one stage is provided as input to the next stage, and each stage has a different power clock. Buffers are used in the absence of circuit to propagate the output of one stage to the next stage.

4 Results and Discussions

The schematic of adders and multipliers is designed and analyzed in Cadence Virtuoso in 180 nm technology. The simulations are carried out in the Cadence Spectre simulator. The basic circuits of FA, HA, and multiplexer are designed using static CMOS and PFAL logic. The schematic of static CMOS-based SQRT CSLA using RCA is as shown in Fig. 7 which is formed by integrating the RCAs and multiplexers. The RCAs occupy more area, thereby increasing the power dissipation. To overcome this limitation, the RCAs in the second stage are replaced by BECs as shown in Fig. 8 which occupies less area and also dissipates less power. The SQRT CSLA using RCA is implemented using PFAL as shown in Fig. 9 which dissipates minimum power compared to the static CMOS design. The SQRT CSLA using BEC

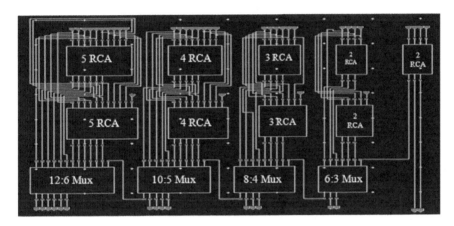

Fig. 7 Snapshot of 16-bit CMOS-based SQRT CSLA using RCA

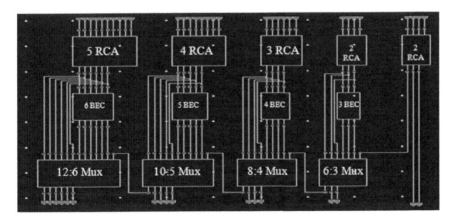

Fig. 8 Snapshot of 16-bit CMOS-based SQRT CSLA using BEC

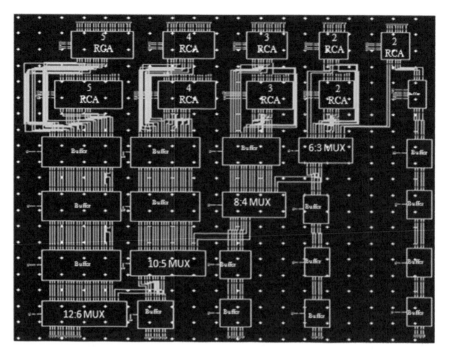

Fig. 9 Snapshot of PFAL-based 16-bit SQRT CSLA using RCA

is also implemented in the same way by replacing second stage of RCAs by BECs. The highest voltage at which the circuit operates is 1.8 V, and the lowest voltage is 0 V. The inputs are the pulse, varying between 1.8 and 0 V. Voltage 1 is considered as 0 V and voltage 2 is 1.8 V for the input to be high and vice versa for the input to be low.

The static CMOS-based WTM is implemented using the concept of carry-save addition as shown in Fig. 10. The input bits are multiplied using AND gates to provide the partial products. The static CMOS-based RCWTM implemented is shown in Fig. 11 which uses fewer HAs as compared to WTM. The RCWTM is implemented using PFAL as shown in Fig. 12 where the FAs and HAs are labeled, and rest are the buffers. The adiabatic structures (PFAL) use different power clocks at each stage, and the output of present stage is provided as the input to the next stage by using buffers wherever necessary. The adders and multipliers are verified by providing different inputs. The PFAL-based SQRT CSLA output is displayed in the 4th phase of the output waveform. The PFAL-based RCWTM output is displayed in the 5th phase. The CMOS circuits use a single power supply which makes the output to appear in the 1st phase, and adiabatic circuits use different power clocks at each stage which results the output to appear in different phase. Waveforms are not included in this paper.

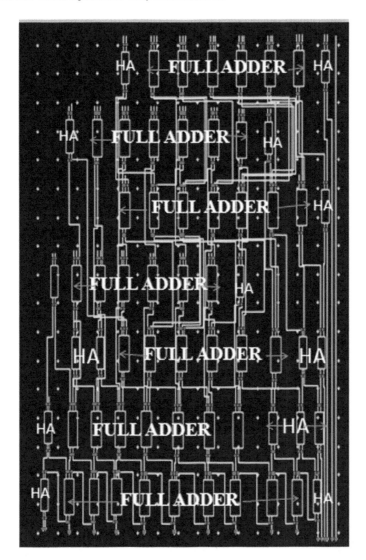

Fig. 10 Snapshot of CMOS-based 8 × 8 WTM

The power dissipation in the WTM and the RCWTM is almost same as listed in Table 1, but they differ in area. The RCWTM uses minimum number of HAs and with marginal increase in the FAs. The number of gates in the RCWTM has reduced by 12.5%, the number of HAs reduced by 52.94%, and number of FAs increased by 2%. RCWTM reduces the complexity of the circuit by employing minimum number of HAs, thereby reducing the area of the multiplier circuit.

Table 2 lists power dissipation of the static CMOS- and PFAL-based 16-bit SQRT CSLA using RCA, 16-bit SQRT CSLA using BEC, and 8 × 8 RCWTM at a frequency

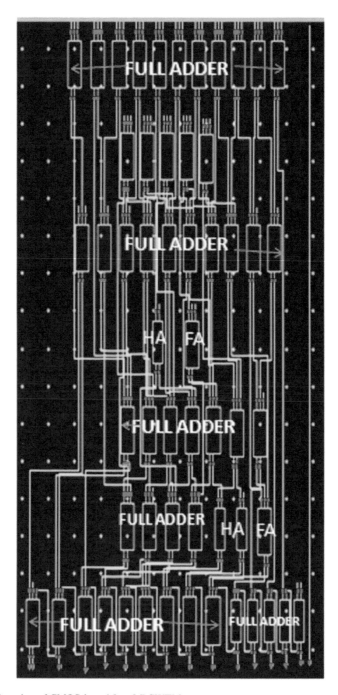

Fig. 11 Snapshot of CMOS-based 8 × 8 RCWTM

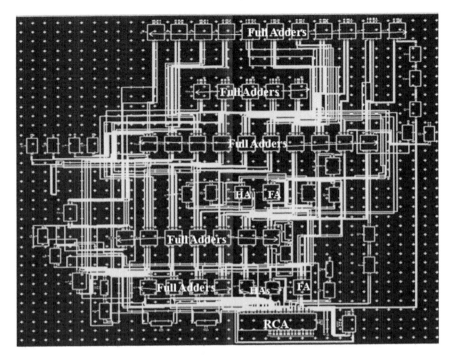

Fig. 12 Snapshot of PFAL-based 8 × 8 RCWTM

Table 1 Power and area analysis of static CMOS-based WTM and RCWTM

Multiplier architectures	Power dissipation (μW)	Number of gates
8 × 8 WTM	22.58	64 (47 FAs and 17 HAs)
8 × 8 RCWTM	22.62	56 (48 FAs and 8 HAs)

of 1 kHz. The static CMOS-based SQRT CSLA using BEC dissipates 50.25% less power as compared to SQRT CSLA using RCA. The PFAL-based SQRT CSLA using RCA dissipates 54.5% less power as compared to static CMOS design; PFAL-based SQRT CSLA using BEC dissipates 83.5% less power as compared to static CMOS design. RCWTM has minimum number of adders as compared to the WTM which reduces the area of the circuit. PFAL-based RCWTM dissipates 81.8% less power than the static CMOS design. The power analysis infers that circuits implemented using PFAL dissipate minimum power as compared to static CMOS circuits with a tradeoff in area.

Table 2 Power dissipation of static CMOS and adiabatic circuits

Architectures	Power dissipation in CMOS (μW)	Power dissipation in PFAL (μW)
16-bit SQRT CSLA using RCA	45.93	20.9
16-bit SQRT CSLA using BEC	22.85	3.77
8×8 RCWTM	22.62	4.11

5 Conclusions and Future Scope

Power optimization is an important criterion in the circuit design although area and delay have their own prominence. The power dissipation and area of the SQRT CSLA using RCA are overcome by replacing the RCAs in the second stage by BEC. The static CMOS-based SQRT CSLA using BEC dissipates 50.25% less power as compared to SQRT CSLA using RCA. RCWTM has minimum number of adders as compared to the WTM which reduces the area of the circuit. Power analysis infers that PFAL proves to be an efficient adiabatic technique in minimizing the power dissipation. PFAL-based SQRT CSLA using BEC dissipates 83.5% less power as compared to static CMOS design. PFAL-based RCWTM dissipates 81.8% less power than the static CMOS design. In future, the multiplier can be implemented using other adders instead of conventional HA and FA. MAC unit can be constructed by designing the accumulator and using the designed adder and multiplier. The designed circuits can be used in applications ranging from DSP, filters, and multimedia applications.

References

1. Dhandapani V (2017) An efficient architecture for carry select adder. World J Eng 1–14
2. Abhiram T, Ashwin T, Sivaprasad B, Aakash S, Anitha JP (2017) Modified carry select adder for power and area reduction. In: Proceedings of the international conference on circuits, power and computing technologies, pp 1–8
3. Biradar VB, Vishwas PG, Chetan CS, Premananda BS (2017) Design and performance analysis of modified unsigned Braun and signed Baugh-Wooley multiplier. In: Proceedings of the international conference on electrical, electronics, communication, computer and optimization techniques, pp 1–6
4. Mandloi A, Agrawal S, Sharma S, Shrivastava S (2017) High-speed, area efficient VLSI architecture of wallace-tree multiplier for DSP-applications. In: Proceedings of the international conference on information, communication, instrumentation and control, pp 1–5
5. Nikil GV, Vaibhav BP, Naik VG, Premananda BS (2017) Design of low power barrel shifter and vedic multiplier with kogge-stone adder using reversible logic gates. In: Proceedings of the 6th IEEE international conference on communication and signal processing, pp 1690–1694
6. Alam S, Ghimiray SR, Kumar M (2017) Performance analysis of a 4-bit comparator circuit using different adiabatic logics. In: Proceedings of the innovations in power and advanced computing technologies, pp 1–5

7. Premananda BS, Chandana MK, Shree Lakshmi KP, Keerthi AM (2017) Design of low power 8-bit carry select adder using adiabatic logic. In: Proceedings of the international conference on communication and signal processing, pp 1764–1768

8. Kumar SD, Thapliyal H, Mohammad A (2018) FinSAL: a novel FinFET based secure adiabatic logic for energy-efficient and DPA resistant IoT devices. IEEE Trans Comput Aided Des Integr Circuits Syst 110–122

9. Bhati P, Rizvi N (2016) Adiabatic logic: an alternative approach to low power application circuits. In: Proceedings of the IEEE international conference on electrical, electronics, and optimization techniques, pp 4255–4260

10. Arunraj GV, Varatharajan R (2016) Design and implementation of low power and efficient adders-a review. Int J Appl Eng Res 7992–7996

11. Patel D, Sinha SRP, Shree M (2016) Adiabatic logic circuits for low power VLSI applications. Int J Sci Res 1585–1589

12. Jaiswal KB, Nithish Kumar V, Seshadri P, Lakshminarayanan G (2015) Low power wallace tree multiplier using modified full adder. In Proceedings of the 3rd international conference on signal processing, communication and networking, pp 1–4

13. Chinnapparaj S, Somasundareswari D (2016) Incorporation of reduced full adder and half adder into wallace multiplier and improved carry-save adder for digital FIR filter. Int J Circuits Syst 2467–2475

Implementation of Doppler Beam Sharpening Technique for Synthetic-Aperture Radars

Peter Joseph Basil Morris, Kunj Dhonde and B. K. Priya

Abstract For the airborne radar systems, resolution has always been a challenge. Fine resolution can be achieved by increasing the aperture of the antenna. The carrying capacity and the streamline structure of the aircraft are the limiting factors. Considering the limitations, the aperture of the antenna cannot be increased after a limit. Therefore, a special category of radars called as Pulse-Doppler radars (PD) are usually used for airborne and spaceborne radar applications. PD radars possess the capability of detecting the targets in the mist of background clutter. Pulse compression is employed at the radar receiver to obtain the fine range resolution. However, it becomes difficult for the radar to resolve two targets present at the same distance. In this scenario, the angular resolution has to be considered for the detection. Doppler Beam Sharpening (DBS) is a technique used to observe and improve the azimuth resolution of the radar. In this paper, the DBS technique is presented to resolve the targets at the same range.

Keywords Doppler Beam Sharpening · Pulse compression · Synthetic-aperture radar · PD radar · Resolution

1 Introduction

Radar signal processing is a method used for the information extraction from the returns of the target. The echoes received at the radar receiver are processed in the digital format. Radars are widely classified on the basis of resolution capability.

P. J. B. Morris
SO-D, FRD Division, Radar-V, LRDE, DRDO, Bangalore, India

K. Dhonde (✉) · B. K. Priya
Department of Electronics and Communication Engineering, Amrita School of Engineering, Amrita Vishwa Vidyapeetham, Bangalore, India
e-mail: kunjdhonde@gmail.com

B. K. Priya
e-mail: bk_priya@blr.amrita.edu

© Springer Nature Singapore Pte Ltd. 2019
V. Sridhar et al. (eds.), *Emerging Research in Electronics, Computer Science and Technology*, Lecture Notes in Electrical Engineering 545,
https://doi.org/10.1007/978-981-13-5802-9_68

Resolution can be defined as the ability of the radar to differentiate between closely spaced targets. Range resolution and azimuth resolution are determined to detect the closely spaced targets in range and angle, respectively. Fine range resolution can be obtained by pulse compression method. Pulse compression includes the use of internally modulated long pulse to obtain high energy which eventually yields the resolution of a short pulse [1].

Doppler Beam Sharpening (DBS) technique can be expressed as the combined product of antenna theory and digital signal processing. Azimuth resolution is improved by DBS technique. In Doppler Beam Sharpening technique, the received signals are pulse compressed to get the desired resolution. The compressed waveforms are then filtered using the matched filter. Matched filters are linear networks which are used to increase the peak signal-to-noise ratio (SNR) of the signal which in turn increases the probability of target detection. DBS takes the advantage of the forward motion of the radar to produce the equivalent large antenna [2]. Increased virtual length of the antenna provides the increase in the resolution in the angular direction.

The concept of synthetic-aperture radar (SAR) was firstly introduced in 1951 by Carl Wiley of Goodyear. SAR was defined as the radar which can analyse the target returns in time domain. Therefore, it was named as Doppler Beam Sharpening technique (DBS). Later, DBS was used to analyse the Doppler-processed echoes to produce better azimuth resolution than that produced by the real beam alone. With the motion of the platform on which the radar is mounted, a synthetic large aperture of the antenna is produced. This, in turn, improves the cross-range resolution. Each time a pulse is transmitted, the radar occupies a position a little farther along on the flight path. By pointing a small antenna out to one side and summing the returns from successive pulses, it is possible to synthesize a very long side-looking linear array [2].

In modern airborne radar systems, Doppler Beam Sharpening technique is used as a mode to get a coarse image of the target region along with fine range and cross-range resolution. In this paper, we have developed a MATLAB code to demonstrate the Doppler Beam Sharpening technique with Doppler diversity.

2 DBS Algorithm

One of the fundamental issues in DBS technique is the selection of pulse repetitive frequency (PRF). The optimal choice of PRF results in finer cross-range resolution and decreases the error probability in detection. With a small physical antenna operating at desirable PRF, DBS can provide azimuth resolution as fine as $0.5°$. The added advantage of DBS is it can work equally well in day or night, through smoke, fog, haze or clouds, rain, etc.

DBS operates in coherent low-PRF mode. Initially, the returns from a target are pulse compressed. The returns from the target have a pre-defined Doppler frequency which in turn is dependent on the relative speed. Lower the speed, lower will be the

Fig. 1 Different scanning regions used in DBS

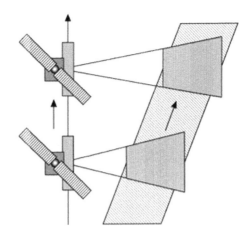

Doppler frequency. Also, the target moving away from the radar imposes a downshift in the frequency and vice versa. Doppler frequency is a function of speed of the radar platform and the measure of the azimuth direction as shown in Fig. 1.

$$f = (2 * v) * \cos \theta / \lambda \tag{1}$$

where,

f   = Doppler frequency
v   = speed
λ = wavelength of signal
Θ = azimuth angle.

2.1 Pulse Compression

Pulse compression is defined as a method which combines the high energy of a long pulse width with the high resolution of a short pulse width [3]. A long pulse is modulated and transmitted to achieve better range resolution. The operation necessarily ignores the involvement of high-power transmission. Long pulses are better for signal reception but contradict to the range resolution as shown in Fig. 2.

In pulse compression technique, usually the signal is frequency or phase modulated. The most commonly used is the linear frequency modulated signal (LFM). LFM is used to achieve wide transmission bandwidth and for the radar receiver. In this paper, we have modulated an up-chirp linear frequency modulation waveform. Mathematically, the up-chirp LFM can be expressed as:

$$S(t) = \sin\{2\pi \left(f * t + \left(k * t^2/2\right)\right)\} \tag{2}$$

Fig. 2 Optimal transmitted
and received signal

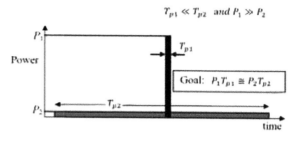

Fig. 3 Linear frequency
modulated waveform

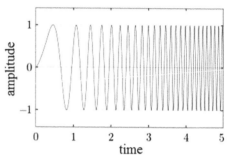

where

S(t) = LFM signal
F   = carrier frequency
K   = chirp rate
T   = time.

Figure 3 illustrates the instantaneous frequency of LFM waveform that sweeps out different time intervals. The input to the pulse compression filter is a weak pulse. The output pulse is, however, a very strong and narrow waveform which increases the detection capacity.

2.2 Matched Filter

The returns from a target are corrupted by additive white Gaussian noise (AWGN). The probability of detection of a target is related to the SNR. Therefore, maximizing the SNR is the primary concern of the filter design than preserving the shape of the waveform. The filter used for this purpose is called matched filter. The filter is matched provided that the signal is the complex conjugate of the time inverse of the filter's impulse response h(τ) [4]. Pulse compression filters are the practical implementation of the matched filter. Mathematically, the output of matched filter is expressed as

$$Y(t) = \int h(\tau) \cdot h * (t - \tau) d\tau \qquad (3)$$

3 Ambiguities in DBS

In DBS, ambiguities arise due to the malfunction of the system or irrelevant parameter selection for the operating radar. Usually, there are two types of ambiguities which occur frequently.

3.1 Range Ambiguity

Range ambiguity occurs when the PRF of the operating radar is high. The time between two successive transmitted pulses is not sufficient for receiving the echoes. For instant, if the echo due to the first transmitted pulse reaches the receiver after the transmission of second pulse, the probability of accurate detection decreases. It may also happen that the first echo coincides with the echo due to the second pulse. This leads to misinterpretation of targets. This phenomenon is called as range ambiguity. For the range to be unambiguous, the PRF chosen should be low. Usually, the low-PRF values lie in the range of 1–30 kHz. Low-PRF operating radar allows the receiver to receive more number of coherent echoes. This decreases the ambiguity and increases the accurate observations as shown in Fig. 4.

3.2 Doppler Ambiguity

Doppler ambiguity arises due to the discontinuous nature of a pulsed signal as shown in Fig. 5. Doppler ambiguities occur at the output due to the imperfections in tuning with the filter response at the receiver of the radar. The received signal passes through a filter which is matched to the frequency of the transmitted signal shifted by the target's Doppler frequency. If the PRF is high, the chances of Doppler ambiguities are negligible. However, if the PRF is low, the rate of Doppler ambiguity increases. The filter at the receiver may be tuned to the transmitted frequency or to the multiples of the frequency shifted by the target's Doppler frequency. These are termed as spectral lines. Greater the difference between the received frequency and the tuned

Fig. 4 Demonstration of range ambiguity

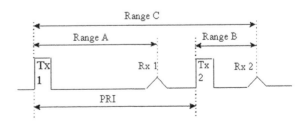

Fig. 5 Illustration of
Doppler effect

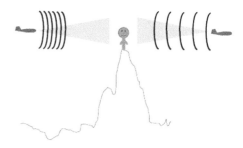

line, deeper will be the effect of ambiguity on the output signal. Hence, depending
on the PRF of the radar, the observed Doppler frequencies may be ambiguous.

4 Simulation Results

The parameters are defined based on the specifications of the real-time radar simulation project. The real-time data is provided by the LRDE based on the echoes
received by the radar, and then the processing of the signal is done using MAT LAB
simulation. Figure 6 shows the pulse compression waveform. The received signal
is swamped by spurious signals and noise (AWGN). Pulse compression detects the
targets even in the presence of the noise.

Figure 7 demonstrates the pulse compression output in 3-D plot. Figure 7 appears
to be more comprehensive than Fig. 6.

In spite of the input signal swamped by the AWGN, the output yields the satisfying
results with respect to the pulse width and peak amplitude. The output possesses a

Fig. 6 Pulse compression
output

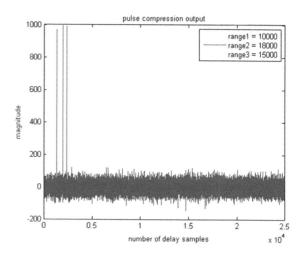

clear visibility of targets. Figure 8 demonstrates the matched filter output after pulse compression. The simulation is done by taking three target echoes that are corrupted by noise. The targets simulated in Fig. 8 are stationary. Thus, there is no Doppler shift imposed on the radar returns.

At the time of the detection of targets, the most important parameter of the targets that has to be known is the range and the velocity of the target. Figure 9 demonstrates the Doppler-range plot used in the real-time radar systems. The plot shows the distance of the target and the relative speed of the target with respect to the radar.

Figure 10 shows the simulation results of moving targets with noise. The different arrangement of target peaks in the plot demonstrates different velocity and range of targets.

The parameters used for simulation are listed as follows (Table 1).

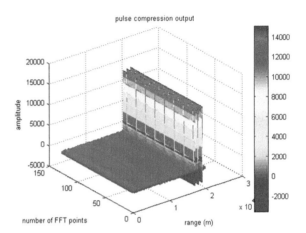

Fig. 7 Detection of stationary targets

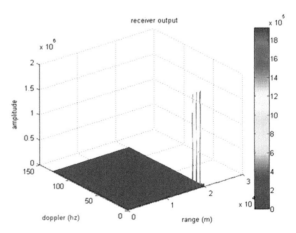

Fig. 8 Matched filter output

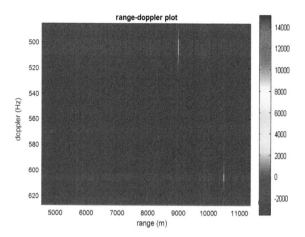

Fig. 9 Range-Doppler plot

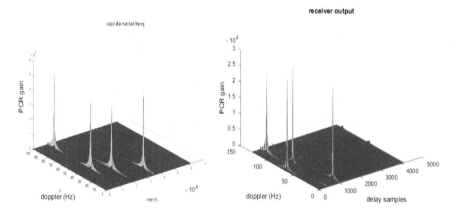

Fig. 10 Detection of moving targets

Table 1 List of parameters used for the simulation

Parameters	Values
Sampling frequency	10 MHz
Pulse width	50 µs
Bandwidth	10 MHz
Wavelength (λ)	0.01818 m
Range resolution	15 m
Pulse repetitive frequency	1 kHz
Number of pulses	128
Total samples	4096

5 Conclusion

The technique of Doppler Beam Sharpening was presented in this paper using the LFM up-chirp pulse modulation. In this method, the received signal is pulse compressed at the initial stages of processing. Further, the waveforms are passed through a matched filter which is tuned to the transmitted frequency. Doppler processing of the signals ensures strong and narrow waveforms with least possible ambiguities. The effectiveness of DBS technique is determined by the PRF of the airborne radar system. In this paper, the effects of PRF on the processing and the respective outputs have been demonstrated. Also, the generation of corresponding ambiguities is demonstrated. The DBS technique is a very important technique used in modern radars especially the SAR where complex signal processing is carried out to resolve range ambiguity and Doppler ambiguity which provides more accuracy to the target detection.

Acknowledgements This project work is carried out in the Electronics and Radar Development Establishment (LRDE) laboratories based on the real-time signals. The authors express their gratitude to the head of LRDE for providing an opportunity to carry out the project work.

References

1. Skolnik Ml (1988) Introduction to radar systems. McGraw-Hill, Sydney, pp 433–435
2. Stimson GW (1998) Introduction to airborne radar. SciTech Publishing Inc, New Jersey, pp 402–404
3. Moreira A, Prats-Iraola P, Younis M, Krieger G, Hajnsek I, Papathanassiou KP (2013) A tutorial on synthetic aperture radar. IEEE Geosci Remote Sens Mag 1(1)
4. Lewis BL, Kretschmer FF (1982) Linear frequency modulation derived polyphase pulse compression codes. IEEE Trans Aerosp Electr Syst AES-18(5):637–641

Capturing Discriminative Attributes Using Convolution Neural Network Over ConceptNet Numberbatch Embedding

Vivek Vinayan, M. Anand Kumar and K. P. Soman

Abstract A semantic representation of text helps us understand the lexical associa-tion between words. Capturing these associations becomes an integral part of perceiv-ing any language. One such fundamental property that expresses these associations is 'similarity.' This property shows consistency in comprehending similar words in the same manner. However, seldom it falls short on specific tasks where the lexical similarity in itself is not sufficient enough to validate the semantic representations. In this paper, the objective is to capture such semantic distinctions. It is based on the shared task 'capturing discriminative attributes' conducted in SemEval-2018. Our team participated in the task and held an F1 score of 0.658 with GloVe representation. An extension to this work is taken up in this paper where a new embedding known as ConceptNet Numberbatch is explored. The ConceptNet word embedding in overall showed improvement in the scores with the previous rule-based feature representa-tion. The model is further tuned over certain hyperparameters, which improved the score to as much as 6%. A comparison is also put forth here with another prominent embedding like FastText. The ConceptNet model achieved a near par score with the state of the art, based only on a simple ensemble of features as representation.

Keywords Discriminative attributes · ConceptNet Numberbatch embedding · Convolution neural network (CNN) · Word-sense disambiguation

1 Introduction

Similarity is one of the most commonly used methods of measure between texts, and semantic similarity in particular is used more often to compare various semantic representations. This metric calculates the distance between terms, based on the likeness of their meaning. Take, for example, these two sentences 'he held an apple'

V. Vinayan (✉) · M. Anand Kumar · K. P. Soman
Center for Computational Engineering and Networking (CEN), Amrita School of Engineering
Coimbatore, Amrita Vishwa Vidyapeetham, Coimbatore, India
e-mail: vivekvinayan82@gmail.com

© Springer Nature Singapore Pte Ltd. 2019
V. Sridhar et al. (eds.), *Emerging Research in Electronics, Computer Science and Technology*, Lecture Notes in Electrical Engineering 545,
https://doi.org/10.1007/978-981-13-5802-9_69

Table 1 Similarity measured for words over GloVe, FastText, and ConceptNet embedding

Words	Word embedding		
	GloVe	FastText	ConceptNet
apple	iphone	apple	red fruit
	ipad	apples	adam_eve
	apple	apple	computer brand
	blackberry	apple	tree_fruits
	ipod	pear	apple john
paris	france	france	ile st louis
	lyon	paris	city of light
	london	paris	In_france
	france	parisian	montmartre
	berlin	london	paris syndrome

and 'he held an orange'; these sentences are similar given the fact that a person is holding a fruit or more generically an edible item, but it does not illustrate the difference between them needless to say it is like 'comparing apples to oranges.' These methods measure a sense of comparison that certain words may carry when used interchangeably, while retaining a similar context. Similarity being implemented over various applications, it has proved to capture common traits among text that have helped attribute it as a feature. The widely considered cosine similarity is one such measure where it is used to calculate the similarity between two vectors in a semantic space of a distributional representation. In Table 1 shown are such similarity words that are generated using commonly used word embeddings like GloVe, FastText, and ConceptNet with gensim [1].

Now, if we take more complex applications like machine translation or chatbot, it becomes a more complicated undertaking with just similarity-based measures as it would require prior knowledge on conversation or data. Let us consider the previous example of apples and oranges; contextually, the text may not have reference to the fruit apple being red or that oranges being round, and without this knowledge, it will become difficulties to attribute them before acknowledging it. Such traits of similarity are also discussed in their work by Faruqui et al. [2] where they showed how similarity could constraint specific applications. This arises a requirement to evaluate such specific semantic representation. Alicia Kerbs and Denis Paperno address in their work [3] how the difference in semantics between a related pair of words can differ contrastingly to that of their similar nature, and capturing these differences can project characteristics that were previously not attributed. The simplistic nature of the similarity generally avoids the need to go in deep, whereas interpreting such semantic intricacies can help in improving the understanding of existing word embedding. Thus, they released a proof of concept dataset which is used in the competition conducted by SemEval-2018's task of 'capturing discriminative attributes' [4].

In the paper [5] presented are the findings by our team for the same competition. Two models are discussed one based of SVM algorithm which is explored earlier for sense disambiguation of a native language (Tamil), presented by Anand kumar et al. [6], and another is a model represented on various features using GloVe embedding [7] evaluated over a simple convolution neural network. There the model is represented over the various dimensions of GloVe embedding, of those the 300 dimensions (trained over a common crawl corpus of size 840B) embedding performed the best for the task. Building on features, a representation is arrived at with a feature length 1203. This model secured an F1 score of 0.6580 posted on their official page.[1] In this paper, we base our representation on a newer method of embedding called the ConceptNet Numberbatch [4] which are pretrained word embedding evolved over data source procured for word2vec [8] and GloVe [7] embedding, combined using extension of retrofitting technique [2]. This is a freely available word embedding[2] which has shown state-of-the-art performance at word similarity, within and across languages at SemEval-2017 [9].

2 Dataset

The dataset being used in this work is a proof of concept dataset provided by [3] for the SemEval-2018 task [4]. The data is split into three sets train, validation, and test. The training set is the largest of the three with over 17 K examples which are automatically constructed examples by a procedure explained in their data creation section of shared task. The test and validation data were manually curated examples which are just over 5 K, where instances are distributed near equally among them. As the validation set is curated similar to that of the test set, it is recommended by the organizers to use validation only for parameter tuning over the trained set model. The interesting part about the feature words is that the ones used in training are mostly not carried over to the validation and test. This is understandable to keep the model from not being hardcoded only to certain categories of attribute words.

Moving to the data in itself, it is binary class classification task with each instance having three words a pivot, compare, and attribute word as shown in Table 2. The original training set having a total 17,782 instances (with few duplicates bringing down the unique set to 17,501). Of which there are 11,171 of a negative instance and 6330 of positive instance this is as provided in their GitHub Page.[3] The validation set contains 2722, where 1364 are positive and 1358 are negative example. The test set has 2340 instances (further details on the individual can be found on their page link given above.). On observing the training data, it can be realized that the data is intentionally kept noisy with the validation set in comparison to the label distribution of each set. The positive instances or label '1' attributes the word having confident association only with the pivot word in the order presented and not the vice

---

Table 2 Snippet of training dataset

Pivot	Compare	Attribute	Label
oven	microwave	control	1
moose	elk	waxing	0
harpoon	missile	inexpensive	0
corn	pineapple	ears	1
panther	elephant	pillows	0
belt	plate	buckles	1
orange	cherry	sections	1
razor	brush	mink	0

verse, e.g., (sailboat, yacht, motor, 1); here, 'motor' is an attribute only associated to 'sailboat' and (yacht, sailboat, motor) will be an invalid entry. The combination (yacht, sailboat) in this order will only be added if concept 'yacht' has a feature that sailboat does not have in this set. On the other hand, the negative examples or label '0' is considered when the attribute is either similar to both pivot and the compare word like (car, tractor, breaks, 0) or are dissimilar to both the words, e.g., (car, tractor, lakes, 0). The work on the dataset is based on a method, that was presented by Lazaridou and team [10] for the prediction of distinguishing feature with use of images as reference for visual discrimination attribute identification task; more prominently, it was related to capturing of lexical information using offset vectors. The data collected by McRae et al. [11] and team was a list of attributes asked to produce by participants on numerous concepts (animate and inanimate). The dataset was created on semantic word pair using random sample words from BLESS [12], where attributes were assigned manually for word pairs.

3 Methodology

In this section, we discuss on rule-based differentiation of representation. Also, the implementation of a recently developed word embedding known as ConceptNet Numberbatch embedding [4]. Further, we show a comparison study over the previous rule-based method and word embedding discussed over from our earlier work, finally concluding with a comparison of accuracies over different pretrained word embedding.

3.1 Representation

As shown earlier, only words are used in datasets and representing them becomes an important part of the objective to capture semantic differences exhibited by the words.

Table 3 Abbreviations for feature used in representation

Legend	
Cos_p	Cosine similarity (Wp, Wa)
Cos_c	Cosine similarity (Wc, Wa)
Dis_p	Kulsinski (Wp, Wa)
Dis_c	Kulsinski (Wc, Wa)
Min_p	Minkowski (Wp, Wa, p = 1)
Min_c	Minkowski (Wc, Wa, p = 1)

These are attributed by using pretrained word embeddings of varied dimension. From the earlier work in [5], it is empirically evident that 300 dimension word vectors are best suitable for this task. Thus, the dataset is represented as follows where Wa denotes attribute word, Wp denotes the pivot word, and Wc denotes the compare word. In Table 3, other commonly used terms are shown that will be discussed ahead.

Using the above nomenclature, we take a simple approach with rule-based representations. As shown in Table 4, conditional representation or CR is derived, where based on certain measure between the words, the first or the second representation is selected. Followed up on these representations, an ensemble of other features is added to further attribute to the representation. This is as shown by representation 3, 4, and 5 in Table 5.

Table 4 Nomenclature for feature representation on rule-based classification

S. no.	Conditional representation (CR)	
	If:	Else:
1	Wp, (Wp + Wa), Wc, Wa	Wp, (Wp − Wa), Wc, (Wc − Wa)
2	Wp, (Wp + Wa), Wc, Wa, (Dis_c − Dis_p)	Wp, (Wp − Wa), Wc, (Wc − Wa), (Dis_c − Dis_p)

Table 5 Validation and testing accuracy using ConceptNet Numberbatch embedding based on Eq. 1

S. no.	Representation	Validation		Testing
		Accuracy	F1 score	F1 score
1	CR1	0.6071	0.5226	0.6373
2	CR2	0.6071	0.5599	0.6516
3	CR1, (cos1 − cos2)	0.6119	0.5929	0.6410
4	CR2, (cos1 − cos2), Min p, Min c	0.5928	0.5267	0.6472
5	CR2, Min p, Min c	0.6001	0.5780	0.6777

3.2 ConceptNet Numberbatch

In the competition, we used GloVe embedding to form our representation which performed considerably well in the competition (although not at par with other systems in the competition). Projecting the specificity of the task, it dealt with only words for representation capitulating further needs for capturing semantic differences intuitively. Thus, we came across another method of embedding called ConceptNet Numberbatch embedding. This embedding has shown to outperform other embeddings like word2vec and GloVe in SemEval-2017 task of extending word embeddings with multilingual relational knowledge [9]. Table 5 shows the accuracy and F1 score of the validation and the test set for a 1D convolution network representation, where the base conditional representation (CR)/rule-based representation is as shown in Table 4 based on the rule of Eq. 1 from Sect. 3.3.

The neural network constitutes a single 1D convolution layer, having twenty convolution kernels of size 3 followed with a single dense layer consisting of thirty-two neurons passed on over 'ReLU' activation function and the output layer with a single neuron classified over sigmoid for the binary classification. It is based on the work presented by Vinayakumar in [13]. From the earlier results that are secured in the work [5], it is noticed that the GloVe embedding evaluated validation accuracy and F1 score have improved considerably with the new ConceptNet embedding. This is also reected in the test score where the labels have been classified considerable better than GloVe embedding.

3.3 Rule-Based Method

As the dataset is of binary class, a simple rule-based approach is taken attributing to the word vector for representation. In our earlier work, a comparison of various distance, similarity, and dissimilarity techniques are implemented on the word embeddings. It is narrowed down to Kulsinski dissimilarity measure expressed using the SciPy [14] library for rule-based differentiation which gave the closest disambiguation between Wp, Wa and Wc, Wa representation from the training label. This is later extended to form representations of the test and validation dataset for evaluation. As the rule-based method is the primary distinguishing task between the classes, another such approach is introduced in this work as the comparison. In the earlier work, only Kulsinski dissimilarity is considered for rule-based representation given in Eq. 1.

$$Dis2 > Dis1 \tag{1}$$

where Dis1 is referred to Dis (Wp, Wa), Dis2 to Dis (Wc, Wa).

Similarity measure like cosine was also tested, but it fetched a comparatively lower validation score over the same set of representations. After the release of the

Table 6 Validation and testing accuracy using ConceptNet Numberbatch embedding based on Eq. 2

S. no.	Representation	Validation		Testing
		Accuracy	F1 score	F1 score
1	CR1	0.6229	0.6435	0.6523
2	CR2	0.6071	0.5599	0.6516
3	CR1, (cos1 − cos2)	0.6086	0.5728	0.6405
4	CR2, (cos1 − cos2), Min_p, Min_c	0.6244	0.6524	0.6617
5	CR2, Min_p, Min_c	0.5884	0.5608	0.6577

gold data, the cosine rule-based feature representation gave an F1 score of 0.6261 on the same representation where Kulsinski ruled based gave 0.6581. In variation to the independent cosine rule, another rule-based representation is formulated by incorporating both the earlier methods shown in Eq. 2.

$$\max(\text{Cos}1, (1 - \text{Dis}1)) > \max(\text{Cos}2, (1 - \text{Dis}2)) \tag{2}$$

where Cos1 is Cos (Wp, Wa) and Cos2 is Cos (Wc, Wa).

Comparing the results of Table 6 with that of the GloVe embedding in [5], the score has improved moderately, whereas compared to the results in Table 5, it is noticeable to see that Eq. 1 rule-based representation gives a better result.

3.4 Hyperparameter Tuning

In further effort of improving on the scores, the model is tweaked around on certain hyperparameters by switching certain optimizer and also by increasing the hidden layer on the neural network. With the change in the optimizer to RMSprop (with default values), we are able to increase F1 score on the test set to as much as 0.6955. This is by far the best score that is gained by the ConceptNet embedding over the model; it is as shown in Table 7.

The neural network is then extended with an additional dense layer of sixty-four neuron with ReLU activation over RMSprop optimizer; the results are as shown in Table 8. The increase in layer did not show any significant improvement over the vious result but on an overall achieved a better result than the GloVe.

It is understandable by now that word representation is the main focus of this work. Capturing the semantic of words plays an important role in forming these representations, and these are captured over well-defined embedding which are openly available. Thus, another such prominently used embedding model is FastText [15].

These use efficient learning models trained over large datasets with a hierarchical softmax approach.

Table 7 Validation and testing accuracy using ConceptNet Numberbatch embedding based on Eq. 1

S. no.	Representation	Validation		Testing
		Accuracy	F1 score	F1 score
1	CR1	0.6141	0.6148	0.6639
2	CR2	0.6115	0.6084	0.6543
3	CR1, (cos1 − cos2)	0.6079	0.5774	0.6691
4	CR2, (cos1 − cos2), Min_p, Min_c	0.6281	0.6391	0.6645
5	CR2, Min_p, Min_c	0.6468	0.6554	0.6955

Table 8 Validation and testing accuracy after increasing the dense layers

S. no.	Representation	Validation		Testing
		Accuracy	F1 score	F1 score
1	CR1	0.6167	0.5882	0.6547
2	CR2	0.6226	0.5867	0.6626
3	CR1, (cos1 − cos2)	0.6046	0.5587	0.6578
4	CR2, (cos1 − cos2), Min_p, Min_c	0.5928	0.5267	0.6472
5	CR2, Min_p, Min_c	0.6119	0.5810	0.6628

Table 9 Validation and testing accuracy over the three embeddings considered for this work

S. no.	Representation	Embedding	Validation		Testing
			Accuracy	F1 score	F1 score
1	CR2, Min_p, Min_c	GloVe	0.6113	0.6023	0.6583
2		FastText	0.6494	0.6653	0.6699
3		ConceptNet	0.6468	0.6554	0.6955

In Table 9, the representation (CR2, Min_p, Min_c) is considered for FastText as this has shown highest accuracy across the embedding with earlier GloVe, ConceptNet embedding. It is evident from the result that ConceptNet is able to capture the semantic differences better among the embedding for the discriminative attribute task.

4 Conclusion and Future Scope

The objective of capturing distinguishing attribute has been evidently supportive of the fact that even with such seemingly simply dataset, similarity measure is not always reliable in distinguishing task. Thus, with such applications, taking a different perspective can contribute in diversifying from the inherent similarity approach and assist in understanding and evaluating the context between words more comprehensively. This added to the fact that capturing discerning feature among perceivable similar words can advocate for attributing to a more profound approach in performing various applications even better. In this paper, we deliberate on how to tackle the problem using a rule-based approach with iterative set of feature representation by using a recently new word embedding called the Concepnet Numberbatch. The new embedding gave the edge in outperforming the earlier GloVe embedding and also over another well-known embedding, FastText. Tuning the model over certain hyperparameter also gained in improving the F1 score to approximately 0.70.

As a future scope of this project, improving the model can be addressed at a rudimentary level by focusing on the rule-based segregation between the binary representation; i.e., the more closer that we are able to bring our rule to the training label, the better we will be able to train the model with the representations. Such evaluation technique can trickle down to help study and evaluate numerous native languages on their morphological structures; ironically, this comes as a double edged sword as this also can pose a bigger challenge when comparing to languages like English. Furthermore, these semantic difference can be attributed not only on multiple Indian languages but also across lingual platform (example, Tamil and Malayalam words resemble in many ways), and understanding such attributes can aid in the application like machine translation.

References

1. Rehurek R, Sojka P (2010) Software framework for topic modelling with large corpora. In: Proceedings of the LREC 2010 workshop on new challenges for NLP frameworks
2. Faruqui M, Dodge J, Jauhar SK, Dyer C, Hovy E, Smith NA (2014) Retrofitting word vectors to semantic lexicons. arXiv:1411.4166
3. Krebs A, Paperno D (2016) Capturing discriminative attributes in a distributional space: task proposal. In: Proceedings of the 1st workshop on evaluating vector-space representations for NLP
4. Krebs A, Paperno D (2018) SemEval-2018 task 10: capturing discriminative attributes. In: Proceedings of international workshop on semantic evaluation (SemEval-2018), New Orleans, LA, USA
5. Vinayan V, Kumar MA, Soman KP (2018) Amrita NLP at SemEval-2018 task 10: capturing discriminative attributes using convolution neural network over global vector representation. In: Proceedings of the international workshop on semantic evaluation (SemEval-2018)
6. Anand Kumar M, Rajendran S, Soman KP (2014) Tamil word sense disambiguation using support vector machines with rich features. Int J Appl Eng Res 9(20):7609–7620
7. Pennington J, Socher R, Manning C (2014) GloVe: global vectors for word representation. In: Proceedings of the 2014 conference on empirical methods in natural language processing (EMNLP), pp 1532–1543
8. Mikolov T, Chen K, Corrado G, Dean J (2013) Efficient estimation of word representations in vector space. arXiv:1301.3781
9. Speer R, Chin J, Havasi C (Feb 2017) ConceptNet 5.5: an open multilingual graph of general knowledge. In: AAAI, pp 4444–4451
10. Lazaridou A, Pham NT, Baroni M (2016) The red one!: on learning to refer to things based on their discriminative properties. arXiv:1603.02618
11. McRae K, Cree GS, Seidenberg MS, McNorgan C (2005) Semantic feature production norms for a large set of living and nonliving things. Behav Res Methods 1;37(4):547–59

12. Baroni M, Lenci A. How we BLESSed distributional semantic evaluation. In: Proceedings of the GEMS 2011 workshop on GEometrical models of natural language semantics, Association for Computational Linguistics, pp 1–10, 31 July 2011
13. Vinayakumar R, Poornachandran P, Soman KP (2018) Scalable framework for cyber threat situational awareness based on domain name systems data analysis. In: Big data in engineering applications. Springer, Singapore, pp 113–142
14. Jones E, Oliphant T, Peterson P (2014) SciPy: open source scientific tools for Python
15. Bojanowski P, Grave E, Joulin A, Mikolov T (2016) Enriching word vectors with subword information. arXiv:1607.04606
16. Speer R, Lowry-Duda J (2017) Conceptnet at semeval-2017 task 2: extending word embeddings with multilingual relational knowledge. arXiv:1704.03560
17. Speer R, Havasi C (2013) ConceptNet 5: a large semantic network for relational knowledge. In: The peoples web meets NLP. Springer, Berlin, Heidelberg, pp 161–176

Prediction of Gold Stock Market Using Hybrid Approach

Vimuktha E. Salis, Akanksha Kumari and Animesh Singh

Abstract Presently, stock market is the most important part of economy of the country and acts as key driver for its growth. Since gold is oldest form of currency, it drives more attention of people to invest in gold stock market. As we know stock market is volatile in nature and risk inevitable. To maximize profit, we need a model which predicts stock in upcoming future. A lot of data have to be dealt for précised prediction, and machine learning will be faultless. This paper uses artificial neural network (ANN) for predicting the fluctuation in gold price. It takes historical data and predicts the price for next day. The aim was to build a model which forecasts price with maximum precision and also helps user to maximize their profit. Model has achieved success but forecasting gold stock market prices is highly complicated and depends on series of events such as festival, political event, and marriage seasons. They also depend on other commodities like Sensex, Nifty, crude oil, and so on. Model will not be capable of taking these events into account as they fall randomly, but people who regularly invest in stock market can give better advice.

Keywords ANN · LSTM · Expert advice · NSE

1 Introduction

The main aim of any investor in stock exchange is to maximize their profit and they can attain it if they know the right time to invest. We have taken gold as our major commodity as it is used as currency worldwide. When major changes occur in stock market, stakeholder tends to invest in gold and considers it as long-term

V. E. Salis (✉) · A. Kumari · A. Singh
BNMIT, Bangalore, India
e-mail: vimuktha_ej@yahoo.com

A. Kumari
e-mail: akanksha5996@gmail.com

A. Singh
e-mail: 04animeshsingh@gmail.com

© Springer Nature Singapore Pte Ltd. 2019
V. Sridhar et al. (eds.), *Emerging Research in Electronics, Computer Science and Technology*, Lecture Notes in Electrical Engineering 545,
https://doi.org/10.1007/978-981-13-5802-9_70

investment. Gold in India has been traditionally and culturally important to people because of their emotions are deeply connected with this commodity. On the other hand, precious metal such as gold historically had a great impact on the prices of other essential commodities. Profit maximization can be done by detailed analysis of present and past situation of the stock market. In this paper, GOLDBEES of National Stock Exchange (NSE) is monitored.

A model is required which predicts next day price with maximum precision. As for detailed analysis, a lot of historical data have to be processed, and machine learning algorithm is required. Previous work shows artificial neural network has the best result. A special case of artificial neural network and recurrent neural network is used for prediction model. Recurrent neural network uses long short-term memory (LSTM) algorithm. A common LSTM unit consists of several cells i.e., input gate, output gate, and forget gate. The cells are responsible for remembering values for certain period of time, and after that some amount of data are removed from memory which is less relevant to approximate the next prediction. These three gates can be considered as conventional artificial neuron as in multilayer of neural network which is used to compute an activation of weighted sum using activation function("reglu," "sigmoid," "softmax," "linear," and so on). Numbers of layer are involved in LSTM algorithm with number of parameters whose value is unknown to user who makes LSTM black box. We provide historical data to LSTM algorithm and it gives prediction for next day by processing internally hiding its parameter details.

This paper also includes expert advice which guides new user when to invest in stock exchange to maximize their profit. There are number of people who invest in stock market on regular basis and can give better advice when to invest as they know effect of various events on stock price which cannot be included in model as event fall randomly. A mathematical model together with expert advice gives us an intelligent model which helps us to predict next day price as well as benefits new user by guiding them when to invest. Second section describes the previous work and research done in this field. Third section includes detailed proposed model design along with bock diagram of both models separately. Fourth section concludes the paper and gives some suggestions for future enhancement which will eventually make the model better.

2   Related Work

There are three techniques related to the information required to make a stock prediction. The techniques are technical analysis, fundamental analysis, and information coming from both (hybrid method). Technical analysis is used within the stock to predict the future stock price and fluctuation in price by examining the historical stock data. Fundamental analysis is based on external influence and factors as political condition in country, GDP growth of country, economic situation of other countries and statements given by economist. This information is taken from unstructured data such as weekly financial report, news articles or even tweets, or blogs by analysts and big investors. Finally, third technique uses information coming from both technical analysis (time series data) and fundamental analysis (textual data).

Xiang and Fu [1] had proposed multiple models of auto-regressive and neural networks to predict S&P 500 price. Multiple models were used to model a particular trend like bear, bull, and choppy. They used decision rule to select one model from multiple models for further prediction. Their result analysis shows that multiple NNs is better than multiple auto-regressive, but it fails to predict value on daily basis.

Budhani et al. [2] had proposed artificial neural network model to predict stock price and suggested that non-linear model performs better than the linear model because of complex nature of stocks. They used feed forward network along with activation function (sigmoid function) to multiply input values to weights of neurons and sum up before sending to output layer and backpropagation algorithm to calculate the error in predicted value.

Somani et al. [3] used hidden markov model to predict stock price. Hidden markov model is very useful to locate patterns from past data that matches the current stock price behavior. They used open, close, high, and low technical indicators of stock for analysis purpose and Buam Welch algorithm used to train data set to develop model. Result analysis and accuracy were done by using MAPE.

Li et al. [4] had proposed long short-term memory (LSTM) neural network which incorporates historical data and sentiments of investor of CSI300 stocks. Naïve Bayes classification is used to categorize the post into positive, neutral, and negative categories, and then investor sentiment index was constructed to measure daily mood of stock market. LSTM model was used to train the past data and sentiment index for better performance. To calculate and compare accuracy from past model, they have taken support vector machine as benchmark.

Li et al. [5] had proposed a model to predict stock price using sentiment analysis and classification technique. They have incorporates—some semi-automatic and manual dictionaries like Harvard, Loughran and McDonald, Cambria—for sentiment analysis. In result analysis, they concluded that this method outperform bag of words architecture in validation and independent testing data sets.

Vivek et al. [6] proposed a hybrid approach where one model takes sentiments of investors and economist from news articles and tweets, and then categorizes the post into positive, neutral, and negative category while other model uses past data of different stock as input which forms positive, neutral, and negative clusters using DENCLUE clustering algorithm. Finally, information from both models were merged and analyzed for future prediction.

3   Proposed System

There were various models that were implemented before, like HMM, SVM, and artificial neural networks. over different models, none of the models considered essential commodities as a major front and sentiment affiliations from experts in the field directly. The key difference between other models and this model is that the method of implementation is incremental learning. The connection of past data and the predicted data together is an incremental form.

A. Model A

Thus Model A illustrates the effect of stock market and events on gold through Goggle feedback form. Each user is allowed to give feedback. They can give their perspective about changes in price of gold due to other commodities and other series of events. They can rate their perspective from 1(denoting less change) to 5(denoting high changes) for each question which will be recorded from each user.

The user is asked to enter his name and whether he/she has ever invested in stock market in "Yes" or "No" whose answers are to be retrieved and analysis is to be performed. This is done by downloading the user feedback in .csv format. Answers about have you ever invested in stock market is passed as query to piece of code written in python to check whether the feedback given by user is appropriate or not to summarize what will be effect of other commodities and events on price of gold (Figs. 1 and 2).

If user does not had have past experience about Stock Market Movement then we are not considering particular feedback on other hand if he has experience then we are combining his/her survey with other surveys and converting into percentage to show the effect of other commodities on price of gold like in our project we have considered the Nifty/Sensex, US Dollar value, Crude Oil, Indian festivals like Diwali/Dushhera/Akashay Tritia.

B. Model B

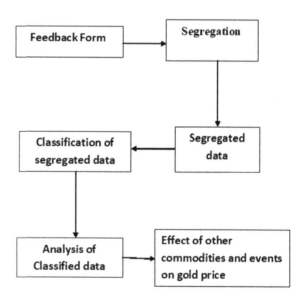

Fig. 1 Model A (feedback form analysis)

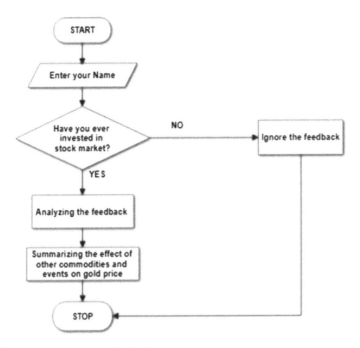

Fig. 2 Flowchart for retrieval of feedbacks by user

Thus Model B illustrates the stock market prediction using LSTM neural network based on technical parameters. As we have explained how LSTM works in brief in introduction part, Jiahong et al. [6] has described the LSTM deep learning approach that we are following here. In this section, we will be describing the methodology we used with help of python artificial neural network library Keras.

1. *Importing the dataset module*

Historical data are downloaded from NSE in .csv format file and imported using pandas library and data are stored in a dataframe named df. To drop the missing values from data set in each row nand column, dropna() function is used. The .csv file contains only open, high, low, close, adjusted close, volume, and corresponding dates data for the stock of RELIANCE GOLDBEES on NSE for the time period from January 1, 2007 to May 8, 2018, but we are building our model only by using open, high, low, and close(OHLC) prices of day (Fig. 3).

2. *Normalizing the data module*

OHLC prices of stock can go to any value, so before building our neural network we need to transform OHLC feature. MinMaxScaler() function is used to scale each feature and here it translates each feature individually such that it is in the given range on training set, i.e., between minus one and one.

Fig. 3 Dataset

Adj Close	open	high	low
1000	1000	1105	940
947.8	957.8	957.8	940.05
942.39	948	948.5	944.1
945.67	950	951.9	946
950.15	950	951	945
947.18	945	945	940
940.71	944.98	948	941.1
943.65	944.86	948.45	942.05
946.9	948	948	945.01
947.05	950	951.4	942.3
944.82	945.82	945.95	930
940.38	941	941	937.75
939.62	949	949	944.9
946.37	945.1	947	944.05
945.82	945.82	952.08	945.82

3. *Splitting the data module*

To train and test data set, we have split the data set into two variables and Split() function. 90% of data is used for train the data and rest of 10% to test the data to do that four different dataframes are used e.g. X_train, X_test, y_train and y_test. The training data is used by the model to arrive at the weights of the model. The test data set is used to see how the model will perform on new data which would be fed into the model.

4. *Building neural network*

To build our neural network, we have used Sequential() function to create a sequential neural network model by passing arguments to its constructor and Dense() function used to build the different layers with different number of neurons, input shape, activation function, etc. (Figs. 4 and 5).

The Dense() function has the following arguments:

Units: This defines the number of nodes or neurons in that particular layer.

kernel_initializer: This defines the starting values for the weights of the different neurons in the hidden layer. We have defined this to be "uniform," which means that the weights will be initialized with values from a uniform distribution.

Activation: This is the activation function for the neurons in the particular hidden layer. In our neural network, we have used to activation functions rectified linear unit function or "relu" for hidden layer and sigmoid function for output layer.

After building network, we cannot directly train the model, you need to configure the learning process; here we have used compile method. It takes three arguments:

Loss: this is the objective that model will try to minimize. This defines the loss to be optimized during the training period. We define this loss to be the mean squared error.

Layer (type)	Output Shape	Param #
lstm_3 (LSTM)	(None, 22, 128)	68096
dropout_3 (Dropout)	(None, 22, 128)	0
lstm_4 (LSTM)	(None, 128)	131584
dropout_4 (Dropout)	(None, 128)	0
dense_3 (Dense)	(None, 32)	4128
dense_4 (Dense)	(None, 1)	33

Total params: 203,841
Trainable params: 203,841
Non-trainable params: 0

Fig. 4 LSTM model building parameters

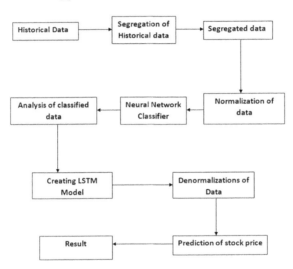

Fig. 5 Model B (LSTM model block diagram)

Optimizer: The optimizer is chosen to be "adam," which is an extension of the stochastic gradient descent.

Metrics: This defines the list of metrics to be evaluated by the model during the testing and training phase. We have chosen accuracy as our evaluation metric.

4   Result Analysis

1. *Performance estimation*

We used mean absolute error and root mean square error (RMSE) as metrics for measuring the performance of mathematical model. Mean absolute error (MAE) is the average difference between actual and predicted value. It is computed using following formula:

$$MAE = \frac{1}{n} \sum_{j=1}^{n} |y_j - y_j|$$ (1)

RMSE value is standard deviation between actual and predicted value and is computed using following formula:

$$RMSE = \sqrt{\frac{\sum_{i=1}^{N} (Predicted_i - Actual_i)^2}{N}}$$ (2)

2. *Plotting the graph of prediction*

Prediction graph is plotted along with actual values of stock. Matplotlib library is used to plot the graph. The plot shown below is the output of the code. The green line represents the actual values and the red line represents the predicted values of stock by the help of legend() and show() functions (Fig. 6; Tables 1 and 2).

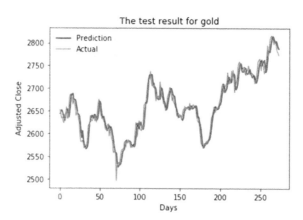

Fig. 6   Actual and predicted values plot

Table 1 Result with performance metrics value

Next day prediction	Actual value	MAE	RMSE
2784.166	2774.95	11.6588	14.5474

Table 2 Actual and Predicted value

Actual value	Predicted value
2652.784	2638.667
2646.985	2646.572
2633.925	2648.517
2635.777	2645.126
2627.59	2638.071
2623.205	2629.857
2642.112	2625.107
2640.163	2646.98
2658.875	2644.484
2634.364	2653.959
2633.34	2643.007
2656.731	2631.844

5 Conclusion and Future Work

In this paper, we have developed LSTM model with four layers which adds significant precision to model prediction. Each layer has 128 neurons and final model was trained with 90% of data and remaining was used for testing the model. For each testing, day prediction was made and along with next day price of gold. This algorithm was chosen as ANN has given précised result in various other research works and stock market prediction requires maximum precision as small change is treated as noise. Each small event has major impact on prediction of stock price.

Along with LSTM model, expert advice is provided. Stakeholder feedback was taken so that user can get advice from regular buyer of stock. This was an attempt to design an intelligent model which guides user to optimize their profit at maximum.

In future to improve accuracy, more index value can be used as getting more data was challenge for us and we used Google feedback to get survey from users, but we faced difficulties in getting feedbacks from regular investors so could not able to give accurate result from investors perspective. We look forward to improve our methodology and gathering more data for further work.

In future work, along with Google feedback survey sentiments of users can be added using tweets from twitter, news articles, weekly business magazines, etc. and as we mentioned we got 11.658 and 14.574 MAE and MRSE respectively so to get better result than this others can try different technical indicators and approach of neural network.

References

1. Xiang C, Fu WM. Predicting the stock market using multiple models, 1-4244-0342-1/06
2. Budhani N, Jha CK, Budhani SK. Prediction of stock market using artificial neural network, pp 1–8, 978-1-4673-9120-7/14
3. Farshchian M, Jahan MV. Stock market prediction using hidden Markov model, 978-1-4673-9762-9/15,473-477
4. Somani P, Talele S, Sawant S. Stock market prediction using hidden Markov model, pp 89–92, 978-1-4799-4419-4/14
5. Rajput V, Bobde S. Stock market prediction using hybrid approach, pp 82–86, 978-1-5090-1666-2/16
6. Li J, Bu H, Wu J. Sentiment-aware stock market prediction: a deep learning method, 978-1-5090-6371-0/17

Analysis of Digit Recognition in Kannada Using Kaldi Toolkit

K. Sundar Karthikeyan, K. Jeeva Priya and Deepa Gupta

Abstract This paper discusses recognition of digits in Kannada language using an open-source speech recognition tool, Kaldi. The system considers small digit corpora with numbers ranging from 0 to 9 and 4480 samples with a set of fourteen speakers. The monophone and triphone models of the corpora for Kannada language are investigated, and a significant decrease in the word error rate is observed while using the triphone modelling using Kaldi toolkit. The feature extraction is done with Mel-frequency Cepstral coefficients (MFCC). The word error rate (WER) is achieved for this corpus and compared with that achieved the HTK toolkit. A WER of 9% and 6%, respectively, is achieved with monophone modelling and triphone modelling using Kaldi toolkit, and with the same corpus, a WER of 10% is applied in HTK toolkit. A preliminary research of the speech recognition using Kaldi toolkit is reported in this paper.

Keywords ASR · Kaldi · Speech recognition · Monophone and triphone models · MFCC · WER

1 Introduction

The world is rapidly changing to digital, and communication between people and their gadgets increase at a greater pace. Speech recognition being one of the major applications of speech processing, is commercially finding wide applications.

K. Sundar Karthikeyan (✉) · K. Jeeva Priya
Department of Electronics and Communication Engineering,
Amrita School of Engineering, Amrita Vishwa Vidyapeetham, Bangalore, India
e-mail: karthikeyan5993@gmail.com

K. Jeeva Priya
e-mail: k_jeevapriya@blr.amrita.edu

D. Gupta
Department of Mathematics, Amrita School of Engineering,
Amrita Vishwa Vidyapeetham, Bangalore, India
e-mail: g_deepa@blr.amrita.edu

© Springer Nature Singapore Pte Ltd. 2019
V. Sridhar et al. (eds.), *Emerging Research in Electronics, Computer Science and Technology*, Lecture Notes in Electrical Engineering 545,
https://doi.org/10.1007/978-981-13-5802-9_71

Automatic speech recognition (ASR) system is the one which understands the spoken speech and converts it into its equivalent textual representation. An ASR system can be classified based on the amount of data or the size of vocabulary used for training the system, the relevance of the speaker and the manner of speech. These three categories can be further classified as:

- Based on data set or the vocabulary size as, small vocabulary which uses less than 100 words, medium vocabulary which uses less than 1000 words and large vocabulary which uses more than 1000 words.
- Based on relevance of the speaker as, speaker dependent and speaker independent.
- Based on the manner of speech as, connected speech recognition, continuous speech recognition, isolated speech recognition and spontaneous speech recognition.

A robust, speaker independent, large vocabulary, continuous speech recognition system is the end goal of any researcher, working on speech recognition, in any language. But the difficulties that come along with this goal are hard to overcome. Especially in a country like India, where no common language is known by all the people, and also each language has various dialects to take into account; the path to the aforementioned goal is further filled with hurdles.

An isolated speech recognition system is a system that has silences or noise between each spoken word. Further, these words can be independent words without any relation to the neighbouring words or can be a part of a sentence with clear silence between them. Ultimately, each word is taken individually for training and recognition. Various open-source toolkits such as HTK, Julius, CMUSphinx and Kaldi are available for speech recognition. We have used Kaldi toolkit [1] to build the automatic speech recognition (ASR) system for the Indian language, Kannada, which is a widely spoken language in the Indian subcontinent, in the state of Karnataka. Kaldi provides a robust and easy to implement environment, wherein the various available recipes can be put together and modified if needed to build the required ASR system. Good results have been achieved in recognition of speech using Kaldi in various languages as Italian [2] and Serbian [3]. Kaldi has been chosen for this work, based on the comparison of various open-source toolkits [4], which has provided a basis based on various parameters to identify that Kaldi is a robust system.

Automatic speech recognition systems have been developed for a few Indian regional languages like Hindi [5, 6], Telugu [7], Assamese [8], Bengali [9] and Odia [10] using various tools such as HTK, CMUSphinx and Kaldi. Thus, we propose an ASR system using Kaldi to recognize digits corpora in Kannada, from shunya (zero) till ombattu (nine).

The paper is organized as follows: we discuss the related works that have been done in the field of ASR for Indian languages (Sect. 2). Then we discuss Kaldi toolkit and its organization (Sect. 3), followed by Sect. 4, which discuss the recognition phases of speech. We start this section with the steps to recognize speech from data preparation, acoustic modelling, feature extraction, language modelling, training and finally testing the data. Section 5 discusses the results followed by discussions and conclusions.

2 Related Work

The research on speech recognition systems for the Indian languages has been going on since a decade now, based on an array of toolkits like HTK, Julius. CMUSphinx, and Kaldi etc. Below mentioned are some of the significant works in the field of speech recognition based on Kaldi toolkit, and a paper published by Gaida et al. [4] gives some proof of superiority of Kaldi toolkit over its peers.

Implementation of a speech recognition system for Hindi using a large vocabulary set of 2007 words forms 100 speakers from the AMUAV corpus discussed in [5].

Recognition is achieved using MFCC and PLP coefficients, and performance based on monophone and triphone using different N-gram quantities is reported. A best WER of 16.09% is achieved.

Speech recognition in Assamese for a spoken query system is described in [8]. A spoken query system which consists of an interactive voice response system and a speech recognition system is designed for retrieving prices of agricultural commodities. A similar system is described in [5] for Kannada language, where they discuss the WER and achieved, while different phoneme levels are used. An asterisk-based system for language Odia is discussed in [10]. A district model and a yes/no model are considered, and a system is built using Kaldi. The district model uses a total of 517 utterances, and the yes/no model uses 91 utterances for training. From these works, we can see that although a robust system can be achieved for Indian languages, major work has to be done with the Indian language Kannada. In this paper, we will be looked at a medium vocabulary speaker-dependent isolated speech recognition system and the results will be compared with a similar work done with HTK toolkit as discussed in [11].

3 The Kaldi ASR Toolkit

Kaldi provides a speech recognition system which is based on weighted finite-state transducers. The source code of Kaldi is written in C++, and the core library supports modelling of arbitrary phonetic-context sizes, acoustic modelling with subspace Gaussian mixture models (SGMM) as well as standard Gaussian mixture models, together with all commonly used linear and affine transforms.

Kaldi is an open-source toolkit which has Apache License v2.0 licensing (Fig. 1).

- Important features [2]

  - Extensive linear algebra support: A matrix library wraps standard BLAS and LAPACK routines.
  - Code-level integration with finite-state transducers (FSTs) compiled against the OpenFst toolkit (using it as a library).
  - Extensible design: As far as possible, algorithms are in the most generic form.

Fig. 1 Block diagram of
Kaldi toolkit

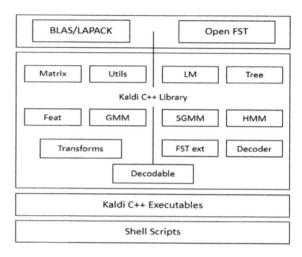

Fig. 2 A simple speech
recognition system

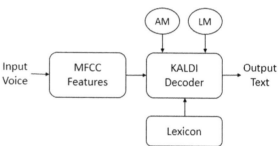

- For instance, the decoders are template on an object that provides a score indexed
  by a (frame, fst-input symbol) tuple. This means that the decoder could work
  from any suitable source of scores, such as a neural net.
- Open licence: The code is licensed under Apache 2.0, which is one of the least
  restrictive licences available.

Kaldi is mainly used for acoustic modelling. Although other tools like RASR
and HTK are available for this purpose, the main advantage of Kaldi over them is
its modern, flexible and neatly structured code. It also has better math and WFST
support.

A block diagram (Fig. 2) of a simple speech recognition system is given below.
Acoustic model (AM), lexicon and the language model (LM) form the basic building
blocks of any speech recognition system.

4 Recognition Phases

The process of speech recognition is not a one-stage process but goes through multiple stages in order to get the system to understand and recognize the speech that has been given as the input. Some of these steps are listed below.

4.1 Voice Data Preparation

In this stage, the voice samples from 14 speakers (8 female and 6 male) are recorded using laptop integrated microphone at a sampling rate of 16 kHz. Samples from different speakers with varying levels of noise in the environment were considered for different training sets. The Kannada digits (shunya to ombattu) were recorded from the speakers, who spoke each word 32 times, i.e. (14 * 10 * 32), resulting in a total of 4480 utterances.

Next, the data were cleaned using the freely available software Audacity v2.1.3. Audacity provides excellent options for noise cancellation without much degradation of the useful signals in the voice samples. Then the data were segmented and indexed; such that the paths and the sample IDs can be easily incorporated into the script of the ASR.

4.2 Acoustic Data Preparation

In this stage, the recorded, cleaned, segmented and indexed voice samples are documented in a predefined format such that the ASR script can identify the voice samples and can consequently advance to the further stages. For the transcription of the words to their respective phones, the phoneme list that has been utilized in [12] has been taken as listed below in Table 1.

4.3 Feature Extraction

The main aim of feature extraction is to extract Mel-frequency Cepstral coefficients (MFCC) and perceptual linear prediction (PLP) features and to set defaults and making certain options that may need modifications like number of Mel bins. Some of the feature extractions supported by Kaldi are VTLN, CMVN, LDA, STC/MLLT and HLDA. In this case, we extract only MFCC components and using that generate CMVN statistics. The procedure to find MFCC features is given in Fig. 3.

Table 1 I: Alphabet to phoneme map

Label	Kannada Phoneme	Label	Kannada Phoneme	Label	Kannada Phoneme	Label	Kannada Phoneme
a	ಅ	oo	ೂ	txh	ಠ್	Ph	ಫ್
aa	ಆ	au	ೌ	dx	ಡ್	B	ಬ್
i	ಇ	k	ಕ್	dxh	ಢ್	Bh	ಭ್
ii	ಈ	kh	ಖ್	nx	ಣ್	M	ಮ್
u	ಉ	g	ಗ್	t	ತ್	Y	ಯ್
uu	ಊ	gh	ಘ್	th	ಥ್	R	ರ್
e	ಎ	c	ಚ್	d	ದ್	L	ಲ್,ಳ್
ee	ಏ	ch	ಛ್	dh	ಧ್	W	ವ್
ai	ಐ	j	ಜ್	n	ನ್	Sh	ಶ್,ಷ್
o	ಒ	tx	ಟ್	p	ಪ್	S	ಸ್

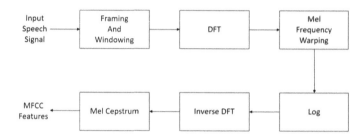

Fig. 3 MFCC extraction procedure

4.4 Language Data Creation

In this stage, we check the validity of the given phone list in the documentation and also check for duplicates and missing phones. Once the validation is successful, then the tool goes on to create a segmented lexicon, in which four states are defined, namely Beginning (_b), Ending (_e), Intermediate (_i) and Singleton (_s), based on the position of the phone in the uttered word.

4.5 Language Model Creation

As Kaldi uses a framework based on FST; so in theory, any system based on FST model can be used by Kaldi. OpenFst is used to convert the standard ARPA format of language models into the .fst format required by Kaldi. SRILM toolkit is used in this implementation for pruning the language model. Here, an ARPA trigram model file is created to generate the probabilities of each phone. Then we create a grammar file based on finite-state transducers to define the grammar rules of the language in use. OpenFst is used for this task.

4.6 Training

In the training stage, the voice samples are intended for training the system in order to extract the features from the voice samples with the knowledge of the samples such that the probability density function for each phoneme can be classified and the segmentation of the voice samples according to the segmented lexicon is done.

A word can be broken into individual units of sound. These are called "phonemes" or "phones." When only one phone is considered, it is called as monophone, as only one phone in the voice sample is considered while training and the adjacent phones are omitted. When three phones are considered in the form of "L – X + R", it is called as triphone. "L" indicates the left phone, and "R" indicates the right phone of the phone under test "X". In triphone training, the adjacent phones are taken into consideration such that the accuracy of the phoneme detection increases as there are some phones that are never adjacent to some other phones. The training data set considered in this work consists of 10 speakers and 4 speakers are used for testing.

4.7 Decoding

In decoding stage using the trained data, the test set of data is compared and the list of phonemes that may be present in the given voice sample is approximated. The samples are decoded using monophone and triphone models in this stage. The monophone decoding model will only try to identify the current phone, one after the other without considering any of the adjacent phones; whereas in triphone decoding model, with the help of the grammar file, both left and right phones are considered while identifying the current phonemes.

5 Experimental Results

The system had been trained with 10 speakers and tested with 4 speakers (2 male and 2 female). The performance analysis of an ASR system is identified with word error rate (WER). Word error rate is calculated as the ratio of sum of insertions (I), substitutions (S) and deletions (D) to that of the total number the phones (N).

$$WER = (I + S + D)/N \qquad (1)$$

The training of the models is done by monophone, the first (tri1) and second (tri2) triphone using MFCC's and delta and delta–delta features. The WER for the data set used with Kaldi toolkit is provided in Table 2.

Table 2 WER performance using monophone and triphone model

Feature	Training Model	Word error Rate (%)
MFCC	Mono	9
MFCC	Tri1	7
MFCC	Tri2	6

The tri2 training model gives a better performance with a high recognition accuracy compared with the tri1 and monophone models. Thus, we observe that the word error rate decreases as we progress from monophone to triphone models, and this is because of the context dependency of the phonemes which is least in monophone models and increases with tri1 and tri2 models.

The paper [11] describes a system for isolated speech recognition using the same database using HTK toolkit. The paper describes the system in terms of accuracy of recognition rate. Although various fronts are explored in the aforementioned work, the most relatable part of this work is the isolated speaker-dependent system using MFCC coefficients. An accuracy of 90% (WER 10%) for triphone recognition is achieved, whereas our system using Kaldi has achieved a WER of 6% using the same dataset, thus giving a superior and a more robust system for speech recognition.

6 Conclusion

The Kaldi toolkit has been explored, and a preliminary analysis of speech recognition in Kannada for numbers has been done in this work. The word error rate for the speech recognition obtained has been satisfactory given the limited set of data and environmental situations, as the recording was done purely in-house and the age group of the speakers was mainly in the range of 18–25. This work has been done with phoneme level of Kannada speech. Further, the research will be continued to make it a robust and spontaneous speech recognition system, with increased corpus and to increase the recognition accuracy of the ASR system. During this project, linking the sample IDs to the audio sample path was time-consuming. Further down the line, we plan on automating this process by using scripting languages.

Acknowledgements Authors have obtained all ethical approvals from appropriate ethical committee and approval from the subjects involved in this study. Authors also thank the speakers for their contribution.

References

1. Povey D, Ghoshal A, Boulianne G, Burget L, Glembek O et al. The Kaldi speech recognition toolkit. In: IEEE 2011 workshop on automatic speech recognition and understanding. IEEE Signal Processing Society, Dec 2011
2. Cosi P (2015) A Kaldi-DNN-based ASR system for Italian. In: IEEE international joint conference on neural networks IJCNN 2015, pp 1–5
3. Popović B, Ostrogonac S, Pakoci E, Jakovljević N, Delić V (2015) Deep neural network based continuous speech recognition for Serbian using the Kaldi toolkit. In: SPECOM 2015. LNCS, vol 9319. Springer, Heidelberg, pp 186–192
4. Gaida C, Lange P, Petrick R, Proba P, Malatawy A, Suendermann-Oeft D (2014) Comparing open-source speech recognition toolkits
5. Upadhyaya P, Farooq O, Abidi MR, Varshney YV (2017) Continuous Hindi speech recognition model based on Kaldi ASR toolkit. In: 2017 international conference on wireless communications, signal processing and networking (WiSPNET), Chennai, pp 786–789
6. Dua M, Aggarwal RK, Biswas M (2017) Discriminative training using heterogeneous feature vector for Hindi automatic speech recognition system. In: 2017 international conference on computer and applications (ICCA), Doha, pp 158–162
7. Kumar AP, Kumar N, Kumar CS, Yadav AK, Sharma A (2016) Speech recognition using arithmetic coding and MFCC for Telugu language. In: 2016 3rd international conference on computing for sustainable global development (INDIACom), New Delhi, pp 265–268
8. Shahnawazuddin S, Thotappa D, Dey A et al (2017) J Sign Process Syst 88:91. https://doi.org/10.1007/s11265-016-1133-6
9. Reza M, Rashid W, Mostakim M, Prodorshok I (2017) A Bengali isolated speech dataset for voice-based assistive technologies: a comparative analysis of the effects of data augmentation on HMM-GMM and DNN classifiers. In: 2017 IEEE region 10 humanitarian technology conference (R10-HTC), Dhaka, pp 396–399
10. Karan B, Sahoo J, Sahu PK (2015) Automatic speech recognition based Odia system. In: 2015 international conference on microwave, optical and communication engineering (ICMOCE), Bhubaneswar, pp 353–356
11. Sneha V, Hardhika G, Jeeva Priya K, Gupta D (2018) Isolated Kannada speech recognition using HTK—a detailed approach. In: Progress in advanced computing and intelligent engineering. Advances in intelligent systems and computing, vol 564. Springer, Singapore
12. Yadava TG, Jayanna HS (2017) Int J Speech Technol 20:635. https://doi.org/10.1007/s10772-017-9428-y

Real-Time Traffic Management Using RF Communication

Prajwal Prakash and Mahabaleshwar Bhat

Abstract Clogging of traffic in streets is one of the biggest challenges faced in all huge and growing urban areas. To solve this quagmire of vehicular transit control at pathway crossings, an intelligent fully automatic real-time traffic control system is proposed in this paper. It uses RF and GPS technology to detect congestion by determining the average velocity of the vehicles and the vehicle count and GSM module to communicate the level of congestion with the central traffic kiosk which changes the traffic signal based on the level of congestion.

Keywords Tag · Reader · Co-ordinator · RF transceiver · GPS · GSM

1 Introduction

Traffic lights play an important role in transit management. The working of typical traffic lights which are deployed at present in numerous junctions is built on pre-calculated timing patterns, which are decided initially itself and remain like that until further resetting. Most of the current smart traffic systems are sensor based and use some algorithms to control switching operation of lights. This system works fine when vehicles transit smoothly but when some unpredictable instances occur, or during the occurrence of jams, there is no right way of handling such an undertaking. A more didactic method has been presented to circumscribe such difficulties. This technique utilizes real-time transit monitoring system with tracking of images [1]. This method has several limitations, even though it gives quantitative report of the traffic flow. The handing out of such large-scale data dynamically may extant exorbitant necessities. False acceptance rate (FAR) and false rejection rate (FRR) are

P. Prakash · M. Bhat (✉)
Department of Electronics & Communication Engineering, PES University, Bangalore 560085, India
e-mail: maba1081396@gmail.com

P. Prakash
e-mail: prakash.prajwalp@gmail.com

© Springer Nature Singapore Pte Ltd. 2019
V. Sridhar et al. (eds.), *Emerging Research in Electronics, Computer Science and Technology*, Lecture Notes in Electrical Engineering 545,
https://doi.org/10.1007/978-981-13-5802-9_72

some of the common problems faced in image processing. Another approach used in real-time traffic management is to fly drones over an intersection with the purpose of identifying and tracking automobiles to extract statistical models and apply computer vision algorithms to the gathered footage [2, 3]. This approach has the problems of image processing as well as erroneous detection in case of jam-packed traffic. On the other hand, the sensor-based transit management [4] needs sensors which use line of sight detection, but still won't be efficient as it fails to spot automobiles that pass through blind spots detection range [5].

But in the space of automatic clogging detection, radio frequency is a technology that still remains largely uncharted [6, 7]. Automobile discovery and totaling can be done commendably using RF technology [8]. A mutiny in the traffic management and control systems can be generated using RF together with GSM technology.

In this paper, we have attempted to create a hardware system which can efficiently identify the amount of automobiles at a traffic junction, compute the mean velocity of the automobiles, and make intelligent decisions regarding congestion at that junction. The system is further capable of communicating with a central traffic kiosk and nearby detection systems and thus help in providing information for manipulation of signals depending on traffic density. Through our simulation model, we intend to highlight the difference in the performance of static and dynamic traffic management systems. In addition to the above, the system can potentially track vehicles at all times, help in theft management and tackle emergency scenarios.

2 Proposed Scheme

The system block diagram is revealed in Fig. 1. The structure as a whole comprises of a Tag (present in the vehicle), a Reader and a Co-ordinator (both on the side of the lane).

The Tag when passes the Reader sends the GPS timestamp (say t1) and the unique registration number of the vehicle it is present in. The Reader checks for the validity of the data and sends it to the Co-ordinator which is present at a prefixed distance (Δd). Now when the same vehicle passes the Co-ordinator, it sends its current timestamp (say t2) and its registration number. The Co-ordinator computes the velocity of the vehicle using the timestamps sent by Reader and the Tag.

The velocity will be computed as

$$v = \Delta t / \Delta d$$

where $\Delta t = (t2 - t1)$.

The Co-ordinator also keeps count of the number of vehicles that have passed by (N). Now if N exceeds a threshold value, say N0, and the average velocity (V) of the vehicles is underneath the optimal value, say V0, implies absolutely that a higher level of congestion has taken place in that particular lane. N0 and V0 are quantified

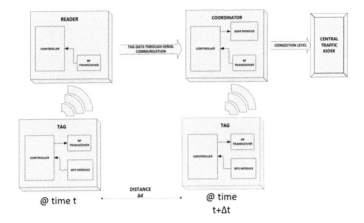

Fig. 1 System block diagram

by parameters like breadth and length of a road stretch for a particular road stretch. Thus, compulsory and adequate circumstances for determining whether a high level of congestion exists are:

$$N > N0 \text{ and } V < V0$$

The level of congestion is then sent to the central traffic kiosk which takes action to relieve the congestion from the lanes with the higher level of congestion. The Tag sends the information to the Reader and the Co-ordinator through RF communication and the message passing between the Reader and the Co-ordinator happens with the help of serial communication. The Co-ordinator sends messages to the central traffic kiosk through GSM.

3 Proposed Design

3.1 Tag

The device in the vehicle consists of an RF transceiver along with a GPS module integrated with microcontroller. The GPS module is used to determine the present location in terms of coordinates. The RF transceiver is capable of sending this information to its nearest Reader. The Tag sends the GPS time (in Universal Time Coordinated (UTC) format) along with its unique registration number. The Tag will not depend on Reader to initiate communication. The Tag is battery operated. When a vehicle is reported stolen, its current location can be determined by RF Tag detection. This tracking can also be used for ensuring uninterrupted flow through the traffic for

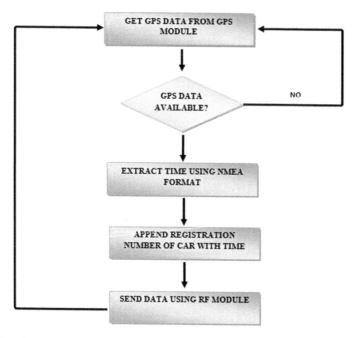

Fig. 2 Vehicle tag flowchart

emergency vehicles like ambulances, fire engines, etc. Figure 2 shows the flowchart of a typical Tag in the vehicle.

3.2 Reader

The Reader is an RF transceiver integrated with microcontroller. It will interrogate the RF tags. It functions in the industrial, scientific, and medical (ISM) band (2.45 GHz). It communicates with the Co-ordinator through serial communication. It receives Tag data, makes comparison and stores relevant information and sends the same to Co-ordinator. The Reader acts as an intermediary node between Co-ordinator and Tag (Fig. 3).

3.3 Co-ordinator

A Co-ordinator is an RF Reader integrated with a GSM modem. It is adept of getting and dispatching a text message to Co-ordinators in further adjoining intersections. Every Co-ordinator has a clock assimilated in it. Co-ordinator quantifies the extent

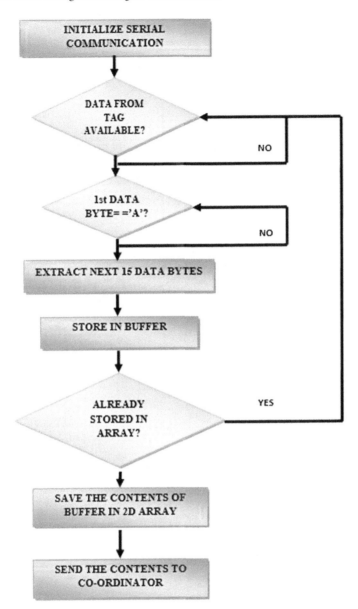

Fig. 3 Reader flowchart

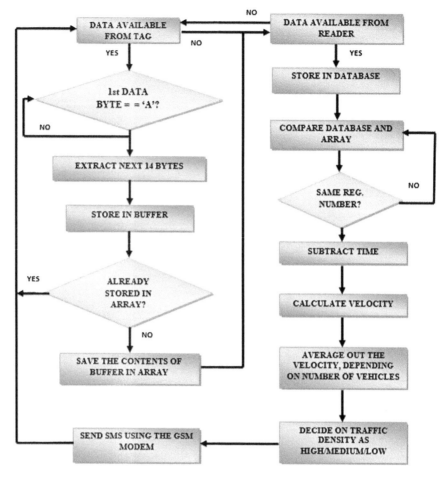

Fig. 4 Co-ordinator flowchart

of clogging based on certain parameters upon procuring the total number and mean speed of all vehicles. The same information is sent to other Co-ordinators and the central network by messages using a GSM modem (Fig. 4).

The Co-ordinator makes the decision on the level of congestion based on the vehicle count and the mean velocity of the vehicles. An example is shown in Table 1 which was used for our design.

If the congestion level sent by the Co-ordinator to the central kiosk is *High,* that particular lane is given the highest priority; i.e., the traffic light of the lane is turned green immediately. Likewise, if the congestion level is *Medium*, it is given next priority and the traffic light in that lane is turned green after the one on the *High* congestion lane. If the congestion level is *Low,* then that particular lane is given the least priority and the traffic light on that lane is the last one to be turned green.

Table 1 Conditions for determination of the level of congestion	Average velocity (m/s)	Vehicle count	Level of congestion
	≤0.3	>40	High
	≤0.5	>30	Medium
	≤1	>20	Low

4 Results

4.1 Results Obtained from Prototype Model

The data sent by the Tag which is received at the Reader is shown in Fig. 5. The Tag sends its current timestamp, GPS location, and the vehicle registration number through the RF transceiver.

The velocity calculation using the timestamp obtained from the Reader as well as the Tag and the message depicting the level of congestion sent to the central kiosk by the Co-ordinator is shown in Fig. 6.

The messages sent by the Co-ordinator and received by the central traffic kiosk through the GSM module is shown in Fig. 7.

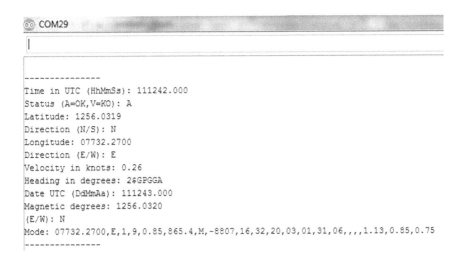

```
COM29

----------------
Time in UTC (HhMmSs): 111242.000
Status (A=OK,V=KO): A
Latitude: 1256.0319
Direction (N/S): N
Longitude: 07732.2700
Direction (E/W): E
Velocity in knots: 0.26
Heading in degrees: 2$GPGGA
Date UTC (DdMmAa): 111243.000
Magnetic degrees: 1256.0320
(E/W): N
Mode: 07732.2700,E,1,9,0.85,865.4,M,-8807,16,32,20,03,01,31,06,,,,1.13,0.85,0.75
----------------
```

Fig. 5 Tag data

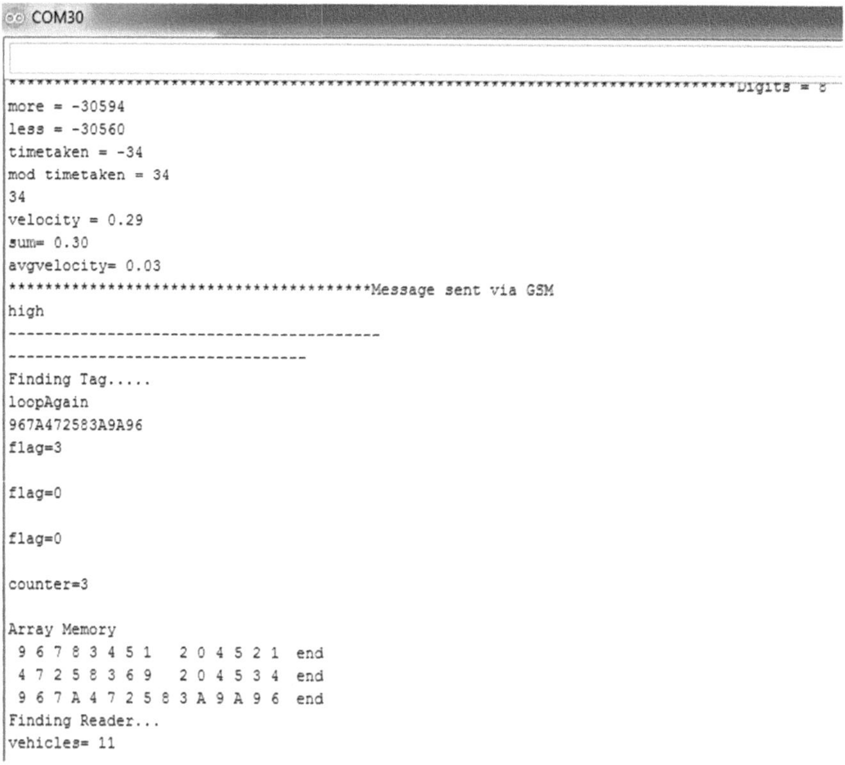

```
⊙ COM30

*****************************************************************Digits = 8
more = -30594
less = -30560
timetaken = -34
mod timetaken = 34
34
velocity = 0.29
sum= 0.30
avgvelocity= 0.03
*************************************************Message sent via GSM
high
-------------------------------------------
-------------------------------
Finding Tag.....
loopAgain
967A472583A9A96
flag=3

flag=0

flag=0

counter=3

Array Memory
 9 6 7 8 3 4 5 1    2 0 4 5 2 1   end
 4 7 2 5 8 3 6 9    2 0 4 5 3 4   end
 9 6 7 A 4 7 2 5 8 3 A 9 A 9 6   end
Finding Reader...
vehicles= 11
```

Fig. 6 Congestion determination

4.2 Simulation Analysis

Simulation of Urban Mobility (SUMO) is an open-source transportation imitation set. SUMO facilitates modeling of inter-modal transit schemes containing automobiles, civic transport, and pedestrians [9]. This paper has used SUMO to simulate the proposed real-time traffic management.

The model submitted here intends to regulate the transit signal dynamically on the basis of the level of vehicle clogging and speed of the vehicle.

The proposed algorithm is applied to a virtual junction J with different congestion levels on different lanes. The yellow-colored triangles depict cars and the longer blue rectangle depicts a longer vehicle, like a bus.

In the junction J, the traffic signal in the lane on the east side is green and is red on the other lanes (Fig. 8). Now the vehicles start accumulating in all the lanes. The Co-ordinators from all the lanes send the message containing the level of congestion in their respective lanes to the central kiosk. The congestion is highest in the west lane compared to the rest of the lanes. Hence, the signal in the east lane is turned red and the west lane is given the green signal (Fig. 9). As the congestion level in the

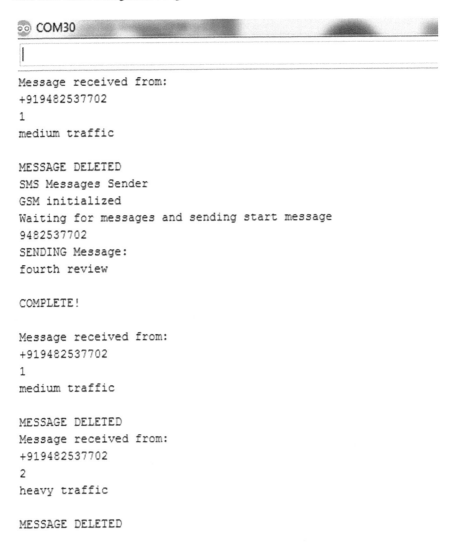

Fig. 7 GSM module communication

west lane decreases, the lane with the highest level of congestion is given the green signal next, which is the south lane. Similarly, the signal in the east lane is made green next rather than the north lane since the congestion is higher in the east lane compared to the north lane (Fig. 11). Thus, the congestion level is kept in check in every lane, thereby preventing a standstill of vehicles (Fig. 10).

Fig. 8 SUMO simulations

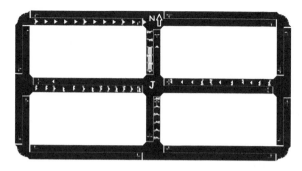

Fig. 9 SUMO simulations

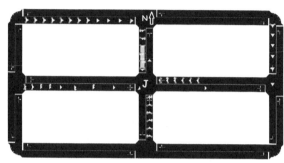

Fig. 10 SUMO simulations

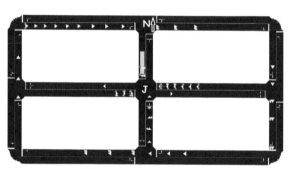

Fig. 11 SUMO simulations

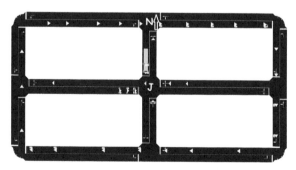

Consider the situation depicted in Fig. 8. Without the proposed traffic management model, i.e., in static traffic signal model, assuming the duration of the green signal to be two minutes, the vehicles in the west lane will have to wait for a total of four minutes (two minutes each for east and south lanes), thereby leading to further increase in congestion.

Using our proposed model, the traffic in the west lane is allowed to move first because of the detection of high congestion. The signal is green until the congestion in the lane comes down to medium level. Then the central kiosk checks for the congestion in other lanes. If there is high or medium level congestion in any other lane, say south lane, then the signal is turned green in the south lane. But if the congestion levels in other lanes are low, then the traffic in the west lane is allowed to move till the congestion there becomes low or nil. Thus, the congestion level is kept in check in every lane, thereby preventing a standstill of vehicles.

The average waiting time of the vehicles without applying our method is shown in Fig. 12. The mean time is computed by subtracting the timestamps obtained at the Co-ordinators before and immediately after the traffic signal. This procedure is repeated for each duty cycle and the graph of it is plotted.

We observe a significant reduction in mean waiting time when we use our method as shown in Fig. 13. The mean halting time saturates to a value of 113-time units constant gradually after a few iterations.

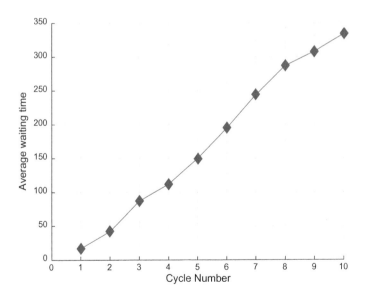

Fig. 12 Average waiting delay without our method

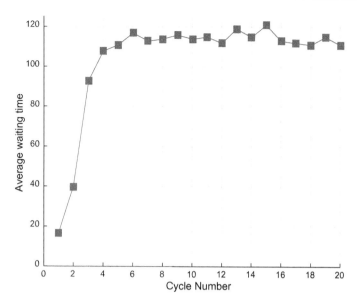

Fig. 13 Average waiting delay using our method

5 Conclusion and Scope for Further Improvement

This paper has proposed a new background for a real time and spontaneous traffic light control system to reduce traffic clogging. The algorithm developed was simulated showing drastic improvement in reducing traffic congestion as compared to conventional traffic control model. This model will make the traffic management system more automatic, reducing costly human involvement. Traffic violations like speeding can be easily tracked and more electronic regulations can be imposed. In the case of vehicle theft, the vehicles can be easily tracked and the concerned authorities can be alerted.

The proposed model can be further improved by using RF transceivers having better range and error-free transmission to have a smoother system. The Readers and the Co-ordinators can be made solar powered and weatherproof making them maintenance-free and eco-friendly. The communication method between the Co-ordinators and the central traffic kiosk can be changed from GSM to a more reliable network solely devised for this purpose. Applications of the proposed system include uninterrupted flow for emergency vehicles like ambulances and fire engines, automatic billing in toll booths and parking lots and finding the best route or a second optimal route between two places in real time.

References

1. Piyush P, Rajan R, Mary L (2016) Vehicle detection and classification using audio-visual cues. In: 3rd international conference on signal processing and integrated networks (SPIN)
2. Lira G, Kikkinogenis Z, Rossetti RJF (2016) A computer-vision approach to traffic analysis over intersections. In: IEEE 19th international conference on intelligent transportation systems (ITSC)
3. Karnadi FK, Mo ZH, Lan K (2007) Rapid generation of realistic mobility models for VANET. In: Wireless communications and networking conference, 2007. WCNC 2007. IEEE, pp 2506–2511
4. Rahman M, Ahmed NU, Mouftah HT (2014) City traffic management model using wireless sensor networks. In: IEEE 27th Canadian conference on electrical and computer engineering (CCECE)
5. Singh SK, Duvvuru R, Thakur SS (2013) Congestion control technique using intelligent traffic and vanet. Int J Comput Eng Appl IV(I/III). arXiv:1311.4036
6. Bajaj D, Gupta N (2012) GPS based automatic vehicle tracking using RFID. Int J Eng Innov Technol 1:31–35
7. Roy S, Das SBM, Batabyal S, Pal S. Real-time traffic congestion detection and management using active RFID and GSM technology. faculty live.iimcal.ac.in
8. Wen W (2008) A dynamic and automatic traffic light control expert system for solving the road congestion problem. Expert Syst Appl 34(4):2370–2381
9. Krajzewicz D, Hertkorn G, Rössel C, Wagner P (2002) Sumo (simulation of urban mobility). In: Proceedings of the 4th middle east symposium on simulation and modelling, pp 183–187
10. Chattaraj A, Bansal S, Chandra A (2009) An intelligent traffic control system using RFID. Potentials IEEE 28(3):40–43

SDN Security: Challenges and Solutions

J. Prathima Mabel, K. A. Vani and K. N. Rama Mohan Babu

Abstract Recently, the need for programmable networks has drawn the interest of industrialists and academicians to develop a programmable networking paradigm called software-defined network (SDN). It is an effort made to separate network intelligence (control plane) from forwarding hardware (data plane). This paper provides a clear perspective of working of SDN and an open interface protocol called OpenFlow(OF). Researchers provide a broad insight into the working of SDN and various challenges faced while implementing it such as scalability, controller bottleneck, load balancing in distributed controller environment, routing and security. This paper focuses on security issues of SDN. We discuss different scenarios at which SDN is vulnerable to attacks and solutions to such attacks. Possible security attacks in the data plane, control plane and the interface between them are elaborated.

Keywords Software-defined network (SDN) · OpenFlow (OF) · Control plane · Data plane · Security

1 Introduction

In a traditional computer network connected by links and nodes, routing is carried out through the routers, switches and gateways. These are the network elements which make routing decision based on Quality of Service (QoS) parameters such as shortest path, network traffic load, bandwidth, delay and jitter. These network elements are vendor dependent. Therefore, the programmability of these elements is limited to the

J. Prathima Mabel (✉) · K. A. Vani · K. N. Rama Mohan Babu
Department of Information Science and Engineering,
Dayananda Sagar College of Engineering, Bangalore, India
e-mail: prathimamabel@gmail.com

K. A. Vani
e-mail: vaniram.reddy@gmail.com

K. N. Rama Mohan Babu
e-mail: rams_babu@hotmail.com

© Springer Nature Singapore Pte Ltd. 2019
V. Sridhar et al. (eds.), *Emerging Research in Electronics, Computer Science and Technology*, Lecture Notes in Electrical Engineering 545,
https://doi.org/10.1007/978-981-13-5802-9_73

specifications of the network vendor and their interoperability. To cut down on this limitation and make networks easily programmable, a new networking paradigm called software-defined network was introduced. In this approach, the network is divided into two planes: control plane and data plane. Control plane is the heart of the network from where the entire network can be programmed according to the needs of the application irrespective of vendor specifications. Data plane is the forwarding plane which forwards data as directed by the control plane.

This paper gives an overview of SDN, OpenFlow and security issues of SDN. Section 2 gives a clear insight into working of SDN and OpenFlow, Sect. 3 emphasizes on the security issues in SDN and proposed solution and Sect. 4 concludes the paper.

2 Software-Defined Network

The idea of SDN was first incubated in Stanford University around 2005 [1]. The main intension of SDN was to make networks easy to programme by separating the network intelligence from forwarding hardware as shown in Fig. 1. This separation divides the network into two planes called the data plane and control plane. Control plane

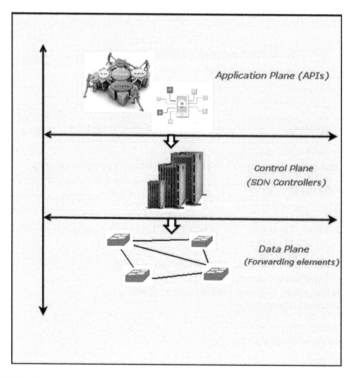

Fig. 1 SDN architecture

consists of controller which is responsible for managing flow control, routing, error control, transmission control, security and other vital functionalities of the network. The controller is the prime element which houses the entire network intelligence. It provides programmable interface to configure the network's QoS parameters and define the rules for routing, flow control, error control mechanisms, security policies, etc. POX, NOX, Maestro, Trema, Beacon, Floodlight, Flowvisor, RouteFlow and OpenDay Light are example of controllers [2].

Deploying new policies and rules in a traditional network is a tedious task as each network element needs to be reprogrammed or reconfigured. This task is made easy in SDN-based networks as controller is the single point of control for the entire network. Adding a new policy or functionality can be done at the controller with the help of application programming interface (API). APIs are designed based on the requirements of the applications and installed at the controller. The network starts functioning as dictated by the controller. The software-based controller acts like the brain of the network in computing routing topologies and updating forwarding tables of the data plane.

Data plane consists of forwarding devices (switches) which mainly forward data from a source to destination as programmed by the controller. Data plane is configured by the controller as per the rule set defined for a specific application. Communication between the control plane and data plane is enabled by an open interface protocol called OpenFlow (OF) [3–6].

Internet Engineering Task Force (IETF) initially designed the OpenFlow protocol. It provides an open interface for communication between the control plane and data plane. Forwarding element in the data plane are mainly OpenFlow switches. These switches support OpenFlow protocol. They consist of Flow tables and a secure channel for communication with the controller. Flow table of each OF switch consists of entries like match, counter and action. *Match* field *matches* the incoming packet with one of the flow entries, *counter* field keeps track of the number of bytes for each flow and the time elapsed since last match, *action* field specifies the action to be taken on the matched/unmatched packet.

Following are the possible set of actions taken on a matched packet

- Forward the packet through all the ports except for the one on which it arrives.
- Encapsulate the packet and forward it to the controller. This happens when it is either the first packet of a flow or there is no match for the packet in the flow table.

If there is no match for a packet in the flow table then it follows action specified by the table miss entry. Table miss entry specifies to drop the packet or to forward it back to the controller.

OF switches communicate with the controller for over a secure communication channel. Controller is responsible for installing the flow table entries based on the rule set, routing and security policies defined by the APIs. Therefore, SDN-based networks are flexible and programmable through the single centralized interface, the controller.

3 Vulnerabilities in the Open Interface

SDN-based networks have to preserve network characteristics such as availability, integrity, confidentiality and performance. Though the open interface and centralized control increases the programmability of the network, it opens up opportunities for attacks and illegal access at various points. The controller is the major network element that can be easily attacked in such architecture. A faintly secured controller provides a major pathway for the attacker to gain access to the entire network. Similarly, hacking the data plane or the secure channel between the data plane and the control plane can give chance for attackers to introduce fraudulent flows and disrupt the working of the network. A security compromise switches makes it easy for an attacker can introduce unwanted flows into the flow tables and divert data to unintended destinations. This may lead to denial-of-service (DoS) attacks, man-in-the-middle attack, eavesdropping, etc. [2, 5, 7–24].

An example of attack is shown in Fig. 2 where a attacker can gain control over the controller and modify the flow table. In this example, flow table of switch 4 can be modified such that a copy of data destined to host B is sent to hacker. The figure also shows another attack scenario. The network administrator defines the route from host H1 to H2 as H1 -> S2 -> S4-> H2. An attacker who gains access to the controller or switches on data plane can modify the route to H1 -> S2 -> S3 -> S1 -> S4 -> H2. This makes the route between H1 and H2 longer introducing unnecessary delays. Further in [25], a SDN scanner can be used to study whether a network is SDN-based or not. This scanner sends ping messages at different times by modifying the header fields. The response times for these messages are noted and analyzed to know the flow rule of the network. Attacker further uses this information to perform a resource consumption attack by flooding packets and utilizing the network resources to carry the flooded traffic instead of the authentic traffic.

OpenFlow protocol highlights certain vulnerabilities in connection and configuration management. The exchange of credentials during connection set up and maintenance have to be secured as the TLS does not provide any information about securing credential details like keys and certificates. Further, the switches on the data plane can be replaced or modified by attackers. This issues needs to be addressed.

The following sections discuss the existing security measures in the control plane and the data plane. This paper also proposes a solution for securing the controller from being compromised.

3.1 Securing the Controller

It is of prime importance to develop effective methods for preventing and recovering from attacks. Hu, F. et al. explain various schemes that are available for intrusion detection, fault isolation and failure recovery running on the controller. NICE (network intrusion detection and countermeasure selection) [26] is a scheme which

Fig. 2 Attack scenarios

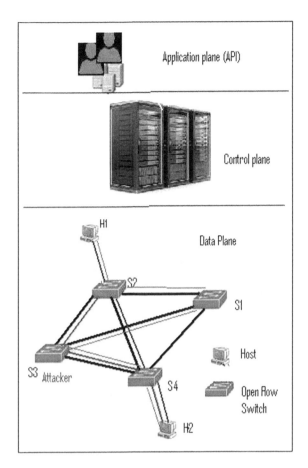

provides intrusion detection in SDN. An intrusion detection agent called NICE runs on the controller which analyzes the first packet of the flow. Packet's traffic compliance is verified and forwarded to attack analyzer. All possible paths that might be taken by the packet is analysed and Scenario Attack Graph (SAG) is updated. Further decision of routing the packet is taken based on the SAG entry.

The NOX controller runs FRESCO an OpenFlow security application development tool. It consists of an application layer and security enforcement kernel. Application layer includes python modules using which secure OpenFlow applications can be programmed. Security enforcement kernel plays an important role in authenticating OpenFlow API which user installs.

Xitao Wen et al. define a permission-based security framework called PermOF which verifies the authenticity of an API by verifying a set of permissions and rules. If the application suffices the rule set, it is allowed to be installed on the controller. It is an overhead to verify the rules each time a new API is to be installed. This is an overhead which affects the performance of the network. Hu et al. address the causes of flow entry conflicts. Occurrence of flow entry conflict might be by an attack or by entries made by operators of different levels. An attacker can get control of the application or controller and modify flow entries in such a way that a copy of data is forwarded to the attacker. Security architecture is proposed to address these challenges. A naming system to prioritize and differentiate users into categories like security administrator, general administrator, user, and guest is designed. Highest priority to modify the flow table is given to security administrator. A packet data scan mechanism is proposed which scans the content of the packet to detect spams and viruses. Action to be taken for this packet is modified according to the packet scan mechanism's analysis.

Abnormality in traffic in OpenFlow can also be detected by algorithms such as Rate Limiting, Threshold Random Walk with Credit Based Rate Limiting, Maximum Entropy Detector and NETAD. Rate Limiting detects attacks by analyzing the number of connection requests in a stipulated time period. Threshold Random Walk with Credit Based Rate Limiting detects a server attack by analyzing each link. Maximum Entropy Detector is used to categorize traffic as authentic or anomalous based on baseline distribution and NETAD acts as a firewall.

Kreutz, D et al. suggest solutions to counter controller attacks to prevent the entire network from being compromised. Here, access to a controller is verified by two different users. This approach provides double credential verification. This can be a better approach to secure the controller from being compromised. Replication and recovery are measures which can be taken to detect and eliminate unusual behaviour. Diversity of controllers, protocols, programming languages etc. can be employed to ensure detection of attacks on controller. Confidentiality of data stored in the controller also needs to be maintained with atmost importance. C. Schlesinger et al. propose a language-based security model. Here, programming models are designed to such that traffic can be sliced. Slicing is done by establishing virtual connections to ensure that traffic from one connection does not interfere with another. If a wary flow is identified then that slice can be excluded. Applications using these models affect performance of SDN as they require an additional set up time which adds up to the delay.

3.2 Securing the Data Plane

Security at the data plane level is of atmost importance since it carries vital data and control information in the network. An external attacker can eavesdrop on the data flowing in the network. Once this information is gathered, the attacker might perform a resource consumption attack, denial-of-service (DoS) or man-in-the-middle (MITM) attack by replaying data or injecting unauthentic data or control messages into SDN network.

Even though proprietary southbound protocols implement security by TLS, an internal hacker can still gain access into the device's flow tables [27]. A hacker may change the switch or modify if to gain access over the flow tables. Unauthentic flow entries can be inserted resulting in malicious data flow in the network. Distrustful flows are a threat and can slow down the network.

3.3   Securing the Channel

A well-defined controller switch interface needs to be defined to prevent attacks. The existing TLS [8] confines to address only limited types of attacks. There is no mention about securing the authentication data such as certificates and keys. A well-defined mechanism to protect the data travelling between the control and data plane is essential. Kreutz D et al. suggest methods such as threshold cryptography and multiple certification authorities which require a certain number of parties to cooperate with the decryption of encrypted data to ensure that data exchanged between the control plane and data plane is trustworthy.

3.4   Security in Virtual Environments

Another significant issue that is to be addressed is security in SDN-based virtual environment. DoS, spoofing attacks and malicious injection are some of the common attacks on virtual networks. OpenVirtex is a controller which is used to set up virtual networks. Though OpenVirtex is used with POX controller, it is vulnerable to such attacks. Security in distributed environment is another open issue. It is vital to keep the policy enforcement, inter controller communication and data transfers secure in distributed environments. OpenFlow actions need to be defined for diversified types of attacks in such scenario.

3.5   Security in Wireless Environment

Wireless architecture takes a leading role in today's networking needs. Building SDN for wireless networks has been a popular research area in the current trend. [28] proposes SDN solutions for wireless networks.

- CellSDN is a project for managing cellular data networks. Here, the subscriber policies are installed on the switches as rules and the access to the switches and overall network intelligence is moved to the controller.
- Softcell is another architecture designed towards addressing scalability of wireless networks. It extends both the control plane and data plane to achieve scalability. It uses local software agents to handle packets in the control plane thus reducing load on the controller software. In the data plane, switches use multi-dimensional forwarding rules to classify the different types of packets from different flows.
- SoftRAN is a core solution used for managing edge access in cellular networks. Multiple base stations are virtually combined to a big base station to enable easy handover between cells.
- OpenRoad is a solution which makes SDN applicable in WLAN. This was deployed in campus networks. Odin and OpenAPI are other approaches to make SDN work for WLANs. Odin is suitable to be deployed in enterprise architecture and OpenAPI is used for edge access.

Security is a predominant issue in wireless and mobile networks where SDN is applied. It is a major concern to secure communication while the host is moving from one cell to another. The authentication and registration messages sent between the access points and hosts must be secured. [28] proposes a enhanced security framework for mobile wireless networks where a security sub layer on the northbound interface implements security features. Security policies programmed into this layer safeguards the wireless communication.

Flow Tracer: Proposed Solution

This paper proposes a solution to the problem of securing the controller from being misused by an attacker. It suggests a method to identify and isolate fraudulent flow entries that may be injected by the hacker. Flow tracer is a proposed module that lies in the controller which performs the job of fraudulent flow isolation. It performs the task of analysing the type of data and control messages that arrive at the controller. It reads the header to gather packet details and updates a table called Flow tracker. After detailed scrutiny of the packet, the controller updates the flow table entries, encrypts the packet using symmetric key encryption technique and forwards the packet to the data plane. Any subsequent packet belonging to the same flow is forwarded to the data plane after encryption (Fig. 3).

Fig. 3 Flow tracer

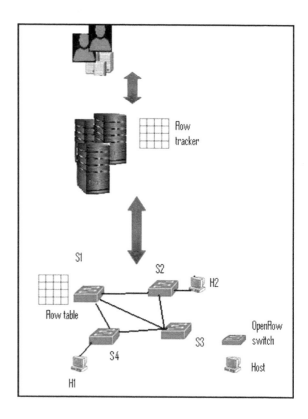

Any new flow that arrives at the controller is first verified against the entries already in the flow table. If an entry exists it is forwarded to the data plane without any further verification. If there is no entry found, an entry is made if and only if the packet seems authentic after scrutiny. If the packet seems to be suspicious it is dropped and an entry is made in the table to mark it as an attack. If the same kind of flow arrives several times it can be from an attacker who is trying to flood the network. Such flow can be isolated and further verified for its authenticity. Such methods can minimize DoS attacks.

PseudoCode for the same is given below

```
Event =Packet_arrives
If (first packet of flow)
{ perform thorough verification of identity and content of the packet
If (scrutiny ==true)
        { update flowtracker table Update flowtable entries in switch
        Encrypt the packet and send
        }
If(scrutiny == false)
        { mark the packet as attack
        Make an entry in the flowtracker table
        Drop the packet
        }
}
```

DoS attack is simulated as a part of this work using mininet emulator. The topology used for simulation is shown in Fig. 4. It consists of two controllers C0 and C1, hosts h1, h2, h3, h4, h5, h6 and OpenFlow switches s1, s2, s3. Switches s1 and s2 are connected to C0, s2 and s3 are connected to C1. Host h3 is considered to be the

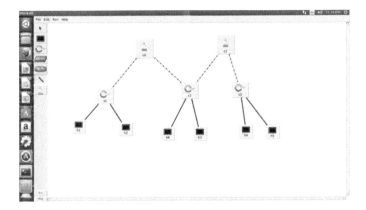

Fig. 4 Simulation topology

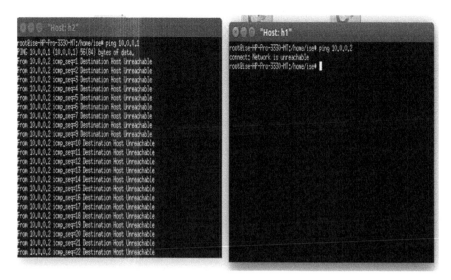

Fig. 5 H1 and H2 reachability result

hacker who floods in malicious traffic and jams the switch s1. Since h1 and h2 are connected to s1 reachability of nodes h1 and h2 is affected as shown in Fig. 5.

4   Conclusion

This paper gives a brief insight into the different types of attacks on an SDN network. It describes the vulnerabilities of an open interface and the countermeasures designed to detect and resolve these attacks. A novel approach to detect and isolate fraudulent data flow on the controller is proposed. In our future work, we will simulate and set up a real SDN environment, implement and improve the proposed technique to attain good success rate of attack detection and isolation.

References

1. Feamster N, Rexford J, Zegura E (Dec 2013) The road to SDN. Queue 11(12):20:20–20:40
2. Astuto BN, Mendonça M, Nguyen XN, Obraczka K, Turletti T (2014) Survey of software-defined networking: past, present, and future of programmable networks. IEEE Commun Surv Tutor PP(99):1–18, ISSN 1553-877X
3. Gude N, Koponen T, Pettit J, Pfaff B, Casado M, McKeown N, Shenker S (2008) NOX: towards an operating system for networks. ACM SIGCOMM Comput Commun Rev 38:105–110
4. McKeown N, Anderson T, Balakrishnan H, Parulkar G, Peterson L, Rexford J, Shenker S, Turner J (2008) Openflow: enabling innovation in campus networks. ACM SIGCOMM Comput Commun Rev 38(2):69–74

5. Yeganeh SH, Kandoo YG (2012) A framework for efficient and scalable offloading of control applications. In: Proceedings of the first workshop on hot topics in software defined networks, HotSDN'12. ACM, New York, NY, USA, pp 19–24
6. Tootoonchian A, Ganjali Y (2010) Hyperflow: a distributed control plane for OpenFlow. In: Proceedings of the 2010 internet network management conference on research on enterprise networking, pp 3–3
7. Caraguay ALV, Peral AB, López LIB, Villalba LJG (Jan 1999) Software-defined networking: evolution and opportunities in the development IoT applications. Int J Distrib Sens Netw 2014(2014):10, Article ID 735142
8. Valdivieso A, Barona L, Villalba L (Nov 2013) Evolution and challenges of software defined networking. In: Proceedings of 2013 workshop on software defined networks for future networks and services. IEEE, pp 61–67
9. Trivedi KDB (July 2013) SDN issues—a survey. Int J Comput Appl (0975–8887) 73:18
10. Gupta L, Jain R (2013) SDN: development, adoption and research trends (A survey of research issues in SDN). In: Thesis of recent advances in networking—data center virtualization, SDN, big data, cloud computing, internet of things course
11. Boucadair M, Jacquenet C (March 2014) Software-defined networking: a perspective from within a service provider environment. RFC: 7149France Telecom. ISSN 2070-1721
12. Hegr T, Bohac L, Uhlir V, Chlumsky P (2013) OpenFlow deployment and concept analysis. Inf Commun Technol Serv 11(5)
13. www.opennetworking.org/images/stories/downloads/sdn-resources/onf-specifications/openflow/openflow-spec-v1.3.0.pdf
14. Wen X, Chen Y, Hu C, Shi C, Wang Y (2013) Towards a secure controller platform for openflow applications. In: Proceedings of the second ACM SIGCOMM workshop on hot topics in software defined networking. ACM, New York, NY, USA ©2013, pp 171–172
15. Lara A, Kolasani A, Ramamurthy B (First 2014) Network innovation usingOpenFlow: a survey. IEEE Commun Surv Tutor 16(1):493–512
16. Lantz B, Heller B, McKeown N (2010) A network in a laptop: rapid prototyping for software-defined networks. In: Proceedings of the ninth ACM SIGCOMM workshop on hot topics in networks
17. Schlesinger C. Language-based security for software—defined networks. http://www.cs.princeton.edu/cschlesi/isolation.pdf
18. Hu F, Hao Q, Bao K (Fourth quarter 2014) A survey on software defined networking (SDN)and openflow: from concept to implementation. IEEE Commun Surv Tutor 16(4)
19. Sezer S, Scott-Hayward S, Chouhan PK, Fraser B, Lake D, Finnegan J, Viljoen N, Miller M, Rao N (2013) Are we ready for SDN? Implementation challenges for software-defined networks. IEEE Commun Mag 51:36–43
20. Shin S, Porras P, Yegneswaran V, Fong M, Gu G, Tyson M (April 2013) FRESCO: modular composable security services for software-defined networks. In: Proceedings of network distributed system security symposium
21. Choi T, Lee B, Song S, Park H, Yoon S, Yang S (April 2015) IRISCoMan: scalable and reliable control management architecture for SDN-enabled large scale networks. J Netw Syst Manag 23(2):252–279
22. Hu Z, Alcatel-Lucent Shanghai Bell Co. Ltd., Shanghai, China, Wang M, Yan X, Yin Y (2015) In: 18th IEEE international conference on intelligence in next generation networks (ICIN), Paris, pp 30–37
23. Kreutz D, Ramos F, Verissimo P (2013) Towards secure and dependable software-defined networks. In: Proceedings of the second ACM SIGCOMM workshop on hot topics in software defined networking, pp 55–60
24. Batista DM, Blair G, Kon F, Boutaba R, Hutchison D, Jain R, Ramjee R, Rothenberg CE (2015) Perspectives on software-defined networks: interviews with five leading scientists from the networking community. J Internet Serv Appl (2015)
25. Shin S, Gu G. Attacking software-defined networks: a first feasibility study. In: HotSDN '13 Proceedings of the second ACM SIGCOMM workshop on hot topics in software defined networking, pp 165–166

26. Chung C-J, Khatkar P, Xing T, Lee J, Huang D (2013) NICE: network intrusion detection and countermeasure selection in virtual network systems. IEEE Trans Dependable Secure Comput 10(4)
27. Open Networking Foundation. https://www.opennetworking.org/
28. Ding AY, Crowcroft J, Tarkoma S, Flinck H (June 2014) Software defined networking for security enhancement in wireless mobile networks. Comput Netw Elsevier 66:94–101

Comparative Performance Analysis of PID and Fuzzy Logic Controllers for 150hp Three-Phase Induction Motor

H. Sathishkumar and S. S. Parthasarathy

Abstract In this paper, comparative performance analysis of fuzzy logic controller and PID controller for space vector pulse width modulation (SVPWM)-based inverter-fed 150hp (horse power) three-phase induction motor which is used in the cable industry (Ravicab Cables Private Limited) at Bidadi is presented. In this cable industry, 611 Nm load torque is considered as full load and 305.5 Nm load torque is considered as half load for the three-phase induction motor. Proportional–integral–derivative (PID) controller-based voltage frequency drive (VFD) is used in this industry to control the speed of 150hp induction motor. Since VFD used in this industry is affected by several disturbances, robust speed controller is needed to be interfaced with the three-phase induction motor. In order to interface and identify the robust controller, this paper deals with simulation and comparison chart. As a part of the simulation, initially PID controller with real-time data which is used in this industry is interfaced with the 150hp induction motor under disturbance environment. Besides, the performance of this PID controller is analysed. Then, the proposed fuzzy logic controller is interfaced with the 150hp induction motor under disturbance environment. Moreover, the performance of this fuzzy logic controller is analysed. At the end, to identify the robust controller, the comparison chart is made.

Keywords Cable industry · 150hp · VFD · PID controller · Fuzzy logic controller

H. Sathishkumar (✉)
Department of Electronics, PET Research Foundation, PES College
of Engineering, Mandya 571401, India
e-mail: gangulysathish@gmail.com

S. S. Parthasarathy
Department of Electrical and Electronics, PES College of Engineering,
Mandya 571401, India
e-mail: vsarathypartha@yahoo.com

© Springer Nature Singapore Pte Ltd. 2019
V. Sridhar et al. (eds.), *Emerging Research in Electronics, Computer Science and Technology*, Lecture Notes in Electrical Engineering 545,
https://doi.org/10.1007/978-981-13-5802-9_74

1 Introduction

Induction motor is necessary in controlling various industrial operations. This paper deals about induction motor and its controller which is used in the cable industry at Bidadi. In this industry, 1hp, 3hp, 5hp, 15hp and 150hp three-phase induction motors are mainly used for various operations. In order to control these induction motors, PID-controller-based variable frequency drive is used in this industry [1]. This PID controller is severely affected by voltage and load variations [2]. Voltage variations deal about voltage sag and voltage swell. Since PID controller is affected by voltage variation, it is very difficult to operate this controller for the speed controlling purpose [3]. Therefore, in this paper, fuzzy-logic-controller-based speed controller is proposed for the three-phase induction motor [4, 5, 6]. Robustness of the proposed fuzzy controller is checked by doing comparative performance analysis with PID controller [4, 3, 7]. Moreover, superior performance of the proposed fuzzy controller is identified at three reference speeds [8, 9, 10]. In order to do the analyses in the effective manner, control system parameters, namely rise time, peak time and steady-state error, are used for the study.

2 Background Information

The cable drawing process is shown in Fig. 1. This cable drawing process is comprised of the various blocks, namely pay-off, wire drawing and annealing process. In this cable drawing process, cable pay-off is used to deliver various diameter level bare copper, namely 4.75, 7.25 and 10.35 mm diameter. These cables (i.e. bare copper) with various diameters are pulled by the cable drawing machine. The pulling force for the cable drawing machine is offered by three-phase induction motor and its VFD. A PID-controller-based VFD is used here to control the speed of this three-phase induction motor. This VFD is suffering from various disturbance signals and nonlinear load. Moreover, this PID-controller-based VFD is not directing the motor to provide sufficient pulling force to pull the cable. For example, a 4.75-mm-diameter cable is not pulled by sufficient pulling force (i.e. torque); then, the cable will not be pulled. Therefore, sufficient pulling force is to be given by the robust controller instead of this PID controller. Similarly, other diameter cables also will not get sufficient pulling force when PID-controller-based VFD is used. Therefore, in this paper, PID-based VFD is simulated with real-time cable industry data. Then, the proposed fuzzy-logic-controller-based VFD is simulated. At last, robust controller for this cable industry is found by doing comparison chart between PID and fuzzy controller simulations.

A cable pay-off process in real time is shown in Fig. 2. In this block, there may be one (or) two bobbins. If one bobbin is there, then it delivers cable from one bobbin. Suppose two bobbins are there, then dual cable pay-off can be done from

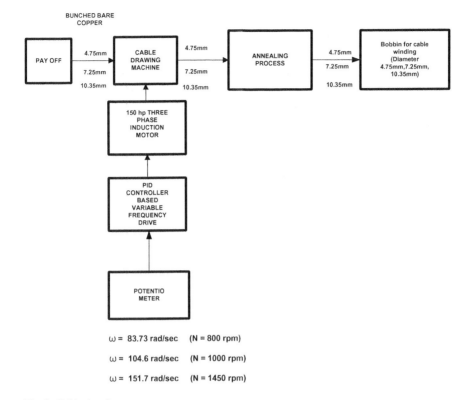

Fig. 1 Cable drawing process

two individual bobbins. In Fig. 2, single bobbin is used for making pay-off (i.e. cable delivery) process.

3 Existing PID Controller in Cable Industry

Block diagram of PID controller for three-phase induction motor is shown in Fig. 3.

A PID controller is used in this cable industry as a VFD. This PID controller is not able to direct the motor to deliver sufficient pulling force. This problem makes this PID controller as obsolete. To replace this PID controller, initially simulation of this existing PID controller is attempted with real-time cable industry data. Moreover in this block diagram, PID controller is the controller unit for the three-phase induction motor. This PID controller gets two inputs. One input is reference speed, and another one input is actual speed. Based on the error signal generated between these signals (i.e. actual speed and reference speed), SVPWM is operated. This SVPWM unit gives the required pulses to the three-phase inverter. Three-phase 150hp squirrel

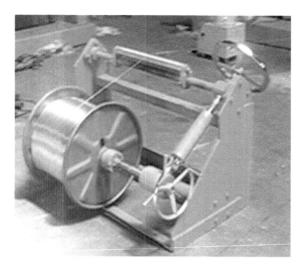

Fig. 2 Cable pay-off process

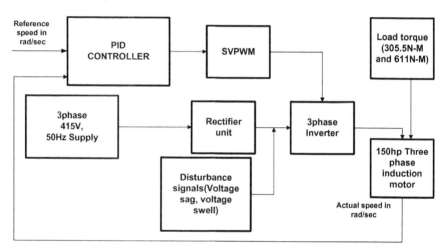

Fig. 3 Block diagram of PID controller for three-phase induction motor

cage induction motor gets the variable stator voltage from this inverter. Actual speed of the motor is measured and fed back to the one of the inputs to the PID controller. Moreover, three-phase, 415 V, 50 Hz AC supply is used as input supply. This supply is converted as DC supply via rectifier. Afterwards, rectified DC is added with the disturbance signals which is in the form of voltage sag and voltage swell. Then, this mixed rectified and disturbance signal is given to the input terminals of the inverter.

PID controller with speed selection unit is shown in Fig. 4. In this speed selection unit, there are four different reference speeds. Based on the control input, any one of the reference speed is selected. For example, if control input is 1, then reference

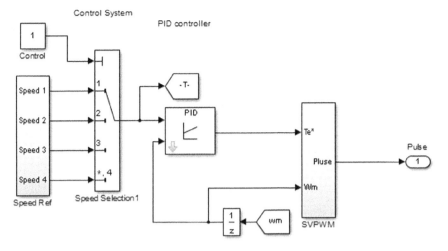

Fig. 4 PID controller with speed selection unit

speed1 (i.e. $\omega = 83.73$ rad/s) is connected with the PID controller via speed selection block.

Equation of the PID controller is of the following form:

$$u(t) = K_p e(t) + K_i \int e(t)dt + K_d(de/dt) \tag{1}$$

The required electric torque is

$$T_e = 1.5(p/2)(Lm/Lr)\psi_r i_{qs} \tag{2}$$

Stator reference flux linkage space vector position is

$$\theta_e = \int \omega_e dt = \int (\omega_{sl} + \omega_r)dt = \theta_r + \theta_{sl} \tag{3}$$

$$\omega_{sl} = K_s i_{qs} \tag{4}$$

$$\omega_{sl} = (L_m R_r / \Psi_r L_r) i_{qs} \tag{5}$$

$$\Psi_r^* = L_m i_{ds}^* \tag{6}$$

$$\theta = \tan^{-1}(\Psi_{qs}/\Psi_{ds}) \tag{7}$$

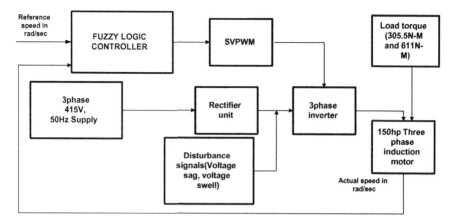

Fig. 5 Block diagram of fuzzy logic controller for three-phase induction motor

4   Proposed Fuzzy Logic Controller for Three-Phase Induction Motor

Block diagram of fuzzy logic controller for three-phase induction motor is shown in Fig. 5. The PID controller used in this cable industry is affected by voltage fluctuations (i.e. voltage sag and swell) and nonlinear load. Therefore, in this paper, fuzzy logic controller is used as a proposed controller. This fuzzy logic controller overcomes the problems (i.e. voltage fluctuations, nonlinear loading) which are predominant in the PID-controller-based speed controller. Hence, fuzzy-logic-based speed controller is simulated.

In this block diagram, fuzzy logic controller is the controller unit for the three-phase induction motor. This fuzzy logic controller gets two inputs. One input is reference speed, and another one input is actual speed. Based on the error signal generation between these signals (i.e. actual speed and reference speed), SVPWM is operated. This SVPWM unit gives the required pulses to the three-phase inverter. Three-phase 150hp squirrel cage induction motor gets the variable stator voltage from this inverter.

4.1   Implementation of the Fuzzy Logic Controller

The relationship between input variable and output variable is shown in Fig. 6. There are two input variables used in this fuzzy logic controller. Error is the first input variable which is formed by using the difference between actual speed (ωm) and reference speed (ω^*). Change in error is the variable. Electric torque reference is the output variable. These input and output variables are connected by using rule-based membership function.

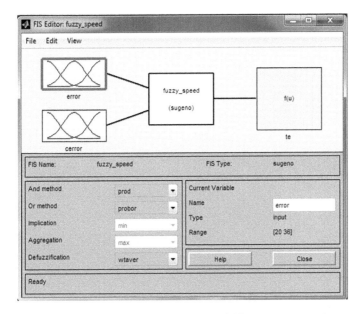

Fig. 6 Relationship between input variable and output variable

Table 1 Rule-based reference electric torque

Error	Change in error		
	Mf1	Mf2	Mf3
Not Mf1	Mf1	–	–
Mf1	Mf1	–	–
Mf2	Mf3	Mf2	Mf3
Mf2	–	Mf1	–
Mf3	–	Mf1	Mf3
Not Mf3	–	–	Mf3

Gauss2 member-function-based error variable is shown in Fig. 7. It comprises of three membership functions, namely membership function 1(Mf1), membership function 2 (Mf2) and membership function 3 (Mf3). Range of this membership function is limited between 20 to 36 in the x-axis and 0 to 1 in the y-axis.

Rule-based reference electric torque can be achieved by using Table 1.

(i)   If error is not Mf1 or change in error is Mf1, then reference electric torque from the fuzzy logic controller is Mf1.

(ii) If error is Mf2 or change in error is Mf2, then reference electric torque from the fuzzy logic controller is Mf2.

(iii) If error is Mf3 or change in error is Mf3, then reference electric torque from the fuzzy logic controller is Mf3.

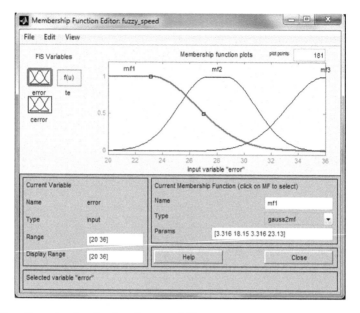

Fig. 7 Gauss2 member-function-based error variable

(iv)   If error is not Mf3 or change in error is Mf3, then reference electric torque from the fuzzy logic controller is Mf3.

 (v)   If error is Mf2 or change in error is Mf2, then reference electric torque from the fuzzy logic controller is Mf1.

(vi)   If error is Mf1 or change in error is Mf1, then reference electric torque from the fuzzy logic controller is Mf1.

(vii) If error is Mf2 or change in error is Mf1, then reference electric torque from the fuzzy logic controller is Mf3.

(viii) If error is Mf2 or change in error is Mf3 then reference electric torque from the fuzzy logic controller is Mf3.

(ix)   If error is Mf3 or change in error is Mf2, then reference electric torque from the fuzzy logic controller is Mf1.

These nine rules are sufficient to operate this induction motor in a correct manner.

Surface viewer for the rule-based reference electric torque is shown in Fig. 8. For example, if change of error is 6 and error is 20, then reference electric torque is 0.6. Similarly, various reference electric torques can be achieved for various errors and changes in error.

Rule-based reference electric torque is shown in Fig. 9. In this figure, error and change in error are varied with the help of ruler which is shown in red line. Reference electric torque is varied w.r.t the variation of error and change in error by using ruler.

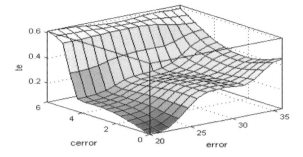

Fig. 8 Surface viewer for the rule-based reference electric torque

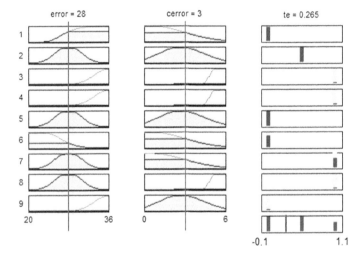

Fig. 9 Rule-based reference electric torque

5 Results and Discussion

Actual speed of the three-phase induction motor for various reference speeds is shown in Figs. 10, 11 and 12. Actual speed values taken from these figures are listed out in Table 2. For instance, in Table 2, reference speed $\omega = 83.73$ rad/s is taken into validation. In this reference speed $\omega = 83.73$ rad/s, PID controller directs the induction motor to produce $\omega = 80.3$ rad/s at half load. However, for the same half load fuzzy logic controller directs the induction motor to produce $\omega = 80.6$ rad/s. During the time of voltage sag disturbance, PID controller directs the induction motor to produce $\omega = 79.5$ rad/s. However, for the same voltage sag disturbance, fuzzy logic controller directs the induction motor to produce $\omega = 80.2$ rad/s. During the time of full load, PID controller directs the induction motor to produce $\omega = 75.1$ rad/s. However, for the same full load, fuzzy logic controller directs the induction motor to produce $\omega = 76.2$ rad/s. During the time of voltage swell disturbance, PID controller

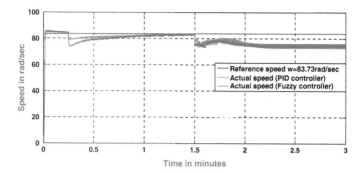

Fig. 10 Actual speed of the three-phase induction motor when reference speed $\omega = 83.73$ rad/s

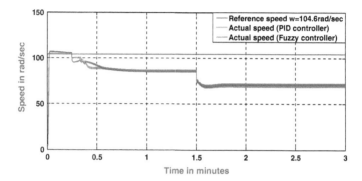

Fig. 11 Actual speed of the three-phase induction motor when reference speed $\omega = 104.6$ rad/s

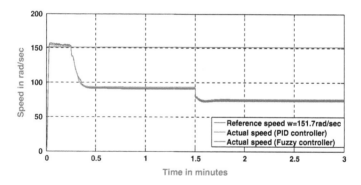

Fig. 12 Actual speed of the three-phase induction motor when reference speed $\omega = 151.7$ rad/s

directs the induction motor to produce $\omega = 75.8$ rad/s. However, for the same voltage swell disturbance, fuzzy logic controller directs the induction motor to produce $\omega = 76.5$ rad/s. Similarly, for other reference speeds, PID and fuzzy logic controllers' comparative performance analysis can be made.

Table 2 PID and fuzzy controllers for the various reference speeds in rad/s

Disturbance signals	Actual speed of the motor at various reference speeds					
	PID (ω = 83.73 rad/s)	Fuzzy (ω = 83.73 rad/s)	PID (ω = 104.6 rad/s)	Fuzzy (ω = 104.6 rad/s)	PID (ω = 151.7 rad/s)	Fuzzy (ω = 151.7 rad/s)
Half load (305.5 Nm) is applied to the motor at 0.25 min	ω = 80.3 rad/s (N = 766.80 rpm)	ω = 80.6 rad/s (N = 769.67 rpm)	ω = 88.3 rad/s (N = 843.20 rpm)	ω = 88.7 rad/s (N = 847.022 rpm)	ω = 92.8 rad/s (N = 886.17 rpm)	ω = 93.6 rad/s (N = 893.81 rpm)
Voltage sag = 27 V is occurring between the time 0.7 min and 0.95 min	ω = 79.5 rad/s (N = 759.16 rpm)	ω = 80.2 rad/s (N = 765.85 rpm)	ω = 86.1 rad/s (N = 822.19 rpm)	ω = 87.8 rad/s (N = 838.42 rpm)	ω = 91.45 rad/s (N = 873.28 rpm)	ω = 93.1 rad/s (N = 889.03 rpm)
Full load (611 Nm) is applied to the motor at 1.5 min	ω = 75.1 rad/s (N = 717.15 rpm)	ω = 76.2 rad/s (N = 727.65 rpm)	ω = 69.4 rad/s (N = 662.72 rpm)	ω = 71.1 rad/s (N = 678.95 rpm)	ω = 74.4 rad/s (N = 710.46 rpm)	ω = 75.8 rad/s (N = 723.83 rpm)
Voltage swell = 38 V is occurring between the time 2.3 min and 2.5 min	ω = 75.8 rad/s (N = 723.83 rpm)	ω = 76.5 rad/s (N = 730.52 rpm)	ω = 69.8 rad/s (N = 666.54 rpm)	ω = 71.5 rad/s (N = 682.77 rpm)	ω = 74.8 rad/s (N = 714.28 rpm)	ω = 76.1 rad/s (N = 726.70 rpm)

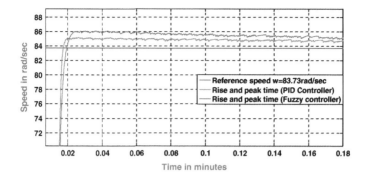

Fig. 13 Rise time and peak time of the actual speed when reference speed ω = 83.73 rad/s

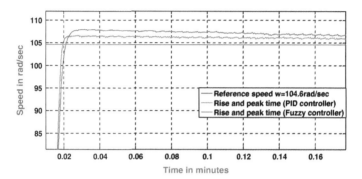

Fig. 14 Rise time and peak time of the actual speed when reference speed ω = 104.6 rad/s

Hence, it is found that from Table 2, the actual speed values are higher for fuzzy-logic-based speed controller over PID controller for the various disturbance signals and nonlinear loads.

Rise time and peak time of the actual speed of the three-phase induction motor are shown in Figs. 13, 14 and 15. Rise time and peak time values taken from these figures are listed out in Table 3. For instance, in Table 3 reference speed ω = 83.73 rad/s is taken into validation. In this reference speed ω = 83.73 rad/s, PID-controller-based speed controller directs the motor to produce 0.0174 min as rise time and 0.020 min as peak time in actual speed. For the same reference speed ω = 83.73 rad/s, fuzzy logic controller directs the motor to produce 0.0192 min as rise time and 0.024 min as peak time in actual speed. Similarly, for other reference speeds, comparison of rise time and peak time can be made between PID and fuzzy controllers.

Therefore, it is found that from Table 3, rise time and peak time values are low for PID-based speed controller compared to fuzzy logic controller.

Steady-state error of the actual speed of the three-phase induction motor is shown in Figs. 16, 17 and 18. Steady-state error taken from these figures is listed out in Table 4. For instance, in Table 4 reference speed ω = 83.73 rad/s is taken into validation. In this reference speed ω = 83.73 rad/s, PID-controller-based speed controller

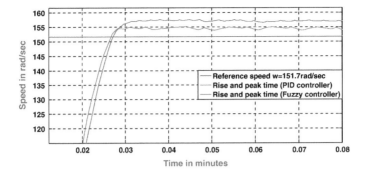

Fig. 15 Rise time and peak time of the actual speed when reference speed ω = 151.7 rad/s

Table 3 Transient state analysis at various speeds in rad/s

Parameters	PID controller (83.73 rad/s)	Fuzzy controller (83.73 rad/s)	PID controller (104.6 rad/s)	Fuzzy controller (104.6 rad/s)	PID controller (151.7 rad/s)	Fuzzy controller (151.7 rad/s)
Rise time in minutes	0.0174	0.0192	0.019	0.021	0.0268	0.0273
Peak time in minutes	0.020	0.024	0.023	0.030	0.035	0.038

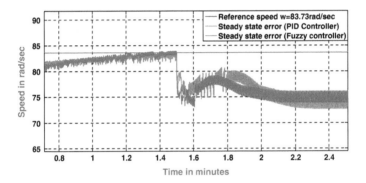

Fig. 16 Steady-state error of the actual speed when reference speed ω = 83.73 rad/s

directs the motor to produce 2.53 rad/s as steady-state error (i.e. reference speed − actual speed) at half load. For the same reference speed ω = 83.73 rad/s, fuzzy logic controller directs the motor to produce 0.93 rad/s as steady-state error at half load. In the full load, PID-controller-based speed controller directs the motor to produce 8.28 rad/s as steady-state error. For the same reference speed ω = 83.73 rad/s, fuzzy logic controller directs the motor to produce 7.58 rad/s as steady-state error at full load. Similarly, for other reference speeds, steady-state error comparison can be made between PID and fuzzy controllers. Hence, it is found that fuzzy-logic-controller-based speed controller reduces the steady-state error significantly over PID controller.

Table 4 Steady-state analysis at various speeds in rad/s

Parameters	PID controller (83.73 rad/s)	Fuzzy controller (83.73 rad/s)	PID controller (104.6 rad/s)	Fuzzy controller (104.6 rad/s)	PID controller (151.7 rad/s)	Fuzzy controller (151.7 rad/s)
Steady-state error at half load (before 1.5 min) (rad/s)	2.53	0.93	16.7	16.4	56.6	56.4
Steady-state error at full load (after 1.5 min) (rad/s)	8.28	7.58	32.8	31.8	76.3	75.5

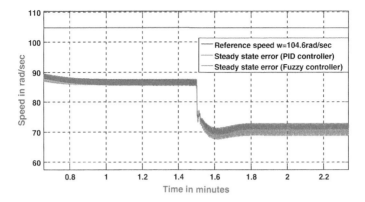

Fig. 17 Steady-state error of the actual speed when reference speed $\omega = 104.6$ rad/s

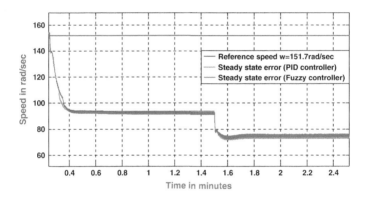

Fig. 18 Steady-state error of the actual speed when reference speed $\omega = 151.7$ rad/s

Therefore, from Tables 2, 3 and 4, it is observed that fuzzy-logic-controller-based speed controller is the suitable robust controller for this cable industry over PID-based variable frequency drive.

6 Conclusion

Cable industry (Ravicab Cables Private Limited) at Bidadi is taken into study. In this industry, various three-phase induction motors are used. However, only 150hp motor which is used for the cable drawing purpose is taken into study. PID-based VFD is used still now in this industry. This PID-controller-based VFD is affected by nonlinear load and disturbance signals. Therefore, in order to make the replacement of this drive, real-time data which is taken from this cable industry (i.e. PID-based VFD) is used for simulation. Then, the proposed fuzzy-logic-controller-based speed controller is simulated. Both controller simulations are done with the help of MAT-LAB software. Moreover, comparison chart (i.e. Tables 1, 2 and 3) is made between these PID and fuzzy logic controllers. From the comparison chart, it is found that the fuzzy logic controller delivers excellent performance over PID-based VFD for this 150hp induction motor.

Appendix

Cable Drawing Motor Name Plate Details

HP	150	kW	111.855
Rated voltage	415 V	Full load current	286.05 A
Power factor	0.85	Efficiency	80%
Frequency		50 Hz	
Poles		4	
Stator resistance R_s		0.435 Ω	
Stator inductance L_s		0.004 H	
Rotor resistance R_r		0.816 Ω	
Rotor inductance L_r		0.002 H	
Mutual inductance L_m		0.06931 H	
Inertia		0.089	

References

1. Ajangnay MO (2010) Optimal PID controller parameters for vector control of induction motors. In: IEEE conference on power electronics electrical drives automation and motion, Italy, pp 959–965
2. Uddin MN, Nam SW (2009) Development and implementation of a nonlinear-controller-based IM drive incorporating iron loss with parameter uncertainties. IEEE Trans Ind Electron 56:1263–1272
3. Bhushan B, Kumar Bairwa G (2010) Performance analysis of indirect vector control induction motor using PI, fuzzy and neural network predictive control. J Electr Syst 6:361–376
4. Dongale TD, Uplane MD (2012) Performance comparison of PID and fuzzy control techniques in three phase induction motor control. Int J Recent Trends Eng Technol 7:101–105
5. Sathishkumar H, Parthasarathy SS (2017) A novel fuzzy logic controller for vector controlled induction motor drive. Energy Procedia 138:686–691
6. Zadeh Lotfi A (2015) Fuzzy logic—a personal perspective. Fuzzy Sets Syst 281:4–20
7. Tran DK (2018) Extending fuzzy logics with many hedges. Fuzzy Sets Syst 345:126–138
8. Shaukat N, Ali SM (2016) Takagi-sugeno fuzzy logic based speed control of induction motor. In: International conference on in frontiers of information technology. IEEE, Pakistan, pp 280–285

9. Vengatesan V, Chindamani M (2014) Speed control of three phase induction motor using fuzzy logic controller by space vector modulation technique. Int J Adv Res Electr Electron Instrum Eng 3:2320–3765
10. Zhang R, Liu X, Zeng D, Zhong S, Shi K (2017) A novel approach to stability and stabilization of fuzzy sampled-data Markovian chaotic systems. Fuzzy Sets Syst 344:108–128

A Hybrid Progressive Image Compression, Transmission, and Reconstruction Architecture

H. K. Ravikiran and Paramesha

Abstract Image compression and progressive transmission (PIT) is a technique used as an alternative solution to the communication problem, where there is a need to transmit huge data such as in medical image transmission. The technique divides image that is to be transmitted into several phases and effectively provides a fairly accurate reconstruction of the original image in every phase. This paper proposes a novel architecture that combines bit-plane slicing, DD-dual-tree DWT, and SPIHT. The bit-plane slicing separates the image into eight planes; each bit plane is then decomposed with wavelet. The wavelet coefficients in different sub-bands are then encoded using SPIHT and transmitted progressively and reconstructed by combining the data received in each phase with the previous phase data. Experimental results have shown that the proposed technique has better efficiency. Even at the lowest SPIHT rate of 0.1 bits/pixel for a 512×512 gray scale medical image, the reconstructed image shows higher quality at third phase itself, which makes it an efficient choice for transmission of medical images even at low speed communication channel.

Keywords Bit-plane slicing · DD-DT DWT · SPIHT

1 Introduction

In most of the developing and under developing countries, rural health is a major issue due to the lack of facilities and experts. A way out to the problem is to allow the experts to treat the patients from where they reside. Hence, a large amount of data is to be sent

H. K. Ravikiran (✉)
Department of Electronics and Communication Engineering, Rajeev Institute of Technology, Hassan 573201, Karnataka, India
e-mail: ravikiranhsn@gmail.com

Paramesha
Department of Electronics and Communication Engineering, Government Engineering College, Hassan 573201, Karnataka, India

© Springer Nature Singapore Pte Ltd. 2019
V. Sridhar et al. (eds.), *Emerging Research in Electronics, Computer Science and Technology*, Lecture Notes in Electrical Engineering 545,
https://doi.org/10.1007/978-981-13-5802-9_75

to diagnose a patient. Another issue over here is transmission bandwidth. The best solution to this is to combine image compression and progressive transmission and reconstruction. Progressive image coding techniques encode the image and generate an embedded bit stream, and the fidelity at the receiver is to reconstruct the image depending on the number of bits received, i.e., the compressed bit streams are sent in a different phase. Progressive image compression and transmission is the innate choice since the transmission can be terminated at any phase of time, if the reconstruction image is found to be irrelevant for the study. This technique is very effective as it reduces the wastage of resources in terms of price and time.

Many techniques are available for image compression and transmission that depend on the type of transformation and encoding techniques that are used. Some of the popular transformations to decorrelate the image pixels are discrete cosine transform (DCT), discrete Fourier transform (DFT), Walsh–Hadamard transform (WHT), Karhunen–Loeve transform (KLT), and discrete wavelet transform (DWT), etc. With these transformations, DCT and DWT are the most popular techniques. JPEG is a first International standard accepted for still image compression, which is based on the DCT and is appropriate for continuous tone images with a broad range of applications. An important drawback with JPEG is blocking artifacts in the reconstructed image at low bit rate. DWT is an excellent energy compaction and superior reconstruction technique; it eliminates blocking artifacts at low bit rates that may occur in DCT-based JPEG. Though algorithms based on DWT offer high coding efficiency for images, it has some major disadvantages such as lack of shift invariance, a poor directional selectivity that deteriorates its use in many applications. By forming dual-tree discrete wavelet transform, a remarkable improvement can be obtained in wavelet-based image analysis by utilizing a pair of wavelet transforms, where the wavelets form a Hilbert transform pair. Such a wavelet transform has several advantages, including near shift-invariance, significantly improved denoising capability, and the implementation of directional 2D DWTs using separable filter banks. A wavelet transform based on oversampled filter banks develops a shiftable multiscale transform with advantages such as very smooth wavelets, near shift-invariance, improved time–frequency bandwidth product, and approximation to the continuous wavelet transform, hence the term double-density DWT. Both dual-tree DWT and double-density DWT are similar in some aspects. A Hilbert transform pairs combing the advantages of both the types is called as the double-density dual-tree DWT [1–5].

There are several types of wavelet-based encoding schemes that support progressive image transmission. A well known such technique is set partitioning in hierarchical trees (SPIHT) which is an improved version of Embedded Zerotree Wavelet Coding technique and has shown better performance for image encoding [6, 7]. EZW uses wavelet transform as the transformation technique. SPIHT is considered better than EZW technique because SPIHT gave a much better performance by reducing the mean square error and increased the peak signal-to-noise ratio which gave a much-improved performance. SPIHT was highly appreciated for its fast and simple algorithm along with its efficiency. Several advancements came to improve the performance of SPIHT and to reduce the complexity of the SPIHT algorithm.

1.1 Need for Progressive Compression

An image could be compressed in one pass, i.e., sequential or progressive. In sequential compression, the entire image bits are encoded in one pass and reconstruction is performed after receiving and decoding all the transmitted bits. While in progressive image compression, the entire image is not encoded in a single phase, instead of in multiple phases generating a layered bit stream. During reconstruction, the images are reconstructed as each phase bits are received. The image is reconstructed as a coarse approximation with the first-phase bit stream, and subsequent image quality is enhanced by adding later phase details.

As telemedicine and modern imaging technique evolved, huge volume of data are generated and exchanged between the doctors for better analysis of the image. The images are transmitted over wireless networks or Internet over band-limited channels, and the cost incurred is directly related to transmission time. When an image is transmitted and reconstructed in phase, it allows the user to decide whether the rest of the data is required to be transmitted or not, thus eliminating wastage of bandwidth and resources. Thus, the progressive coding and reconstruction scheme are attractive for telemedicine application.

2 Implementation

The simplest way to implement progressive image transmission in the spatial domain is to use bit-plane slicing [8]. Figure 1 shows complete flow of the implementation.

Suppose a gray image consists of 8-bit pixel representation, then we can split a gray image into eight different bit planes using bitplane slicing, where the bit plane 0 represents the pixel from LSB and bit plane 7 represents the pixel from MSB. Figure 2 shows the bit plane for 8-bit image data [9]. The bit plane 7 contains more detailed information of an image, and the last bit plane contains fewer details of the image. So, the first phase of transmission consists of only the most significant bit of each pixel in an image followed by reaming bit planes until the final image is

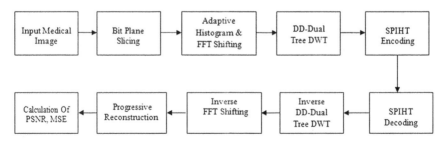

Fig. 1 Block diagram

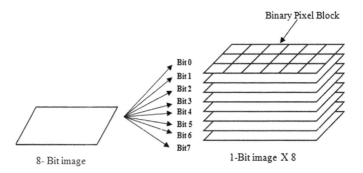

Fig. 2 Bit plane for 8-bit image data

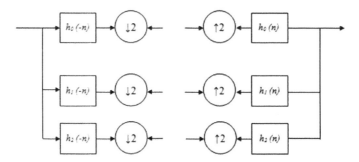

Fig. 3 Oversampled analysis and synthesis filterbank

lossless or until the receiver does not need the image quality to be further improved. These bit planes are subjected to adaptive histogram followed by FFT shifting as a pre-processing stage, to convert the bit planes to continuous function from discrete function. Then these bit planes are processed by double-density dual-tree DWT for image compression.

The double-density dual-tree DWT implemented here is based on concatenating two oversampled DWTs. The filter bank structure corresponding to the double-density dual-tree DWT consists of two oversampled iterated filter banks operating in parallel, similar to the dual-tree DWT. Each iterated filter bank is redundant by a factor 2. The oversampled filter bank is illustrated in Fig. 3 [4]. The iterated oversampled filter bank [4], corresponding to the implementation of the double-density dual-tree, is illustrated in Fig. 4. The analysis filter bank is represented by $h_i(n)$ and the synthesis filters banks by $g_i(n)$, for $i = 0, 1, 2$. The synthesis filters are the time-reversed versions of the analysis filters. The six FIR filters formed here should satisfy perfect reconstruction property and should form Hilbert transform pairs.

Let $H_i(Z)$ be the Z-transform of $h_i(n)$

$$H_i(z) = ZT\{h_i(n)\} = \sum_n h_i(n)Z^{-n} \qquad (1)$$

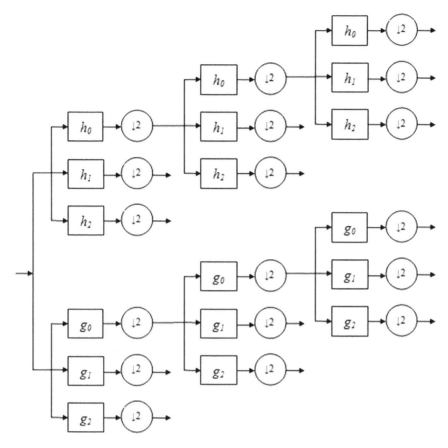

Fig. 4 Iterated filter bank for the DD-dual-tree DWT

and $G_i(z)$ is similarly defined. From the identities of basic multirate, the perfect reconstruction condition is as follows:

$$\sum_{i=0}^{2} H_i(z)H_i\left(\frac{1}{z}\right) = 2 \tag{2}$$

$$\sum_{i=0}^{2} H_i(z)H_i\left(-\frac{1}{z}\right) = 0 \tag{3}$$

$$\sum_{i=0}^{2} G_i(z)G_i\left(\frac{1}{z}\right) = 2 \tag{4}$$

$$\sum_{i=0}^{2} G_i(z)G_i\left(-\frac{1}{z}\right) = 0 \tag{5}$$

The scaling and wavelet functions are implicitly defined through the dilation and wavelet equations as:

$$\phi_h(t) = \sqrt{2} \sum_n h_0(n)\phi_h(2t - n) \tag{6}$$

$$\psi_{h,1}(t) = \sqrt{2} \sum_n h_1(n)\phi_h(2t - n) \tag{7}$$

$$\psi_{h,2}(t) = \sqrt{2} \sum_n h_2(n)\phi_h(2t - n) \tag{8}$$

The image is thus decomposed into sub-bands. The sub-bands which are gradient basis are neglected; only the sub-band that has more information is picked and forwarded for progressive SPIHT transmission model and remaining sub-bands are stored in order to reconstruct back along with modified sub-band.

The SPIHT groups the decomposed wavelet coefficients into sets called as spatial orientation tree [7], which is then encoded progressively from MSB bit planes to LSB bit planes, starting from the coefficient with the highest magnitude. Before the encoding procedure takes place, the budget bits or SPIHT rate is to be initialized, i.e., a number of bits per pixel. So that encoding procedure allocates a number of bits available for encoding procedure. SPIHT uses two coding passes: the refinement pass and the sorting pass. In the sorting pass, the significant and insignificant coefficients are separated based on the thresholds' value. Later, the precision bits of the significant coefficients are sent during the refinement pass. After each scan pass, i.e., with one sorting and refinement pass, the threshold is halved and the coding procedure is repeated until required bit rate is achieved.

At the receiver side, decompression takes place by performing inverse computation of each encoding block.

3   Experimental Results

Based on precision rate, PSNR, and MSE, the performance of the methodology is evaluated. Following formulas are used to calculate MSE and PSNR.

$$\text{MSE} = \sum_{i=1}^{M} \sum_{j=1}^{N} \frac{(x - x1)^2}{M*N} \tag{9}$$

$$\text{PSNR} = 10\log_{10}\left(\frac{255*255}{MSE}\right)\text{dB} \tag{10}$$

Here we have considered medical images represented by 256 gray levels, and each image has 512×512 pixels. The PSNR and MSE values of the each phase for the tested image are shown in Table 1. We can observe an increase in the image

Table 1 PSNR and MSE for each decoding level

Decoding level	Performance parameters	SPIHT rate-0.1	SPIHT rate-1
Decoding level 1	PSNR	14.67	16.74
	MSE	2214.15	1375.49
Decoding level 2	PSNR	16.26	20.72
	MSE	1535.52	550.46
Decoding level 3	PSNR	17.60	25.32
	MSE	1127.57	190.69
Decoding level 4	PSNR	18.32	28.94
	MSE	957.21	82.98
Decoding level 5	PSNR	18.77	32.90
	MSE	862.48	33.33
Decoding level 6	PSNR	18.98	35.17
	MSE	821.70	19.74
Decoding level 7	PSNR	19.08	36.19
	MSE	802.61	15.61
Decoding level 8	PSNR	19.13	36.59
	MSE	793.53	14.24

Fig. 5 Input medical image

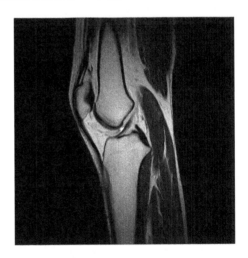

quality in each phase. Figure 5 shows the input medical image. Figure 6 illustrates the progressive reconstructed image. In our experiment, we have used eight planes to transmit, i.e., transmission of MSB bit plane to LSB bit plane. Since the quality image can be obtained in earlier transmission, the person at the receiver side can decide the further transmission required or not.

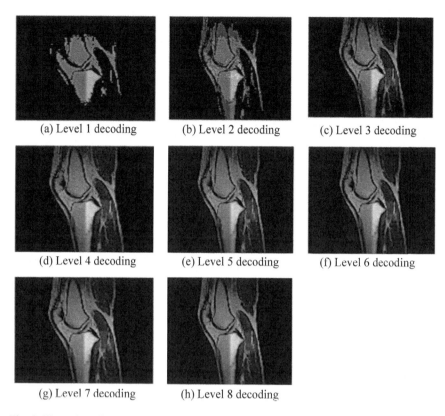

(a) Level 1 decoding   (b) Level 2 decoding   (c) Level 3 decoding

(d) Level 4 decoding   (e) Level 5 decoding   (f) Level 6 decoding

(g) Level 7 decoding   (h) Level 8 decoding

Fig. 6 Illustration of progressive reconstruction for SPIHT rate of 0.1

4 Conclusions

In this paper, a hybrid efficient progressive image compression, transmission, and reconstruction technique is implemented. According to the experimental results, our scheme shows better performance even in the lower SPIHT rate. Hence, the technique is suitable for low-bandwidth application. Also significant better image quality can be obtained in the earlier phase itself, which allows the receiver side to decide whether further transmission is required or not.

References

1. Kingsbury NG (1998) The dual-tree complex wavelet transform: a new technique for shift invariance and directional filters. In: IEEE digital signal processing workshop, vol 86. Bryce Canyon, pp 120–131

2. Kingsbury N (2001) Complex wavelets for shift invariant analysis and filtering of signals. Appl Comput Harmonic Anal 10(3):234–253
3. Selesnick IW (2001) The double density DWT. In: Wavelets in signal and image analysis: from theory to practice. Kluwer, Boston, MA
4. Selesnick IW (2004) The double-density dual-tree DWT. IEEE Trans Signal Process 52(5):1304–1314
5. Selesnick IW, Baraniuk RG, Kingsbury NC (2005) The dual-tree complex wavelet transform. IEEE Signal Process Mag 22(6):123–151
6. Shapiro JM (1993) Embedded image coding using zerotrees of wavelet coefficients. IEEE Trans Signal Process 41(12):3445–3462
7. Said A, Pearlman WA (1996) A new, fast, and efficient image codec based on set partitioning in hierarchical trees. IEEE Trans Circuits Syst Video Technol 6(3):243–250
8. Chang C-C, Shiue F-C, Chen T-S (1999) A new scheme of progressive image transmission based on bit-plane method. In: Fifth Asia-Pacific conference on communications, APCC/OECC'99 and fourth optoelectronics and communications conference, vol 2. IEEE, pp 892–895
9. Sun S (2015) A new information hiding method based on improved BPCS steganography. Adv Multimed 2015:5

Design and Development of Non-volatile Multi-threshold Schmitt Trigger SRAM Cell

L. Nikitha, N. S. Bhargavi and B. S. Kariyappa

Abstract Memory is one of the fundamental components of the modern computers. The need for low-power, faster non-volatile memories has been increasing due to compact and increased chip density. In this paper, the faster volatile Schmitt trigger SRAM cell with improved read and write operation is made non-volatile by inclusion of memristors. Multi-threshold CMOS (MTCMOS) technique is applied to reduce the overall power consumption of the circuit. The Schmitt trigger (ST) implementation improved the switching characteristics, reduced the leakage power, and gave improved static noise margin (SNM). The addition of memristor to the Schmitt trigger SRAM cell made the cell non-volatile and further increased the SNM. The MTCMOS non-volatile ST SRAM reduced average power consumption by 56.67% and increased SNM value by 58.65%.

Keywords SRAM · Schmitt trigger · Non-volatile · Memristor · MTCMOS

1 Introduction

Memories form an important part of computers and are used to store data required for computing operations. Memories are broadly classified into two types, i.e., volatile and non-volatile memories. Volatile memories such as static random-access memory (SRAM) and dynamic random-access memory (DRAM) tend to lose data stored in them as soon as the power supply is turned off. However, volatile memories tend to be faster and hence find applications in high-speed memories of the computers such

L. Nikitha (✉) · N. S. Bhargavi
R.V. College of Engineering, Bangalore 560059, India
e-mail: lokarajunikitha@gmail.com

N. S. Bhargavi
e-mail: janavi.bhargavi@gmail.com

B. S. Kariyappa
Department of ECE, R.V. College of Engineering, Bangalore 560059, India
e-mail: kariyappabs@rvce.edu.in

© Springer Nature Singapore Pte Ltd. 2019
V. Sridhar et al. (eds.), *Emerging Research in Electronics, Computer Science and Technology*, Lecture Notes in Electrical Engineering 545,
https://doi.org/10.1007/978-981-13-5802-9_76

as cache. Non-volatile memories do not need power supply to retain data hence tend to retain data even after power supply variations [1, 2]. A sense amplifier was also designed and integrated along with the SRAM array for read and write operations. The various design challenges involved in the design of SRAM cell and the effective optimization methods to overcome the leakage power during SRAM cell operation were discussed in [3]. A Schmitt-trigger-based SRAM cell that has improved read and write noise margin and also has very less leakage power is designed in [4, 5]. The non-volatile characteristic was introduced by using a combination of memristor and complemented metal oxide semiconductor. A binary logic was introduced in the paper for better read and write ability of the memory cell. Low-power-based multi-threshold CMOS(MTCMOS) technique was implemented on 12T SRAM cell, and power analysis was done in [6]. There was dynamic power reduction and overall power reduction using the MTCMOS technique. Design of 7T SRAM cell using improved self-voltage-level method was done in [7, 8]. The proposed method showed a great reduction in the leakage power of the SRAM cell. A comparative study of the various 7T SRAM cells was done in [9, 10].

Section 1 gives brief introduction about the project, and the literature survey is carried out. Section 2 explains the proposed cell design, the working principle, and procedure. The third section explains the results, analysis of the proposed cell, and comparison of area, power, and SNM parameters for the various designed cells. Section 4 gives the conclusion, future research work, and limitations of the proposed cell design.

2 Proposed Cell

A basic 6T SRAM cell is designed and analyzed in terms of power, area and static noise margin. To avoid the destructive read operation happening in the conventional 6T SRAM, a Schmitt-trigger-based SRAM cell is realized to improve the switching inverter characteristics and also to reduce the leakage power [10]. However, the 6T SRAM and the 10T Schmitt trigger SRAM are volatile. To allow the SRAM to retain data even after power supply is switched off, the Schmitt trigger SRAM is made non-volatile by adding a non-volatile memristor component to it. The memristor has a very small piece of a transition metal oxide placed between two electrodes. The electrical resistance of the memristor dramatically decreases or increases by applying a negative or positive voltage pulse. This behavior allows the memristor to be used as a non-volatile computer memory that is quite similar to a flash memory as it is capable of retaining its state without the need for being refreshed with extra power. The addition of memristor to the Schmitt trigger SRAM increased the power consumption of the non-volatile SRAM. Hence, to decrease the overall power consumption of the circuit, multi-threshold CMOS (MTCMOS) logic was applied to the non-volatile Schmitt trigger SRAM.

Figure 1 shows MTCMOS-based memristor ST SRAM cell schematic. It is integrated with the test signals to form a test circuit. Two memristor components are

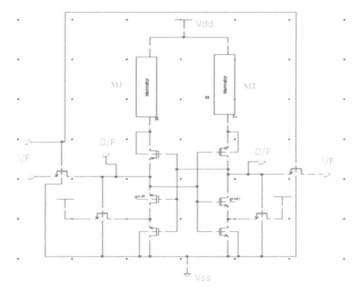

Fig. 1 MTCMOS and memristor-based Schmitt trigger SRAM Cell

added to the ST SRAM cell, and critical path transistors are replaced with low threshold voltage transistors. A Vpulse signal is given as input to the word line with appropriate pulse width and period. The outputs Q and Qb (Qbar) are considered to check the bit values stored in the memory.

The write-driver circuit will control the current flow through the circuit to make sure the designed cell is operating properly. The word line defines operational modes. When WL is low, both access transistors are off and cell is isolated. To undergo read or write operation, the word line is made high which turns on both access transistors.

When the power is switched off for Schmitt trigger SRAM cell and then switched on, the data stored is lost and operation must start from the beginning again. In order to solve this problem, a memristor symbol is synthesized and used in addition to the Schmitt trigger SRAM cell. The input is given through bit and bit_bar. If data to be written is '1', bit is raised to Vdd and bit_bar is pulled to the ground. If data to be written is '0', bit is pulled to the ground and bit_bar is raised to Vdd. Initially, word line is made high to write the data and write-driver circuit is used to write the data into the ST-based SRAM cell. During read operation, initially, bit and bit_bar are precharged to Vdd/2. Depending on the values stored in the cell, there will be an increase or decrease of voltage in bit and bit_bar. If bit is at a higher voltage than bit_bar, it means data read is '1'. If bit is at lower voltage than bit_bar, then the data read is '0'. During the write 1 operation, the resistance of M1 memristor is higher than the resistance of M2 memristor. Then the bit and bit_bar will be precharged to a value of Vdd/2. The drop in voltage is high across memristor M1 because of the high resistance of M1, and the drop across M2 is very less. During the write 0 operation, the resistance of M2 memristor is higher than the resistance of M1 memristor. Then

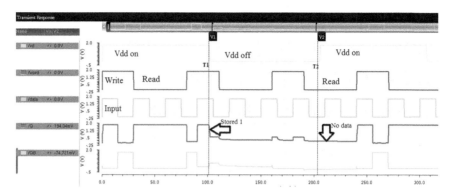

Fig. 2 Transient plot for ST SRAM with Vdd variations

the bit and bit_bar will be precharged to a value of Vdd/2. The drop in voltage is high across memristor M2 because of the high resistance of M2, and the drop across M1 is very less [5].

In the proposed cell design, bit and bit_bar lines are connected to two voltage sources. This reduces the voltage swing at the output lines, and it will result in dynamic power reduction when switching activity is taking place. The transistors present in the critical path are replaced with these LVT transistors which reduce the total average power [6].

3 Results and Analysis of the Proposed Cell

The transient analysis of the SRAM cells during read and write operations is described. Following this are the performance analysis like average power and SNM and comparative analysis between SRAM and Schmitt-trigger-based SRAM cell, Schmitt-trigger-based SRAM cell with Memristor and MTCMOS ST-based SRAM cell with Memristor. All schematics are drawn in virtuoso ADE of Cadence version 6.1.6, and all simulations are carried out using Cadence Specter analyzer with 45 nm technology library files at 1.8 V Vdd.

Figure 2 indicates the output of the ST SRAM cell with Vdd variations. To check the data retention capability, the Vdd supply is switched off and on for a finite duration. When power is switched off and on, the data stored is lost in the ST SRAM cell. Two memristor components are added to the ST SRAM cell, and the transistors present in the critical path are considered and are replaced with low threshold voltage transistors to form the MTCMOS-based memristor ST SRAM cell.

To check the data retention capability of the memristor, the Vdd supply is switched off and on for a finite duration. We make use of write-driver circuit to check the circuit operation during the on and off period. Figure 3 represents the plot of output and input waveforms performed using transient analysis. When power is switched off and

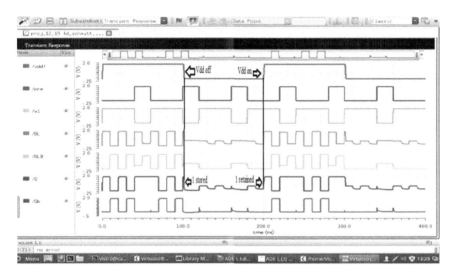

Fig. 3 Transient plot for MTCMOS-based memristor ST SRAM cell with Vdd variation

on in the MTCMOS-based memristor ST SRAM circuit, the data stored is retained and displayed.

The butterfly curve or VTC curve is obtained by superposing the voltage transfer characteristics (VTC) of one cell inverter to the inverse VTC of the other cell inverter. The resulting two-lobed graph is called a butterfly curve, and it is used to determine the SNM. The SNM that affects the read and write noise margins of the SRAM cell is dependent on the threshold voltage of the CMOS transistors. Typically, to increase the SNM, the threshold voltages of the NMOS and PMOS devices need to be increased. Figure 4 shows the SNM plot of the MTCMOS memristor ST SRAM, and the SNM value is 825 mV.

The 6T SRAM consumes a considerable amount of power of 30 μW. Schmitt trigger-based SRAM helps in reduction of leakage power. Hence, the power consumption was found to be lower than conventional 6T SRAM. The Schmitt-trigger-based SRAM consumed power of 15 μW. It reduced the average power consumption by 50%. The non-volatile Schmitt-trigger-based SRAM due to the presence of memristors consumed a power of 460 mW. Thus the non-volatile advantage was acquired at the cost of power. Hence, MTCMOS technique applied to the circuit reduced the power consumption of the non-volatile Schmitt-trigger-based SRAM to 13 μW. Hence the device is a very low power-consuming device.

The conventional 6T SRAM occupies the least area consisting of only six transistors. The number of transistors increases to ten in case of Schmitt-trigger-based SRAM. The presence of memristors further increases the chip area due to the presence of registers in the memristor circuit. The use of MTCMOS technique reduces the area consumed as the size of transistor decreases. In ST SRAM cell, the number

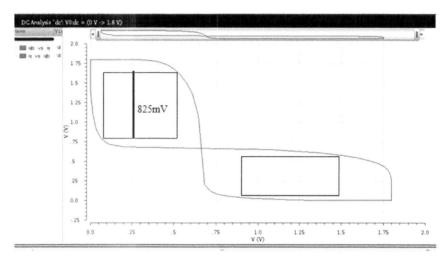

Fig. 4 SNM plot for MTCMOS memristor-based Schmitt trigger SRAM cell

of transistors is less but two pull down transistors are of large size, whereas in ST SRAM cell the size is reduced for pull down transistors.

The conventional 6T SRAM allowed a noise margin of around 520 mV. The implementation of the Schmitt-trigger-based SRAM cell increased the noise immunity of the circuit giving an SNM of 690 mV. Further, the memristor and MTCMOS-based memristor Schmitt trigger SRAM cell gave a higher static noise margin of 839 mV and 825 mV, respectively. The addition of memristor further increased the static noise margin of the circuit by over 58%. Hence, the designed circuit has improved noise margin compared to the conventional 6T SRAM cell.

A comparative tabulation of the above results is given in Table 1.

4 Conclusion

A non-volatile low-power Schmitt trigger SRAM was realized. The inclusion of memristor made the cell non-volatile, and the MTCMOS technology resulted in a low power memory cell inspite of the memristor component introduced. The Schmitt trigger realization further decreased the leakage power and improved the SNM. Memristor component is added to make the designed cell non-volatile and also improved the SNM value. The average power consumption in the design non-volatile multi-threshold Schmitt trigger SRAM cell reduced by 56.67%, and the SNM value improved by 58.65%.

The main limitations and drawbacks of the approach followed are increase in area due to addition of memristor components to make it non-volatile. This will require careful placement and routing of the designed cell to reduce the area and improve

Table 1 Comparison of area, power, and SNM parameters for the various designed cells

Device	Power (μW)	Area	SNM value (mV)
SRAM using 6T [1]	30	6T	520
Schmitt trigger SRAM using 10 T [2]	15	10T	690
Memristor-based ST SRAM	460	10 T + 2 memristor	839
MTCMOS memristor-based ST SRAM	13	10 T + 2 memristor (Low Vt transistors)	825

efficiency. The proposed MTCMOS memristor SRAM cell speed is a bit less. To improve the speed of the SRAM cell, a supply voltage scaling method can be used. By improving the speed of the cell, the speed of the memory can be improved. For future scope of work, different types of non-volatile components available can be compared with memristor and implemented. The array of memory can be built for a definite size using the proposed MTCMOS memristor-based Schmitt trigger SRAM cell. The array design helps in storing of data in large quantity.

References

1. Rohit P, Anjaneyulu G (July 2017) Analysis and performance comparison of different SRAM cells. Int J Adv Res Electron Commun Eng (IJARECE) 6(7)
2. Preeti Bellerimatha S, Banakar RM. Implementation of 16X16 SRAM memory array using 180 nm. Int J Curr Eng Technol. ISSN 2277-4106
3. Birla S, Shukla NK, Pattanaik M, Singh RK (Dec 2010) Device and circuit design challenges for low leakage SRAM for ultra low power application. Canadian J Electr Electron Eng 1(7)
4. Ahmad S, Gupta MK, Alam N, Hasan M (Aug 2016) Single-ended schmitt-trigger-based robust low-power SRAM cell. IEEE Trans Very Large Scale Integr (VLSI) Syst 24(8)
5. Saminathan V, Paramasivam K (Nov 2016) Design and analysis of low power hybrid memristor-CMOS based distinct binary logic non-volatile SRAM cell. Circuits Syst 7
6. Upadhyay P, Ghosh S, Mandal D, Ghoshal SP (May 2013) Low static and dynamic power MTC-MOS based 12T SRAM cell for high speed memory system. In: International joint conference on computer science and software engineering, vol 2, issue 5
7. Kumar NS, Sudhanva NG, Shreyas Hande V, Sajjan MV, Hemanth Kumar CS, Kariyappa BS (July 2017) SRAM design using memristor and self-controllable voltage (SVL) technique. In: International conference on computational intelligence & data engineering (ICCIDE 2017), 978-981-10-6318-3

8. Hemanth Kumar CS, Kariyappa BS (Dec 2017) Analysis of low power 7T SRAM cell employing improved SVL (ISVL) technique. In: International conference on electrical, electronics, communication, computer and optimization techniques (ICEECCOT-17), 978-1-5386-2361-9
9. Kariyappa BS, Madiwalar B (July 2013) A comparative study of 7T SRAM cells. Int J Comput Trends Technol (IJCTT) 4(7):2231–2803, page 2188
10. Madiwalar B, Kariyappa BS (2013) Single bit-line 7T SRAM cell for low power and high SNM. In: International multi conference on automation, computing, control, communication and compressed sensing (IMAC4S-13), pp 223–228, 978-1-4673-5089-1

Intelligent Phase-Locked Loops for Automotive Applications

Mukunda Byre Gowda, R. C. Biradar and Mohan Kumar Kotgire

Abstract To meet the time-critical and fail-safe requirements of automotive applications, there are several hardware and software components which are implemented on multiple electronic control units (ECU). With the recent trends in automotive technology, the vehicular functions are increasing, especially the advanced powertrain control demands more sophisticated intelligent hardware and software algorithms to be integrated into the electronic control units. The complex timing systems of advanced powertrain/e-powertrain requires maximum accuracy and precision with synchronization, especially while processing the complex sensors and actuators. In this paper, we will discuss about the implementation of innovative—intelligent phase-locked loops (IPLL) VHDL model for the advanced engine control applications. The IPLL module is designed to provide the high-resolution sensor output in normal operating mode and in addition, it shall retain the synchronization among the systems during the disturbance or loss of high-frequency sensor signal. This is achieved by generating the IPLL output through the self-learning hardware, even though when there is no valid sensor signal available. Hence the virtual synchronization with accurate positions of the engine is maintained.

Keywords Powertrain · VHDL · Automotive · ECU · Sensor · Phase-locked loop

M. B. Gowda (✉) · R. C. Biradar
REVA University, Bangalore, India
e-mail: mukunda.ec16@gmail.com

R. C. Biradar
e-mail: dir.ece@reva.edu.in

M. K. Kotgire
Hochschule Darmstadt, Darmstadt, Germany
e-mail: mohan.k.kotgire@stud.h-da.de

© Springer Nature Singapore Pte Ltd. 2019   885
V. Sridhar et al. (eds.), *Emerging Research in Electronics, Computer Science and Technology*, Lecture Notes in Electrical Engineering 545,
https://doi.org/10.1007/978-981-13-5802-9_77

1   Introduction

Timer IP's are the core of powertrain—engine control applications. Powertrain relies on the timing/angle information derived from the engine positioning system. The real-time sensor signals and actuator control are dynamic in nature. The sophisticated sensor data which derives continuous engine position depends on various drive conditions and the dynamics of the engine. Continuous engine position is derived from the phase-locked loop, which is a core of engine control, where all the complex functions starting from the fuel injections or ignition till the exhaust control is dependent on the said phase-locked loop output.

There are several literatures on implementation of digital phase-locked loops [1–7] and their realization using MATLAB Simulink models, FPGA models, etc. The phase-locked loops designed for automotive applications are considered as one of the powerful modules, which can generate a very high-resolution continuous engine position. However, these phase-locked loops generate continuous engine position as long as the complex sensor data is valid. As we know that the engine compartment is noisy and prone to interference, leading to loss of sensor data or interference in the signal. In such cases, the engine losses synchronization among the system and the fuel engine/ignition is shutoff, leading to deceleration in the vehicle speed also the engine stalling at lower speeds.

There are no any prior-arts or literatures exist to handle such scenarios, especially during the transition from normal operating mode to the secondary mode of operation. In this paper, the novel IPLL design provides the solution to the existing problems in the vehicle during loss of sensor signal and the transition phases (secondary-mode transition).

2   Overview of Automotive Systems

The vehicular technology can be classified into different domains as listed below.

(a) Powertrain electronics
(b) Chassis electronics
(c) Active safety
(d) Body electronics
(e) Driver assistance
(f) Passenger comfort
(g) Entertainment systems
(h) Electronic Integrated Cockpit systems, etc.

Powertrain electronics will be the focus area in our paper. The powertrain contains the subsystems like engine control, transmission control, and e-powertrain for hybrid and electric vehicles as shown in Fig. 1.

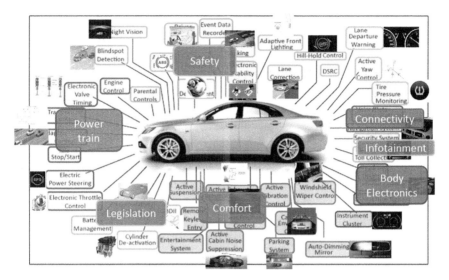

Fig. 1 Overview of automotive systems [8]

3   Powertrain Sensor-Signal Processing

The powertrain subsystems contain several complex sensor modules like (a) cylinder pressure sensor (b) manifold pressure and temperature sensors (c) crankshaft sensors (d) camshaft sensors (e) exhaust gas sensors (f) throttle position sensor (g) fuel pressure sensor, and (h) engine knock sensor which must be processed at accurate timelines

Figure 2 shows the electronic engine control unit with multiple sensors and actuators connected, where the fuel injection, throttle position control and complex engine position management, etc. needs to be controlled/processed at higher accuracy and resolution.

Figure 3 illustrates a schematic of an engine position sensor. For each cylinder, there exists at least one inlet and one outlet valves. These valves are operated with the help of camshaft lobes. The camshaft is mechanically coupled with the crankshaft through drive-chain mechanism. The engine has at least two position sensors, i.e., a crankshaft position sensor and a camshaft position sensor and associated flywheels with defined teeth patterns. The accuracy of the continuous engine position depends on the number of hard teeth on the trigger wheel and the accuracy of estimated frequency.

In case of sensor errors or failures, the system enters limp home mode/backup mode. In this paper, we will focus on the position sensor failures and its associated hardware IPLL mechanisms for handling such failures.

The high-frequency crank position sensor may fail or stop transmitting the digital signal indicating the position or speed of the engine. For example, hardware of

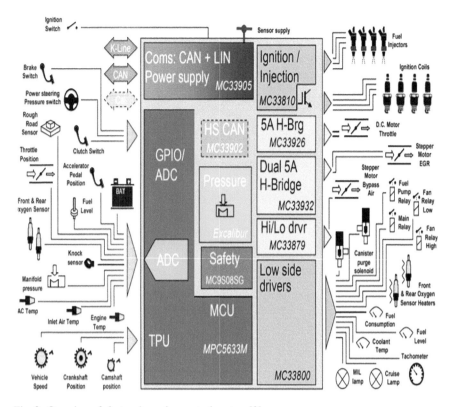

Fig. 2 Overview of electronic engine control system [9]

position sensor may fail, connections can short or open, etc. In addition, the position sensor failure may be caused due to physical wear or damage due to extreme heat at the engine compartment, or the damaged ASIC in the sensor. Alternatively, for example, the failure may be a result of a fluid or wear over long period. A secondary or backup sensor may be implemented for such failure instances. Implementing an additional position sensor will be expensive.

One or more camshafts of the engine rotate in relation to the crankshaft, and crankshaft gear drives a timing belt which drives a gear coupled to the camshaft. The camshaft position, therefore, is in relation to the crankshaft position. Also, a camshaft position sensor measures a position/speed of the camshaft. Therefore, the camshaft position sensor is used when there is a failure of crankshaft position sensor. Specifically, the camshaft position sensor can be used to predict the crankshaft position (limp home mode) and can control the fuel injection and spark delivery.

Possible problems during the entry of limp home mode are as listed below.

1. The major problem seen during the entry of limp home mode is that the system takes larger time to get synchronized with the engine.

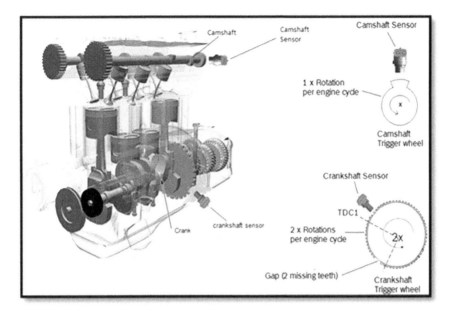

Fig. 3 Crankshaft and camshaft sensors [10]

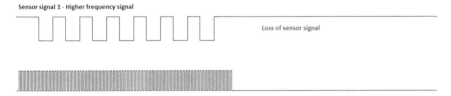

Fig. 4 Stopped PLL during loss of high-frequency crank signal

2. The engine position is not maintained until it successfully enters secondary crankshaft mode.
3. The injections/ignitions are missed till the synchronization with the position is achieved
4. A lot of resynchronization attempts are observed.
5. With lower engine speed the engine may stall, the transition to limp home mode takes longer time.

In the general, the continuous engine position or the output of phase-locked loop is stopped as soon as the no signal time-out occurs as shown in Fig. 4. The synchronization takes place once the obtained CAM sensor values match with the expected CAM values.

4 Implementation of Intelligent Phase-Locked Loops—IPLL

The legacy PLL module is designed to provide the high-resolution output when the proper sensor signal is applied to the module. In the new IPLL design methodology, whenever the proper high-frequency sensor-trigger signal is lost, or any disturbance is observed, the generation of microticks is not stopped, immediately the microtick generation is continued based on the calculated or the predicted values of sub-incremental frequency (past sensor data—stored sensor frequency) and low-frequency sensor signals. This process is active until the reception of first valid low-frequency sensor signal. After that, the valid low-frequency sensor signal is used for next increment frequency calculation. Hence, the virtual synchronization is maintained from the point of higher-frequency signal loss till the synchronization of lower-frequency signal is achieved.

This technique can be implemented by two approaches.

1. **Hardware approach**—In this method, the VHDL model for the IPLL is implemented along with the VHDL test bench (simulating sensor signals). In this methodology, let us say the high-frequency sensor signal 1 (crank) fails then the system enters temporary limp mode/urgency mode, the output of IPLL is not stopped instead it is continued by the IPLL hardware module. On the loss of signal, the time-out signal drives the IPLL to limp home or temporary urgency mode thus generating the continuous engine position based on the calculated values from the learnings of sensor signal frequencies, until the next sensor signal 2 edge is seen. After that, it considers the sensor signal 2 information (tooth time/frequency) for generating IPLL output—continuous engine position as shown in Fig. 5.

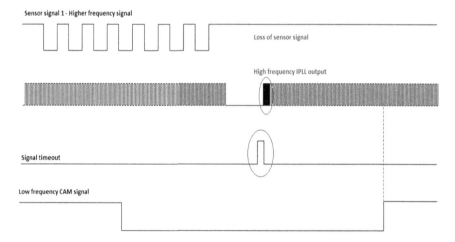

Fig. 5 Working of IPLL module—hardware approach

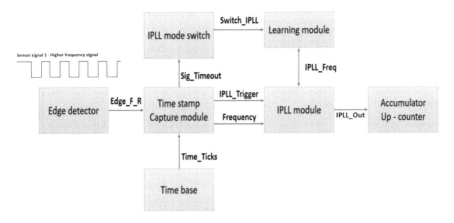

Fig. 6 Block diagram of IPLL module—hardware approach

In this paper, IPLL learning is implemented considering only the past sensor patterns of three cycles, trends in overall signal frequency, and the observations derived from the last five to eight valid signal frequencies.

The IPLL is simulated using the ModelSim—a multi-language HDL simulation environment by Mentor Graphics. The IPLL is modeled in VHDL at RTL level. Figure 6 shows the block diagram of IPLL and its associated modules.

2. **Software approach**—With the conventional PLL—During the loss of proper sensor signal 1, the virtual signal pattern can be simulated via PWM generator and fed through the timer input module of the complex timer. As soon as an edge transition is detected, the timer input module captures the time stamps of the signal and triggers frequency multiplier/phase-locked loop, an output of the frequency multiplier is the high-resolution engine position, which can be further be used to control accurate fuel injections/ignitions. However, our study is focused on the hardware approach.

3. **Special technical points to be considered**—The limp home mode has a speed limitation, say 2000/3000 RPM. If the vehicle loses the crank signal at higher RPM, then the IPLL must provide TEMP_LIMP_BIT to high as a notification to the system indicating the speed is above the threshold.

The application/hardware near software modules shall get an information that it is a temporary signal or position, till the proper diagnostics, and the synchronization is obtained.

Fine tuning of IPLL output takes place, after receiving at least one valid low-frequency sensor signal 2 from the point of sensor signal 1 failure/loss, delta mismatch during missing IPLL output in time-out correction + Fine-tuned correction will be completed upon the first valid low-frequency signal.

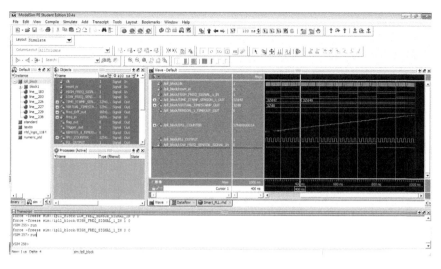

Fig. 7 IPLL simulation results—normal operating mode

Onboard diagnostics regulation conveys that switching to limp home mode should take place only after the proper diagnostic entries are registered. To handle this issue, we should maintain an interface signal informing that it is a temporary system synchronization by IPLL.

5 Simulation Results—IPLL VHDL Model

We were successfully able to simulate the intelligent behavior of our VHDL model—IPLL module during the normal operating mode and during the transition phase—proper operating mode to secondary operating mode (sensor signal 1 back up mode) at different real-time scenarios like loss of signal or disturbed sensor signal and vehicle dynamics. The VHDL—IPLL_test bench is used to simulate the above-said inputs. We observed the accurate IPLL outputs—continuous positions at the above cases with the learned frequencies as shown in Figs. 7 and 8.

6 Summary with Conclusion

With the intelligent phase-locked loop design, we were able to gauge the behavior and performance of the IPLL by subjecting it to various real-time scenarios like the loss of signal or interference in the position signal with engine dynamics. The learning mechanism of the IPLL leads to improved IPLL output—continuous engine position, especially during the transition phase from normal operating mode to limp

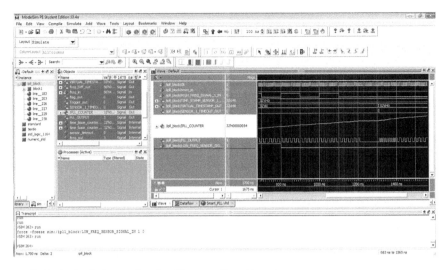

Fig. 8 IPLL simulation results—Intelligence—Transition phase

home mode. This IPLL design also reduces the engine stall by unnecessary resynchronization attempts, by driving the IPLL output during the signal loss. Further, this IPLL can be extended to support different automotive application domains.

References

1. Lindsey WC, Chie CM (April 1981) A survey of digital phase-locked loops. In: Proceedings of the IEEE, vol 69, no 4, pp 410–431
2. Levantino S (2013) Advanced digital phase-locked loops. In: Proceedings of the IEEE 2013 custom integrated circuits conference, San Jose, CA, pp 1–95
3. Singhal A, Madhu C, Kumar V (2014) Designs of all digital phase locked loop. In: 2014 recent advances in engineering and computational sciences (RAECS), Chandigarh, pp 1–5
4. Kumm M, Klingbeil H, Zipf P (2010) An FPGA-based linear all-digital phase-locked loop. IEEE Trans Circuits Syst I Regul Pap 57(9):2487–2497
5. Zhang Q, Huang K, Liu Z, Li Z (2009) Research and application of all digital phase-locked loop. In: 2009 second international conference on intelligent networks and intelligent systems, Tianjin, pp 122–125
6. Wang X, Choi YB, Je M, Yeoh WG (2007) A simulink model for all-digital-phase-locked-loop. In: 2007 IEEE international workshop on radio-frequency integration technology, Rasa Sentosa Resort, pp 70–73
7. BOSCH (2012) Application note AN011 DPLL micro tick generation, BOSCH semicondictors and sensor, GTM-IP application note
8. Karthikeyan R, Mithun BR (2014) Virtual hardware setup for automotive software testing. DVCON India

9. Freescale Semiconductor (2009) Small engine reference design user manual. NXP, User's Guide KT33812ECUUG

10. Gowda MB, Ramachandran K (2017) Co-simulative verification of a complex automotive IP(GTM) at pre-silicon phase. In: 2017 design and verification conference and exhibition, Bengaluru

Design and Implementation of Logarithmic Multiplier Using FinFETs for Low Power Applications

Vaishnavi Kumbargeri, Anusha Mahale and H. V. Ravish Aradhya

Abstract In all processing systems, multiplication is one of the computation-intensive operations demanding more resources. Hence, multiplication operations demand more time, power and resources. One of the better solutions is Mitchell's algorithm. Mitchell-based logarithmic multiplier is used as alternative approach which improves the speed, at the cost of accuracy. This paper presents the logarithmic multiplier implementation using the FinFETs. The hardware level simulation is done in Cadence Virtuoso using 18 nm technology. Comparison of power consumption of logarithmic multiplier using MOSFETs and FinFETs is presented. A 93.69% power reduction is seen in the proposed design as compared with the previous work.

Keywords Logarithmic multiplier · FinFET · Mitchell algorithm

1 Introduction

One of the power, time and area hungry arithmetic operations, especially for large bit-length operands is multiplication. When a huge number of operations are involved, for example, in Digital Signal Processing (DSP) applications, this bottleneck is even more highlighted [1]. The conventional multipliers consume more power and large area. Instead of binary number system multipliers, we can use logarithmic number system multipliers [8]. Logarithms have been used in mathematics for simplification of multiplication and division operations. But a trade-off between the computational speed and low accuracy is inevitable. Hence, the usage of such multipliers is limited

V. Kumbargeri (✉) · A. Mahale · H. V. Ravish Aradhya
Department of ECE, R.V. College of Engineering, Bangalore, Karnataka, India
e-mail: vaishnavik.lvs17@rvce.edu.in

A. Mahale
e-mail: anushapramodmh.lvs17@rvce.edu.in

H. V. Ravish Aradhya
e-mail: ravisharadhya@rvce.edu.in

© Springer Nature Singapore Pte Ltd. 2019
V. Sridhar et al. (eds.), *Emerging Research in Electronics, Computer Science and Technology*, Lecture Notes in Electrical Engineering 545,
https://doi.org/10.1007/978-981-13-5802-9_78

to signal processing applications (DSP) where very high accuracy is trivial. Also, it is ensured that limit on the error accepted is higher.

Logarithmic Number System (LNS) multipliers are of two types: Mitchell algorithm (MA) based and Look-up table (LUT) based. Due to less hardware complexity MA based, LNS multipliers are used predominantly. The building blocks of such multipliers are encoders, shifters, adders and decoders [10].

This paper is structured as follows: Sect. 2 discusses the literature study on Mitchell algorithm, logarithmic multiplier concept and the advanced devices. Section 3 is concerned with the design and implementation of logarithmic multiplier using FinFETs. Section 4 contains simulation results for the designed MA-based logarithmic multiplier. Finally, paper is concluded in Sect. 5.

2 Background

This section briefs about the motivation for the research along with a literature survey. The Mitchell algorithm is summarized. Also, FinFET device level equations and conceptual diagrams are depicted.

2.1 Motivation

Speed of operation of a multiplier is the principal criterion for its implementation. But for higher order multipliers, along with the speed, power consumption is a major factor. Conventional multipliers such as Array multipliers and Booth's multipliers use adders and shifters extensively. On the other hand, logarithmic multipliers use the combination of adders, shifters and encoders such that the overall power consumption is reduced.

In many systems, this balance is required for achieving the system productivity. Furthermore, FinFETs can be proposed to unanimously decrease the power consumption.

2.2 Mitchell Algorithm and Logarithmic Multiplier

In MA-based LNS multiplier, logarithmic values of two numbers are computed, summed up and then, the antilogarithm of this sum is calculated, i.e., the product of two numbers.

$$log_2(N_1 \cdot N_2) \approx k_1 + k_2 + x_1 + x_2. \tag{1}$$

The approximated log value of the product of two numbers is given by (1), where k_1 and k_2 are denoted as the characteristic number representing the position of most significant bit with value '1'.

$$P_{MA} = (N_1 \cdot N_2)_{MA} = \begin{cases} 2^{k_1+k_2}(1 + x_1 + x_2) \\ 2^{k_1+k_2+1}(x_1 + x_2) \end{cases}. \tag{2}$$

The end product approximation of the inputs depends on the carry bit of sum of mantissa with '1' [1]. The error percentage of the log multiplier can be further reduced by iterative process and pipe lining concept.

2.3 FinFETs

Nowadays, computer chips are packed with more number of transistors than approximated by the Moore's law. Also, the different short channel effects associated with such transistors are dominant in drain current equations of MOSFETs, for channel length reduction. Alternatively, FinFETs can be bright adaptations instead of the conventional MOSFET technology [2]. This ensures uninterrupted pace of device scaling, without any hindrance by issues such as parasitic resistances, gate oxide capacitances etc. An informative review of FinFETs can be found at [5] (Fig. 1).

FinFETs provide improved short channel and sub-threshold behavior. This results in improved Drain Induced Barrier Lowering (DIBL) [3], effectively improving the leakage currents. Low operating voltages due to scaling in channel length reduces the dynamic power consumption. The detailed current model and along with the solutions of the Poisson's equation can be referred from [4].

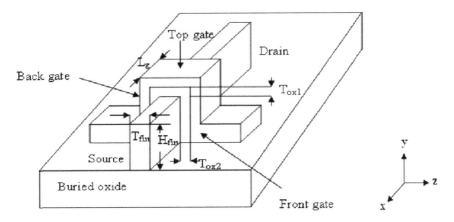

Fig. 1 Schematic diagram of FinFET

3   Design and Implementation

The algorithm for the MA-based log multiplier is described in this section. This section also presents the block diagram for log multiplier and its implementation using encoders, barrel shifter [9] and adders. Mitchell's algorithm can be elucidated as in algorithm 1.

The block diagram for MA-based log multiplier is shown in Fig. 2. At first, the number N1 is fed to Leading One Detector (LOD) circuit and leading one position k_1 is detected. The output k_1 is XORed [6] with input N_1 to get $N_1 - 2k_1$ and it is then left shifted. Similarly for number N_2, both k_2 and $N_2 - 2k_2$ are found. Both the left-shifted numbers are added. Further, the encoded values k_1 and k_2 are added using 3-bit adder and then decoded using 4×16 decoder. Here, the output carry bit is given as MSB input to the decoder. Finally, the decoder output and the sum of shifted values are added which produces the final approximated product of two numbers.

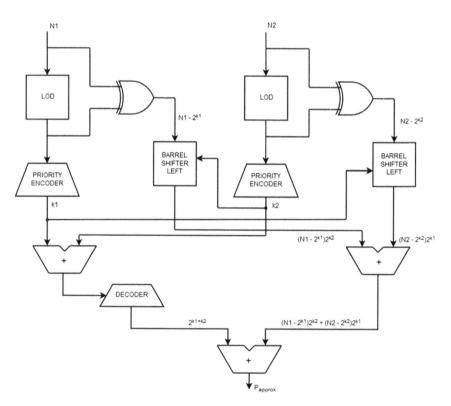

Fig. 2 Block diagram of logarithmic multiplier

Algorithm 1 Mitchell's algorithm

1: **procedure** $MA(N_1, N_2)$ ▷ The product of N_1 and N_2
2:     $k_1 \leftarrow$ first '1' position of N_1
3:     $k_2 \leftarrow$ first '1' position of N_2
4:     $x_1 \leftarrow N_1 \ll N_1 - 2^{k_1}$ ▷ Left shift using barrel shifter
5:     $x_2 \leftarrow N_2 \ll N_2 - 2^{k_2}$
6:     $k_{12} = k_1 + k_2$
7:     $x_{12} = x_1 + x_2$
8:     **if** $x_{12} \geq 2^N$ **then**
9:        $k_{12} = k_1 + k_2$
10:       Decode k_{12} and append x_{12} in the position of P_{apporx}
11:     **else**
12:       Decode k_{12} and enter 1 in the same position of P_{apporx}
13:       Append x_{12} immediately next to 1 in P_{apporx}
14:     $P_{MA} \leftarrow N_1 \cdot N_2$
15:     **return** P_{MA} ▷ The product is P_{MA}

4 Results and Discussion

Figure 3 provides the simulation results of MA-based log multiplier. Here, the multiplier is designed for 8-bit inputs and 16-bit output. Verilog HDL is used for functional verification of the design. The simulation is carried out using Xilinx 14.2 ISIM simulator.

(a)

(b)

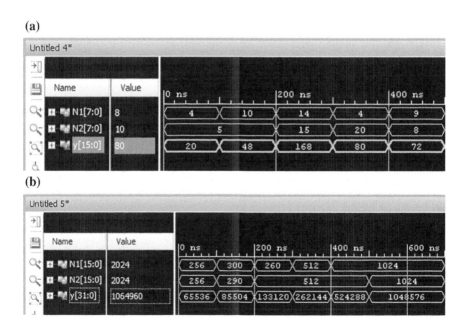

Fig. 3 Functional verification of **a** 8-bit, **b** 16-bit logarithmic multiplier

From the results, it can be observed that the numbers nearer or equal to the power of 2 tend to produce less error as compared to the other numbers. For example, in Fig. 3a, the numbers 4 and 5 produce 20 as output, which is accurate, where as 10 and 5 produce output as 48, which should have been 50. The error percentage is 4%. But for the numbers 14 and 15, product obtained is 168, as opposed to the real product 210. Thus, the error percentage is 20%.

Also in Fig. 3b, simulation of log multiplier with 32-bit output is shown. The higher bit numbers of the power of 2 are given as input and similar behavior is seen. The numbers deviating from powers of 2, such as 300 and 290 produce error percentage of 1.72%.

This behavior is seen because the Mitchell algorithm applies piecewise linear approximation to the logarithmic curves. Improvising the accuracy of the Mitchell algorithm can be done using various methods as proposed in [7].

The overall schematic implemented in Cadence is shown in Fig. 4. Since the multiplier is designed for 16-bit output, a 16-bit adder is utilized at the output. Along with that 8-bit barrel shifters (for left shifting), 8:3 priority encoders, 4:16 decoder and 8-bit LOD and XOR gates are used. 3-bit and 8-bit adders are used for lower bit addition.

For realizing the circuit using FinFETs and power analysis, the circuit is implemented using FinFET technology library in Cadence. 18 nm devices with low V_t, i.e., lvt models are used for this purpose. The lvt models provide higher switching time accuracy as compared to hvt models, which are power critical. Even then, the power consumption is 35.09 μW, which is lower compared to [10], noting that the multiplier is designed for 16-bit output in both the cases. The results are tabulated in Table 1. The logic implemented in the paper is conventional CMOS logic, which may be replaced by other logic families.

Thus, the available headroom for power consumption can be utilized to improve the accuracy of the design.

5   Conclusion

The advent of FinFETs has a huge impact on the low power design approaches. Even without applying fine adjustments in the design methodology, reduction in power consumption is considerable. At the same time, better performance in terms of speed is observed. As compared with the SCRL logic in [10], 93.69% of power dissipation is reduced in the proposed design.

Improvements can be done at architectural and logic level of abstraction, as the future work. At architectural level, better adder circuits such as Carry save adder, Kogge Stone adders can be implemented. Also, barrel shifters with better perfor-

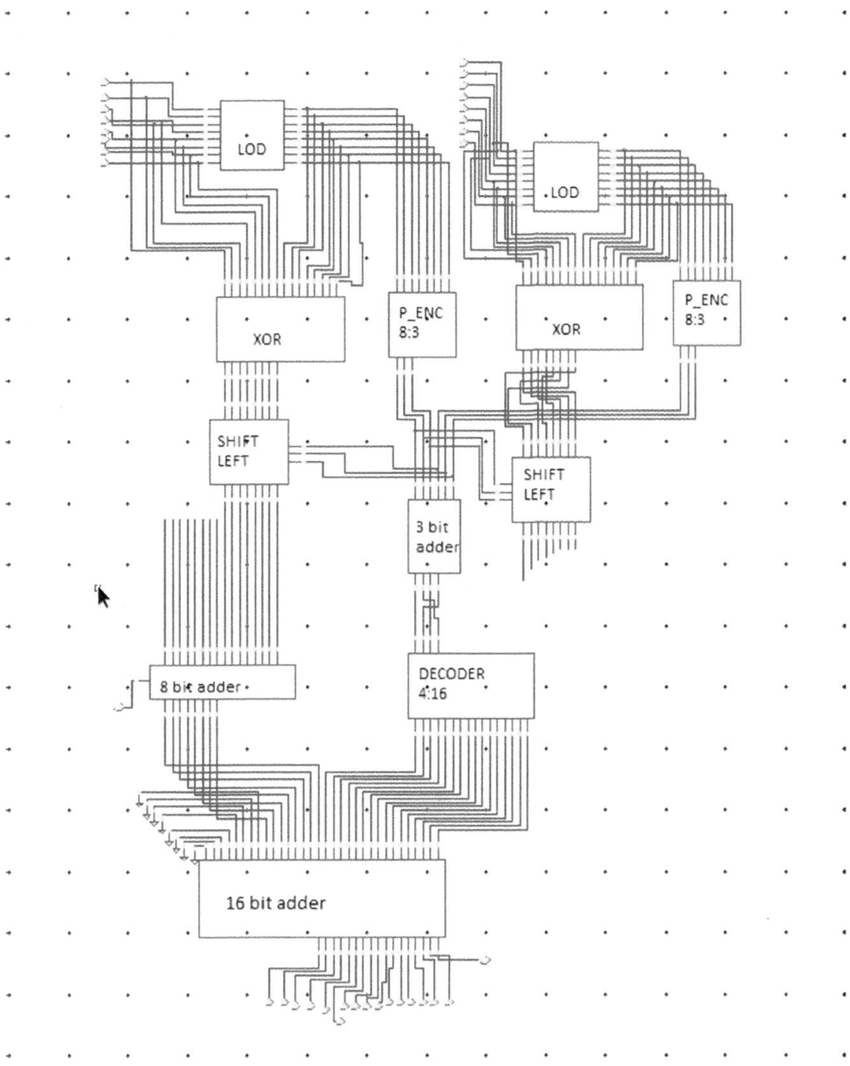

Fig. 4 Final schematic of logarithmic multiplier implemented using FinFETs

Table 1 Power consumption comparison for 16-bit output. Energy Charge Recovery Logic (ECRL) and Switch Rail Charge Recovery Logic (SCRL) are favored adiabatic logic systems for low power designs

Design	Power consumed (mW)
CMOS logic [10]	2.979
ECRL logic [10]	1.984
SCRL logic [10]	0.555
Proposed design	0.035

mance [11] can be adopted. Low-power logic families may be applied to obtain ultra-low power multipliers. Error correction logic [7] may be realized for increasing the reliability of the design.

References

1. Babić Z, Avramović A, Bulić P (Feb 2011) An iterative logarithmic multiplier. Microprocess Microsyst 35(1):23–33. https://doi.org/10.1016/j.micpro.2010.07.001
2. Fahad HM, Hu C, Hussain MM (Jan 2015) Simulation study of a 3-d device integrating FinFET and UTBFET. IEEE Trans Electron Devices 62(1):83–87. https://doi.org/10.1109/ted.2014.2372695
3. Guo D, Shang H, Seo K, Haran B (Oct 2014) 10 nm FINFET technology for low power and high performance applications. In: 2014 12th IEEE international conference on solid-state and integrated circuit technology (ICSICT). IEEE. https://doi.org/10.1109/icsict.2014.7021207
4. Havaldar D, Katti G, DasGupta N, DasGupta A (April 2006) Subthreshold current model of FinFETs based on analytical solution of 3-d poisson's equation. IEEE Trans Electron Devices 53(4):737–742. https://doi.org/10.1109/ted.2006.870874
5. Jurczak M, Collaert N, Veloso A, Hoffmann T, Biesemans S (Oct 2009) Review of FINFET technology. In: 2009 IEEE international SOI conference. IEEE. https://doi.org/10.1109/soi.2009.5318794
6. Khandekar PD, Subbaraman S (2008) Low power 2:1 MUX for barrel shifter. In: 2008 first international conference on emerging trends in engineering and technology. IEEE. https://doi.org/10.1109/icetet.2008.47
7. Mahalingam V, Ranganathan N (Dec 2006) Improving accuracy in Mitchell's logarithmic multiplication using operand decomposition. IEEE Trans Comput 55(12):1523–1535. https://doi.org/10.1109/tc.2006.198
8. Mitchell JN (Aug 1962) Computer multiplication and division using binary logarithms. IEEE Trans Electron Comput EC-11(4):512–517. https://doi.org/10.1109/tec.1962.5219391
9. Rajalakshmi R, Priya PA (May 2014) Design and analysis of a 4-bit low power universal barrel-shifter in 16 nm FinFET technology. In: 2014 IEEE international conference on advanced communications, control and computing technologies. IEEE. https://doi.org/10.1109/icaccct.2014.7019141
10. Ranjitha HV, Pooja KS, Ravish Aradhya HV (May 2017) Design and implementation of low power mitchell algorithm based logarithmic multiplier. In: 2017 2nd IEEE international conference on recent trends in electronics, information & communication technology (RTEICT). IEEE. https://doi.org/10.1109/rteict.2017.8256828
11. Ravish Aradhya HV, J L, KN M (Feb 2012) Design optimization of reversible logic universal barrel shifter for low power applications. Int J Comput Appl 40(15):26–34. https://doi.org/10.5120/5057-7379

Design of Ternary SRAM Cell Based on Level Shift Ternary Inverter

N. Shylashree, Amruta Hosur and N. Praveena

Abstract In terms of memory, multivalued logic can be the fitting logic for the existing binary logic. Ternary logic contains three symbols in place of two symbols used in the binary logic, i.e., 0, 1, 2. More information can be stored with the help of these three symbols. SRAM cell is widely used in the digital circuit. The SRAM cell designed using the ternary logic can be used in the design of large memory arrays designed using ternary logic. The traditional ternary inverter which is used in the design of the traditional ternary SRAM cell is unable to store the proper values for the second state, there is a voltage level drop, which in turn affects the data read/write value of the SRAM cell designed using this traditional ternary inverter. Hence there is a need to design the ternary inverter cell which can give the proper output voltage level of all three states of the ternary logic. The level shift ternary inverter is designed to fulfill this disadvantage. The ternary inverter is designed in order to achieve the ideal DC characteristics, and the same level shift ternary inverter is used in the design of level shift ternary SRAM. This ternary SRAM stores the data properly at read/write signal. The traditional ternary inverter and traditional ternary SRAM, level shift ternary inverter and level shift ternary SRAM are implemented in Cadence 45 nm technology. The traditional ternary inverter consumes 2.37 µW power, and the level shift ternary SRAM consumes 2.43 µW power. The traditional ternary SRAM consumes 3.012 µW and level shift ternary SRAM consumes 3.14 µW. At the cost of a little bit increased power and the number of transistors, the traditional ternary SRAM can be replaced with level shift ternary SRAM. This level shift ternary SRAM stores all the voltage levels at all three levels. The same level shift ternary SRAM cell can be used for the design of large memory arrays.

Keywords Ternary memory · Ternary inverter · Ternary SRAM

N. Shylashree · N. Praveena
Department of ECE, Rashtreeya Vidyalaya College of Engineering, Bangalore 560059, India

A. Hosur (✉)
VLSI Design and Embedded Systems, Rashtreeya Vidyalaya College of Engineering,
Bangalore 560059, India
e-mail: amruta.hosur1@gmail.com

© Springer Nature Singapore Pte Ltd. 2019   903
V. Sridhar et al. (eds.), *Emerging Research in Electronics, Computer Science and Technology*, Lecture Notes in Electrical Engineering 545,
https://doi.org/10.1007/978-981-13-5802-9_79

1 Introduction

The digital logic system usually uses the radix two, and hence it has two symbols to represent the logic levels. If the digital system has the radix greater than two, then it is called as a multivalued logic system [1]. If the radix used is three, then it is called as ternary system. In ternary logic system there are three logic states or symbols, i.e. 0, 1, and 2. In ternary system log3 (2n) bits are required for the representation of binary number with n-bits.

The truth table of ternary inverter is as shown in Table 1.

Multivalued logic helps in dealing with the serious pin out problems in complex VLSI circuits [2]. This kind of logic is more helpful in the design of memories [3, 4]. Ternary memories are also implemented using CNFET [5].

The SRAM cell contains the back-to-back connected inverters which act as a latch and helps in storing the information. Along with this latch, SRAM cell also has bit lines and select lines. If the select line is active, then the bit line will have access to the SRAM cell to read or write the data [6]. In the binary SRAM cell, by replacing the inverters with the ternary inverters, ternary SRAM cell can be designed.

In [6] authors explain about the problem with the traditional ternary inverter and its effects when such inverter is used in the design of the ternary SRAM cell. When traditional ternary inverter is used in the design of SRAM, the voltage at the second level will not restore properly. The authors also gave the solution to the problem by designing the level shift ZV ternary inverter. When the level shift ternary inverter is used in the design of ternary SRAM, the voltage values at the data read and write values at the ternary SRAM will restore with proper values. In [6], authors use the standard ternary inverter (STI). In [7], the authors concentrate on the design of ternary SRAM array. The authors designed the ternary SRAM in three variations like negative ternary inverter (NTI), positive ternary inverter (PTI), and standard ternary inverter (STI).

In this work, the voltage level at the second state of the ternary inverter is retained at the proper voltage levels by designing level shift circuit.

2 Traditional Ternary Inverter

The traditional ternary inverter is designed using the CMOS inverter. In the CMOS inverter the voltage of the second state is achieved by using the voltage divider circuit having the resistor network. This circuit is implemented in 45 nm technology. The circuit is shown in Fig. 1.

Table 1 Truth table of ternary inverter

Input state	Output state
0	2
1	1
2	0

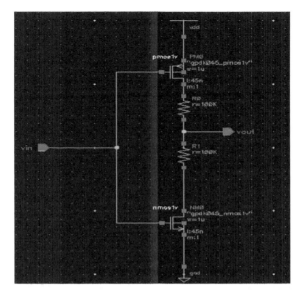

Fig. 1 Traditional ternary inverter

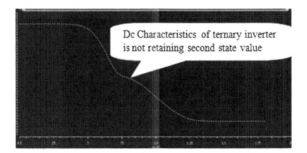

Fig. 2 Traditional ternary inverter DC characteristics

The DC characteristic of traditional ternary inverter is as shown in Fig. 2.

3 Traditional Ternary SRAM

The SRAM circuit using the traditional ternary inverter can be implemented as shown in Fig. 3.

In the design of traditional ternary inverter and the SRAM circuit designed using the same, the MOS transistor values are chosen such that they should be in saturation region. All the circuits in this work are implemented in Cadence Virtuoso 45 nm technology.

The SRAM circuit designed using the traditional ternary inverter does not restore the values properly at read/write signals. The results of the transient analysis of

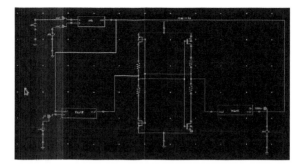

Fig. 3 Ternary SRAM

traditional ternary inverter and the SRAM circuit designed using the same ternary inverter are shown the Figs. 12 and 14, respectively.

The disadvantage of this SRAM cell is the voltage levels after voltage division at ternary inverters is not constant; this is because the ternary inverter is having the MOS transistors which are operating in saturation region. In saturation region MOS transistors behave as current sources. But for the proper voltage division MOS transistors should work as linear resistors. For the proper voltage division Vout of the inverter should be exactly half of the supply voltage (Vdd), when both NMOS and PMOS in the inverter are in saturation region. This is possible when current at PMOS (Ipmos) and current at the NMOS (Inmos) are exactly equal. The current at the MOS transistors depends on the voltage values at the gate and source of respective MOS transistors. If we design the inverter with the proper values of W/L of NMOS as well as PMOS to overcome the mobility issues of the PMOS and NMOS and to get the exactly equal NMOS and PMOS current, this current will be equal only for certain voltages and will vary for some different voltages. This difference in the voltages will produce the voltage drop at the rds of other transistor.

Because of this reason, when such ternary inverter is used in the design of SRAM, a slight decrease in voltage at the time of switching will cause an increase in voltage values of the inverter slightly. This voltage is given as an input to the other inverter, which will produce the decreased voltage value at the output. Because of this reason, the SRAM cell designed using traditional ternary inverter fails to hold the stored data.

4 Level Shift Ternary Inverter

The traditional ternary inverter can be modified to achieve the proper output voltage values. This can be done by designing the ternary inverter to yield the ideal DC characteristics. The ideal DC characteristics of the ternary inverter are as shown in Fig. 4.

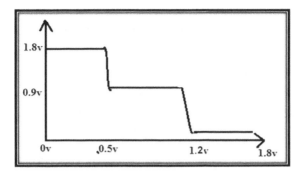

Fig. 4 Ideal DC characteristics of ternary inverter [6]

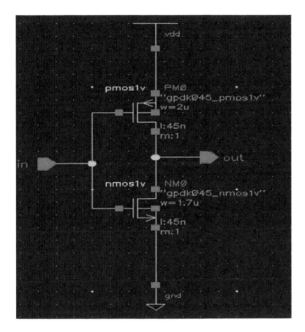

Fig. 5 CMOS Inverter with higher transition voltage

The ideal DC characteristics can be achieved simply by averaging the DC characteristics of CMOS inverter with higher transition voltage and DC characteristics of CMOS inverter with lower transition voltage.

Figures 5 and 6 show the CMOS inverter with higher and lower transition voltages, respectively. The DC characteristics of these inverters are shown in Figs. 7 and 8, respectively.

By averaging the DC characteristics shown in Figs. 7 and 8, the DC characteristics of ideal ternary inverter as shown in Fig. 4 can be achieved. These DC characteristics can be averaged using the averaging circuit shown in Fig. 9. This averaging circuit has the resistor network.

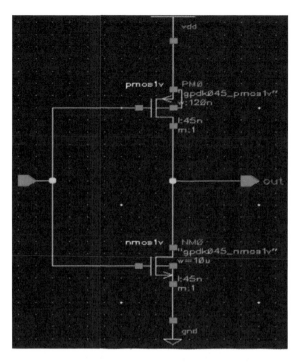

Fig. 6 CMOS Inverter with lower transition voltage

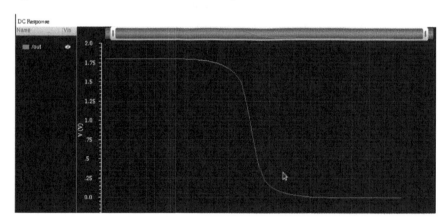

Fig. 7 DC characteristics of CMOS inverter with higher transition voltage

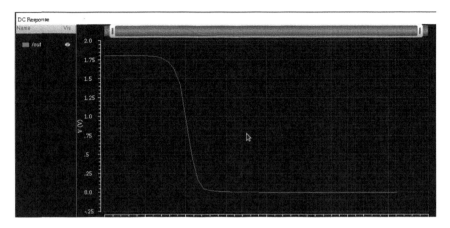

Fig. 8 DC characteristics of CMOS inverter with lower transition voltage

Fig. 9 Averaging circuit

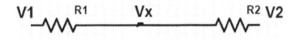

The nodal analysis of this averaging circuit results in the Eq. (2), which shows that Vx is the average of V1 and V2.

$$\frac{V_x - V_1}{R} = \frac{V_x - V_2}{R} \tag{1}$$

$$Vx = \frac{V_1 + V_2}{R} \tag{2}$$

The level shift ternary inverter to get the ideal characteristics of the ternary inverter is obtained by using the inverters in Figs. 5 and 6 and the averaging circuit in Fig. 9.

Figure 10 shows the level shift ternary inverter. P-level shifter and n-level shifter blocks in the circuit contains CMOS inverter with the higher and the lower transition voltages.

5　Level Shift Ternary SRAM

The level shift ternary SRAM cell can be implemented by using the level shift ternary inverter, along with the transmission gate having bit and bit-bar signals of the SRAM and the AND gate giving the data read/write signal by logical ANDing the row select and the column select signals. The level shift SRAM circuit is as shown in Fig. 11.

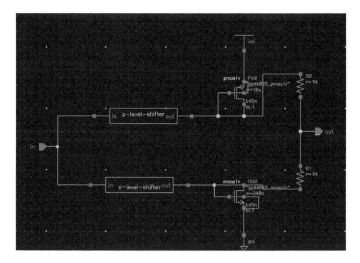

Fig. 10 Level shift ternary inverter

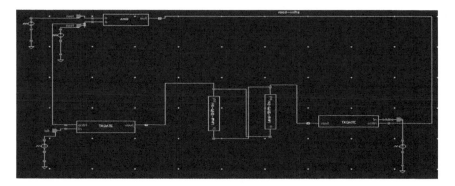

Fig. 11 Level shift ternary SRAM

The level shift ternary SRAM circuit is having two back-to-back connected level shift ternary inverters, which forms the latch to store 1 bit of memory.

6 Results and Discussion

In this section, the results of the above implementations are listed. The results contain the transient behavior of traditional ternary inverter, traditional ternary SRAM, level shift ternary inverter, level shift ternary SRAM circuits, and the comparison of power and area in terms of number of transistors.

Figure 12 shows the result of traditional ternary inverter. Here X-axis shows the time and Y-axis shows the voltage level of input and output signals. Here the output

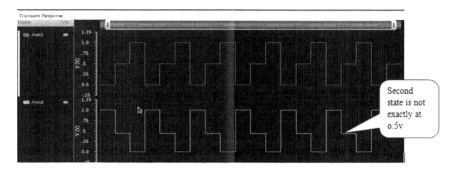

Fig. 12 Result of traditional ternary inverter

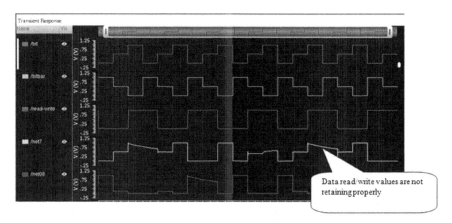

Fig. 13 Result of traditional ternary SRAM

voltage for input value 0.5 is not exactly 0.5, it is below that value and hence needs level shifter.

Figure 13 shows the result of traditional ternary SRAM. The X-axis shows the time and Y-axis shows the voltage values at the various signals. Signals 1 and 2 are the bit and bit-bar signals, respectively. Signal 3 shows the read/write. When it is 1 it implies write signal, and when zero it represents read signal. Here the read/write values of the SRAM are not retaining properly.

Figure 14 shows the result of transient analysis of level shift ternary inverter. The voltage level of the output for input value of 0.5 V is shifted up by nearly up to 0.5 V at the output. The X-axis of Fig. 14 shows time and the Y-axis shows the voltage levels of the signals.

Figure 15 shows the result of the level shift ternary SRAM, where the data at the SRAM is retained properly for all the three levels. Signals 1 and 2 are the bit and bit-bar and signal 3 shows the read/write signal. Signal 4 shows the read data from the SRAM.

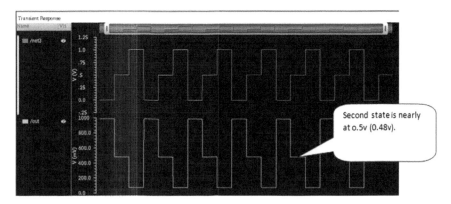

Fig. 14 Result of level shift ternary inverter

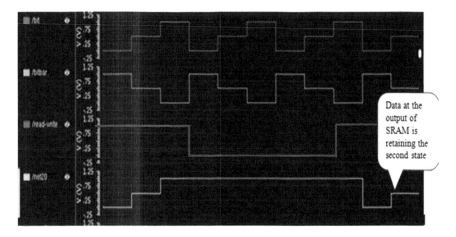

Fig. 15 Result of level shift ternary SRAM

a. **Comparison Between Traditional Ternary Inverter and Level Shift Ternary Inverter**

Traditional ternary inverter and level shift ternary inverter are compared for power, delay, area in terms of the number of transistors and the level of middle state among the three states of the ternary inverter. The comparison is given in Table 2.

Table 2 shows that the power consumed by the traditional ternary inverter and level shift ternary inverter almost remain the same, and at the cost of area, the second state voltage level can be maintained to nearly ideal (0, 0.5, 1).

b. **Comparison Between Traditional Ternary SRAM and Level Shift Ternary SRAM**

Table 2 Comparison of traditional ternary inverter and level shift ternary inverter

	Traditional inverter (45 nm)	Level shift ternary inverter (45 nm)
Power (μW)	2.37	2.43
Area (# of transistors)	2	4
Voltage levels (in V)	(0, 0.44, 1)	(0, 0.48, 1)
Delay (ps)	45.85	68.56

Table 3 Comparison of traditional ternary SRAM and level shift ternary SRAM

	Traditional ternary SRAM (45 nm)	Traditional ternary SRAM (180 nm)	Level shift ternary SRAM (45 nm)
Power (μW)	3.012	16.8	3.14
Area (# of transistors)	14 (4T: transmission gate, 6T: AND gate, 4T: traditional ternary inverter)	14 (4T: transmission gate, 6T: AND gate, 4T: traditional ternary inverter)	18 (4T: transmission gate, 6T: AND gate, 8T: level shifted ternary inverter)
Delay (ns)	4.079	195.13	11.047

The traditional ternary SRAM and level shift ternary SRAM are compared for the power and area in terms of the number of transistors. This comparison is shown in Table 3.

Table 3 shows that the power consumed by the traditional ternary SRAM and level shift ternary SRAM remains almost the same, at the cost of area, delay, the data at the SRAM can be retained as shown in Fig. 15. The number of transistors, power, delay values for the traditional ternary SRAM in 18 nm is also listed in Table 3.

This section contains the implementation results of the design of ternary SRAM Cell using traditional ternary inverter and level shift ternary inverter. All these circuits are implemented in Cadence Virtuoso with 45 nm technology.

Compared to level shift ternary inverter in [6], the number of transistors required for level shifting operation is less by 6 transistors, by using the CMOS inverter with higher transition voltage and lower transition voltage for level shifting.

7   Conclusion

Multivalued logic is more helpful in the design of memories, because it offers reduced complexity of interconnections. Ternary SRAM cell with the standard ternary inverter (STI) is most commonly used variation of ternary memory cell. Because of the problem in achieving proper output level at the ternary inverter, sometimes data may not be retained properly at the ternary SRAM cell. To overcome this problem, the level shift ternary SRAM is considered.

The level shifting can be achieved by simply varying the transition voltage of the two CMOS inverters and averaging the results of those inverters. By doing so, the value at the SRAM is retained. With the proper retained values at the SRAM cell, the complete array of the SRAM can be implemented. At the cost of number of transistors, with almost same power, traditional ternary inverters can be replaced with level shift ternary inverter in the ternary SRAM to form level shift ternary SRAM.

Even though the power and area increase in the individual SRAM cell, when the entire chip having the ternary SRAM array is considered, the pin count will be decreased and more information can be stored as well as communicated with the use of ternary memories.

a. **Future Scope**

The low power techniques can be incorporated in the design to restore all three states of the ternary SRAM cell without consuming more power. The level shift ternary SRAM cell can be used in the design of large ternary memory arrays. The same design can be implemented using CNFET, FINFET, etc.

References

1. Srinivasa Raghavan B, Kanchana Bhaaskaran VS. Design of novel multiple valued logic (MVL) circuits. In: 2017 International conference on nextgen electronic technologies: silicon to software (ICNETS2), Chennai, India, pp 371–378
2. Vasundara Patel KS, Gurumurthy KS (2009) Quaternary CMOS combinational logic circuits. In: 2009 international conference on information and multimedia technology, Jeju Island, pp 538–542
3. Shanmugavadivu P, Sugunadevi S, Sukanya B (2016) Study of static noise margin of SRAM based on supply voltage and topologies. IJAR. ISSN Print 2394-7500, ISSN Online 2394-5869
4. Srinivasan P, Bhat AS, Murotiya SL, Gupta A (2015) Design and performance evaluation of a low transistor ternary CNTFET SRAM cell. In: 2015 international conference on electronic design, computer networks & automated verification (EDCAV), Shillong, pp 38–43
5. Moaiyeri MH, Mirzaee RF, Doostaregan A, Navi K, Hashemipour O (2013) A universal method for designing low-power carbon nanotube FET-based multiple valued logic circuits. IET Comput Digital Tech 7(4):167–181
6. Jahangir MZ, Narasimha KV. Design of a new ternary SRAM cell (ZV-SRAM) based on innovative level shift based ternary inverter (ZV-Inverter). In: Annual India conference (INDICON). IEEE, New Delhi, India, 17–20 Dec 2015
7. Jayashree HV, Sai Shruthi VP. Ternary SRAM for low power applications. In: International conference on communication, information & computing technology (ICCICT), Mumbai, India, Oct 2012

Machine-Vision-Assisted Performance Monitoring in Turning Inconel 718 Material Using Image Processing

Y. D. Chethan, H. V. Ravindra and Y. T. Krishne Gowda

Abstract Machining performance monitoring is the utilization of different sensors to determine the condition of processes. Machine vision system has been used to monitor the state of both cutting tool and workpiece during turning process. The turning experiments on Inconel 718 material have been performed in a precision lathe using coated carbide cutting tool in dry conditions. Cutting tool and machined surface images were acquired using machine vision. Image features of machined surface and cutting tool were extracted by processing the images. Image features such as wear area and perimeter have been considered to characterize tool wear state; consequently, machined surface state was characterized by means of image histogram frequency. Further, trends have been plotted with image features extracted from both tool and machined surfaces. Results indicate that monitoring of turning performance could be effectively accomplished by plotted trends.

Keywords Machine vision · Image processing · Image histogram · Cutting tool wear

1 Introduction

Metal cutting operations like milling, drilling, and turning play a significant role in today's industrial production process. Lots of efforts have been made to automate condition monitoring system of machine tools; since it reduces idle time, production costs, and lower the scrap rate. A primary benefit of machine vision system is to facilitate condition monitoring of process. Machine vision-based monitoring involves the monitoring of certain machine elements related to machine tool while machining

Y. D. Chethan (✉) · Y. T. Krishne Gowda
Maharaja Institute of Technology Mysuru, Srirangapatna Tq, Mandya 571438, Karnataka, India
e-mail: ydcgowda@gmail.com

H. V. Ravindra
Department of Mechanical Engineering, PES College of Engineering, Mandya 571401, Karnataka, India

© Springer Nature Singapore Pte Ltd. 2019
V. Sridhar et al. (eds.), *Emerging Research in Electronics, Computer Science and Technology*, Lecture Notes in Electrical Engineering 545,
https://doi.org/10.1007/978-981-13-5802-9_80

and the subsequent corrective actions could be taken prior to machine tool failure which is in a closed-loop control system.

The practicality of using machine vision system as investigated by Pfeifer and Wiegers [1] has proved to be advantageous, but integration of such measurement systems in industrial systems is under continuous scrutiny. For this to happen, quality of measurement results, tool handling, and advanced techniques of lightning for obtaining better images for different cutting tools have been presented as basic requirements. Li and An [2] have presented a micromachine vision system for automated monitoring of cutting tool status. Wear land area has been divided into segments by means of watershed transform. The gray values of entity pixel in each segment are then replaced with mean gray value of subsequent region. The sum-modified-Laplacian (SML)-focusing evaluation has been utilized to search focal plane using hill climbing algorithm. To segment every region of tool wear, they have implemented an adaptive Markov random field (MRF) algorithm. Finally, results show that these algorithms could enhance robustness and accuracy of proposed system. Fernandez-Robles, et al. [3] have developed an automated insert breakage monitoring system using machine vision. The developed system is capable of detecting inserts breakage automatically during end-milling operation. Garcia-Ordas et al. [4] have reported an approach to classify the wear levels of cutting tool. Shape descriptors are extracted from the tool wear image using machine vision and machine learning techniques. The dataset with more than 200 tool wear images were created to assess proposed approach. Luk et al. [5] have developed a technique for surface roughness assessment using microcomputer-based vision system. To derive a roughness parameter, they have adopted a vision system capable of analyzing the pattern of scattered light from the surface. In the current study, a new machine-vision-assisted monitoring technique is employed to monitor performance of turning process in terms of cutting tool and workpiece status through processing the image features.

2 Experimental Details

Due to the extreme toughness and work-hardening characteristic of the Inconel 718, the problem of turning this alloy is one of growing magnitude. The experiments have been conducted for 450 rpm speed, 0.2 mm depth of cut and feeds considered are 0.05, 0.06 and 0.07 mm/rev. The chemical compositions of Inconel 718 materials are mentioned in Table 1. Nikon D-90 digital camera used to acquire images of cutting tool and workpiece. Table 2 gives the specification of Nikon D-90 digital camera.

Table 1 Composition of Inconel 718

Substance	Ni	Cr	Fe	Ni	Mo	Al	C
%	53	19	18.5	5.1	3	0.5	0.08

Table 2 Specification of NIKON D-90 Digital camera

Sensor in effective pixels	12.3 million
Image sizes, no. of pixels, vertical x horizontal	4288 × 2848, 3216 × 2136, 2144 × 1424
Sensor cleaning	Image sensor cleaning, image dust off
Auto focus	Nikon multi—CAM1000
Lens servo	Single, continuous, automatic manual focus (M)
Continuous in frame/second	4.5
White balance	Automatic

3 Performance Monitoring

Performance monitoring could be carried out by capturing the information given by cutting tool and the workpiece. Flow chart of performance monitoring using image processing is as shown in Fig. 1.

A series of tool images and corresponding machined surface samples are taken during performance monitoring in turning nickel-based super alloys is as shown in Fig. 2. The initial status of both tool and workpiece is as shown in Fig. 2a, which corresponds to the original unused state. With usage, the tool worn out and hence produces unacceptable, deteriorated machined surface as shown in Fig. 2d. It is also observed that worn tool causes irregularities such as microparticle deposits and feed marks on machined surface are as shown Fig. 2b, c.

3.1 Characterizations of Cutting Tool Wear Using Image Processing

Machine vision system was utilized to capture cutting tool images, and processing of acquired images was done using view flux software. Extraction of image feature that accurately characterizes the tool wear state is made, i.e., wear area and perimeter. Wear Area = Area of the cutting tool wear region, the number of pixels within the wear region as shown in Fig. 3.

3.2 Machined Surface Characterization Using Image Histogram

Histogram of an image is defined as the graphical depiction of gray-level intensity variations as per the roughness of the machined surface. Left side of image histogram represents smaller intensities, and right side represents large value of intensities. To

Fig. 1 Flow chart of
performance monitoring
using image processing

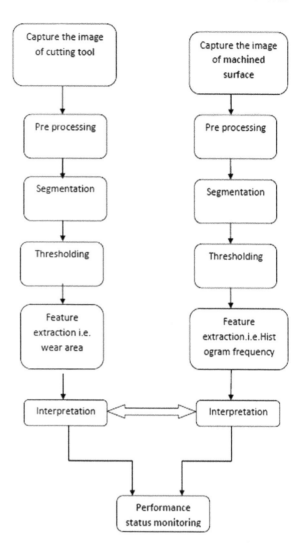

monitor the machined surface roughness, right side of histogram is preferable as the
metal surface exhibits high reflectivity and hence gray level 125 has been considered
as reference point to compute the histogram frequencies. In Fig. 4, smooth-machined
surface having surface roughness Ra $= 0.5\ \mu$m, gray level 125 approximately having
frequency 600.

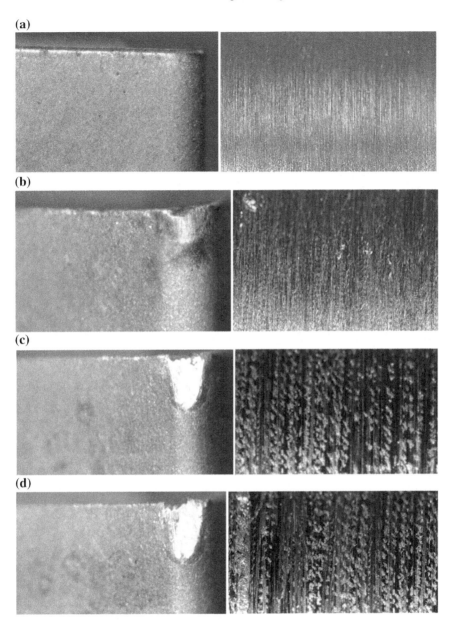

Fig. 2 A series of tool images and corresponding machined surface samples are taken during performance monitoring in turning nickel-based super alloys (Speed = 450 rpm, DOC = 0.2 mm and feed = 0.07 mm/rev)

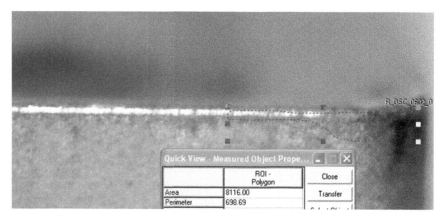

Fig. 3 Wear area and perimeter of cutting tool image

Machined surface image having Ra=0.5µm   Gray scale image of machined surface

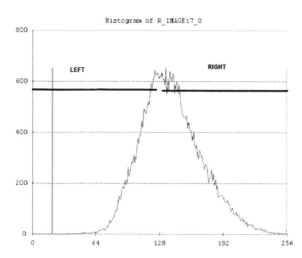

Fig. 4 Histogram of machined surface of initial run having Ra = 0.5µ, with the speed 710 rpm, feed 0.05 mm/rev and depth of cut 0.2 mm for Inconel 718 material

4 Result and Discussion

Machine vision parameters could be used as performance indicators. Progressive wear studies and their effect on surface roughness have been carried to assess their role as a factor of increasing tool wear state. The tool wear status is characterized in terms of machine vision features such as wear area and perimeter. The machined surface characterization has been done in terms of machine vision and traditional stylus method such as image histogram frequency and Ra. Performance of machining is monitored in terms of surface finish obtained which varies with respect to the status of the tool. In order to keep track of this machining process, the tool status is as important as that of keeping track of the machined surface. Both the tool and the machined surface of the workpiece carry the information about overall performance of the turning process. Hence, monitoring both the cutting tool and machined surface status at the interaction zone, which is called as performance monitoring, is a key to obtain the desired state of the machining process. Tool status is being evaluated in terms of run-in-wear, steady wear, and rapid wear. Work status is evaluated in terms of surface roughness.

It is clearly observed from Figs. 5 and 6 that machine vision features such as wear area and perimeter follow the trend till the measured flank wear of 0.3 mm. As the flank wear measurement crosses 0.3 mm, due to rapid wear of the tool, the values of the measured features increase drastically. Since the behavior of the measured features follows the established trend, the features themselves are potentially dependable information carriers of performance status during machining of Inconel 718 work material using coated carbide inserts.

Increase in feed rate increases the interface between tool and work material. This causes more friction and hence more heat is generated. Increase in cutting force and temperature leads to the formation of microwelds at the interface which decreases the strength of the cutting edge. This phenomenon occurs even at relatively low spindle speeds of about 280 to 450 rpm. Reduction in strength leads to plastic deformation and built-up-edge formation, as a result increasing tool wear area and perimeter. As the speed further increases, the BUE gets dislodged and the process continues and flank wear thus increases to intolerable levels.

Image histogram frequency presents machined surface status in terms of surface roughness as depicted in Fig. 7. The image histogram frequency plots at different feed rates are observed to be almost constant until the flank wear of 0.3 mm and beyond which they dropped to alarming levels indicating the deterioration of machined surface roughness. Arithmetic mean of surface deviation, Ra, captured using stylus method has been adopted to ascertain the surface roughness. By observation, it is inversely related to the image histogram values. Ra has been plotted against machining time as shown in Fig. 8. Beyond flank wear of 0.3 mm, Ra increases rapidly more or less at the same instance at which the image histogram plot drops.

Image histogram frequency of the machined surface plays a major role with respect to tool status measured in terms of wear area as is evident from Fig. 9 for different conditions of machining. When the measured flank wear is beyond 0.3 mm, the

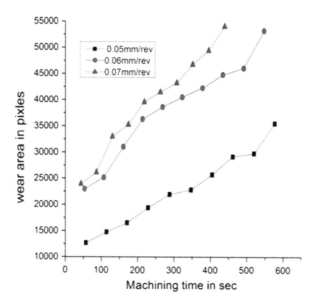

Fig. 5 Wear area versus machining time for Inconel 718 material

Fig. 6 Wear perimeter
versus machining time for
Inconel 718 material

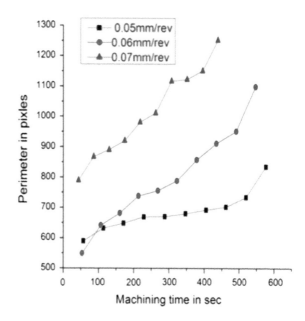

Fig. 7 Histogram frequency versus machining time for Inconel 718 material

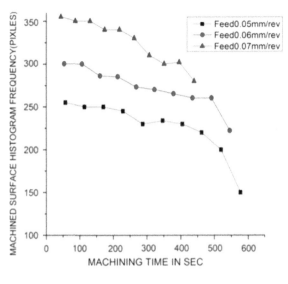

Fig. 8 Ra versus machining time for Inconel 718 material

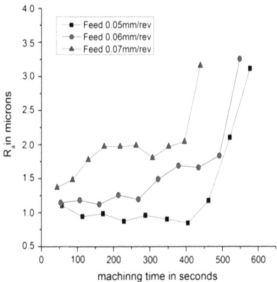

image histogram values drops, termed as last values, indicating the tool unworkable life. Wear area and flank wear are higher at feed of 0.07 mm/rev than 0.05 mm/rev and 0.06 mm/rev. The wear area of the insert grows faster at 0.07 mm/rev, and the generated surface is very rough. The same trends have been observed for all considered cutting conditions.

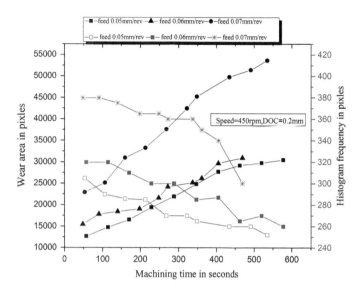

Fig. 9 Correlation of histogram frequency and wear area progression with machining time for Inconel 718 material

5 Conclusion

The tool status has been assessed through the machine vision image features: wear area and perimeter and simultaneously the machined surface roughness is monitored through machine vision image feature: the histogram frequency. The performance parameters such as wear area, perimeter, and histogram frequency record higher values when the feed of 0.07 mm/rev. The tool tends to wear less at lower feed due to reduced component forces, reduction in chip-tool contact time thereby leading to reduced temperature and stresses acting on the tool. Flank wear alone is not the only dependable information carrier of surface roughness. Also notch wear and crater wear which occur as a result of increased friction at higher speeds and feeds are major components in causing variations in surface roughness.

References

1. Pfeifer T, Wiegers L (2000) Reliable tool wear monitoring by optimized image and illumination control in machine vision. Measurement 28:209–218
2. Li L, An Q (2016) An in-depth study of tool wear monitoring technique based on image segmentation and texture analysis. Measurement 79:44–52
3. Fernández-Robles L, Azzopardi G, Alegre E, Petkov N (2017) Machine-vision-based identification of broken inserts in edge profile milling heads. Robot Comput Integr Manuf 44:276–283

4. Garcia-Ordás MT, Alegre E, González-Castro V, Alaiz-Rodriguez R (2017) A computer vision approach to analyze and classify tool wear level in milling processes using shape descriptors and machine learning techniques. Int J Adv Manuf Technol 90:1947–1961
5. Luk F, Huynh V, North W. Measurement of surface roughness by a machine vision system. J Phys E Sci Instrum 22(12)

Improved WEMER Protocol for Data Aggregation in Wireless Sensor Networks

K. K. Thashrifa and R. Bhagya

Abstract The wireless sensor networks are the decentralized and self-configuring network in which sensor nodes can sense the surrounding environment and pass the information to the base station. Due to decentralized nature and distant deployment, the consumption of energy is one of the major issues of wireless sensor networks. To reduce consumption of energy in wireless sensors, hierarchal clustering is the efficient type of clustering technique. In this research work, WEMER protocol is implemented and improved to increase lifetime of sensor networks. In the improved WEMER protocol, whole network is divided into many clusters, and for each cluster, one cluster head is selected. The proposed WEMER protocol is implemented in MATLAB. The simulation results show that proposed WEMER protocol has less number of dead nodes send more number of packets and less energy consumption.

Keywords Improved WEMER · LEACH · Gateway · Leader node · Energy consumption

1 Introduction

The recent developments made in the wireless sensor networks have provided great innovations and applications that involve such as the mechanical monitoring, traffic monitoring, and cropping. Advance creative and productive thoughts are to be generated within this area such that their usage can be more helpful. Various methods have been introduced in the recent years in the field of information routing, compression as well as network aggregation [1]. Sensor node is the vital part of the network since all the operations occur based on the information given by these nodes as shown in Fig. 1.

K. K. Thashrifa (✉) · R. Bhagya
Department of Telecommunication Engineering, R.V. College of Engineering, Bangalore, India
e-mail: thashukk@gmail.com

R. Bhagya
e-mail: bhagyar@rvce.edu.in

© Springer Nature Singapore Pte Ltd. 2019
V. Sridhar et al. (eds.), *Emerging Research in Electronics, Computer Science and Technology*, Lecture Notes in Electrical Engineering 545,
https://doi.org/10.1007/978-981-13-5802-9_81

927

There are numerous nodes deployed within specific area to monitor the surrounding area of those nodes. To provide communication within the nodes present in the network, the sensor hub is present which consists of sensors, memory, actuators, and processor. There is no wired connection present within these networks [2]. The battery in the sensor nodes is of smaller size. Also the nodes are placed at far distances where human is not able to reach. So the major concern within the WSNs is the usage of energy within them. This also affects the overall lifetime of the nodes and thus the deployment of the network [3].

The major problem that arises in the wireless sensor networks is limited energy in battery of nodes [4]. There are limited constraints such as size of battery, processors, and memory present within the sensor nodes of the network. Thus, the major concern here is to upgrade the amount of energy being consumed by these networks. In order to provide solution to this problem, regular time constraints are provided within the network such that the data that is gathered can be transmitted to the destination with minimal energy consumption.

Organization of the paper includes literature review of some of the existing routing techniques in Sect. 2. Overview of the proposed algorithm is listed in Sect. 3. The results are discussed in Sect. 4 and conclusions in Sect. 5.

2 Literature Review

The recent work on the routing algorithm in WSN has been studied. Various routing algorithms used to reduce the energy consumption and to provide the stability in the network are reviewed.

The segmented LEACH is an improvement on basic LEACH protocol is discussed and the results are compared [3]. The corresponding protocol has segmentation phase

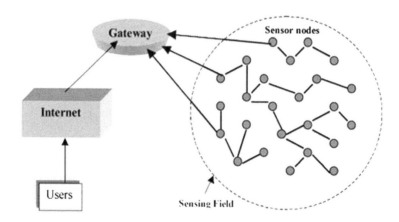

Fig. 1 Wireless sensor network

which is the beginning step. Then setup phase where each node calculates its probability function followed by steady state phase. In the comparison result, it is observed that the first dead node is seen at the 1400 round in segmented LEACH but at 1026 in LEACH.

In the coronas hierarchical model [4], the Dijkstra shortest path algorithm is used to calculate the optimal sequence of transmission distance from the source node to the sink node. The dynamic multi-path routing algorithm helps in energy balance of the network. In addition, when the nodes transmit information from outer coronas to inner the q-switch algorithm is used, which allows each node have many number of nodes available to choose one with the maximum energy to keep the balance of the network. When the nodes from a corona run out of energy, one can search the remaining distance sequence to achieve the optimal energy of the nodes through the dynamic routing method.

To overcome the limited energy problem in WSN, a clustering-based routing algorithm known as KACO (K-means and Ant Colony) [5] is studied. In this scheme, it deploys the nodes as an ant colony and uses K means algorithm to form a cluster. In order to select the cluster head for each cluster, it considers the energy ratio, node location, and distance. Dynamic hybrid routing is adopted in the transmission phase to create the shortest path between nodes to reduce the node energy consumption. The experimental results show that the KACO has optimal performance in terms of node energy consumption, number of transmitted packets, and lifetime of the network

An adaptive priority [6] based hop selection to enhance the network lifetime. This technique presents an ideal transceiver optimization strategy which fully capitalizes the minimum remaining energy. Simulations were conducted to evaluate lifetime of the network. An average lifetime improvement of 90.5% is achieved

The literature review gives a brief knowledge about different routing techniques. The important factor here is the energy consumption factor. So there exists a need for a scheme with minimal energy consumption.

3   Proposed Algorithm

The wireless sensor networks are self-configuring network and size of the sensor nodes is very small. Due to which energy consumption is the major issue in wireless sensor networks. The LEACH is the energy efficient which is used to reduce energy consumption of the network. The various improvements in the LEACH protocol are done in the recent times to reduce energy consumption. In the proposed improvement, three levels of architecture are proposed in which leader nodes, cluster heads, and gateway nodes are involved in the data communication. The proposed technique involved following phases.

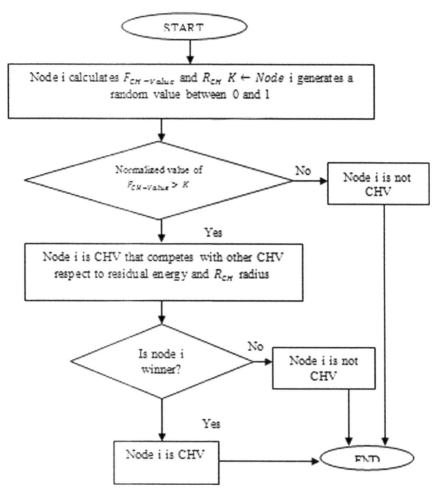

Fig. 2 Flowchart of cluster head selection

3.1 Cluster Head Selection

The cluster head selection is the first phase in the network as shown in Fig. 2. The network is deployed with the finite number of sensor nodes. The base station is deployed at the center of the network. The base station broadcasts the message in the network. The base station calculates the signal strength and nodes which have signal strength above threshold value will be eligible to be selected as the cluster head. The threshold value will be defined by the equation.

$$R_{CH} = R_{min} * \left[1 + \left(\frac{d_{BS} - d_{BSmin}}{d_{BSmax} - d_{BSmin}} \right) \right] \qquad (1)$$

In the given equation R_{min} is the radius of the cluster, d_{BS} is the node distance from the base station, d_{BSmin} is the minimum distance from the base station, and d_{BSmax} is maximum distance from the base station.

$$F_{CH-value} = \alpha * N_{deg} + \frac{\beta}{MSD_{deg}} + \frac{\gamma}{d_{BS}} \qquad (2)$$

In Eq. 2, the N_{deg} is the number of neighbor nodes of the particular node, MSD_{deg} is the mean distance of all nodes in the network, α, β, and γ is the threshold values whose total is 1.

A random value which lies between 0 and 1 is generated by each node. Any node is selected as cluster head when it satisfies the condition given in Eq. 3.

$$K(i) > F_{CH-value} \qquad (3)$$

The K(i) is the random value generated by the sensor node individually.

3.2 Leader Node Selection

The second phase of the proposed technique is the selection of leader nodes as shown in Fig. 3. The nodes except cluster head will be selected as the leader nodes. The leader nodes are responsible to collect the data from the normal sensor nodes and then pass the sensed data to the cluster head. The volunteer leader node will be selected by Eq. 4

$$F_{LN-value} = \eta * M_{deg} + \frac{\lambda}{K_{LN}} \qquad (4)$$

M_{deg} is the number of leader nodes which volunteer to select as leader node. K_{LN} is the number of nodes which comes under the defined radius. η and λ are the two constants whose total will be 1. The nodes which are the volunteer to be selected as leader node will generate random number from 0 to 1 and nodes which satisfy condition 5 will be selected as leader node.

$$K(i) > F_{LN-value} \qquad (5)$$

3.3 Gateway Node Selection

In the last phase, the gateway nodes are deployed as shown in Fig. 4. The gateway nodes depend upon the total number of nodes which is described by Eq. 6.

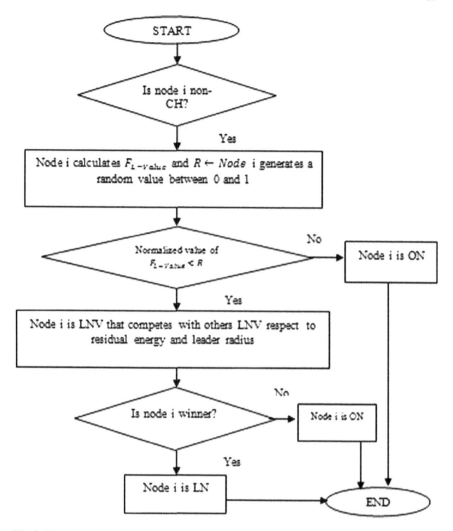

Fig. 3 Flowchart of leader node selection

$$\text{Gateway}_{\text{nodes}} = \text{total number of nodes}/4 \tag{6}$$

The gateway nodes are the fourth part of the total nodes. The best nodes in terms of energy are selected from overall gateways nodes to send data to the base station. The distance from base station to the gateway node calculated using Eq. 7

$$\text{Distance} = \sqrt{(x(i) - x)^2 + (y(i) - y)^2} \tag{7}$$

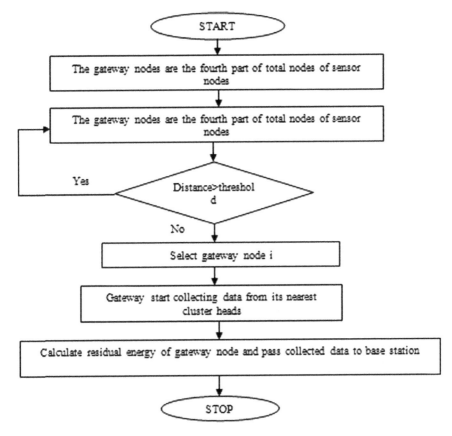

Fig. 4 Flowchart for gateway node selection

In the improved technique, the leader nodes help in aggregation of data from the normal sensor nodes. The aggregated data is now sent to the cluster head by the leader nodes. The gateway node which is nearest to the base station will pass the data to the base station.

The energy values for the sensor nodes are taken and the system parameters are shown in Table 1.

4   Results and Discussions

The improved WEMER technique is implemented in MATLAB and the results are evaluated by making comparisons with the existing approach in terms of packet transmission and number of dead nodes.

Table 1 System parameters

Parameters	Value
Deployed area	100×100 Square Area
Number of sensor nodes	100 Nodes
Data packet	4000 bits
Initial energy	0.5 J
Transmission energy	50×10^8 J
Reception energy	50×10^8 J
Energy for processing	5×10^8 J

Fig. 5 Residual energy comparison

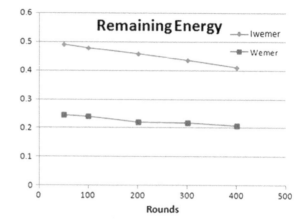

The residual energy of the network for different number of rounds for both the techniques is shown in the Fig. 5. The WEMER and IWEMER protocols are compared in terms of residual energy. It is analyzed that improved technique has more residual energy compared to the existing technique. The residual energy of the existing technique is 0.2986 J and that of improved WEMER technique is 0.4896 J. Thus due to the less energy consumption, the network lifetime increases, and the performance improves.

Figure 6 shows the dead node comparison of WEMER and IWEMER protocol for various numbers of rounds. It is observed that due to gateway node deployment in the network the number of dead nodes is reduced in IWEMER protocol as compared to existing protocol. It is also evident from the graph shown.

5 Conclusions

Proposed modified wedge merging technique prevent the network from energy hole problem, consumes less energy, and increase network lifetime. The proposed modified WEMER scheme is compared with existing technique. Simulation is performed

Fig. 6 Number of dead nodes comparison

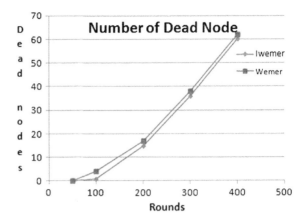

using Matlab version R2017b. Simulation results prove that improved WEMER performs better compared to existing work in terms of network lifetime, remaining energy, and number of node dead nodes.

References

1. Jia H, Fan X, Liu K, Qian Y (2017) An energy efficiency routing algorithm for wireless sensor network. In: 2017 IEEE international conference on computational science and engineering (CSE) and IEEE international conference on embedded and ubiquitous computing (EUC), Guangzhou, pp 735–739
2. Yadav MK, Daniel AK (2017) A study of energy conserving adequate coverage protocol for maximizing the lifetime of wireless sensor network. In: 2017 international conference of electronics, communication and aerospace technology (ICECA), Coimbatore, pp 394–398
3. Sharmin N, Alam MS, Moni SS (2016) WEMER: an energy hole mitigation scheme in wireless sensor networks. In: 2016 IEEE international WIE conference on electrical and computer engineering (WIECON-ECE), Pune, pp 229–232
4. Brindha N, Vanitha S (2017) The data aggregation approach to enhance the lifetime of wireless sensor network. In: 2017 international conference on innovations in green energy and healthcare technologies (IGEHT), Coimbatore, pp 1–5
5. Kakhandki AL, Hublikar S, Kumar P (2017) An efficient hop selection model to enhance lifetime of wireless sensor network. In: 2017 innovations in power and advanced computing technologies (i-PACT), Vellore, pp 1–5
6. Basu SV, Ashwin KP, Neti NK, Premananda BS (2017) Improving the network lifetime of a wireless sensor network using clustering techniques. In: 2017 2nd IEEE international conference on recent trends in electronics, information & communication technology (RTEICT), Bangalore, pp 1872–1877

Analysis of Speckle Diminution in Ultrasound Images—A Review

N. Tilakraj and K. M. Ravikumar

Abstract Ultrasound is used imaging modality for the diagnosis and diseases. In past decades, the advances in technology have become crucial imaging modality, due to its suppleness and non-invasive. Ultrasound image uses high-frequency sound waves to contrasting reflection signals created when a light emission is anticipated into the body the convenience of ultrasound image is corrupted by the noise identified as dot (speckle). The speckle model depends on the image tissue and different image parameters. The noise shows in ultrasound picture influences edges and subtle elements contain the differentiation and determination. The reasons for speckle noise reduction in ultrasound image (i) The ultrasound images are improved for human interpretation (ii) The speckle noise reduction is the preprocessing step for segmentation and registration in ultrasound image processing tasks. The objective of paper is to give different techniques have been used to decrease speckle noise in ultrasound image.

Keywords Speckle noise · Ultrasound imaging · Region of interest · Filter

1 Introduction

Ultrasound image plays important role in therapeutic image because of its non-obtrusive nature, ease and framing ongoing imaging. Ultrasound waves which are created by transducer from body tissues, achieves a surface with various surface or acoustic in nature. The transducer is used to receive the echoes and converted

N. Tilakraj (✉) · K. M. Ravikumar
Department of ECE, S J C Institute of Technology,
Chikkaballapur, Karnataka, India
e-mail: tilakrajn86@gmail.com

K. M. Ravikumar
e-mail: kmravikumar75@gmail.com

N. Tilakraj
VTU-RRC, Belgaum, India

© Springer Nature Singapore Pte Ltd. 2019
V. Sridhar et al. (eds.), *Emerging Research in Electronics, Computer Science and Technology*, Lecture Notes in Electrical Engineering 545,
https://doi.org/10.1007/978-981-13-5802-9_82

into electric current. These signals are improved and shown on a display device in real time. The image generated using ultrasound imaging commonly known as Ultra sonogram. The resolution of the image is increased by using higher frequencies. There are several methods of ultrasound imaging. The regular modes are (1) B-mode—2-D intensity mode, (2) M-mode to assess moving body parts from the echoed sound and (3) Color mode pseudo coloring based on detected cell motion.

Ultrasound imaging is a generally for restorative indicative system because of its non-intrusive nature, minimal effort and framing ongoing imaging. To accomplish the most ideal determination, the medicinal pictures to be pointed, accurate and gratis of commotion and ancient rarities. However, the spot noise is an issue with ultrasound imaging caused by impedance of vitality from haphazardly appropriated scrambling. Spot commotion it's a tendency to lessen picture determination, complexity and obscure essential points of interest, consequently diminishing indicative estimation of the imaging methodology. In this way, spot commotion decrease is a critical essential in ultrasound imaging. The ultrasound image is adjustable, moveable and moderately safe, these kind of image consists of speckle noise and artifacts, which degrades the organ and reduces the contrast. It affects the human perception to recognize pathological tissue.

This paper is described as follows: Sect. 2 presents the related work. Section 3 describes different noise models. The methods and results to filter the speckle noise are described in Sects. 4 and 5 and conclusion in Sect. 6 are as follows.

2 Related Work

The ultrasound-based investigative medicinal imaging method used to outline muscles and inner organs, size, structure and neurotic wounds with continuous tomographic pictures. It is used to imagine an embryo amid routine and crisis pre-birth mind. Obstetric ultrasonography is generally used amid pregnancy. It is a standout among the most generally utilized demonstrative instruments in present-day prescription. The state of art is moderately cheap and solid, particularly when contrast and other imaging methods, for example, attractive reverberation imaging and figured tomography.

Speckle noise [1] influences all intelligent imaging frameworks including therapeutic ultrasound. The determination cell is a variety of basic diffuses mirror the occurrence wave toward the sensor. The backscattered cognizant waves with a variety of stages experience a productive or in an irregular way. The obtained picture is in this way tainted an irregular granular example, called spot that postpones the translation of picture content. The ultrasound image of kidney is used to assess kidney size, position and help to analyze auxiliary variations from the norm and the nearness of sores and stones. Nonetheless, because of the nearness of spot commotion in these, playing out the division strategies for the kidney pictures were extremely testing and thusly, erasing the muddled foundation will accelerate and builds the exactness of the division procedure [2]. Accordingly, this examination proposes a programmed region of interest (ROI) age for kidney ultrasound pictures.

The picture handling can be utilized to naturally recognize the centroid of human kidney. For the outcome, middle channel has been picked as speckle commotion diminishment systems is quicker and identify kidney centroid enhanced contrasted with wiener channel and wavelet channel. This product can be distinguishing centroid up to 96.4% of precision [3].

A calculation is depicted for clean-up speckle noise in ultrasound therapeutic pictures. Scientific morphological activities are utilized as a part of [4]. This calculation depends on Morphological Image Cleaning calculation (MIC). The calculation utilizes distinctive systems for remaking the highlights that are lost while expelling the commotion. In ultrasound pictures, the noise can able to prevent data for the common professional. A wavelet-based thresholding technique is utilized for noise concealment in ultrasound images. Quantitative and subjective examinations of the outcomes are obtained by the wavelet-based thresholding and approach accomplished from spot commotion decrease strategies show its higher execution for speckle diminishment [5].

3 Noise Models

Speckle noise is an subjective and deterministic in a image. Speckle is negative effect on ultrasound image. Radical diminishment might be in charge of the poor powerful purpose of ultrasound when contrasted with MRI.

If there is an occurrence of therapeutic written works, spot noise is or else called surface. The representation of the speckle is given by

$$a(n, m) = b(n, m)\,c(n, m) + \xi\,(n, m) \tag{1}$$

where a, b, c and ξ stand for the observed image, new image, multiplicative element and preservative element of the speckle noise. Here (n, m) identifies the axial and lateral indices of the image sample. In ultrasound images, the multiplicative element of the noise is to be considered and it can be model by disregarding the additive term, so that the Eq. (1) given by

$$a(n, m) = b(n, m) * c(n, m) \tag{2}$$

The speckle denoising methods take benefit of the logarithmic transformation, where it converts the multiplicative noise to additive noise. The logarithms of a, b and c by a_1, b_1 and c_1, respectively, the Eq. (2) becomes

$$a_1(n, m) = b_1(n, m) * c_1(n, m) \tag{3}$$

The method of despeckling is to reduce the additive noise, and different types of noise-suppression techniques are considered in order to carry out denoising.

A. *Speckle Noise in Ultrasound Medical Images*

In ultrasound medical image processing is very important to achieve the correct images, which facilitate the accurate interpretation for the given application. Usually, medical images are corrupted by speckle noise. The quality of the images is decreases where the feature extraction, recognition, analysis and quantitative measurement become difficult.

B. *Noise in Ultrasound Images*

Ultrasound imaging framework is broadly utilized demonstrative instrument for present-day solution. The ultrasound image is used for the representation of muscles, inner organs of the human body, size and wounds. In an ultrasound image, the speckle noise shows its subsistence in visualization process [6].

C. *Medical Ultrasound Speckle Pattern*

Natures of speckle design rely upon the quantity of scrambles per determination cell. Spatial conveyance and the attributes of the image framework can be isolated into three classes:

- The full-grown spot design happens when numerous irregular dispersed scrambling exists inside the determination cell of the image framework. Platelets are the case of this class.
- Tissue disseminates is no haphazardly dispersed with long-extend arrange.
- A spatially invariant reasonable structure is available inside the irregular disperse locale like organ surfaces and veins [7].

4   Various Methods

There are numerous speckle diminishment channels accessible which give enhanced visual understandings while others have great noise decrease capacities.

A. *Averaging*

The speckle noise can be reduced by using averaging as large as possible. The scanning under exactly same conditions one obtains identical speckle patterns.

There are two amplitude values independent of each other if the transducer is translated by partly of its bandwidth between sizes [8]. The main drawback of this method is that the blurring of de-noised image and loss of details.

B. *Median Filter*

Median filter [9] obtains the average of pixels with in a adjacent window and replaces the middle pixel with this average value. This method is efficient for the cases of noise model consist of conserved edges. The main disadvantage of the median filter is that additional time required to place the intensity value of the every one position.

The adaptive weighted median [10] is a median filter through the introduction of weight coefficients and accordingly the smoothing uniqueness of the filter according to the neighborhood information in the region of each pixel of the image. The other approach of obtaining this is to decide a family of weights reduces when moving left from the midpoint of the window. The weights are in sync according to local information of image given by

$$p(i, j) = [p(l + 1, l + 1) - cd\sigma^2/m] \tag{4}$$

$cs\sigma^2/m$ is small so that maximum noise is reduced.
Where c is scaling factor, m, σ^2 is the mean and variance inside the $2\,l + 1 \times 2\,l + 1$ window and d is the distance of point (i, j) from center of window $(l + 1, l + 1)$. For uniform areas, constant c should be selected in such a way that. In case of boundary, c should be selected such that $c\sigma^2/m$ should be high to preserve image details. The drawback of this method is that the computation is more when image divided into more number of angles.

C. Wiener Filter

The Wiener Filter [11], also called as LMS filter and the subsequent expression is given by.

$$F(u, v) = \left[\frac{H(u, v)^*}{H(u, v) + \left[\frac{S_n(u,v)}{S_f(u,v)} \right]} \right] G(u, v) \tag{5}$$

$H(u, v)$ is the degradation function and $H(u, v)^*$ its complex conjugate. $G(u, v)$ the degraded image. Functions $S_f(u, v)$ and $S_n(u, v)$ represent the power spectra and noise of original image.

D. Frost Filter

Frost filter [12] is a spatial and it is based on multiplicative noise; it adapts the variance of noise inside the filter window by weighting factors M as:

$$M = \exp(-(DAMP * (S/Im)^2) * T) \tag{6}$$

The weight aspect decreases as the filter windows reduces. DAMP is a characteristic that is used to find the level of damping exponential for the image. The value of DAMP is put to one. 'S' is the standard deviation, 'Im' is the value of mean and 'T' is the total value of the pixel. The weighted value of the image as:

$$Im\, g(i, j) = \frac{\sum P_n * M_n}{\sum M_n} \tag{7}$$

The Frost filter is used to organize the difference in all area. Area difference is small, and then the filtering will effect smoothing. Tiny smoothing occurs and edges are retained in high variance.

E. *Anisotropic Diffusion*

An isotropic filter is capable to smoothen the image and decreases the clearness in features of interest. Anisotropic diffusion [13] applies to smooth an image while preserving features edges and improves the false edges introduced by the speckle pattern. Speckle reducing anisotropic diffusion (SRAD), developed incorporate speckle statistics into the established anisotropic diffusion framework.

SRAD is based on a nonlinear partial differential equation. The continuous-domain version of this PDE is

$$\frac{\partial}{\partial t} I(x, y; t) = div[c(q)\nabla I(x, y; t)] \tag{8}$$

where (x, y) are image coordinates, t is diffusion time, $I(x, y; t)$ is the image intensity function, and $c(q) \in [0, 1]$ is the diffusion coefficient. The SRAD diffusion coefficient is given by

$$c(q) = \left[1 + \frac{[q(x, y; t)^2 - q_0^2(t)]}{q_0^2(t)[1 + q_0^2(t)]}\right]^{-1} \tag{9}$$

F. *Adaptive Nonlinear Filters*

The recursive median filter [14] reduces the noise, which is efficient than a non-recursive median filter. In contrast to a recursive linear filter, the recursive median filter is naturally stable since the value of the median is per definition equal to one of the input samples. Hence, the median value is bounded while the input signal is bounded by an appropriate window size 'w', the effects must be taken into account. The noise inhibition increases with growing window size 'w'; conversely, the space resolution decreases with increasing window size.

A median filter removes all objects on a flat environment which is less than (w + 1)/2 pixels. To solve this difficulty, usually a small window is used, and the median filtering is repetitive, until no further changes occur. In this manner, the performance of smoothing and space resolution is controlled by an weighting factor as a function of the local signal-to-noise ratio, which is predictable from the noisy image.

5 Results

The following figures exhibit the comparison of all the filters defined above for an input ultrasound images of fast trauma (a–b) and kidney (c) shown in Fig. 1a–c [15]. The corresponding output of each filter is shown in Fig. 2a–c through Fig. 7a–c.

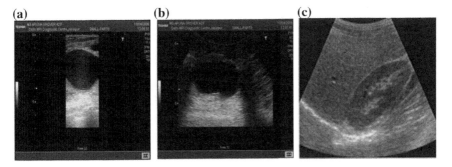

Fig. 1 Input US images of fast trauma (**a–b**) and kidney(**c**)

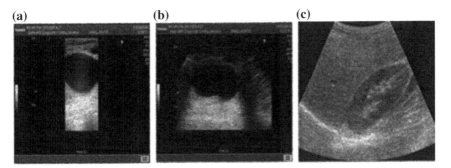

Fig. 2 Output images for average filtering

Table 1 shows the mean square error, peak signal-to-noise ratio, correlation and SSIM (Index which has values between 0 and 1) for all the speckle noise filters.

6 Conclusion

Some of the filter techniques used to minimize speckle noise is analyzed. Table 1 summarizes the output from all filters used to minimize speckle noise for three input ultrasound images. The MSE, PSNR, correlation of input and output images, SSIM are compared. The limitations of these algorithms are approachable to the dimension and contour of the window. If the size of window is big then smoothing will occur, if the window size is small the smoothing capability of the filter will not reduce speckle noise. The existing despeckle filters do not improve the edges; it will reduce the smoothing near the edges. If the edge is enclosed to the filtering window, the coefficient of variation will be high and smoothing is introverted. The selection of despeckling filter and speckle model plays an essential role in the design of speckle noise reduction methods and it differs from one application to other. With above analysis and review of this work, our future work will be development of a

Table 1 Comparison of all filters for speckle noise

Method/Parameter	Ultrasound image 1				Ultrasound image 2				Ultrasound image 3			
	MSE	PSNR	Correlation	SSIM	MSE	PSNR	Correlation	SSIM	MSE	PSNR	Correlation	SSIM
Average filter	18.25	35.52	0.96	0.89	17.27	35.76	0.97	0.89	22.84	34.54	0.98	0.83
Median filter	20.51	35.01	0.87	0.88	21.40	34.83	0.92	0.88	39.66	32.15	0.96	0.71
Wiener filter	17.51	35.70	0.98	0.88	19.23	35.29	0.98	0.86	27.08	33.80	0.97	0.76
Frost filter	16.80	35.88	0.98	0.90	18.96	35.35	0.97	0.88	33.49	32.88	0.97	0.69
Anisotropic diffusion	16.84	35.87	0.98	0.90	18.21	35.53	0.98	0.88	21.26	34.86	0.98	0.83
Adaptive filter	19.53	35.22	0.90	0.84	20.52	35.01	0.86	0.83	25.70	34.03	0.96	0.81

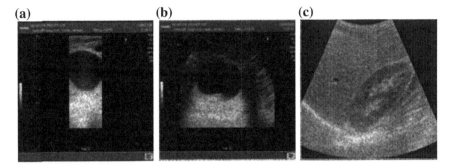

Fig. 3 Output images for median filtering

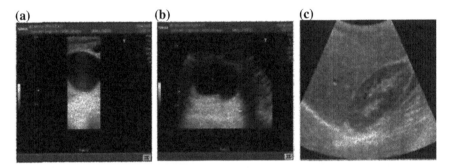

Fig. 4 Output images for Wiener filtering

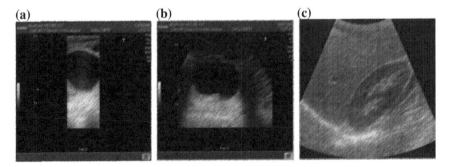

Fig. 5 Output images for frost filtering

robust and efficient algorithm to minimize speckle noise in the edge of the image by maintaining the smoothing in edges (Figs. 3, 4, 5, 6 and 7).

(a)   (b)   (c)

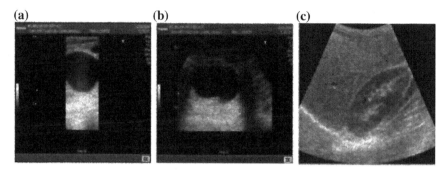

Fig. 6 Output images for anisotropic diffusion filtering

(a)   (b)   (c)

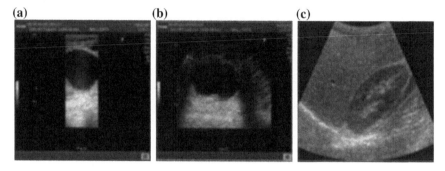

Fig. 7 Output images for adaptive filtering. Courtesy: Input US Images from ultrasoundidiots.com

References

1. Gupta N, Swamy MNS, Plotkin E. Despeckling of medical ultrasound images using data *and rate adoptive lossy compression*. IEEE Trans Med
2. Hafizah WM, Supriyanto E (2012) Automatic generation of region of interest for kidney ultrasound images using texture analysis. Int J Biol Biomed Eng 6(1)
3. Hafizah WM, Tahir NA, Supriyanto E, Arooj A, Nooh SM (2012) New technique towards operator independent kidney ultrasound scanning. Int J Comput 6(1)
4. Ratha Jeyalakshmi T, Ramar K (2010) A modified method for speckle noise removal in ultrasound medical images. Int J Comput Electr Eng 2(1)
5. Sudha S, Suresh GR, Sukanesh R (2009) Speckle noise reduction in ultrasound images by wavelet thresholding based on weighted variance. Int J Comput Theory Eng 1
6. Sarode MV, Deshmukh PR (2011) Reduction of speckle noise and image enhancement of images using filtering technique. Int J Adv Technol 2
7. AbdElmoniem KZ, Kadah YM, Youssef AM. Real time adaptive ultrasound speckle reduction and coherence enhancement. 078032977/00/$10© 2000 IEEE, pp 172–175
8. Burckhardt CB (1978) Speckle in ultrasound B-mode scans. IEEE Trans Sonic Ultrason SU-25:1–6
9. Ritenour ER, Nelson TR, Raff U (1984) Applications of the median filter to digital radiographic images. In: Proceedings of IEEE international conference on acoustics. speech, signal processing, San Diego, CA, pp 23.1.1–23.1.4
10. Loupas T, McDicken WN, Allan PL (1989) An adaptive weighted median filter for speckle suppression in medical ultrasonic images. IEEE Trans Circuits Syst 36(1):129–135

11. Lee J-S (1980) Digital image enhancement and noise filtering by use of local statistics. IEEE Trans Pattern Anal Mach Intell pami-2(2)
12. Frost VS, Stiles JA, Shanmugam KS, Holtzman JC (1982) A model for radar image & its application to Adaptive digital filtering for multiplicative noise. IEEE Trans Pattern Anal Mach Intell PMAI 4:175–166
13. Yu Y, Acton ST (2002) Speckle reducing anisotropic diffusion. IEEE Trans Image Process 11:1260
14. Bernstein R (1987) Adaptive nonlinear filters for simultaneous removal of different kinds of noise in images. IEEE Trans Circuits Syst cas-34
15. https://www.ultrasoundidiots.com

Comparative Study of g_m/I_D Methodology for Low-Power Applications

Namboodiri Akhil M. M. Krishnan, K. S. Vasundhara Patel
and Manjunath Jadhav

Abstract This paper provides a detailed analysis of the g_m/I_D design methodology for low-power applications. A systematic procedure is proposed to fix the current and transistor dimensions of analog circuits so as to meet specifications such as gain–bandwidth while optimizing power and area. The paper also provides an explanation as how short channel effects are taken into consideration when designing analog circuits. A simple differential amplifier is used to illustrate the methodology.

Keywords Transconductor efficiency (g_m/I_D) · Week inversion · Moderate inversion · Transit frequency (f_T) · Sub-threshold

1 Introduction

Traditional analog design methodologies typically require iterative design. The "square law" design equations, which are used in larger channel devices, are inaccurate for submicron devices due to dependency on poorly defined parameters like process transconductance (g_m), threshold voltage (V_{th}), saturation voltage (V_{dsat}). It is difficult to achieve an optimum power in the design. Square law design fails in sub-threshold region. This paper illustrates the g_m/I_D design method to achieve optimum power in the circuit and design circuits in sub-threshold region.

Due to increase in the application of CMOS technology [1], more analog blocks are needed on chips which increases the overall power consumption. The different papers [2–6] shows different methods to address this issue, such as knowledge database [2], qualitative reasoning [3] and circuit optimization [4] and analog block reuse are proposed. In real-world portable commercial systems such as mobile phones, high-quality audio devices, and hearing systems are increasing the demand for low-power data converters.

N. A. M. M. Krishnan (✉) · K. S. Vasundhara Patel · M. Jadhav
Department of Electronics and Communication, BMS College of Engineering,
Bull Temple Road, Basavanagudi, Bangalore 560019, Karnataka, India
e-mail: akhil.krishnan1405@gmail.com

© Springer Nature Singapore Pte Ltd. 2019
V. Sridhar et al. (eds.), *Emerging Research in Electronics, Computer Science and Technology*, Lecture Notes in Electrical Engineering 545,
https://doi.org/10.1007/978-981-13-5802-9_83

In paper [7], an automated synthesis tool for design of pipelined ADC using g_m/I_D design method is presented. Use of the automated tool helps to reduce the design time considerably. In paper [8], an UWB distribution amplifier has been designed using the g_m/I_D method. Use of this method allows the designer to optimize the transistor dimensions and to achieve the best possible trade-off between DC power consumption, gain, noise figure, and I/O matching.

Scaling down of MOSFET requires V_{DD} to be scaled down but V_{th} does not scale down by the same factor due various reasons. This causes devices to be operated in sub-threshold region. Paper [9] discusses the concept of inversion coefficient (IC) that is used to define the three operating regions of a MOSFET. Inversion coefficient is the measure of level of channel inversion.

Paper [10] explains the effect of small geometry effects on g_m/I_D. The paper also depicts how design of "unit-sized" transistors can reduce the short channel effects on parameters such as current density and self-gain. Paper [11] provides the design methodology for integrated CMOS instrumentation amplifier. The paper makes use of g_m/I_D analysis for sizing of the critical transistors so that they operate in the appropriate region of operation. Paper [12] introduces a method for design of cascode LNA using scattering parameters together with g_m/I_D for transistor sizing. The authors make use of g_m/I_D to get maximum gain without much difficulty. Paper [13] talks about a fully automated design flow for design of fully differential switched capacitor differential amplifier. It makes use of g_m/I_D methodology in the form of lookup tables from pre-generated simulation models.

This paper gives in-depth analysis of g_m/I_D method for design of analog circuits targeting low-power applications. Section 2 talks about transistor figure of merits; in Sect. 3, we give a systematic procedure for design of circuit using g_m/I_D method. Section 4 explains design of differential amplifier using both square law and g_m/I_D method. Section 5 gives the experimental results for comparison of these two methods. Section 6 provides conclusions, and Sect. 7 provides the future scope.

2 g_m/I_D Figure of Merits

The following parameters of transistors can be considered as FOM of a transistor.

1. Transistor transconductance efficiency (g_m/I_D)
2. Transit frequency (f_T)
3. Intrinsic gain ($g_m * R_o$)

2.1   Transconductor Efficiency (g_m/I_D)

Transconductance efficiency is the parameter that tells the designer how much current needs to be burnt to obtain a particular g_m. By choosing a larger value of g_m/I_D, one

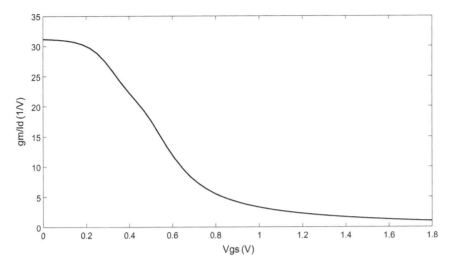

Fig. 1 Plot of g_m/I_D versus V_{gs}

can ensure that the value of g_m is obtained by burning as minimum current as possible. Figure 1 shows a plot of g_m/I_D versus V_{gs}.

g_m/I_D or transconductance efficiency is given by

$$\frac{g_m}{I_D} = \frac{2}{V_{ov}} \tag{1}$$

As seen, g_m/I_D is maximum when V_{gs} is minimum. This is because as gm/ID is inversely proportional to V_{ov} (=$V_{gs} - V_{th}$) as seen in Eq. (1). Based on the value of V_{gs}, we can have a MOSFET operation in three regions—weak inversion, moderate inversion, and strong inversion. In weak inversion, the value of gm/ID is maximum, and in strong inversion, g_m/I_D is minimum. Conversely, current is maximum in strong inversion and minimum in weak inversion as shown in Fig. 2.

2.2 Transit Frequency (FT)

Transit frequency is the frequency beyond which the transistor stops acting as an amplifier. This is the parameter that governs the speed of the amplifier. Higher the transit frequency, higher the speed and higher the bandwidth. Figure 3 shows the variation of transit frequency with V_{gs}.

Transit frequency is given by

$$f_T = \frac{3}{4\pi} \frac{\mu V_{ov}}{L^2} \tag{2}$$

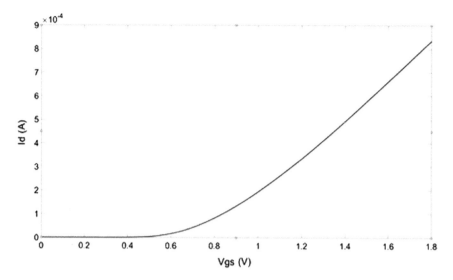

Fig. 2 Input characteristics showing current in strong and week inversion

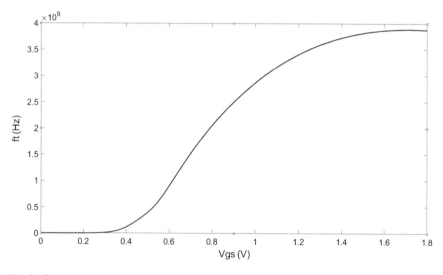

Fig. 3 Curve showing variation of frequency versus V_{gs}

Transit frequency is directly proportional to V_{ov}. As seen in Fig. 3, f_T is low for lower values of V_{gs} but increases with V_{gs}. Thus, transistors operating in strong inversion are faster than those operating in weak inversion. Thus, there is always a trade-off between g_m/I_D and f_T.

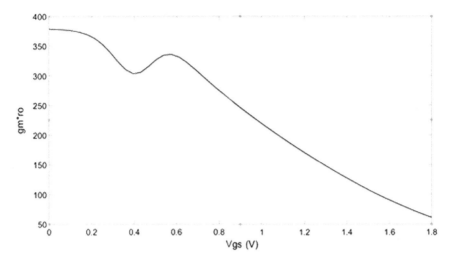

Fig. 4 Variation of intrinsic gain with V$_{gs}$

2.3 *Intrinsic Gain (g$_m$* R$_o$)*

Intrinsic gain of a transistor represents the maximum possible gain of a transistor regardless of the bias point. Figure 4 shows the variation of intrinsic gain with V$_{gs}$.
    Intrinsic gain is given by

$$g_m r_o = \frac{2}{\lambda V_{ov}} \tag{3}$$

As V$_{gs}$ increases the intrinsic gain decreases. This is because as intrinsic gain is inversely proportional to V$_{ov}$ (=V$_{gs}$ − V$_{th}$) as seen in Eq. (3). Thus to have higher gain, the MOSFET must be operated in weak inversion region.

2.4 *g$_m$/I$_D$ Versus f$_T$ Trade-Off*

The plot in Fig. 5 shows the variation of f$_T$ * g$_m$/I$_D$ with V$_{gs}$.
    The plot peaks at moderate inversion. Thus, if the design has to be optimized for both gain and frequency, then operating the MOSFET in moderate inversion would be preferable.

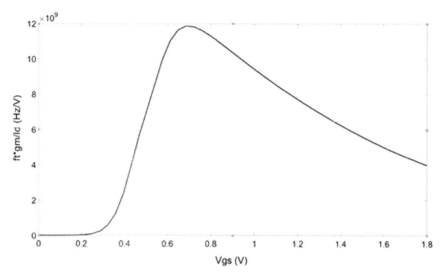

Fig. 5 Variation of $f_T * g_m/I_D$ with V_{gs}

3 g_m/I_D Design Methodology

In g_m/I_D design methodology, we treat g_m/I_D as a design parameter as V_{ov} in square law design. Here the objective is to find the W/L of a transistor using transistor models and graphs rather than the inaccurate square law equations. Figure 6 shows the various graphs needed for this design (Figs. 7, 8 and 9).

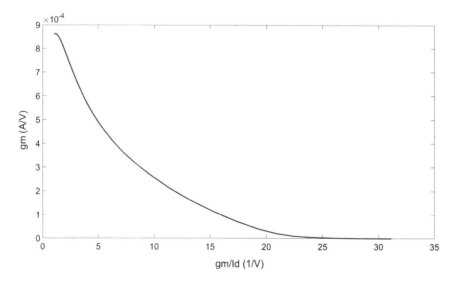

Fig. 6 Variation of g_m with g_m/I_D

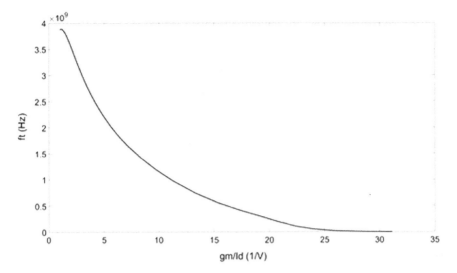

Fig. 7 Variation of f_T with g_m/I_D

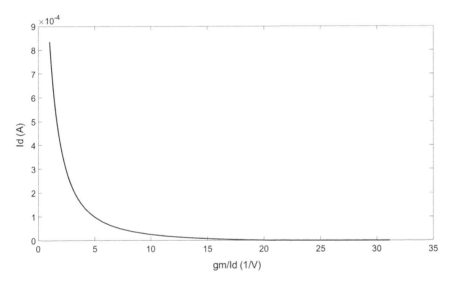

Fig. 8 Variation of I_D with g_m/I_D

Generic steps for design using g_m/I_D method are given below

1. From the specifications, extract the value of g_m/I_D. This could be done in a number of ways.

   i. Given f_T (unity gain bandwidth), plot f_T versus g_m/I_D, and find the value of g_m/I_D for given f_T.

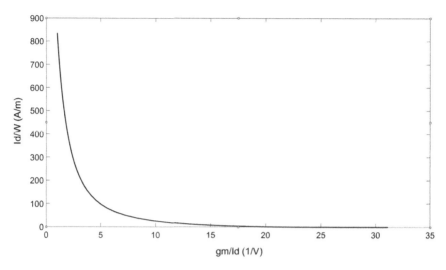

Fig. 9 Variation of I_D/W with g_m/I_D

    ii.   Given gain, calculate the value of g_m. Then plot g_m versus g_m/I_D and find the value of g_m/I_D for calculated g_m.

2. Once the value of g_m/I_D is selected, plot g_m/I_D versus I_D to obtain the value of I_D. If I_D can be derived from the specification itself, then there is no need to plot this graph.

3. Then plot g_m/I_D versus I_D/W to find the current density for selected g_m/I_D. The value of W can be obtained from the values of I_D and I_D/W.

Note: When selecting the value of g_m/I_D, we have to take into consideration the region of operation (weak, moderate, or strong). For weak, moderate, and strong inversion, we must choose a high, medium, and low value of g_m/I_D, respectively.

4 Design of Differential Amplifier

A differential amplifier is one of the basic building blocks used in analog design. It offers a variety of advantages like noise immunity, reduction of second-order harmonics, and high gain.

We have designed the differential amplifier using the square law method where we have used the I_D, g_m, and f_T equations. From these equations, we calculated the W/L of the transistors in the circuit. The circuit is designed in saturation region.

We have designed the same circuit in strong, moderate, and weak inversion regions using the g_m/I_D design method. In this method, we first found the g_m/I_D from the desired gain. Then we plotted variation of I_D and I_D/W with g_m/I_D to calculate W. We assumed $L = 1 \, \mu m$ for weak and moderate inversion design. For design in strong

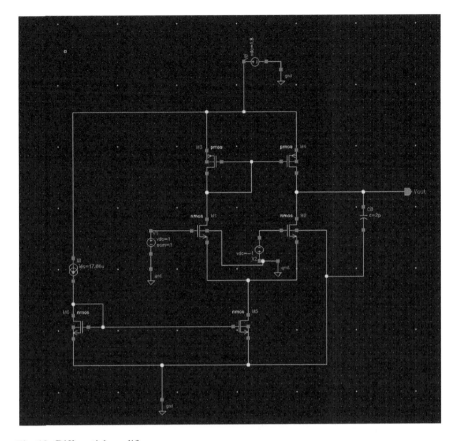

Fig. 10 Differential amplifier

inversion region, we have taken $L = 3$ μm. The differential amplifier is designed in saturation region for strong and moderate inversion regions and in sub-threshold region for weak inversion region.

The circuit of the differential amplifier is shown in Fig. 10.

5 Experiment Result

Table 1 shows the results of design of the differential amplifier using square law and g_m/I_D method. It can be seen that to obtain the same gain the amount of current we have to burn is 64.54% lower when the device is designed using g_m/I_d method in strong inversion. The bandwidth and the GBW also increase. When the differential amplifier is designed in weak inversion, the power consumption reduces by 96.49% but the bandwidth and the GBW product reduce considerably. When the circuit is

Table 1 Comparision table

Parameter	Square law method	g_m/I_D method		
		Strong inversion	Moderate inversion	Weak inversion
V_{DD}	1.8	1.8	1.8	1.8
I_{SS}	17.06 μ	5.7 μA	3.2 μA	200 μA
g_m/I_D	–	5	15	25
$(W/L)_{1,2}$	1.22	1/3	1	4
$(W/L)_{3,4}$	2.44	2/3	2	8
$(W/L)_{5,6}$	4.5	4.5	4.5	4.5
Gain (dB)	40.71	44.52	43.07	42.9
f_{3db} (kHz)	51.84	62.69	54.772	5.907
GBW	5.7 MHz	2.8 MHz	2.37 MHz	254.672 kHz

designed in moderate inversion, we get a 43.86% reduction in power consumption. The bandwidth and GBW product are also comparable to that obtained when the circuit was designed for strong inversion.

6   Conclusion

This paper we present a differential amplifier design using g_m/I_D method in all three regions of operation and compared with square law method. Gain variation is not observed throughout the experiment. To achieve low-power consumption without affecting bandwidth and GBW, analog circuits are to be designed in moderate inversion using g_m/I_D method, whereas week inversion region is suitable for low-frequency and low-power application. g_m/I_D method is the tool to achieve lowest power without sacrificing the gain.

7   Future Scope

Currently, there is no automated way for design of analog circuits. Making use of g_m/I_D design methodology to make lookup tables from accurate simulation models one can automate the design of analog circuits. This will save a lot of time in designing accurate circuits that meet given specification by burning minimum current.

References

1. Yang T et al (2010) A new reuse method of analog circuit design for CMOS technology migration. J Clerk Maxwell A Treatise Electr Mag, 3rd ed, vol 2. Clarendon, Oxford, 1892, pp 68–73. IEEE 978-1-4244-6734-1/10
2. Neff RR, Gray PR, Sangiovanni-Vincentelli A (1996) A module generator for high-speed CMOS current output digital/analog converters. IEEE J Solid-State Circuits 31:448–451
3. Francken K, Gielen G (1999) Methodology for analog technology porting including performance tuning. IEEE Int Symp Circuits Syst 1:415–418
4. Phelps R, Krasnicki MJ, Rutenbar RA, Carley LR, Hellums JR (June 2000) A case study of synthesis for industrial-scale analog IP: redesign of the equalizer/filter frontend for an ADSL CODEC. In: IEEE design automation conference, pp 1–6
5. Funaba S, Kitagawa A, Tsukada T, Yokomizo G (2000) A fast and accurate method of redesigning analog subcircuits for technology scaling. Anal Integr Circ Signal Process 25(9):299–307
6. Hammouda S, Dessouky M, Tawfik M, Badawy W (Oct 2004) Analog IP migration using design knowledge extraction. In: IEEE custom integrated circuits conference, pp 333–336
7. Shyu Y, Lin C, Lin J, Chang S (2009) A g_m/I_D-based synthesis tool for pipelined analog to digital converters. In: 2009 International Symposium on VLSI Design, Automation and Test, Hsinchu, pp 299–302
8. Piccinni G, Avitabile G, Coviello G, Talarico C (2016) G_m over I_D design for UWB distributed amplifier. In: 2016 IEEE 59th International Midwest Symposium on Circuits and Systems (MWSCAS), Abu Dhabi, pp 1–4
9. Enz C, Chalkiadaki M (2015) Nanoscale MOSFET modeling for low-power RF design using the inversion coefficient. In: 2015 Asia-Pacific Microwave Conference (APMC), Nanjing, pp 1–3
10. Ou J, Ferreira PM. Implications of small geometry effects on gm/I_D based design methodology for analog circuits. In: IEEE transactions on circuits and systems II: express briefs
11. Hernández Sanabria E, Amaya Palacio J, Herrera HH, Van Noije W (2017) A design methodology for an integrated CMOS instrumentation amplifier for bioespectroscopy applications. In: 2017 CHILEAN conference on electrical, electronics engineering, information and communication technologies (CHILECON), Pucon, pp 1–7
12. Castagnola JL, García-Vázquez H, Dualibe FC (2018) Design and optimisation of a cascode low noise amplifier (LNA) using MOST scattering parameters and g/Iratio. In: 2018 IEEE 9th Latin American symposium on circuits & systems (LASCAS), Puerto Vallarta, pp 1–4
13. Hillebrand T, Hellwege N, Taddiken M, Tscherkaschin K, Paul S, Peters-Drolshagen, D (2016) Stochastic LUT-based reliability-aware design method for operation point dependent CMOS circuits. In: 2016 MIXDES—23rd International Conference Mixed Design of Integrated Circuits and Systems, Lodz, pp 363–368

Vehicle Speed Warning System and Wildlife Detection Systems to Avoid Wildlife-Vehicle Collisions

S. R. Bhagyashree, T. Sonal Singh, J. Kiran and Likhitha S. Padmini

Abstract One serious problem that all the developing nations are facing today is injuries and death of animals due to road accidents. Report says that, there are around 300,000 collisions per year. However, many of the databases exclude accidents that have vehicle damage less than $1,000 (https://apiar.org.au/wpcontent/uploads/2017/07/23_APJCECT_ICT-268-281.Pdf, [1]). Accidents lead to the reduction in wildlife. Eventually, this may lead to reduction and endangered of rare species. A system has to be designed to overcome this problem. In this paper, the problem is addressed by focusing on designing an IoT-based system which will perform two functions one is alerting the driver whenever an animal is nearer to the vehicle and the second one is alerting the driver whenever he exceeds the speed limit, especially in the forest region.

Keywords Injuries · Accidents · IoT-based system

1 Introduction

In the current scenario, India accounts for 10% of global road accidents. Of which around 1.46 lakh fatalities are being observed annually and this happens to be the highest in the world. The collision between wildlife and vehicles is more severe in forest regions. Administrative Departments working for public safety, road security and wildlife protection aspire for a stable solution. Structures like fences and underground passages are used for protecting the wildlife. The problem with this is it cannot be used for the whole forest region. In addition to the usage of expensive fences and underground passages for animals, other devices like light reflectors or ultrasound noise generators are also used. However, usage of these devices tuned out to be ineffective. To acquire more knowledge about the behavior of wild animals RFID, thermal cameras and other devices are being used. Incidentally, these devices

S. R. Bhagyashree (✉) · T. Sonal Singh · J. Kiran · L. S. Padmini
Department of ECE, ATME College of Engineering, Mysuru, India
e-mail: bhagyashreeraghavan@gmail.com

© Springer Nature Singapore Pte Ltd. 2019
V. Sridhar et al. (eds.), *Emerging Research in Electronics, Computer Science and Technology*, Lecture Notes in Electrical Engineering 545,
https://doi.org/10.1007/978-981-13-5802-9_84

are not used as assistive devices in the prevention of wildlife collision. When cost becomes the parameter of concern, GPS and ultrasonic proximity technology find huge applications [2].

The movement and the presence of wildlife are estimated, using simple and less expensive ultrasonic proximity sensors integrated into small wireless devices installed in automobile vehicles. The work provides a solution to wildlife-vehicle collisions problem by providing an audio indication to the driver whenever the wildlife approaches near the vehicle. The challenge of this system is the sensor integration in a low-power and low-cost hardware platform [3]. The proposed work addresses the above-mentioned challenges and provides a cost effective, user-friendly solution. Organization of paper is as follows. In this paper, Sect. 1 speaks about introduction. Section 2 focuses on literature survey. Section 3 gives an insight on design methodology. In Sect. 5, results are discussed. Conclusion and future work are discussed in the last section.

2 Literature Survey

In India, in Bandipur National park, accidents occurred due to over speed, have led to the death of wild animals. Around 20 spotted deer, 2 leopards, 2 tigers and 6 elephants have been killed due to road accidents [4]. The representation in Fig. 1 indicates the number of animals killed and injured between the years of 1990 and 2017.

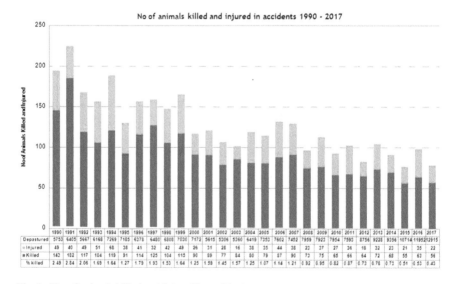

Fig. 1 No. of animals killed and injured in accidents

In New Forest of southern England 132 ponies, 43 cattle, 2 sheep were killed in 2013. In 2015, 80 ponies, 26 cattle were killed. In 2016, 92 ponies, 34 cattle were killed.

From the graph, it is clear that large number of animals are being killed due to road accidents. This paper focuses on alerting the driver whenever the speed exceeds the limit in the forest range and alarming him until he brings the speed to the normal [5].

Between January and June 2007, around 423 animals belonging to 29 different species have died on NH212 and NH67 of Karnataka. Now with increased number of vehicles and increased travelers, the road accidents will also eventually increase [6].

GPS and GSM based system is designed for tracking the vehicles moving from one place to another place. GPS (Global Positioning System) provides the current location of the vehicle. GPRS sends the tracking information to the server. The device mounted in the interior of the vehicle whose location is to be determined on the Web page is supervised on real-time basis. Whenever the driver is on the wrong path and whenever he feels drowsy, an intimation is sent to the owner. In addition to that, the buzzer produces sound and that will make the driver to become alert [4].

The safety of vehicle is very essential in case of public transport. Authors considered over speed as one of the main reasons of increasing accidents. They have mentioned that, though good number of techniques is available for monitoring the excess speed; most of them need lot of workforce. Hence, they have a proposed a system that continuously monitors the location of the vehicle using GPS coordinates. From the data that are gathered, speed of the vehicle is calculated. Using the same information, they have even identified the location and the maximum speed that is allowable in that particular region. Whenever the driver exceeds the limits, an information will be sent to the vehicle owner. The disadvantage of this system is, it requires two power supplies [5].

Bhagyashree et al. have discussed using GPS and GSM for identifying the location patients suffering from Alzheimer's disease and giving intimation to the caregivers about their location [7].

Dhinakaran K, Srinath S, Sriram S and Venkateshwar R proposed Global Positioning System-based system for finding the location of the people. The system keeps track of people who are traveling and informs the preferred contacts, whenever the traveler is off the route. Contacts of highest preference will have highest priority. This work will save the life of the people during unpredicted situations [8].

3 Design Methodology

The representation in Fig. 2, indicates the block diagram of the vehicle tracking system using proximity sensor. The proposed road-crossing early-alert system uses multiple ultrasonic proximity-sensing unit integrated into a small, low-power and low-cost WSN architecture.

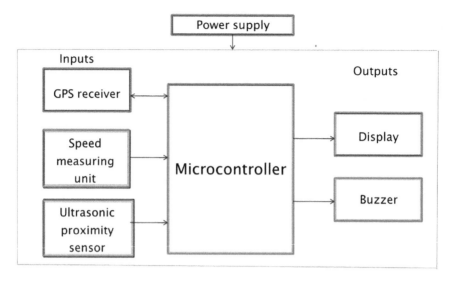

Fig. 2 Block diagram

More in detail, the network is equipped with ultrasonic proximity sensors with different orientations. GPS receiver keeps updating the microcontroller regarding the coordinates. Microcontroller compares the read coordinates with the coordinates stored in memory that are identified as forest coordinates. When they match, it infers the driver with both audio and visual alert regarding the forest region. In the forest region, the speed-measuring unit keeps track of the speed and whenever the speed exceeds the limit, the driver will be intimated through buzzer. While moving in the forest region if the proximity detector detects any wildlife then the microcontroller has to send a message to the display and a signal to the buzzer. This helps the driver to take appropriate action.

4   Flowchart

The representation in Fig. 3 indicates the flowchart of speed warning system and wildlife detection systems to avoid wildlife-vehicle collision.

At first, the system initializes the GPS receiver and controller and then it receives the geolocation of the vehicle. If the vehicle is in the forest region, then the controller by means of LCD and buzzer intimates the driver to say that he is in the forest region. Then the system will check for the speed of the vehicle. If the speed of the vehicle is above the limit specified, then the driver will be alerted through the buzzer. The proximity sensor will help in detecting the obstacles. If an obstacle is detected, then the driver will be alerted through the buzzer.

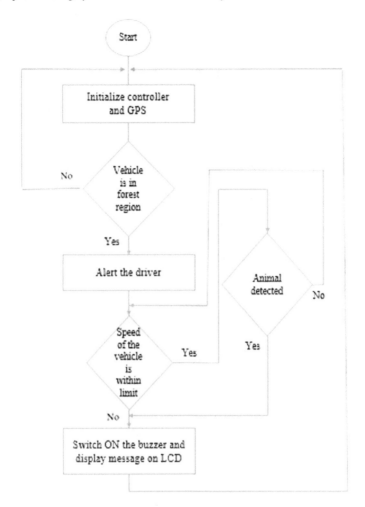

Fig. 3 Flowchart of vehicle tracking system

5 Result

This topic includes the obtained result of each step. Initially, when the power is switched on, the LCD displays as below. Figure 4 shows the GPS receiver setup.

GPS receiver is interfaced with Arduino Uno and LCD. Figure 5 shows the Latitude and longitude of location of interest.

Figure 6 shows the setup, comprises of proximity sensor, GPS receiver and LCD interface. Figure 7 shows the output of the proximity sensor.

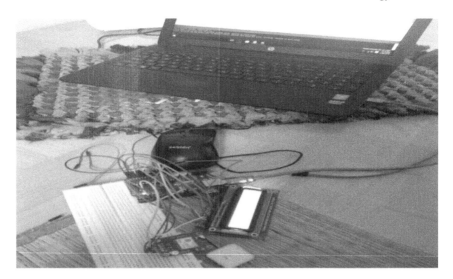

Fig. 4 Setup of the GPS receiver

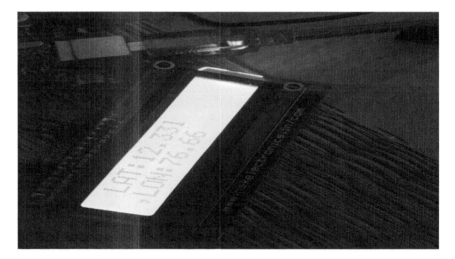

Fig. 5 Latitude and longitude of location of interest

6 Conclusion and Future Work

An accident in the forest region leads to reduction in wildlife. Driving the vehicle with limited speed and taking necessary action when the wildlife is close by will provide solution to the above problem. In this work, in both the situations, the driver is alerted through buzzer and display. In this work, proximity sensors are used to sense the obstacle. The disadvantage in this work is that proximity sensors have limitation

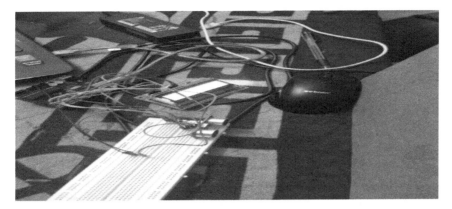

Fig. 6 Setup

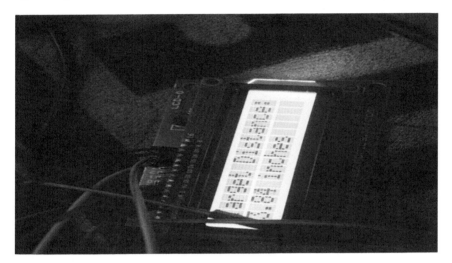

Fig. 7 Display when the obstacle is nearby

with respect to range. In future work, the proximity sensors can be replaced by radar sensors. The future work may also include applying automatic brake system whenever the wildlife is nearby. As of now, this system does not provide any information during the occurrence of accidents. In future, this can be implemented with ease of coding by using raspberry pi processor or any conventional microcontroller and GSM.

Acknowledgements The authors are thankful to Principal and Management of ATMECE, Mysuru.

References

1. https://apiar.org.au/wpcontent/uploads/2017/07/23_APJCECT_ICT-268-281.Pdf
2. https://www.globalspec.com/learnmore/sensors_transducers_detectors/proximity_presence_sensing/ultrasonic_proximity_sensors
3. Anusha A, Ahmed SM. Vehicle tracking and monitoring system to enhance the safety and security driving using IOT. In: 2017 international conference on recent trends in electrical, electronics and computing technologies
4. Jyothi P, Harish G. Design and implementation of real time vehicle monitoring, tracking and controlling system. In: 2016 international conference on communication and electronics systems (ICCES)
5. Kodali RK, Sairam M. Over speed monitoring system. In: 2016 2nd international conference on contemporary computing and informatics (ic3i)
6. Selvan KM, Sridharan N, John S (2012) Roadkill animals on national highways of Karnataka, India. J Ecol Nat Environ 4(14):363–365
7. Bhagya Shree SR, Sheshadri HS, Shivakumar R, VinayKumar HS. Design of embedded system for tracking and locating the patient suffering from Alzheimer's disease. In: 2014 IEEE international conference on computational intelligence and computing research, pp 1–5, 18 Dec−20 Dec 2014
8. Dhinakaran K, Srinath S, Sriram S, Venkateshwar R. GPS based tracking system for transit objects. In: 2017 third international conference on science technology engineering & management (ICONSTEM)

Camera Raw Image: A Study, Processing and Quality Analysis

K. Murugesh and P. K. Mahesh

Abstract RAW is a digital file contains the camera-captured image data regarding the sensor pixels values and text information. The raw is being highlighted as digital negative and varies with the formats, which depend on hardware manufacturer. The raw processing is significant to ignore the duplication of data, to economize the space needed, to ease image file operations, and to have an uninterrupted capturing. The image quality is the substantial parametric quantity which determines the visual of the captured raw. The most extreme resolution with no inbuilt compression (raw) results in high image from any digital camera. The proposed workflow is to extract the contents of raw sensor information from the raw files and processing and displaying the information in image format. The raw test files were gathered from cameras by different manufactures. The MATLAB R2016a has been used for executing the workflow and analysis purpose. The display quality is ensured by the performance parametric—Quality of Image Improvement (QOII), and also the file size reduction ratio was analyzed.

Keywords Raw image · Sensor information · QOII · Reduction ratio

1 Introduction

RAW file carries the camera sensor pixel data, and uncompressed and image text information of a captured image. The hardware (camera) manufacturer decides a file format/extension of digital negative (raw); a commonly used format for raw is .dng file format. Raw information from the sensor clearly contains data about a scene; however, it is not characteristically conspicuous to human eye. Raw image file's image intensity is a single channel, conceivably with a nonzero least incentive to denote the black that contains 10–14 bits information for digital cameras. Instead of discussing regarding a white value, no pixel values of raw will be larger than the

K. Murugesh (✉) · P. K. Mahesh
Department of ECE, ATME College of Engineering, Mysuru 570028, India
e-mail: muru.global@gmail.com

© Springer Nature Singapore Pte Ltd. 2019
V. Sridhar et al. (eds.), *Emerging Research in Electronics, Computer Science and Technology*, Lecture Notes in Electrical Engineering 545,
https://doi.org/10.1007/978-981-13-5802-9_85

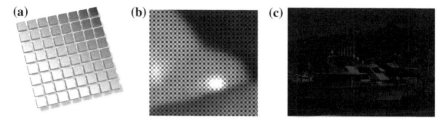

Fig. 1 **a** An area array, **b** detail of raw sensor data image, and **c** Nikon—raw test image

max value that indicates the pixel CCD's saturation point. The camera sensor's pixel dimensions may be smaller than obtained raw result pixel measurements, including a fringe of unexposed pixels to one side (left) and above the significantly exposed ones. Various diverse advances were incorporated in different makes of "computerized camera," yet about those that shoot raw are of the sort known as "mosaic sensor" or CFA cameras. The CFA cameras utilize the 2D array to gather the photons which are captured in the picture. The cluster is comprised of lines and sections of photosensitive identifiers commonly utilizing either charge-coupled device (CCD) or complementary metal oxide semiconductor (CMOS) innovation to shape the picture [1]. The physical view of the sensor area array, sensor raw data of a captured image and a sample test raw image from the Nikon camera are displayed in the Fig. 1a, b, and c respectively.

The JPEG conversion parameters can be varied depending on the make of the camera. But raw capturing is different comparing to JPEG image capturing; the user may get the full access control of raw file through the previously mentioned parts of the conversion. When we shoot raw, the main on-camera settings that affect the caught pixels are ISO speed, the screen speed, and the variable-sized opening (aperture) setting. The other sections of the paper are framed as follows: Sect. 2 and its subsections explain the proposed method of reading, processing, and displaying the raw image; Sect. 3 briefs our experimental results yield from the proposed workflow, and Sect. 4 comments the remarks on results and conclusion.

1.1 Color Filter Array (CFA)

CFA is a spatial multiplexing of RGB channels over the picture-sensor surface. Presently, CCD is broadly utilized as a sensor in the most customer-advanced items, for example, computerized camera, advanced camcorder, and cell phone. Be that as it may, the picture sensor itself does not look about the hues at the procedure of photoelectric change. Consequently, a layer of CFA is used to obtain the color information from the sensor image data. This process is presented in Fig. 2 from which we can see that there is just a single of three essential hues at all pixel. Raw (digital negative) data normally comes as a color filter array (CFA). This is m-by-n

(a)   **(b)**

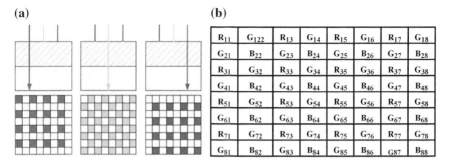

R$_{11}$	G$_{122}$	R$_{13}$	G$_{14}$	R$_{15}$	G$_{16}$	R$_{17}$	G$_{18}$
G$_{21}$	B$_{22}$	G$_{23}$	B$_{24}$	G$_{25}$	B$_{26}$	G$_{27}$	B$_{28}$
R$_{31}$	G$_{32}$	R$_{33}$	G$_{34}$	R$_{35}$	G$_{36}$	R$_{37}$	G$_{38}$
G$_{41}$	B$_{42}$	G$_{43}$	B$_{44}$	G$_{45}$	B$_{46}$	G$_{47}$	B$_{48}$
R$_{51}$	G$_{52}$	R$_{53}$	G$_{54}$	R$_{55}$	G$_{56}$	R$_{57}$	G$_{58}$
G$_{61}$	B$_{62}$	G$_{63}$	B$_{64}$	G$_{65}$	B$_{66}$	G$_{67}$	B$_{68}$
R$_{71}$	G$_{72}$	R$_{73}$	G$_{74}$	R$_{75}$	G$_{76}$	R$_{77}$	G$_{78}$
G$_{81}$	B$_{82}$	G$_{83}$	B$_{84}$	G$_{85}$	B$_{86}$	G87	B$_{88}$

Fig. 2 **a** Color filter array (CFA) and **b** Bayer-patterned CFA image with size 8×8

cluster of pixels (where m and n are the measurements of the sensor) where every pixel conveys data about a solitary color channel: red–green–blue. The light which falls on any photo-sensor of the CCD is saved as a no. of electrons in single capacitor, and it can be recorded as scalar esteem (value); a solitary pixel cannot hold the 3D nature of perceptible light.

CFAs over a trade-off where information/values about the specified color channels are pictured at different areas by methods for range-specific filters are placed over every pixel. While we may just know a color esteem at any pixel area, we can estimate the other color esteems from close-by neighbors of those hues are known, called as demosaicking and produce the m-by-n-by-3 cluster of RGB esteems at all pixel area we normally anticipate from a color digital image [2].

The well-known Bayer CFA design is presented in Fig. 2. There are twice the same no. of pixels that indicate the green light in a Bayer cluster picture on the grounds that human eye is more sensible to changes in green shades, and it is all the more firmly corresponded with the view of chroma of a scene [3]. The above shown pattern is genuinely standard; sensors from various camera producers may have an alternate "phase." That is, the "first" color on the upper left pixel might be different. The four choices, normally indicated as "RGGB," "BGGR," "GBRG," and "GRBG," demonstrate the raster-wise introduction of the foremost "four array" of the picture. It is important for a demosaicking calculation to know the right level of the cluster.

2 Proposed Workflow

The proposed approach of converting the raw image to a viewable image and processing the raw image is described in this section with the help of a workflow Fig. 3. So as to work with and show in MATLAB pictures starting from sensory information, we should consider the previously mentioned characteristic of raw information. Figure 3 pictured the work process is a first step in estimating, how to get a correct displayable yield picture from the raw sensor information. The array of two-dimensional

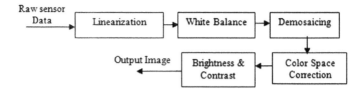

Fig. 3 Proposed workflow of displaying the raw sensor data to an image

raw is not yet a linear image. It is conceivable that the camera employed a nonlinear transformation to the sensor information for saving the data.

2.1　Linearization

A two-dimensional array raw is not a linear image. The possibilities are there for applying a nonlinear transformation to sensor information for storing requirements in the camera. Additionally, the raw information from the camera's imaging sensor contains plenty of meta-data about the pixel esteems and exposing itself. If that case, the digital negative meta-data carries a table of values in a subimage file directory which is created from the image information.

The linearization is a process of representing the raw array data with the meta-information with ten to fourteen bits. The operation is to locate the dark-level pixel value and saturation pixel value as below and complete a relative change to the pixels of the raw data to make it standardized and linearized to [0, 1]. Likewise, as a result of sensor clamor, it is conceivable that there exist esteems in the cluster which are over the hypothetical extreme esteem or underneath the dark level. These ought to be cut off. There may exist an alternate dark level or saturation level for all the four Bayer color channels which is assumed as a single level.

2.2　White Balancing

The scaling of individual c-channel in the CFA by a suitable add up to white adjust the picture is being executed in white-balancing process. Since just the proportion of three hues matters, we can subjectively set one channel's multiplier to 1; this is normally improved the situation for green pixels. The value of the multipliers for another two channels (red and blue) can be fixed to any esteem as the user need. The Exif data present in raw file contains standard multiplier esteems for various standard illuminants; here we utilize the multipliers the camera figured at the season of shooting. Once the values are identified, multiply each red-area pixel inside the picture by the red multiplier and each blue-area pixel by the blue multiplier [4].

(a)   **(b)**

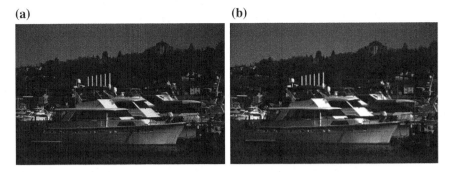

Fig. 4 **a** Linearized raw image and **b** white-balanced raw image

The segments are adjusted to guarantee that dark tones are not seen with any shading tint in the created picture. To this end, the RGB segments are duplicated by camera-subordinate constants kr, kg, and kb, separately. More often, these constants are standardized so that kg = 1. A number of the inverses of the multiplier esteems, for [R G B], are found in meta-information subdirectory. Along these lines, we reverse the qualities and after that rescale them all so the green multiplier is 1. The Linearized and White balanced raw image through the proposed work were displayed in the Fig. 4a, b respectively.

2.3 Demosaicking

A demosaicking (likewise demosaicking or debearing) calculation is a procedure employed for recreating a full RGB image from incomplete color tests yield from an image sensor covered with a CFA. Later by applying a demosaicking algorithm, a three-layer RGB (image) variables can be generated. The current RGB picture is perceptible with standard MATLAB displaying procedure. In any case, its pixels have not aligned with the right RGB space that is normal by the working framework or operating systems. The RGB values of pixels which indicate a color basis vector described by the sensor of the camera should be changed to the monitor expected color basis. This can be handled by applying linear transformation, by applying 3 × 3 lattice transformation to all the pixels.

After applying the transformation, we presently have a 16-bit RGB image that has been color amended and exists in the correct color space for displaying. But still it is an image contains values identifying with what was detected, which may not be in a range to display. Scaling the image may brighten it by adding some constants just make it to look gray or by implementing the nonlinear transformation, and this can be handled by gamma and brightness correction. In the typical demosaicking process, the (N × M) red pixels from the mosaic picture are introduced to make a red segment of size 2N × 2M. In particular, the red pixels are duplicated from

(a)   **(b)**

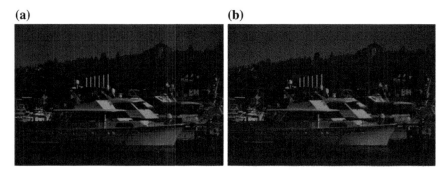

Fig. 5 **a** Demosaicked raw image and **b** color-space-converted raw image

their unique positions in the mosaic picture to the same areas in the red part. The subsequent red segment at that point has pixels just at positions $\{(2i, 2j): 0 = I < N, 0 = j < M\}$.

So also green and blue segments of size $2N \times 2M$ are made from the green and blue pixels of the mosaic picture, individually. The 3NM missing pixels in all the red and blue segments (and also the 2NM missing pixels in the (green part) are then captured by means of interjection. In this approach, four segments are made. Pixels indicated as r, G, g, and b are utilized to make main, second, third, and fourth parts, individually [5]. A case of this option demosaicking with $M = N = 2$ is given by

$$\begin{vmatrix} r(0,0) & G(0,0) & r(0,1) & G(0,1) \\ g(0,0) & b(0,0) & g(0,1) & b(0,1) \\ r(1,0) & G(1,0) & r(0,1) & G(1,1) \\ g(1,0) & b(1,0) & g(1,1) & b(1,1) \end{vmatrix} = \begin{bmatrix} r(0,0) & r(0,1) & G(0,0) & G(0,1) \\ r(1,0) & r(0,1) & G(1,0) & G(1,1) \\ \\ g(0,0) & g(0,1) & b(0,0) & b(0,1) \\ g(1,0) & g(1,1) & b(1,0) & b(1,1) \end{bmatrix} \qquad (1)$$

Interpolation is then connected to every part independently to obtain four parts of size $2N \times 2M$. It is significant that before interpolation, the first mosaic picture can be recovered from the yield parts coming about because of either approach [6]. However, contingent upon interpolation calculation utilized, the first pixel esteems may not be recoverable after the interpolation. The demosaicked raw test image is presented in Fig. 5a.

2.4   Color Space Conversion

The demosaicked RGB image is distinguishable with a standard image processing tools' displaying function. In all cases, its pixels may not be in right RGB space that is anticipated by the working framework. As mentioned earlier, any given pixel's RGB esteems, which indicates a vector in the color base is determined by the camera's sensors, must be changed over to some color base which the screen anticipates [7]. The linear transformation can be used for performing the same, so there is a need for applying 3×3 matrix transmutations to each pixel. But right matrix to apply can be hard to find. The color coordinates of a RGB system (xrxr, yryr), (xgxg, ygyg) and (xbxb, ybyb) and its reference white (XWXW, YWYW, ZWZW), a strategy to calculate the 3×3 lattice for RGB—XYZ conversion.,

$$\begin{bmatrix} X \\ Y \\ Z \end{bmatrix} = [M] \begin{bmatrix} R \\ G \\ B \end{bmatrix} \tag{2}$$

where,

$$[M] = \begin{bmatrix} S_rX_r & S_gX_g & S_bX_b \\ S_rY_r & S_gY_g & S_bY_b \\ S_rZ_r & S_gZ_g & S_bZ_b \end{bmatrix}; \; X_r = \frac{x_r}{y_r}; \; Y_r = 1; \; Z_r = \frac{\left(1 - x_r - y_r\right)}{y_r}$$

$$X_g = \frac{x_g}{y_g}; \; Y_g = 1; \; Z_g = \frac{\left(1 - x_g - y_g\right)}{y_g}; \; X_b = \frac{x_b}{y_b}; \; Y_b = 1; \; Z_b = \frac{\left(1 - x_b - y_b\right)}{y_b}$$

$$\begin{bmatrix} S_r \\ S_g \\ S_b \end{bmatrix} = \begin{bmatrix} X_r & X_g & X_b \\ Y_r & Y_g & Y_b \\ Z_r & Z_g & Z_b \end{bmatrix}^{-1} \begin{bmatrix} X_w \\ Y_w \\ Z_w \end{bmatrix} \tag{3}$$

To implement this matrix properly, the RGB esteems should be in the normal and linear range of [0.0, 1.0]. In particular, RGB esteems need the transformation (for instance, partitioning by 255 and after that raising them to exponent). The backward lattice (i.e., the lattice changing over XYZ to RGB) is figured by inverting lattice [M] above. The color-space-converted raw test image is presented in Fig. 5b.

2.5 Brightness and Gamma Correction

We currently have a 16-bit RGB image that has been demosaicked and exists in the correct space to display. But, yet it is a linear image with values denoting with what was detected, which may not be in a range suitable for being shown. We can increase the brightness level of image by scaling it (introducing a constant would simply influence it to look gray), or something more difficult, e.g., using a transformation (nonlinear). As a measure of simple brightness increment, we can find the mean luminance of the picture and afterward scale it; hence, the mean luminance is some more sensible esteem. In this theme, we (reasonably) scale the image with the goal that the mean luminance is one-fourth the most extreme.

The picture is as yet linear, which will nearly conviction not be the best to display (dull areas will show up excessively dim, and so on). Let us use a "gamma correction"

(a)   **(b)**

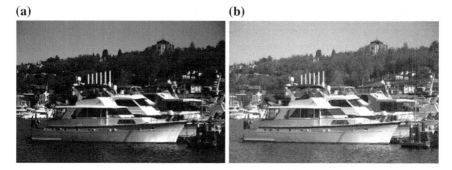

Fig. 6 **a** Brightness-corrected raw image and **b** gamma-corrected raw image

power factor to this picture as a basic method to fix the issue. Regardless of the way that the conventional sRGB compression method utilizes a power factor with $\gamma = 1/2.4$ and a linear toe area for the most reduced qualities, this is regularly approximating $\gamma = 1/2.2$ compression. Note that, it is needed to apply a function to the image that has been scaled to be in the range [0, 1]. Gamma correction can be implemented to remove the GC which has the capacity to evacuate lack of clarity in color-corrected image to some level, yet it is hard to accomplish an ideal exchange off between the over-saturation of close-extend areas and the complete dehazing of long-extend areas.

With the increment in the correction factor, the blurred area in long-range region gets clearer but the close-range region becomes darker. The conventional GC [8] is expressed by

$$I_g = I^\tau \tag{4}$$

The brightness-corrected raw image displayed in Fig. 6a shows clearly that the dark regions in Fig. 5b have been corrected to a viewable image. The next step is to further correction with respect to the gamma power factor; hence, the raw image can be displayed with more clarity. Figure 6b shows the gamma-corrected raw image in which the clarity of the image is still better than the brightness-corrected raw image.

3 Experimental Results

The blocks from Fig. 3 have been executed using MATLAB (R2016a), and the respective results of each block were presented in the corresponding sections. The raw test images had been collected from different camera brands like NIKON, SONY, CANON; the processed file size and its reduction ratio are listed for different raw files in Table 1. Figure 7 displays the block-wise results for the proposed workflow using the collected raw test images. Also an analysis was performed, in which the

Table 1 Raw image size versus proposed image size with size reduction ratio

Raw image	Raw size (Mb)	Proposed size (Mb)	[a]Reduction ratio (%)	Raw image	Raw size (Mb)	Proposed size (Mb)	[a]Reduction ratio (%)
A550	27.33	4.13	6.62	CAL	15.66	1.10	14.19
NEX3N	31.19	3.43	9.08	RX10	38.94	2.48	15.71
A77V	46.80	4.93	9.50	GPS	25.97	1.64	15.87
NEX-5R	31.25	2.96	10.55	NEX7	46.83	2.88	16.29
1DX	36.96	3.50	10.56	ISO100	31.38	1.91	16.45
D1	5.33	0.50	10.72	P7100	19.53	1.12	17.49
NEX-6	31.24	2.87	10.87	A58	38.70	2.01	19.27
D7000	31.18	2.69	11.60	NX100	28.37	1.43	19.87
D3	23.62	1.96	12.04	A35	31.14	1.55	20.09
P340	23.68	1.97	12.05	NX300	40.23	1.93	20.89
1S2	27.77	2.15	12.89	NTI	23.95	1.14	21.06
SHIP	15.63	1.21	12.89	D5100	31.31	1.20	26.03
A350	27.16	1.97	13.78				

[a]Reduction Ratio (%) in hundreds

(a) **(b)** **(c)** **(d)** **(e)** **(f)** **(g)** **(h)**

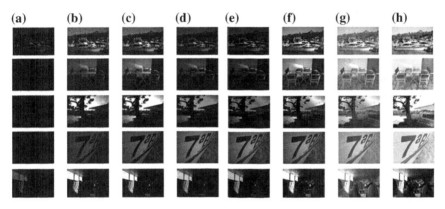

Fig. 7 **a** Raw test images, **b** linearized raw images, **c** white-balanced image, **d** demosaicked image, **e** color-space-converted image, **f** brightness-corrected image, **g** gamma-corrected image, and **h** unprocessed raw image

file size reduction ratio between the raw and the processed image files was compared and plotted in Fig. 8.

The file size reduction ratios have been calculated by using the concept of compression ratio. Thus, the reduction ratio is calculated from the below-mentioned formula.

$$\text{Reduction Ratio} = \frac{\text{Raw Image File Size}}{\text{Processed Image File Size}} \quad (5)$$

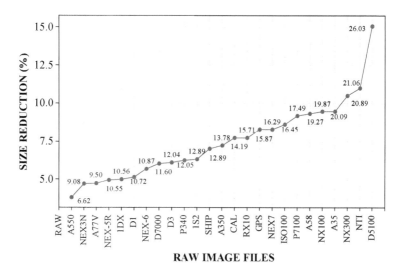

Fig. 8 Raw image files versus size reduction ratio

Table 2 Quality of Image Improvement (QOII) in % for raw test images

Raw	SNR raw	SNR	QOII (%)	Raw	SNR raw	SNR	QOII (%)
SHIP	13.14	16.35	24.42	P7100	11.04	11.98	8.56
NX3N	12.57	14.96	19.07	NEX7	12.65	13.71	8.39
A35	11.74	13.79	17.46	NTI	10.54	11.33	7.50
RX10	11.35	13.25	16.68	D3	12.32	13.16	6.88
5R	11.02	12.74	15.65	CAL	12.22	12.91	5.62
1S2	9.17	10.48	14.29	A77V	12.91	13.55	4.93
GPS	9.92	11.26	13.48	A58	15.31	16.06	4.90
D5100	9.46	10.69	12.99	NX100	11.96	12.46	4.19
A350	11.47	12.86	12.12	1DX	14.46	14.58	0.83
P340	11.60	12.98	11.96	D1	14.65	14.62	−0.14
D7000	16.78	18.68	11.30	A550	12.10	11.60	−4.08
ISO100	11.48	12.64	10.15	NX300	10.28	8.92	−13.24
NEX-6	11.41	12.42	8.85				

The signal-to-noise ratio (SNR) is a significant parameter which describes the quality of the image. The performance analysis based on the SNR for the raw and processed image is listed in Table 2.

In this work, the SNR of unprocessed raw test images and the images obtained as a result of proposed method has been compared. The Quality of Image Improvement (QOII) in percentage was calculated using the following expression.

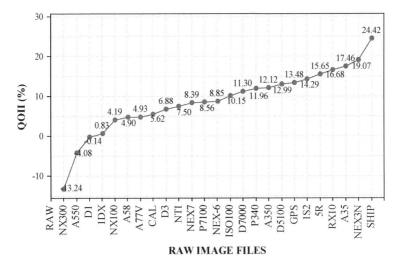

Fig. 9 Quality of Image Improvement (QOII %) for raw test images

$$\text{QOII } (\%) = \left(\frac{\text{SNR of Processed Image}}{\text{SNR of Raw Image}} - 1 \right) \times 100 \qquad (6)$$

The SNR comparison between raw test images and the images obtained as a result of implementing the proposed workflow was done, and the comparison results have been presented in Fig. 9. The proposed method yields good results in the size reduction ration metrics up to 25%. In case of QOII metrics, the proposed workflow yields an efficiency of 88%. The QOII varies with respect to the different camera manufactures. Figure 9 displays the QOII percentage with respect to the raw test Images. The experimental result briefs that the proposed workflow is capable handling the raw images from any camera manufacture.

4 Conclusion

The proposed workflow was implemented as a step-by-step process using the MAT-LAB R2016a. The raw test images were collected from the different cameras of various manufactures. The displayable image was obtained from the proposed workflow from the raw test images, and the comparison analyses were done based on the size reduction ratio and the Quality of Image Improvement percentage with respect to SNR. The workflow was executed, the data yielded as output was tabulated along with the above-mentioned space saving and image quality analysis metrics. The proposed workflow yields good reduction ratio for all the test images. The image quality improvement metrics also yields 88% percentage of results and still need to improve further in the future works. This proposed workflow with further more improvement will gain more storage space saving comparing along with the improved QOII % to the traditional image displaying methods.

References

1. Sumner RC (2014) Processing raw images in image processing tools. Department of Electrical Engineering, UC Santa Cruz, pp 1–15
2. Fraser B (2004) Understanding of digital raw capture. White paper of Adobe Systems Incorporated
3. Koh C, Mukherjee J, Mitra SK (Nov 2003) New efficient methods of image compression in digital cameras with color filter array. IEEE Trans Consum Electron 49(4):1448–1456
4. Nikitenko D, Wirth M (2007) White-balancing algorithms in colour photograph restoration. In: IEEE international conference on systems, man and cybernetics, pp 1037–1042
5. Khashabi D, Nowozin S, Jancsary J, Fitzgibbon AW (2014) Joint demosaicing and denoising via learned nonparametric random fields. IEEE Trans Image Process 23(12):4968–4981
6. Hernandez-Cabronero M, Marcellin MW, Blanes I, Serra-Sagrista J (2018) Lossless compression of color filter array mosaic images with visualization via JPEG 2000. IEEE Trans Multimed 20(2):257–269
7. Takeuchi M, Saika S, Sakamoto Y, Matsuo Y, Katto J (2018) A study on color-space conversion method considering color information restoration. In: IEEE international conference on consumer electronics (ICCE), pp 1–2
8. Ju MY, Ding C, Zhang DY, Guo YJ (2018) Gamma correction based visibility restoration for single Hazy images. IEEE Signal Process Lett (Early Access) 1–5

An Image Processing Approach for Compression of ECG Signals Based on 2D RLE and SPIHT

M. B. Punith Kumar, T. Shreekanth, M. R. Prajwal and N. S. Shashank

Abstract This paper proposes an image processing approach for compression of ECG signals based on 2D compression standards. This will explore both inter-beat and intra-beat redundancies that exist in the ECG signal leading to higher compression ratio (CR) as compared to 1D signal compression standards which explore only the inter-beat redundancies. The proposed method is twofold: In the first step, ECG signal is preprocessed and QRS detection is used to detect the peaks. In the second step, baseline wander is removed and a 2D array of data is obtained through the cut-and-align beat approach. Further beat reordering is done to arrange the ECG array depending upon the similarities available in the adjacent beats. Then ECG signal is compressed by first applying the lossless compression scheme called the 2D Run Length Encoding (RLE), and then a variant of discrete wavelet transform (DWT) called set partitioning in hierarchical trees (SPIHT) is applied to further compress the ECG signal. The proposed method is evaluated on the selected data from MITs Beth Israel Hospital, and it was conceded that this method surpasses some of the prevailing methods in the literature by attaining a higher compression ratio (CR) and moderate percentage-root-mean-square difference (PRD).

Keywords CR · DWT · PRD · RLE · SPIHT

1 Introduction

An ECG signal is an imperative wellspring of data for cardiologist for the diagnosis of cardiovascular patients. Long-haul ECG observing is prescribed when patients are determined to have gentle cardiovascular issue or disorder, yet at the same time

M. B. Punith Kumar (✉)
PES College of Engineering, Mandya, India
e-mail: punithpes@gmail.com

T. Shreekanth · M. R. Prajwal · N. S. Shashank
Sri Jayachamarajendra College of Engineering, Mysuru, India
e-mail: shreekanth_t@sjce.ac.in

© Springer Nature Singapore Pte Ltd. 2019 981
V. Sridhar et al. (eds.), *Emerging Research in Electronics, Computer Science and Technology*, Lecture Notes in Electrical Engineering 545,
https://doi.org/10.1007/978-981-13-5802-9_86

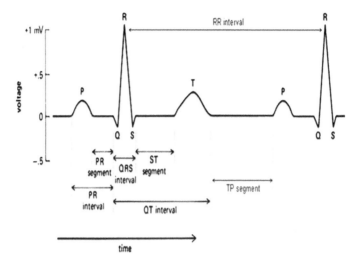

Fig. 1 ECG signal representing P-, Q-, R-, S-, T-, and U-peaks

keeping up with their dynamic way of life [1]. ECG is utilized as a vital signal that gives data about electrical activity of the heart. The standard ECG for clinical applications and vector cardiogram of ECG signals are recorded to screen the variations from the normal value. Because of consistent observation of ECG signals with 24-h checking, the data storage necessity increases within the ambulatory framework. It expands the storage cost. Rather than directly transmitting the stored information, the ECG signal is compressed and then transmitted through normal correspondence channels like telephone line or versatile station. The compression of ECG signals diminishes the cost of transmission and storage. The compression is done to calculate the reduction in data to its maximum value. In the meantime, vital elements of an ECG signal must be protected and then reconstructed. Figure 1 represents an ECG signal with peaks.

The ECG signal comprises P, Q, R, S, T, and U waves. P-wave is primary positive wave. Q, R, and S waves together form a QRS complex. After ventricular activation, the wave is being received. The result of the ventricular depolarization is the T-wave forming a smooth dome. A U-wave takes after the T-wave and goes before the P-wave of the following cycle.

The compression approaches can be divided into three different approaches: time-domain approach, parametric approach, and transform-domain approach. In a typical transfer-domain approach, diverse wavelet-based compression methods are employed. Many data compression applications utilize wavelets because of its time–frequency localization property. This work proposes the application of wavelet-based coding using SPIHT. A 2D approach is more useful because both inter-beat and intra-beat redundancies can be taken as advantage, whereas 1D approach explores only the inter-beat redundancy. Hence, this work proposes a 2D approach for ECG compression.

There are various progressive coding-supported methods proposed for efficient compression of ECG signals. DCT is used in JPEG image compression to remove the unwanted components on image, whereas in SPIHT, wavelet transform is preferred [2]. If signal quality upgrades over time, then bit rate of compressed signal will increase further. After we get the required signal quality, the encoding will stop [3]. A few ECG data compression techniques using RLE and SPIHT encoding and their alterations have been exhibited. Zhitao et al. demonstrated 1D ECG SPIHT coding for signal and multi-lead compression of ECG [4]. Pooyan and others decomposed ECG signals into non-overlapped frames, and on each frame, 1D SPIHT coding is applied [5]. Goudarzi et al. proposed wavelet-dependent SPIHT encoding after transform is applied over multi-wavelet-based 2D array of ECG data [6]. Rezazadehet al. implemented sub-band energy compression before wavelet SPIHT coding equivalent method from Goudarzi for building 2D array of ECG [7]. Tai et al. likewise utilized comparative method to develop 2D array of ECG and proposed modified version of SPIHT coding that partitioned into three parts comprising of wavelet-based transformed image [8]. Sharifahmadian et al. showed for compression of multi-lead ECG signals how to limit redundancy in evaluation available during the sorting phase of SPIHT [9]. Sahraeian and Fatemizadeh proposed the residual image acquired from SPIHT coding applied by vector quantization [10]. Shreekanth et al. proposed a 2D compression of ECG signal based on JPEG and region of interest strategy [11]. This is limited to compressing the ROI at higher compression rate and non-ROI at lower compression rate.

The rest of the paper is categorized as follows. Section 2 provides in detail, the methodology of the proposed algorithm. The results of the proposed work obtained by evaluating it on the MIT database and the results of the proposed method in comparison with existing techniques are provided in Sect. 3. Finally, Sect. 4 concludes the proposed work.

2 Methodology

The block diagram depicted in Fig. 2 represents the proposed compression and decompression stages. Initially, for baseline wander isolation, a moving average filtering is applied and an algorithm based on wavelet technique is utilized for denoising [12]. The next step is to detect QRS complex using Pan–Tomkins algorithm. The duration of beats is evaluated from RR interval. Since the time period for individual beat is unique, normalization of beats in view of amplitude and period standardization method is implemented [13]. Next, the 2D array is created using the beat normalization output.

The reordered beats are utilized to upgrade SPIHT coding by making some adjustments in the beat arrangement in a 2D array of ECG based on the view of their identities. Reordering of beats is done by gathering comparable beats in array. RLE is then applied to the 2D array that will reduce the array to the values representing a simple count for every successive runs. Then DWT is applied on the ECG followed by

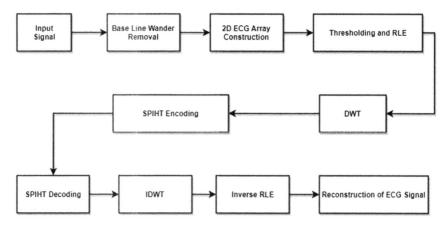

Fig. 2 Block diagram representation for 2D ECG compression using RLE and SPIHT encoding

SPIHT encoding to perform the compression explained below. The proposed method is as shown in Fig. 2.

2.1　Removal of Baseline Wander

This section explains the proposed method implemented to remove baseline wander in ECG. While recording an ECG, the variations in baseline happen when patient respires and are represented in sinusoidal domain specifying the frequency component.

There is a variation in the ECG's amplitude by 15% due to respiration thus resulting in baseline wandering. The baseline wander is removed by performing the moving average filtering on the signal with a span of 150 samples as depicted in Eq. (1). The baseline drift is eliminated by subtracting the original signal with the smoothened version of it.

$$S_{MA} = \frac{1}{n} \sum_{i=0}^{n-1} S_{M-i} \tag{1}$$

where S_M, S_{M-1}, S_{M-2}, ..., $S_{M-(n-1)}$ are the samples of the signal baseline wandered signal S. The above operation results in smoothing of the signal S. Then the difference between the original signal and the moving averaged signal is obtained to arrive at the signal with baseline wander being removed as depicted in the middle plots of Figs. 3 and 4.

$$x = S - S_{MA} \tag{2}$$

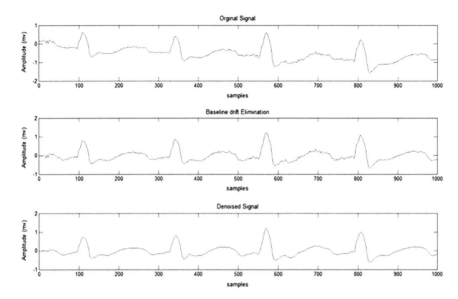

Fig. 3 Baseline wander removal on ECG 109 record of MIT-BIH database

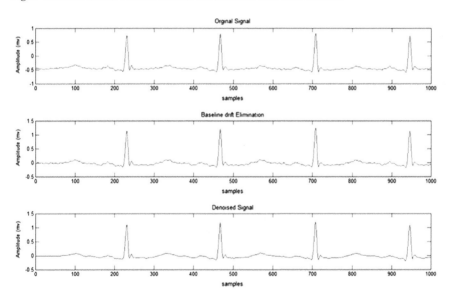

Fig. 4 Baseline wander removal on ECG 205 record of MIT-BIH database

The next step in the process is to remove the noise that has been picked up during ECG acquisition. The original signal $x(n)$ is passed through a low-pass filter $g(n)$ and a high-pass filter $h(n)$. After the filtering, half of the samples will be eliminated according to the Nyquist rule. This constitutes one level of decomposition and can mathematically be expressed as follows:

$$cA(k) = \sum_n x(n)g(2k - n) \tag{3}$$

$$cD(k) = \sum_n x(n)h(2k - n) \tag{4}$$

where $cA(k)$ and $cD(k)$ are the outputs of the low-pass and high-pass filters which represent the approximation and detail coefficients of the signal, respectively, after sub-sampling by 2.

Let $X = \{x(i), 1 \leq i \leq N\}$, be an ECG signal with N samples. The signal is decomposed to eight levels using the db4 wavelet which is applied to calculate the wavelet coefficients $cA8$, $cD8$, $cD7$, ..., $cD1$, where $cA8$ is the coarse signal of eighth level and the detail signals of different levels are $cD8$, $cD7$, ..., $cD1$. The ECG is then reconstructed by keeping only the approximation coefficients through soft thresholding approach. The denoised ECG signal is depicted in the bottom plots as shown in Figs. 3 and 4.

2.2 Detecting QRS Complexes

An ECG comprises P, T, and QRS complexes. The QRS complexes are very weak components of the frequency, and hence, their signal strength is low in P and T waves which are of same frequencies with characteristics as compared with the QRS components which lead to their easy detection. There are various forms of noise that can affect the ECG signal. This may include the contact with testing electrodes, shorting of power rails, contracting of muscles, poor contacts, and respiratory disturbances.

The detection of QRS complexes should be intact and should be able to detect even in the time-varying environment. In this algorithm, the time between the Q to R and R to S is detected. These techniques are utilized for extracting QRS complexes from an actual signal. A normal QRS will be into the form of sine and triangle waves as shifted and scale versions.

The easy method to detect the QRS waves is to pass the ECG to be extracted through the band-pass filter in combination with the high-band-pass filter at frequency 10 Hz. The concentration of the energy is present within 5–15 Hz. Also setting 11 Hz as cut off frequency, the high-frequency components can be removed. The power rail will be operated at 50 Hz frequency, and thus, it can be eliminated.

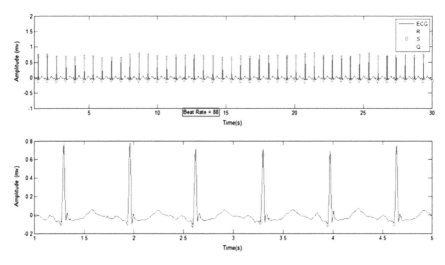

Fig. 5 Detecting QRS complexes for an ECG 109 record of MIT-BIH database

Also for eliminating the components having lower frequency like P/T waves, frequency for HPF is set to 5 Hz as cut off. Therefore, all the frequency components below this cutoff frequency will eliminate the low-frequency components. In this way, the output got is a denoised ECG signal.

Good SNR ratio is obtained at band-pass stage, and thus, threshold values for the signals are decided. Using this threshold, the QRS complexes can be detected. Figure 5 shows the detection of QRS complexes.

2.3 Construction of 2D ECG Array

ECG signals are correlated in two forms, individual ECG cycle called intra-beat correlation and correlation ECG cycles called inter-beat correlation. A suitable technique for compressing a signal is required to perform decorrelation on both types of correlations at very low distortion and for achieving high compression rate. Hence, the ECG signal is arranged into 2D array of ECG data comprising of at least one or more than one normalized heartbeats. In a 2D ECG array, the column indicates the intra-beat correlation, while the rows represent the inter-beat correlation. To obtain the heartbeat duration, the peak intervals among the ECG signals are evaluated. This can be done using various QRS detection complexion techniques.

Due to difference in the time duration between the heartbeats for building 2D data array of ECG, signals should be normalized to a constant value. Here the predictable duration for every heartbeat contains 256 samples, taken from MIT-BIH arrhythmia database. Heartbeat duration is normalized using PAN TOMPKINS method. Interpolation by L factor is done for performing the beat normalization.

Down-sampling of the signal is done by the exact factor, in order to make all the lengths of heartbeat constant. Say x(n) is the interpolation filter's input, up-sampling factor is L, and h(n) is an impulse response, so output Y(n) represented below will be

$$y(n) = \sum_{k=-\infty}^{\infty} x(k)h(n - kL) \tag{5}$$

In between these successive samples, $L - 1$ zeros are inserted by the up-sampler. The inserted zeros are replaced with the interpolated values by the filter h(n) whose operating rate is higher by a factor L over the input. Ensuring of efficient interpolation is done by polyphase filtering. The decimation filter's output y(n) whose impulse is h(n) with down-sampling factor M is given as

$$y(n) = \sum_{k=-\infty}^{\infty} x(k)h(nM_i - kL) \tag{6}$$

The LPF h(n) is responsible for the removal of anti-aliasing effect due to down-sampling of signal. The reverse process is the sampling rate variation. So the resampled bit is brought back to the original one by multi-rate processing. The normalized output is given as

$$Y_j(n) = \sum_{j=0}^{P_j-1} X_k(j)h(nM_j - kL) \tag{7}$$

Here, the jth input beat is $X_k(j)$ and $Y_j(n)$ is the normalized beat output for nth sample and the filter impulse response is h(n), plus samples present in the jth original beat. For the ith beat vector, the up-sampling and down-sampling factors are L and M_j, respectively.

Different techniques are used to build array of 2D ECG data than those implemented in [14]. Every line of array strategy is extracted right after the start of a peak to the next R-wave peak instead of P-wave to P-wave peak of ECG signal. R-wave is the most important compared to Q-wave, because it is simpler to recognize. In some cases of recordings, no P-wave is considered.

DWT is a vital tool for signal processing and also for the compression of the data especially in non-stationary analysis of the signal. In DSP, after inverse wavelet transform is applied, it executes as the tree structures culminate filter banks and reconstruction. In implementation, the factors to be chosen wisely should be the ECG array size, no. of layers of transform, and the pair of filters. The layers will give the resolution of the frequency of the changed and ought to be no less than 4 for sufficient compression. Expanding the layers will be more difficult for evaluation with actual results. Wavelet coefficients are encoded using RLE and SPIHT storing the reconstructed ECG.

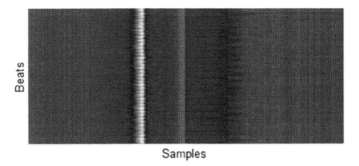

Fig. 6 Mapping of 2D array in gray scale

Detecting P-wave will lead to errors. The array which is 2D type has 256 columns that represent magnitude of ECG with 256 rows specifying the 256 ECG cycles. Mapping of an array representing 2D ECG in gray scale is as shown in Fig. 6 for the MIT-BIH 109 record.

2.4 Run Length Encoding

It is a technique for digital data compression where successive runs are considered as same value data followed by count instead of the original runs. This will definitely decrease the amount of data for storing and transmission. It is a lossless transmission technique.

For example, consider a hypothetical scan line

wwwwwwwwwwbwwwwwwwwwwwbbbwwwwwwwwwwwwwwwwwwbwwwwww

On applying Run Length Encoding compression algorithm to the above hypothetical scan line, the line can be rendered as

10w1b10w3b18w1b6w

The above compressed data can be interpreted as ten w's, one b, ten w's, three b's, eighteen w's, one b, and six w's. The Run Length Encoding algorithm represents the original 49 characters in only 17 characters.

2.5 2D Discrete Wavelet Transform

Wavelet transformation is done when the signal is not stationary. The forward as well as inverse WT is being implemented on the tree structure following reconstruction of the filter banks. The crucial factor for implementation will be the size of the array

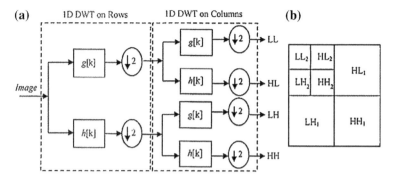

Fig. 7 **a** Level 1 decomposition after 2D DWT and **b** 2D array construction representing wavelet coefficients

with the pair of filters and the number of wavelet layers required for decomposition. The minimum number of layers must be four for determining the closest resolution of frequency. If the number of layers is increased, then the computation will become more difficult. These coefficients are then utilized, and encoding is done using RLE and SPIHT techniques. The level 1 decomposition after 2D DWT and the 2D array construction representing the wavelet coefficients is shown in Fig. 7.

2.6 Thresholding of Wavelet Coefficients

Thresholding of coefficients is defined by

$$T = \sigma\sqrt{2\log(n)} \tag{8}$$

where limit of the threshold is T, n indicates the number samples, and σ is the noise deviation. The threshold or contracting of the wavelet transform will expel the low amplitude noise or, on the other hand undesired signals and accomplish high compression ratio in view of the concentrating ability of the wavelet transform.

2.7 SPIHT

It is the wavelet-depended coding technique that uses the set partitioning algorithm relied on sub-band pyramid for arranging the transformed coefficients. Most important coefficients which are ordered are only utilized by the SPIHT coding which reduces the information required for reconstructing of the original signal.

Desirable bit rate can be achieved on encoded bitstream progressive transmission. Encoding can be stop anytime, permitting the achieved bit rate met precisely or when distortion parameter is achieved. The binary finite representation is achieved in embedded coding. A real number is usually a string of binary digits. To the right of the binary digit are added digit yielding the high precision. The process of encoding can be stopped any time after getting the best real number. Inside the framework, the good signal representation is achieved and the SPIHT encoded can be stopped likewise [8].

After the wavelet transform is performed, the SPIHT develops a quad-tree-like structure on the signal. The low-frequency coefficients will contain the energy of wavelet transformed signal. This gives the view of the parent–child relationship when the coefficients are ordered through the sub-bands' SPIHT uses the relationship for sparing numerous bits, representing unimportant coefficients. The SPIHT calculation depicted as mentioned below:

(i)   Initialization: Firstly, LSP-The significant points which listed are unfilled set. Now, roots are set underlying tree having similarities in the LIP, also that of the list of the LIS (insignificant sets). Let an edge be $T_0 = 2n$ and $n = log2max|(c$ (*i*) (*j*)|, C (i) (j) at(i, j) position of coefficients.
(ii) LIP sorting pass: Within LIP, every coefficient is verified moving to LIP the vital coefficients. The signed bits of coefficients which are critical are encoded.
(iii) LIS sorting pass: A one is sent after two offspring are verified that an entry similar in the LIS, whereas a zero is sent for insignificant entry in LIS.
(iv) Refinement pass: In LSP, every old entry is verified. In the event for an important entry, a one is sent reducing the magnitude of the current threshold. On the off chance that it is unnecessary, a zero is sent.

3   Results

This paper demonstrates 2D DWT-based ECG compression using 2D RLE and SPIHT encoding techniques. The experiments were performed using multiple records of MIT-BIH database. The quality of reconstructed ECG is determined by evaluating performance parameters defined below,

Compression ratio:
It is the ratio of the length of input sequence to that of output sequence multiplied by bits per sample represented as follows:

$$CR = \frac{\text{Length of input stream}}{\text{Length of output stream}} * 11 \tag{9}$$

Percentage-root-mean-square difference:
Reconstructed signal's quality is decided by PRD. In other words, it is the rate of difference between the actual and the reconstructed signals. It defines efficiency of the algorithm. It is represented as

$$\%PRD = \sqrt{\frac{\sum_{n=1}^{N}(x(n) - x'(n))^2}{\sum_{n=1}^{N} x^2(n)}} \qquad (10)$$

where x(n) is the original signal and x'(n) is the reconstructed signal. Also n defines number of samples.

Table 1 shows the results of the proposed technique with their equivalent compression ratio and the PRD. Here the sampling frequency is 360 Hz. The reconstruction of ECG yields better results with minimum percentage of error. The ECG signal is reconstructed at 8 bpp.

Table 2 indicates the comparison of various ECG compression algorithms with the proposed one on the basis of CR and PRD. It can be found that the obtained CR and PRD are comparable with those existing techniques in the literature. Figures 8 and 9 show 1000 samples of original signal, reconstructed and error signal corresponding to record number 102 and 114 of MIT database, respectively.

Table 1 Performance evaluation of the proposed method

MIT-BIII database records	CR	PRD
Record 100	21.9	2.77
Record 102	21.6	3.24
Record 103	21.8	3.08
Record 109	23	2.01
Record 111	22	2.33
Record 113	22	3.17
Record 115	21.8	6.6
Record 117	21.9	1.09
Record 124	21.9	1.25
Average	22	2.84

Table 2 Performance comparison

Compression techniques	CR	PRD
AZTEC [15]	10	28
Improved modified AZTEC [16]	2.76–9.91	4.54–7.99
CORTES [17]	4.8	7.0
JPEG 2000	8	0.86

(continued)

Table 2 (continued)

Compression techniques	CR	PRD
Bilgin [18]	20	3.26
SPIHT [4]	8	1.18
Abo-Zahhad et al. [19]	23.1	1.6
Mukhopadhyay et al. [20]	7.18	0.023
Shreekanth and Shashidhar [11]	10	0.6
Proposed	22	2.84

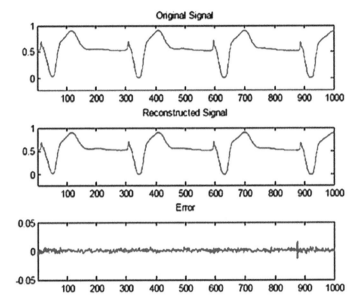

Fig. 8 Waveforms for original ECG, reconstructed ECG after RLE- and SPIHT-based compression, and error signal for record 102

4 Conclusion

In this work, an image processing approach for compression of ECG signals is proposed. The proposed 2D compression of ECG signals has been evaluated using the MIT-BIH arrhythmia database. The improved performance of this method is attributed due to the application of Run Length Encoding scheme prior to the SPIHT coding technique. An average compression ratio (CR) of 22:1 is achieved, and an average percentage-root-mean-square difference (PRD) of 2.84 is reasonable when compared to other techniques in the literature. Also the results indicate that RLE- and wavelet-based compression techniques yield better results when compared to 1D compression techniques. Further, beat reordering and the period normalization of ECG may yield better results in future for achieving good compression rates, and the compression of multi-channel ECG signal is also a challenge.

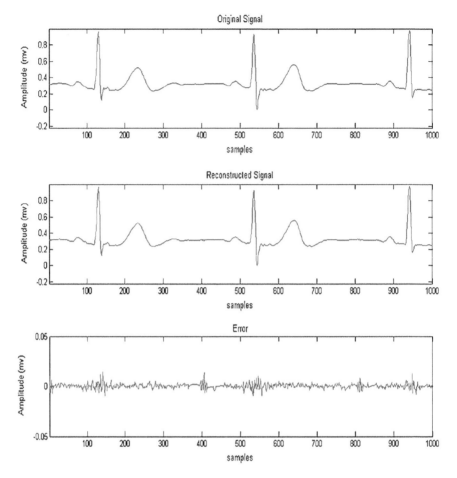

Fig. 9 Waveforms for original ECG, reconstructed ECG after RLE- and SPIHT-based compression, and error signal for record 114

References

1. Chaudhuri S, Pawar TD, Duttagupta S (2009) Ambulation analysis in wearable ECG. Springer Publishing Company, Incorporated
2. Zheyuan X, Xiaping F, Shaoqiang L, Yongzhouand L, Huan Z (2013) Performance analysis for DCT-based coded image communication in wireless multimedia sensor networks. Int J Smart Sensing Intell Syst 6(1)
3. Huang C-Y, Miaou S-G (2001) Transmitting SPIHT compressed ECG data over a next-generation mobile telecardiology testbed. In: Proceedings of the 23rd annual international conference of the IEEE engineering in medicine and biology society, volume 4, pp 3525–3528. IEEE
4. Lu Z, Kim DY, Pearlman WA (2000) Wavelet compression of ECG signals by the set partitioning in hierarchical trees algorithm. IEEE Trans Biomed Eng 47(7):849–856

5. Pooyan M, Taheri A, Moazami-Goudarzi M, Saboori I (2004) Wavelet compression of ECG signals using SPIHT algorithm. Int J Signal Process 1(3):4
6. Moazami-Goudarzi M, Moradi MH, Abbasabadi S (2005) High performance method for electrocardiogram compression using two dimensional multiwavelet transform. In: 2005 IEEE 7th workshop on multimedia signal processing. IEEE, pp 1–5
7. Mohammad Rezazadeh I, Hassan Moradi M, Motie Nasrabadi A (2006) Implementing of SPIHT and Sub-band Energy Compression (SEC) method on two-dimensional ECG compression: a novel approach. In: 27th annual international conference of the engineering in medicine and biology society, IEEE-EMBS 2005. IEEE, pp 3763–3766
8. Tai S-C, Sun C, Yan W-C (2005) A 2D ECG compression method based on wavelet transform and modified SPIHT. IEEE Trans Biomed Eng 52(6):999–1008
9. Sharifahmadian E (2006) Wavelet compression of multichannel ECG data by enhanced set partitioning in hierarchical trees algorithm. In: 28th annual international conference of the IEEE engineering in medicine and biology society, 2006. EMBS'06. IEEE, pp 5238–5243
10. Sahraeian SME, Fatemizadeh E (2007) Wavelet-based 2D ECG data compression method using SPIHT and VQ coding. In: The international conference on" Computer as a Tool", EUROCON 2007. IEEE, pp 133–137
11. Shreekanth T, Shashidhar R. An application of image processing technique for compression of ECG signals based on region of interest strategy. In: International conference on computational vision and bio inspired computing, Coimbatore, Tamil Nadu, India on 21–22 September
12. Sargolzaei A, Faez K, Sargolzaei S (2009) A new robust wavelet based algorithm for baseline wandering cancellation in ECG signals. In: 2009 IEEE international conference on signal and image processing applications (ICSIPA). IEEE, pp 33–38
13. Ramakrishnan AG, Saha S (1997) ECG coding by wavelet-based linear prediction. IEEE Trans Biomed Eng 44(12):1253–1261
14. Houghton AR, Gray D. Making sense of the ECG: a hands-on guide. Hodder Arnold
15. Cox JR, Nolle FM, Fozzard HA, Oliver GC (1968) AZTEC, a preprocessing program for real-time ECG rhythm analysis. IEEE Trans Biomed Eng 2:128–129
16. Kumar V, Saxena SC, Giri VK, Singh D (2005) Improved modified AZTEC technique for ECG data compression: effect of length of parabolic filter on reconstructed signal. Comput Electr Eng 31(4):334–344
17. Abenstein JP, Tompkins WJ (1982) A new data-reduction algorithm for real-time ECG analysis. IEEE Trans Biomed Eng (1):43–48
18. Bilgin A, Marcellin MW, Altbach MI (2003) Compression of electrocardiogram signals using jpeg 2000. IEEE Trans Consum Electron 49(4):833–840
19. Abo-Zahhad M, Al-Ajlouni AF, Ahmed SM, Schilling RJ (2013) A new algorithm for the compression of ECG signals based on mother wavelet parameterization and best-threshold levels selection. Digital Signal Process 23(3):1002–1011
20. Mukhopadhyay SK, Mitra S, Mitra M (2011) A lossless ECG data compression technique using ASCII character encoding. Comput Electr Eng 37(4):486–497

Classification of Service Robot Environments Using Multimodal Sequence Data

P. Saleena and Gopalapillai Radhakrishnan

Abstract The usage of autonomous robots is getting increased day by day. Most of the applications are moving toward automation with the help of robots. This paper mainly focuses on service robots and understanding their working environments. A few robotic scenarios are created using Webots tool, and the data from there are collected as a sequence of images and lidar sensor values. The lidar values are collected with both single layer and multilayer. The environments are analyzed with the help of the collected data. The collected multimodal data are preprocessed in order to reduce the number of features. After that, the collected data are sorted out to suitably characterize each environment, and the machine learning techniques are applied to classify the environments. Different machine learning algorithms like Naive Bayes classifier, support vector machine, decision-tree-like random forest tree, and simple logistic regression are used for the classification, and results are compared with each other.

Keywords Robotic application · Webots · Naïve Bayes · Support vector machine · Decision tree

1 Introduction

Recent developments in robotics are being leveraged in many application areas in the real world. Autonomous robots are conquering most of the applications. Usage of autonomous robots helps to overcome human limitations to a great extent. Each robot is designed for a particular application, and it should have the knowledge about its working environment. Hence, the learning of the environment is a crucial part for

P. Saleena (✉) · G. Radhakrishnan (✉)
Department of Computer Science & Engineering, Amrita School of Engineering,
Amrita Vishwa Vidyapeetham, Bangalore, India
e-mail: saleenaktr@gmail.com

G. Radhakrishnan
e-mail: g_radhakrishnan@blr.amrita.edu

© Springer Nature Singapore Pte Ltd. 2019 997
V. Sridhar et al. (eds.), *Emerging Research in Electronics, Computer Science and Technology*, Lecture Notes in Electrical Engineering 545,
https://doi.org/10.1007/978-981-13-5802-9_87

a robot to be successfully deployed. Each robot's learning behavior is different from each other's according to their application.

Some of the applications of autonomous robots are assisting humans in areas like home, work, assisting in disaster recovery, autonomous vehicles, items delivery from e-commerce sites, etc. This paper focuses on a home service scenario where a robot has to assist humans. In such scenarios, the robot should move through the environment and collect details of that environment continuously. This study focuses on collecting data from the environment and processing the data to get a good understanding of those environments. In order to process the collected environmental details, machine learning algorithms have been used. The data captured from robots are processed as a sequence of data.

Since the size of available data is getting increased day by day, machine learning techniques are getting high priority nowadays. The processing of data becomes easier with machine learning techniques. The methods in machine learning mainly consist of supervised, unsupervised, and reinforcement learning. In supervised, some labels are used to classify the objects in an efficient way. In unsupervised learning, no labels are present. This project mainly focuses on supervised learning with the classification of different environments. If environments are familiar to a robot, then it will classify the objects to that particular environment so that it can work efficiently later.

Remaining sections of this paper are organized as follows. Work related to applications of machine learning technique to discover robot's environments is discussed in Sect. 2. Section 3 discusses the method used in this study to collect and then process the data. The results of the classification and analysis of the results are done in Sect. 4. Conclusions from the study are discussed in Sect. 5.

2 Related Work

This section discusses the works that have been reported in the area of environmental classification. Some of these works for robotics applications have used machine learning techniques.

The application of data mining in the robotics area [1] is investigated by Morteza Moradi et al. by dividing robots in two ways: information collector and systems. The different applications of robots with sundry types of data are discussed in their paper. The paper discusses data mining approaches for robotic data with these two collectors and gathers outlook with some Robocop vision 2050. A related work [2] made an experimental setup with a robot equipped with four sensors that follows a straight-line path to gather information about its working environment.

Vision-based Robot Navigation for Disaster Scenarios [3] discuss how a robot understands a given environment while moving through it and how it can control its gestures appropriately. Principal component analysis with image moments is used for gesture identification in this paper. Analysis of robotic environments done with collected time series data using a set of sensors is discussed in [4]. This work clustered robotic environments with help of sensors.

The work for pedestrian detection uses K-nearest neighbor, Naïve Bayes classifier, and support machine for the analysis [5]. To predict the driver's intent gaze by using lidar or radar data for an autonomous vehicle [6] achieves its goal with artificial neural networks, Bayesian networks, and the Naïve Bayes classifier.

A survey and taxonomy of multimodal machine learning [7] explain the challenges such as representation, translation, alignment, fusion, and co-learning. In this paper, two ways of representation for multimodal data, i.e., joint and coordinated representations are briefly explained. Joint representation uses an early fusion, whereas coordinated representation uses late fusion. For handling lidar type of data, a 3D convolutional neural networks (CNN) for the safe landing of a helicopter [8] make coupling of a volumetric occupancy map with a CNN. Here input is taken from a globally registered lidar points cloud for a predefined area of the region. In this work, the CNN model consists of an input layer followed by one or two convolutional layers, a single dense layer, and a classification output layer.

Pattern identification of robotics environment with help of machine learning techniques using algorithms such as Naive Bayes (NB), logistic regression (LR), multilayer perceptron (MLP), AdaBoost, and support vector machine (SVM) for classification is discussed in [9]. In this paper, a firebird robot is used with two sensors such as an infrared sensor (IR) and thermal imaging sensors. Scenarios created have been classified with an accuracy between 98 and 99%. The proposed work uses image and lidar data for classification.

3   Proposed Method

The work discussed in this paper includes data collection, preprocessing, and classification. Each of these tasks is described below in detail.

3.1   Environmental Setup and Scenario Creation

Data collection for this study is done using Webots simulator. Webots is a robot simulator that provides a complete development environment to model, program, and simulate robots [10]. Webots simulator is used to simulate the robot in different scenarios. An e-puck robot is used for the task. The e-puck robot uses an obstacle avoidance controller for navigation. Each scenario consisted of a rectangle arena of 100 cm × 100 cm. Each scenario encompassed different geometrically shaped objects that have unique colors. The e-puck robot is equipped with an inbuilt camera and a distance sensor. Distance sensors are primarily used for collision avoidance. Additionally, an external lidar sensor is mounted to its turret slot for distance calculation from all the detected objects. Lidar is used for object detection and to calculate its distance from a robot. Preprocessing of the data is done using the R software tool in an efficient manner.

3.2 Data Collection

For the purpose of data collection, four novel scenarios were created using Webots. Each of these scenarios has objects with different shapes and in different colors. The four scenarios used to congregate the data are shown in Fig. 1. For example, Environment-1 contains five objects which are in blue, gray, green, and yellow in color and cylindrical, square, cone, and spherical in shape, respectively.

The e-puck robot has used its inbuilt camera, distance sensor, and an extra lidar sensor. Using the inbuilt camera of an e-puck robot, images of the environment are captured. The position of objects relative to the location of the robot is measured using a lidar sensor that was attached to its turret slot. The lidar collects distance measurements from objects by using light energy emission. In this paper, the data are captured in two distinct ways with lidar. Firstly, lidar squanders data with a single layer which acts as a distance sensor. Secondly, the data collected with 39 layers which retrieve data with the horizontal resolution of 52 and a vertical field of view of 1.17. The robot collects the data in a streamed way. Hence, in real time, the data collected by robots are very huge in volume and comes as a data stream. The data collected has the characteristics of a streamed big data.

For data collection, the robot moves from one corner of the scenario to the other corner, and the data collected during this exploration of the environment are stored

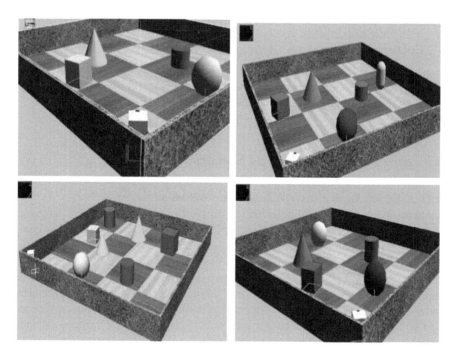

Fig. 1 Scenarios used in simulation

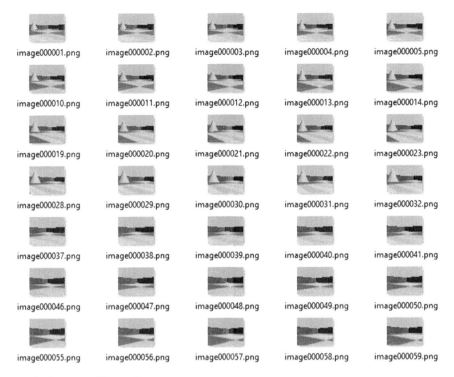

Fig. 2 Sequence of image data

in a file. Samples of image data and lidar data collected are given in Fig. 2 and in Fig. 3, respectively.

Figure 2 consists of a sequence of image data gathered by the e-puck robot. The actual number of images captured by the robot varied between 164 and 190 for one layer. In the given figure, only 35 images are shown out of the total set. Each of the image is captured with respect to robot's basic time step. Webots is configured to set the robot's basic time step as 32 ms. Hence, images of the environment are captured at an interval of 32 ms. The multilayered lidar also collects the data at the same interval.

Figure 3 shows the snapshot of the collected dataset consisting of distance values with respect to x, y, z coordinates and time stamp. This work has initially taken lidar with only one layer so that it acts like a distance sensor. In this case, only x values are getting recorded by lidar since it contains only one layer and with that layer, it can collect only one-dimensional data. The y and z coordinates are stored with zero values. Hence, only x values are used for classification.

Data collection setup was later updated to use multiple layers of lidar beams. Figure 4 shows the lidar data collected with 39 layers. Each lidar point in the cloud is represented by its (x, y, z) coordinates and the depth information of a point in the surface of an object can be calculated with this coordinates value. Each row in the

Fig. 3 Lidar data with
single-layer lidar

```
time=0.752000,x=-0.096299,y=0.000000,z=-0.000000
time=0.880000,x=-0.102829,y=0.000000,z=-0.000000
time=1.008000,x=-0.109301,y=0.000000,z=-0.000000
time=1.136000,x=-0.115692,y=0.000000,z=-0.000000
time=1.264000,x=-0.121990,y=0.000000,z=-0.000000
time=1.392000,x=-0.128204,y=0.000000,z=-0.000000
time=1.520000,x=-0.134332,y=0.000000,z=-0.000000
time=1.648000,x=-0.140375,y=0.000000,z=-0.000000
time=1.776000,x=-0.146332,y=0.000000,z=-0.000000
time=1.904000,x=-0.152210,y=0.000000,z=-0.000000
time=2.032000,x=-0.158003,y=0.000000,z=-0.000000
time=2.160000,x=-0.163711,y=0.000000,z=-0.000000
time=2.288000,x=-0.169345,y=0.000000,z=-0.000000
time=2.416000,x=-0.174885,y=0.000000,z=-0.000000
time=2.544000,x=-0.180291,y=0.000000,z=-0.000000
time=2.672000,x=-0.185608,y=0.000000,z=-0.000000
time=2.800000,x=-0.190852,y=0.000000,z=-0.000000
time=2.928000,x=-0.196017,y=0.000000,z=-0.000000
time=3.056000,x=-0.201109,y=0.000000,z=-0.000000
time=3.184000,x=-0.206198,y=0.000000,z=-0.000000
time=3.312000,x=-0.211220,y=0.000000,z=-0.000000
time=3.440000,x=-0.216173,y=0.000000,z=-0.000000
time=3.568000,x=-0.221060,y=0.000000,z=-0.000000
```

table corresponds to one point in the point cloud, and the first three columns give the x, y, and z coordinates, respectively, and the fourth column gives the layer number. For example, in Fig. 4 first line shows that there is one point of the object which is located at 0.16 m from the x-axis, 0.54 m from y-axis, and 0.82 m from z-axis of the robot's current position. A sequence of points gives a three-dimensional view of objects. The distance to the object is calculated using x, y, and z coordinates and the layer number.

3.3 Preprocessing

Each time when the robot moves from one end to the other, its wheel's speed has minor variations due to the noise factor incorporated in the simulator. Due to this, the data collected have a small variation in the number of samples collected in different trials. In order to use the same number of samples from every trial, some normalization of the data is done. The equation for finding the normalization factor is given in formula (1).

$$NF = \frac{X^1}{X - X^1} \tag{1}$$

Fig. 4 Lidar data with
multilayers

```
x=-0.167172,y=-0.541614,z=-0.823837,distance= 1.000000 layer: 37
x=-0.141722,y=-0.541614,z=-0.828594,distance= 1.000000 layer: 37
x=-0.116138,y=-0.541614,z=-0.832566,distance= 1.000000 layer: 37
x=-0.090444,y=-0.541614,z=-0.835747,distance= 1.000000 layer: 37
x=-0.064664,y=-0.541614,z=-0.838136,distance= 1.000000 layer: 37
x=-0.038823,y=-0.541614,z=-0.839730,distance= 1.000000 layer: 37
x=-0.012945,y=-0.541614,z=-0.840527,distance= 1.000000 layer: 37
x=0.012945,y=-0.541614,z=-0.840527,distance= 1.000000 layer: 37
x=0.038823,y=-0.541614,z=-0.839730,distance= 1.000000 layer: 37
x=0.064664,y=-0.541614,z=-0.838136,distance= 1.000000 layer: 37
x=0.090444,y=-0.541614,z=-0.835747,distance= 1.000000 layer: 37
x=0.116138,y=-0.541614,z=-0.832566,distance= 1.000000 layer: 37
x=0.141722,y=-0.541614,z=-0.828594,distance= 1.000000 layer: 37
x=0.167172,y=-0.541614,z=-0.823837,distance= 1.000000 layer: 37
x=0.192462,y=-0.541614,z=-0.818298,distance= 1.000000 layer: 37
x=0.217571,y=-0.541614,z=-0.811983,distance= 1.000000 layer: 37
x=0.242473,y=-0.541614,z=-0.804898,distance= 1.000000 layer: 37
x=0.267145,y=-0.541614,z=-0.797049,distance= 1.000000 layer: 37
x=0.291563,y=-0.541614,z=-0.788445,distance= 1.000000 layer: 37
x=0.315705,y=-0.541614,z=-0.779092,distance= 1.000000 layer: 37
x=0.339548,y=-0.541614,z=-0.769000,distance= 1.000000 layer: 37
x=0.363068,y=-0.541614,z=-0.758179,distance= 1.000000 layer: 37
x=0.386244,y=-0.541614,z=-0.746639,distance= 1.000000 layer: 37
x=0.409054,y=-0.541614,z=-0.734390,distance= 1.000000 layer: 37
x=0.431475,y=-0.541614,z=-0.721445,distance= 1.000000 layer: 37
x=0.453488,y=-0.541614,z=-0.707816,distance= 1.000000 layer: 37
x=0.475070,y=-0.541614,z=-0.693515,distance= 1.000000 layer: 37
x=0.496202,y=-0.541614,z=-0.678556,distance= 1.000000 layer: 37
x=0.516862,y=-0.541614,z=-0.662953,distance= 1.000000 layer: 37
x=0.537033,y=-0.541614,z=-0.646722,distance= 1.000000 layer: 37
x=0.556694,y=-0.541614,z=-0.629877,distance= 1.000000 layer: 37
x=0.575827,y=-0.541614,z=-0.612435,distance= 1.000000 layer: 37
```

where NF is the normalization factor, X^1 is the least number of images captured from all the environments, and X is the total number of images captured in that particular trial. In our experiments, the least number of images captured in any trial was 164 and hence the value of X^1 was 164. An image is discarded if its sequence number is matching the rounded off multiple of NF value. For example, if the number of images in the current is 190, then the value of NF is approximately 7 and the images at sequence numbers 7, 14, 21, etc., are discarded to make the total number of images selected to 164.

The data collected by the robot has a sequence of images. The normal size of an image is 52 × 39 pixels. Hence, the data extracted from each image consist of 2028 features. In order to reduce the dimensionality of the data, each image is split into four tiles. The average values for red, green, and blue colors in each tile are calculated separately in the next step. Each image is thus reduced to 12 features. In addition to images, at each time step of robot one lidar reading is taken and that value is added to the extracted twelve image features. Lidar was configured to have one layer of a laser beam which collects the depth distance to a particular object which comes within the field of view of the robot. Hence, it acts identically to a distance sensor.

F2	F3	F4	F5	F6	F7	F8	F9	F10	F11	F12	F13	F14	F15	F16	F17	F18	F19	F20	F21
162.4019	199.4788	85.14808	146.4596	205.5596	177.585	166.1437	107.7166	179.4717	155.0425	105.7895	88.37692	162.2558	198.2058	85.15769	146.4462	205.0115	176.0729	164.4798	106.0
163.5154	202.9654	86.93269	149.0288	206.9558	182.4312	167.8664	112.17	188.8704	166.8583	116.5506	94	162.6385	203.8154	87.42692	149.7769	207.1885	180.8684	164.9393	109.5
163.2577	202.9308	86.93462	149.0288	206.9173	182.4555	167.7571	112.1356	188.9028	166.913	116.5547	94.38462	163.3288	203.0635	87.50769	149.8769	206.9481	180.67	165.3117	110.3
163.0135	204.3788	87.29808	149.5077	206.7269	182.5	167.1559	112.5709	189.8097	167.9615	116.9737	95.35385	163.3481	203.325	88.34808	151.0731	207.4481	180.4615	164.7773	110.8
162.8288	203.9423	87.50192	149.8692	206.9404	181.8644	166.7166	112.1255	190.3401	168.5061	117.1134	96.98077	163.6827	204.0635	88.96154	151.9365	207.5846	180.4028	164.6559	112.1
162.5712	203.7385	86.98077	149.1038	206.6308	182.1154	167.0344	111.751	189.2672	167.2632	116.5466	94.50769	163.0365	203.1115	87.80769	150.2788	207.0827	180.4393	164.666	110.0
162.8288	203.9423	87.50192	149.8692	206.9404	181.8644	166.7166	112.1255	190.3401	168.5061	117.1134	96.98077	163.6827	204.0635	88.96154	151.9365	207.5846	180.4028	164.6559	112.1
162.8846	202.9327	87.30769	149.525	206.7538	182.4899	167.33	112.0162	189.7247	167.8381	116.8563	95.24808	163.5462	203.2635	88.02308	150.6558	207.3058	180.3765	165.0121	110.8
163.1538	202.9231	86.93269	149.0327	206.9173	182.4069	167.6721	112.0526	188.8806	166.8988	116.5425	94.35769	163.0346	203.0404	87.49231	149.8673	206.9365	180.5992	165.1235	110.1
162.9731	202.9481	87.31538	149.5346	206.7769	182.4818	167.4069	112.0607	189.6012	167.7146	116.7713	95.29231	163.8904	203.3115	88.03269	150.6442	207.3135	180.3988	165.1174	110.8
154.6865	204.8596	77.08077	125.0846	181.6269	191.5243	162.836	113.4413	182.8785	157.3259	111.67	102.4135	154.3538	204.5904	78.18846	126.4981	183.6212	191.6316	162.5972	113.7
154.7308	204.8019	77.35769	125.6365	182.4269	191.4575	162.8522	113.3846	182.9049	157.3583	111.6781	102.2615	154.5058	204.9038	79.44808	128.3481	185.6788	191.3785	162.3583	113.6
154.6923	204.875	77.10577	125.0827	181.65	191.5789	162.8866	113.4838	182.8725	157.3097	111.664	102.4481	154.3827	204.6269	78.21731	126.5096	183.6481	191.6842	162.6559	113.8
154.3827	204.4615	77.64615	126.2365	182.6192	191.4919	162.9555	113.3198	183.8158	158.2733	112.081	101.7692	154.5712	204.6635	79.35577	128.3731	185.5673	191.2449	162.8441	113.1
154.7308	204.8019	77.35769	125.6365	182.4269	191.4575	162.8522	113.3846	182.9049	157.3583	111.6781	102.2615	154.5058	204.9038	79.44808	128.3481	185.6788	191.3785	162.3583	113.6
154.7308	204.8019	77.35769	125.6365	182.4269	191.4575	162.8522	113.3846	182.9049	157.3583	111.6781	102.2615	154.5058	204.9038	79.44808	128.3481	185.6788	191.3785	162.3583	113.6
154.7308	204.8019	77.35769	125.6365	182.4269	191.4575	162.8522	113.3846	182.9049	157.3583	111.6781	102.2615	154.5058	204.9038	79.44808	128.3481	185.6788	191.3785	162.3583	113.6
154.6038	204.6962	79.44808	128.6192	186.0308	191.0405	162.3219	112.751	184.6984	158.913	113.0769	102.1558	154.5365	204.4615	81.43077	132.5288	190.5308	189.9615	160.7348	111.9
154.7942	205.4962	77.11346	124.6346	181.4769	192.1275	163.3644	113.9028	182.8198	157.0344	111.6862	102.15	154.4385	204.8481	76.98654	124.4923	181.1442	192.0445	163.2794	114.2
154.7308	204.8019	77.35769	125.6365	182.4269	191.4575	162.8522	113.3846	182.9049	157.3583	111.6781	102.2615	154.5058	204.9038	79.44808	128.3481	185.6788	191.3785	162.3583	113.6

output1-data

Fig. 5 Combined lidar and image data

The data obtained from cameras and lidar are combined to form multimodal data, and a part of it exhibited in a tabular form is shown in Fig. 5. Each row of the table corresponds to the features extracted from one trial. Here F1 and F2, etc., indicate simply column names for the features. As discussed earlier, each image contributes 12 features. During the traversal of the robot from one corner of the environment to the other corner, images and lidar readings are taken at every 32 ms. Altogether 164 reading is taken during a traversal. Hence, each row of the table has 12×164 features extracted from images and another 164 features captured by the lidar. Data are collected using 10 trials from each environment making the total number of trials to 40. Hence, the data contain $12 \times 164 + 164$ columns and 40 rows. An additional column indicating the environment number which is used as a class label is added.

The multilayered lidar data contain 52×39 points for each time step. The average of these 2028 values is taken as a single feature. Hence, this dataset also resembles that of a single-layered lidar dataset.

3.4 *Classification*

Since the single modality cannot give the exact details about the environments, this work takes multimodal data to classify the robotic environments. The multimodal data with image and lidar give 2D and 3D information about the robots working environment. With these data, it will be easy for a robot to analyze and to perform appropriate action with the knowledge of the environment.

In order to classify the collected data, Weka [11] tool is used. Weka has a suite of machine learning algorithms for classification, like Naïve Bayes, support vector machine (SVM), AdaBoost, decision trees, and simple logistic regression. In this paper, some of these machine learning algorithms are used and then the classification results are compared among them. The main classical algorithms used for this work are the Naïve Bayes classifier, SVM, decision trees like a random forest, random tree, and simple regression. In the given data, four different scenarios are used so there are four classes to which the data should get classified. The class labels are given as env-1, env-2, env-3, and env-4. Here the training and testing are done with cross-validation of fivefolds.

Classifiers
SVM works by finding out an optimal line between classes so that each object gets grouped into an appropriate class. Here objects from different classes should have maximal margin in between them. Naïve Bayes classifier works based on Bayes' theorem with a probabilistic approach. In a decision tree, it forms tree-structured graphical forms with some conditions as nodes and its consequences as its children. Random forest is a type of decision tree which forms its swarm at training time and gives output as the simple majority class predicted by the individual trees. Regression is a linear approach to modeling the relationship between a scalar variable and one or more independent variables.

4 Results and Analysis

Classification of environments based on the data collected has been done with three different sets of features. First, the classification has been done taking features extracted from images alone. Subsequently, classification has been done using only lidar features. Finally, classification has been done using combined lidar and image data.

4.1 Evaluation

For the analysis of the result of classification, two methods are used.

(1) Accuracy: It is a measure to calculate how many items from the input set is correctly got classified. It is expressed in percentage.
(2) Confusion matrix: It is a tabular representation of the test data which describes the actual and predicted outcomes for it.

4.2 Results

The results achieved for image data are shown in this section. Figure 6 depicts the result and accuracy of image data with Naïve Bayes classification. Here Recall connotes the accuracy of the method. The Naïve Bayes algorithm achieves 100% accuracy with image data. Figure 7 shows the confusion matrix obtained by the

```
=== Summary ===

Correctly Classified Instances          40                100      %
Incorrectly Classified Instances         0                  0      %
Kappa statistic                          1
Mean absolute error                      0
Root mean squared error                  0
Relative absolute error                  0      %
Root relative squared error              0      %
Total Number of Instances               40

=== Detailed Accuracy By Class ===

                TP Rate  FP Rate  Precision  Recall  F-Measure  MCC    ROC Area  PRC Area  Class
                1.000    0.000    1.000      1.000   1.000      1.000  1.000     1.000     env-1
                1.000    0.000    1.000      1.000   1.000      1.000  1.000     1.000     env-2
                1.000    0.000    1.000      1.000   1.000      1.000  1.000     1.000     env-3
                1.000    0.000    1.000      1.000   1.000      1.000  1.000     1.000     env-4
Weighted Avg.   1.000    0.000    1.000      1.000   1.000      1.000  1.000     1.000

=== Confusion Matrix ===

  a  b  c  d   <-- classified as
 10  0  0  0 |  a = env-1
  0 10  0  0 |  b = env-2
  0  0 10  0 |  c = env-3
  0  0  0 10 |  d = env-4
```

Fig. 6 Image classification with Naïve Bayes

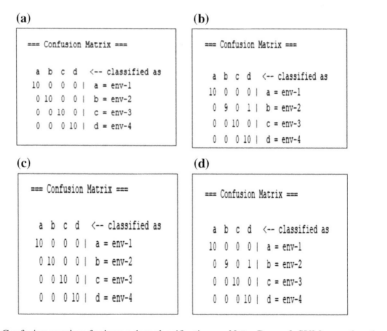

(a)

```
=== Confusion Matrix ===

  a  b  c  d   <-- classified as
 10  0  0  0 |  a = env-1
  0 10  0  0 |  b = env-2
  0  0 10  0 |  c = env-3
  0  0  0 10 |  d = env-4
```

(b)

```
=== Confusion Matrix ===

  a  b  c  d   <-- classified as
 10  0  0  0 |  a = env-1
  0  9  0  1 |  b = env-2
  0  0 10  0 |  c = env-3
  0  0  0 10 |  d = env-4
```

(c)

```
=== Confusion Matrix ===

  a  b  c  d   <-- classified as
 10  0  0  0 |  a = env-1
  0 10  0  0 |  b = env-2
  0  0 10  0 |  c = env-3
  0  0  0 10 |  d = env-4
```

(d)

```
=== Confusion Matrix ===

  a  b  c  d   <-- classified as
 10  0  0  0 |  a = env-1
  0  9  0  1 |  b = env-2
  0  0 10  0 |  c = env-3
  0  0  0 10 |  d = env-4
```

Fig. 7 Confusion matrices for image data classifications. **a** Naïve Bayes, **b** SVM, **c** random forest, and **d** simple logistic

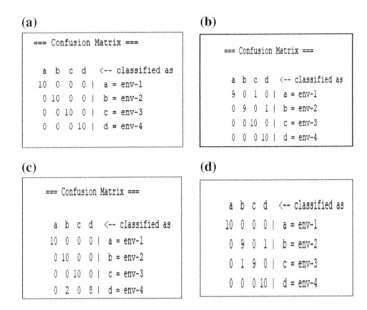

(a)
```
=== Confusion Matrix ===

 a  b  c  d   <-- classified as
10  0  0  0 |  a = env-1
 0 10  0  0 |  b = env-2
 0  0 10  0 |  c = env-3
 0  0  0 10 |  d = env-4
```

(b)
```
=== Confusion Matrix ===

 a  b  c  d   <-- classified as
 9  0  1  0 |  a = env-1
 0  9  0  1 |  b = env-2
 0  0 10  0 |  c = env-3
 0  0  0 10 |  d = env-4
```

(c)
```
=== Confusion Matrix ===

 a  b  c  d   <-- classified as
10  0  0  0 |  a = env-1
 0 10  0  0 |  b = env-2
 0  0 10  0 |  c = env-3
 0  2  0  8 |  d = env-4
```

(d)
```
 a  b  c  d   <-- classified as
10  0  0  0 |  a = env-1
 0  9  0  1 |  b = env-2
 0  1  9  0 |  c = env-3
 0  0  0 10 |  d = env-4
```

Fig. 8 Confusion matrices for multimodal data classifications with single-layered lidar. **a** Naïve Bayes, **b** SVM, **c** random forest, and **d** simple logistic

processing of image data using (a) naïve Bayes method, (b) SVM, (c) Random forest and (d) Simple logistic. In SVM and simple logistic one, data object got misclassified thus giving 97.5% accuracy.

Similarly, Fig. 8 shows the confusion matrices obtained by multimodal data with single-layered lidar. Here Naïve Bayes gives 100% accuracy while other's accuracy got decreased due to misclassification of a few environments. Figure 9 depicts the confusion matrices for the multilayered lidar data. Here only SVM gives 100% accuracy. Figure 10 shows the confusion matrices for multimodal data with multilayered lidar and image. Both random forest and simple logistics show 100% accuracy by this method.

Figure 11 shows the comparison of four classification models in a graphical view for individual modality and for multimodality with single-layered lidar. Here the accuracy of all classification methods for individual modality gets compared with the features of multimodal data. It can be seen that image data give good classification accuracy. The accuracy gets reduced when lidar data are added. Figure 12 depicts the classification of the result of multimodal data with multilayered lidar and image.

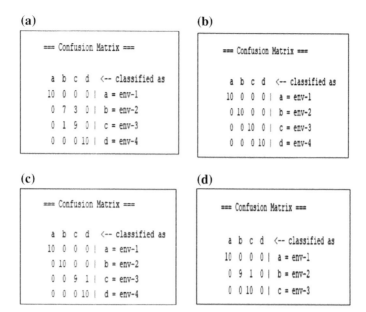

Fig. 9 Confusion matrices for multilayered lidar data classifications. **a** Naïve Bayes, **b** SVM, **c** random forest, and **d** simple logistic

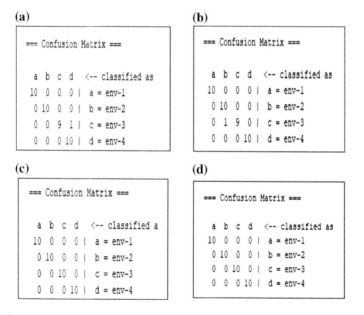

Fig. 10 Confusion matrices for multimodal data classifications with multilayered lidar. **a** Naïve Bayes, **b** SVM, **c** random forest, and **d** simple logistic

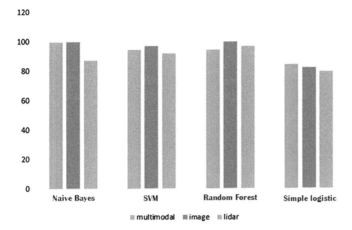

Fig. 11 Accuracy of all classifiers for proposed multimodal data with single-layered lidar

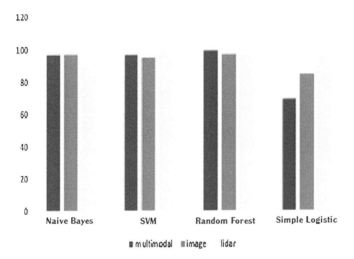

Fig. 12 Accuracy of all classifiers for proposed multimodal data with multilayered lidar

5 Conclusion

The results from the experiments give good classification accuracy of the multimodal data which consist of images and lidar sensor values. These works reduce the number of features by good feature selection and proper preprocessing. The proposed model achieves an excellent result of 100% accuracy by the Naïve Bayes classifier and 95% of accuracy by both SVM and random forest tree with single-layered lidar. The same work extended with multilayered lidar which gives 100% accuracy with both random forest tree and simple logistic. 97.5% accuracy is achieved with both SVM and Naïve Bayes classifiers.

The future work aims to do real-time collection of data. The classification of robot's environments using the collected multimodal data in real time is to be explored. A large amount of data can be collected, then investigate whether classification of complex scenarios can be improved using deep learning techniques.

References

1. Moradi M, Ardestani MA, Keyvanpour MR, Moradi M (April 2016) Applications of data mining in robotics. In: Artificial intelligence and robotics (IRANOPEN), Qazvin, Iran, pp. 18–24
2. Radhakrishnan G, Gupta D, Sudarshan TSB (2014) Experimentation and analysis of time series data for rescue robotics. In: Recent advances in intelligent informatics, pp 443–453
3. Sudheesh P, Gireesh KT (2012) Vision based robot navigation for disaster scenarios. Int J Comput Appl 49
4. Radhakrishnan G, Gupta D, Abhishek R, Ajith A, Sudarshan TSB (2012) Analysis of multimodal time series data of robotic environment. In: 12th international conference on intelligent systems design and applications (ISDA), pp 734–739
5. Navarro PJ, Fernández C, Borraz R, Alonso D (2017) A machine learning approach to pedestrian detection for autonomous vehicles using high-definition 3D range data, vol 17
6. Lethaus F, Baumann MRK, Köster F, Lemmer K (2013) A comparison of selected simple supervised learning algorithms to predict driver intent based on gaze data, vol 121, pp 108–130
7. Baltrušaitis T, Ahuja C, Morency L-P (2017) Multimodal machine learning: a survey and taxonomy. arXiv:1705.09406
8. Maturana D, Scherer S (2015) 3D convolutional neural networks for landing zone detection from LiDAR. In: IEEE international conference on robotics and automation (ICRA), Washington
9. Gopalapillai R, Gupta D, Sudarshan TSB (2017) Pattern identification of robotic environments using machine learning techniques. In: 7th international conference on advances in computing & communications (ICACC-2017), Cochin, India
10. Cyberbotics. https://www.cyberbotics.com/
11. Frank E, Hall MA, Witten IH (2016) The WEKA workbench. Online appendix for data mining: practical machine learning tools and techniques, 4th ed. Morgan Kaufmann

Comparative Analysis of Existing Latest Microcontroller Development Boards

Vidhyotma and Jaiteg Singh

Abstract The embedded system is the combination of electronics hardware and software. Its applications intermingle uninterruptedly with the surrounding environment through different types of sensors and actuators. In electronics market, the plethora of embedded controller boards is available for engineers/developers to automate the world around them. The vision of this paper is to compare three controller boards, e.g., Arduino, Intel Galileo, and mbed LPC1768 through the case studies of implemented projects of automation:

- Automatic Auditorium System Using Arduino Board
- IOT-Based LCD Gadget using mbed LPC1768
- Home Automation using Intel Galileo Board

Analysis performed for the important parameters reliability, efficiency, and the user-friendly nature of latest development boards. It will help to engineers and professional developers to easily choose their microcontroller to develop any project or automation system/device.

Keywords Arduino · Automation · Embedded system · Intel Galileo · LPC1768 · Microcontroller boards · Sensors

1 Introduction

Technological revolution paves twenty-first century to embedded system design which provides the automation. The embedded system is the combination of electronics tool and software [1, 2]. It takes 15 decades that shook the embedded world

Vidhyotma (✉) · J. Singh
Department of Computer Science and Engineering, Chitkara University Institute
of Engineering and Technology, Chandigarh, India
e-mail: Vidhyotma.gandhi@chitkara.edu.in

J. Singh
e-mail: jaiteg.singh@chitkara.edu.in

© Springer Nature Singapore Pte Ltd. 2019
V. Sridhar et al. (eds.), *Emerging Research in Electronics, Computer Science and Technology*, Lecture Notes in Electrical Engineering 545,
https://doi.org/10.1007/978-981-13-5802-9_88

as design and development board. It makes a peaceful revolution to create a violent inevitable embedded world. Remotely controlled devices are a major concern these days. These type of devices and applications are developed by embedded systems and controller boards [3]. The informal definition of embedded systems is the assembly of programmable components such as microcontrollers and digital signal processors fenced by application-specific integration circuits (ASICs) and supplementary standard apparatus or components that intermingle uninterruptedly with the surrounding environment through different types of sensors and actuators [4]. Embedded systems are normally used in life-critical conditions when safety, security, and reliability are more important than other factors [1, 3]. Two major things that required to start with embedded systems are controller development board along with an IDE. A board is a designed printed circuit board (PCB) with specific circuit and hardware to facilitate lots of application-based experiments which are possible with features of that microcontroller board. The combination of a microprocessor, memory, integrated circuits (IC) and involved peripherals, e.g., USB port, ADC, serial port, Ethernet, RTC, voltage regulators, memory chip slot, etc. with reset features [2]. These types of boards not only save engineers or developers from messing with the external connections of jumper leads and also save time [5]. The working phenomena of microcontroller boards are given in Fig. 1. Microcontroller boards should be chosen on the basis of processor used, the type of data bus, memory space, operating system, and I/O ports [6]. In the last decade, we have seen that the Internet is not only used by the human being but also used by the devices, machines or one can say the anything in the universe. By the huge availability of IPV6, an engineer/developer can connect any kind of entity with the Internet. The centroid of all these developments is controller board [5].

This paper presents a comparative analysis of some existing control units on latest design and development boards as in Table 1 and Fig. 3. It also presents three case studies of some real-time applications of embedded system design using different and latest microcontroller-based design and development boards to avoid situations in which energy is being wasted and also provide comfort to human life and design the world of dream (Fig. 2). Through sensors, it senses the surrounding/external world and behaves accordingly to provide automation. Case-I was the implementation of "Automatic Auditorium System using Arduino Board". This project uses different types of sensors to pick data in real time which is processed by Arduino and then provide input to connected output peripherals with Arduino to act as instructed by programmed Arduino for automation. Case-II implemented "IoT-Based LCD Gadget using mbed LPC1768". In this case, a portable device was designed for the university to continuously display a message of updated news/information for students/faculty

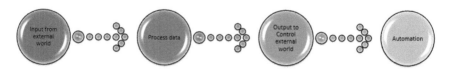

Fig. 1 Working phenomena of microcontroller boards

Table 1 Theoretical comparison of microcontroller boards [7–10]

Parameters	Arduino	LPC1768	Intel Galileo
Operating voltage (V)	5	4.5–9	3.3
Microcontroller	AVR (Atmel ATmega 168/328)	ARM Cortex-M3	Intel® Quark SoC X1000
Word length (bits)	8/16/32	32	32
software compatibility	IDE	Cloud-Based (C/C++)	IDE/Eclipse/Python
Compiler	IDE	Web Based	IDE
Clock speed (MHz)	16	100	400
Flash memory (KB)	–	512	512
SRAM (KB)	2	64 (32 + 32)	512
EEPROM	1 KB	512 KB	11 KB (additional SD card up to 32 GB supported)
Digital I/O pins	14 (6 PWM)	20	14 (6 PWM)
Analog I/O pins	8	8	8
Interrupts	2	4	–
Programmer	USB flash	USB flash	USB flash
Platform independent	Cross platform	Cross platform	Cross platform
Recommended input voltage (V)	7–12	12	7–12
Timers	2	4	4
DC current per I/O PIN (mA)	40	100	80
Ethernet	External shield needed	10/100 Mbps	10/100 Mbps
Wifi	External shield required	External shield required	External shield required
SPI	√	√	√
I2C	√	√	√
USB	√	√	√ (client and host)
Cost (approximate)	Rs. 800/-	Rs. 3000/-	Rs. 6800/-

to update them about institutional activities without visiting their website. Serial interface color LCD was used to display the message. Case-III was a very common concept but with a new feature of IoT that was "Home automation system using Intel Galileo board. Firstly, we automatically control the home appliances, lighting system and then put all the controls on the internet through Ethernet by using the feature of IoT in Intel Galileo board. After the implementations, comparisons of three microcontroller boards were done and shown in Table 2 and Fig. 3.

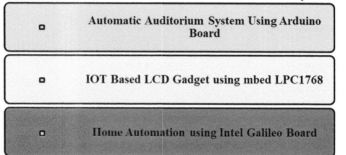

Fig. 2 Case studies

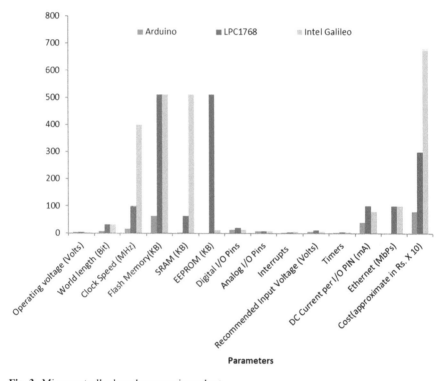

Fig. 3 Microcontroller boards comparison chart

All microcontroller boards are cool design and development platform, and the best part is that they keep getting small in size day by day. Arduino and Intel Galileo microcontroller boards are of credit card-sized single-board computers, and mbed LPC1768 is smaller than others [8–10].

This paper divided in six sections. Introduction and theoretical comparison of three boards on different parameters was covered in Sect. 1. Practical implementations of all three cases: automatic auditorium system using Arduino, IoT-based LCD gadget

Table 2 Practical comparison of microcontroller boards

	Arduino	Intel Galileo	LPC1768
Idle with LED load	6.7 mA (33.5 mW)	4.4 mA (22 mw)	101.9 mA (509.5 mW)
Sleep with LED load	0.043 mA (0.225 mw)	0.031 mA (0.15 mW)	96.5 mA (482.5 mW)
Idle with smoke sensor load (500 mS) (mA)	2.5	1.9	166.8
Sleep with smoke sensor load (10 s) (mA)	0.069	0.8	113.7

using mbed LPC 1768, home automation using Intel Galileo board were presented in Sects. 2, 3, and 4, respectively (Fig. 4). The results of these implementations along with their current and power analysis were given in Sects. 5, and 6 concludes the paper.

2 Case 1: Automatic Auditorium System Using Arduino Board

Embedded systems are required for a life of sensation rather than of thoughts [3]. As one explores phenomena or ideas at the frontiers of technical knowledge, it was the unexpected result that provides clues to guide the further work. By using the idea of embedded systems, the project "Automatic auditorium system using Arduino Board" is designed. Figures 5 and 6 show the block diagram of this application.

This automatic auditorium system consists of Arduino, infrared sensors, relays, LCD displays, actuators, ICs [5], etc. It was aimed to reduce the deliberate efforts and time of man required to open or close doors of the auditorium. This system was highly versatile due to the Arduino microcontroller board. It was an Arduino-based standalone device which can perform many different functions/operations [11]. A variety of sensors was interfaced with Arduino to sense the real-world happenings and provide data to control the light and AC system, door opening, fire safety system, etc. in auditorium [12]. The auditorium was basically divided into four blocks/quadrants in form of a 2 × 2 grid, to make the auto-controlled light system more efficient. Depending on the number of persons sitting in a particular block, the light system and fan/cooler/AC of that particular block were controlled. In the absence of any individual, all the electrical appliances of a block were shut down in order to save electric energy. Apart from this, the auditorium was self-equipped to encounter the situation of fire hazards. Four smoke/heat detectors were deployed to detect the presence of smoke/heat inside the auditorium and trigger a fire alert alarm to warn

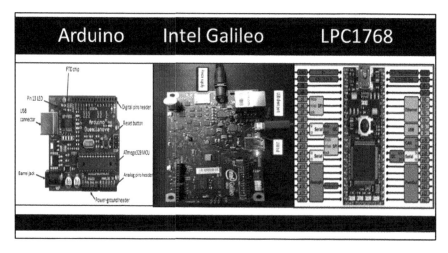

Fig. 4 Latest design and development boards

Fig. 5 Block diagram of
automatic auditorium system
using Arduino

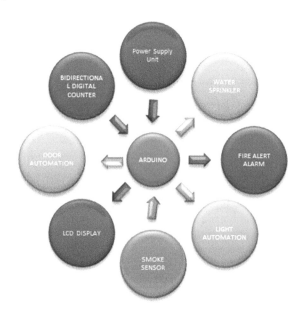

the audience about the possibility of fire [13]. This mitigation strategy allowed early
evacuation of people from the auditorium before the situation goes out of hands
and thus helped in saving many precious lives. The detectors not only the alarm but
simultaneously initiate the working of the water sprinklers inside the auditorium to
suppress the fire inside the hall before it takes any major form. All these automated
tasks of the auditorium were monitored, initiated, stopped, and controlled by the
Arduino, to which all these peripherals are attached, either as an input device or
output device [11].

This embedded system has four modules: First, a digital counter circuit which is used to count the number of persons present going inside and coming out from the auditorium [13]. The first module was in the support to the next module of the auto-controlled light system, which was used to switch on/off the electrical depending on the number of visitors inside the auditorium [1, 2]. The main motive of this module was to reduce power consumption and manpower because electricity was wasted mainly because of negligence; so, there was no need to keep track of unused electrical appliances. The third one was door automation which was used for reducing the manpower and increasing the ease of entry/exit to the auditorium hall. This module was fused by the same sensors which were troop into line for action in the first module. It controls the open/close gates system automatically and keeps the count of the persons toward the inside or leaving the auditorium. This was instigated by means of a pair of infrared sensors [7]. A liquid crystal diode display was placed outside the auditorium hall to display the value of person count which increments when someone enters the auditorium and at that same time the door will be opened automatically and fans and coolers/AC are turned on accordingly. When the auditorium hall is full with its maximum capacity, the doors will remain close automatically so that no other person can enter unless someone left the auditorium hall. The automatic auditorium door opening and closing system efficiently manages and controls the crowd. The fourth was the automatic fire safety system was one step forward in controlling emergency situations. This system should be implemented at many crowded places to control and manage crowd at low power and at low cost and with very few efforts. So, it was true that embedded systems were helpful in reducing the manpower and electricity by providing automation of various processes.

3 CASE 2: IoT-Based LCD Gadget Using MBED LPC1768

In today's busy life, it is the need of conglomerates to display latest news and notices on the organization website. But it is not possible for each and every one to visit the organization's website regularly to check the latest updates. To overwhelm this issue, an Internet of Things (IoT)-based LCD gadget was designed to automatically display the latest news and notices of the organization from the website. The gadget will provide 24×7 updates, and it was portable to carry everywhere; so that it can display conglomerates happenings at most visited places. It can implant at most visited places to make autovisible updated information and happenings of conglomerates. It was useful to make announcements or alerts for the general public. All updating can be handled by the server via online services. 24×7 internet connectivity was required to use these IoT-based LCD gadgets [14]. This gadget was infused with all the features of IoT as explained further.

"Internet of things" is an exhilarating and groundbreaking field that engenders novel applications with the integration of multiple traditional innovative technologies [15]. IoT is the interconnection of uniquely identifiable embedded computing large number of devices within the existing Internet or similar network infrastructure

[16]. Building blocks of IOT are smart devices which are any products built with M2M communication capabilities [6]. Every device is assigned an IP address which provides its ability to transfer data over the network. IPV6's huge availability of addresses is the main factor in the development of this technology [17]. A Project of displaying a web page on handheld device to use the feature of IoT. Block diagram of IoT-based LCD gadget using mbed LPC1768 is illustrated in Fig. 7.

This project was implemented using mbed NXP LPC1768 32-bit ARM cortex low-power microcontroller interfaced with serial-colored uLCD-144-G2 embedded with GOLDELOX processor having 128×128 pixels resolution for display [18]. Ethernet socket RJ-45 is used for web page connectivity [8]. mbed microcontroller has the Web (cloud)-based compiler with online libraries with application interface approach program can be write in C++/C [8].

3.1   Methodology

mbed NXP LPC1768 microcontroller was used to employ this technology. This was one of the mbed ARM Microcontrollers series Philips (originally) but now "NXP". It was designed for rapid prototyping to develop embedded system device with lots of features. It was a low-power ($4.5-9$ V) 32-bit ARM processor. It was a 40-pin Dual-In-Package board with a 0.1-inch pitch. It consists of 100 MHz ARM processor with 64 KB of SRAM, 512 KB of FLASH memory. Lots of interfaces like USB, SPI, I²C,

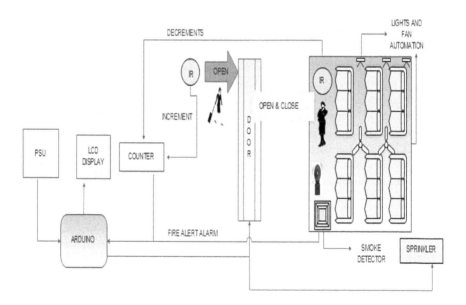

Fig. 6 Design of the automatic auditorium system

CAN, Ethernet, and Serial are supported by mbed LPC1768. Its web (cloud)-based compiler having capabilities to write the program in C/C++ and online mbed library access, which provides API-driven approach. 8-channel DMA controller, 4 UARTs, ADC of 12 bits and 8 channels, DAC of 10-bits, and PWM were its special features. It was having 4 general-purpose timers, quad encoder interface, and general-purpose 6-output PWM [8].

To display message, uLCD-144-G2, a serial LCD having TFT screen was used. It was a low-power, low-cost serial interface with ten pins for connections and 5v operating voltage. It works on GOLDELOX processor with 128 × 128 pixels resolution with having capabilities to display true to life colors; this display module was perfect for animations, slideshows, and other multimedia presentations. Powerful Graphics, 65 K true to life colors, low-cost display solution. Ethernet RJ-45 is used to provide internet connectivity and supports the data transfer rate of 100 Mbps and fetches the IP address through dynamic host configuration protocol [18]. Practical implementation of the project is shown in Fig. 8.

4   Case 3: Home Automation Using Intel Galileo Board

Hollywood cinemas are liked by everyone, especially the ones which have Tony Stark in them. After watching Iron Man, everyone loves to have a house that understands you and acts accordingly. Home automation can offer improved life quality for the disabled and elderly person without any permanent caretakers or institutional upkeep [19]. This project described the design of a house of such type. It was designed using

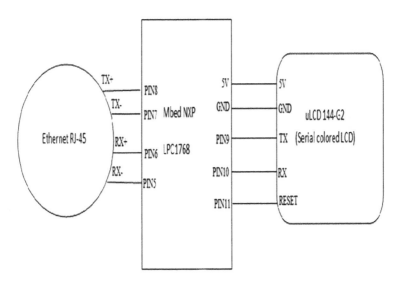

Fig. 7 Block diagram of IoT-based LCD gadget

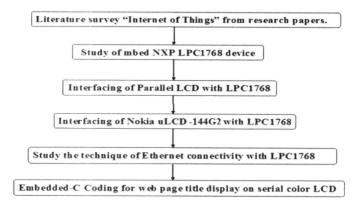

Fig. 8 Methodology adopted for IoT-based LCD gadget

Intel Galileo. It brought a few steps closer to automating and remote controlling the house. A home automation system integrates electrical devices in a house according to the environmental needs. Secure and automate the home remotely using IoT feature of Intel Galileo. The remote commands were sent through laptop, smartphone, or desktop. Scheduling and controlling of all home appliances were done remotely as well as manually [14]. It can be enhanced for live video streaming of home and can be viewed by a web-enabled gadget. Prototype model of a home automation system is shown in Figs. 9 and 10.

The project "Home Automation Using Intel Galileo" was designed with the motive of creating a remotely accessible network with the help of sensors. Home automation gave ability to manage and control the devices in home by a smartphone at location throughout the world. The device can be any programmable, like sprinkler systems and thermostats or any other normal home appliances like lights, electrical outlets,

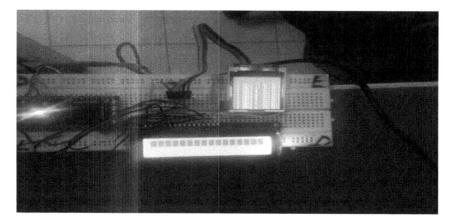

Fig. 9 Practical implementation of IoT-based LCD gadget

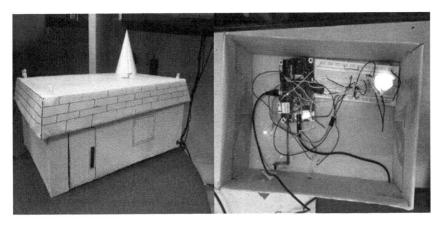

Fig. 10 Model and practical implementation of home automation using Intel Galileo

cooling systems, and heating are hooked up to a remotely controlled network [12, 13]. A home automation system integrates electrical devices in a house according to the environmental needs [19].

In this project, a basic model showing a home with a room having the rainbow lights effect using the RGB LEDs, a room with an IR sensor placed near the door which on sensing the door opening will make the LED inside glow, and a terrace in which the lights glow the moment the LDR sensor senses darkness. All these controls were operative remotely as well as automatically.

Intel Galileo is a cool development platform like the Arduino. The possibilities of building real-time applications with this are endless. The best part of these micro-controller board is that they keep getting smaller day by day. The sketch runs on the Intel Galileo Board, and it communicates with the Linux kernel inside the board's firmware using the Arduino I/O adapter [9]. When the board boots up, two scenarios are possible:

- The execution of an already available sketch in persistent stowage.
- If no sketch is available in persistent stowage, then wait for IDE upload command.

New sketch can be uploaded from IDE during the execution of a running sketch without pressing the reset button. The running sketch was stopped till the uploading of new sketch after that started new sketch automatically. Reset button was used restarts the running sketch or any attached shield [9].

Project model showed a home automated system in which there was a room which has an inlet door and a dome of the house along with the terrace. The home was automated as such the room will light up when the passage door would be opened. The IR sensor senses the value of the door at a distance, and it thus resulted in the lightening of the room. The dome of the house shows the diffusion of the RGB LEDs (i.e., red, blue, and green light-emitting diodes) this adds to the attraction of the house. The LDR sensor in the model senses the light coming from the outside source to auto control the lights of the terrace (Fig. 11).

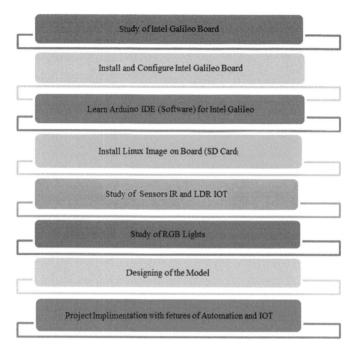

Fig. 11 Methodology adopted for home automation using Intel Galileo

4.1 Methodology

See Fig. 12.

5 Results

After the comparison of three microcontroller-based control unit boards and implementation of three different embedded system projects, the observations for few parameters are:

- **Input Voltage**: For low-power application, one should go with Intel Galileo because it is low-power controlling unit and works on 3.3 V but Arduino works on 5–9 V and mbedLPC1768 works on 5 V.
- **Portable Power source**: Arduino works well with 9 V battery as a portable power source, but Intel Galileo Gen-I and Gen-II do not work with 9 V battery because it needs 5 V/3 A (15 w) power to work properly which cannot deliver by the battery. Although a special circuit can be designed for the portable source for Intel Galileo board power (in this case did not apply). mbed LPC1768 board works properly

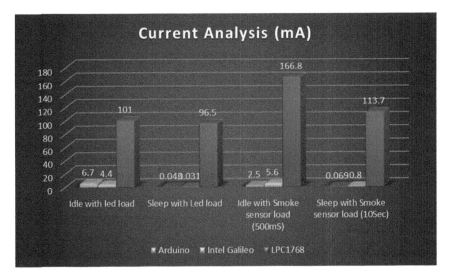

Fig. 12 Current analysis

by detaching it from USB power supply and connecting 5 V supply with Vin pin. (9 V battery and 7805 voltage regulator).

- **Duration of time with Portable Power Supply**: Arduino project time duration increased by 15% with using sleep() function and adding libraries like "avr/sleep.h", "avr/power.h" and "avr/wdt.h". It put the unused peripherals in sleep mode and save power. Although in Arduino case I have not used "avr/wdt.h" because there no such type of sensor is used in my project. mbed LPC1768 project is managed for long-lasting time duration by slow down the clock frequency at the time not in use by adding the libraries "PowerContrl/PowerControl.h" and "Power-Contrl/EthernetPowerControl.h". In this case, I power-down of unused peripherals like UART, PWM, Timers, SPI, CAN, and I2C. It increases the time duration little bit less than double. Without using Power Control libraries, it works for 5 h but with these libraries, it works for 8 h. When the Lpc1768 was run in normal mode, it consumes power 7 mW; by power-down mode of unused peripherals, it consumes 6 mW; and in sleep mode, it consumes 5 mW. All these readings are taken by calibrated Protech digital multimeter N5010(4000 counts, 10 MHz frequency counter). By managing power consumption of board, we increase 20% the running duration time of LPC1768 project.

- **DC Current per I/O PIN**: If more output current is needed for output peripherals, then go ahead with mbed LPC1768 because its output current is 100 mA but for Arduino is 40 mA and for Intel Galileo is 80 mA. So according to a device like led consumes 20 mA and DC motor requires 100 mA IR sensor needs 50 mA one should choose controller board.

- **IoT**: If someone wants to put data on the Internet after processing or want to implement IoT, then choose Intel Galileo board; because, there is no need for

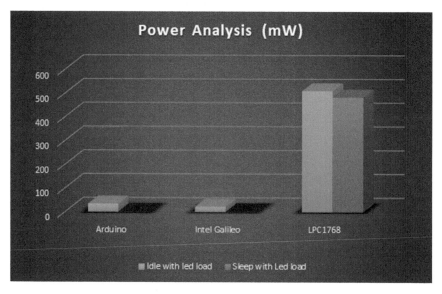

Fig. 13 Power analysis

external Ethernet shield. But for Arduino, one needs an Ethernet shield to interface with a board. In the case of mbed, I do not use any shield in my project; it is done by simply giving web link for the site of which message is displayed on serial-colored LCD display.

- **Programming Ease**: To program an Arduino one should be comfortable with C because IDE programming is in embedded C and at the back end, its header files are defined in C/C++ with gcc compiler. For mbed, LPC almost language proficiency is required but it uses the cloud-based compiler. But Intel Galileo provides language flexibility; it can be programmed in IDE, C, C++, Python, and Java. It provides Eclipse platform for programming and compiler is Linux-based. In my case, I tried IDE and C++ programming for Intel Galileo. Both are equally good (Figs. 12 and 13).

6 Conclusion

This paper compares some existing control units on latest design and development board and elaborates their specifications/parameters, e.g., operating voltages, output current for the digital and analog pin, their software platform, hardware specifications, communication protocols, etc. Here, three different project implementations using different control units are also explained. According to the application implementation, controller boards are chosen. Other major factors for choosing board is the cost of project and expertise or comfort level with the software and hardware of implementer. Arduino can be programmed with IDE only, but Intel Galileo provides

Eclipse platform and can also be programmed in python, C/C++, java, and Arduino IDE, whereas mbed LPC1768 uses embedded C in cloud environment editor. So, there are a lot of factors to be considered to choose the perfect and most suitable design and development board according to the application.

References

1. Marwedel P (2006) Embedded system design, vol 1. Springer, New York
2. Wolf W, Yen T-Y (2013) Hardware-software co-synthesis of distributed embedded systems. Springer Science & Business Media
3. Gajski D, V ahid F, Narayan S, Gong J (1994) Specification and design of embedded systems. Prentice Hall, pp 355–370
4. Liu B, Wang B (2014) Embedded reconfigurable logic for ASIC design obfuscation against supply chain attacks. In: Design, automation and test in Europe conference and exhibition (DATE)
5. https://www.elprocus.com/different-types-of-microcontroller-boards/, May 2018 [Online]
6. https://circuitdigest.com/microcontroller-projects/web-controlled-iot-notice-board-using-raspberry-pi, May 2018 [Online]
7. https://www.arduino.cc/en/Guide/HomePage, Arduino [Online]. Accessed Dec 2017
8. http://www.nxp.com/documents/data_sheet/LPC1769_68_67_66_65_64_63.pdf, July 2016 [Online]
9. http://www.arduino.cc/en/ArduinoCertified/IntelGalieo, [Online]. Accessed Dec 2016
10. https://www.arduino.cc/en/Main/ArduinoBoard101, [Online]. Accessed May 2016
11. https://www.arduino.cc/en/Main/Tutorials, [Online]. Accessed June 2016
12. McGrath MJ, Scanaill CN, Nafus D. Sensor technologies healthcare, wellness and environmental applications
13. Bahrudin MSB, Kassim RA, Buniyamin N (2013) Development of fire alarm system using Raspberry Pi and Arduino Uno. In: International conference on electrical, electronics and system engineering, ICEESE 2013
14. Huq SM, Rahman MA, Sabbir M (2017) Application for integrating microcontrollers to Internet of Things. In: 2017 20th international conference of computer and information technology (ICCIT)
15. Vallez N (2017) Eyes of things. In: IC2E Proceedings of IEEE international conference on cloud engineering
16. Madakam S, Ramaswamy R, Tripathi S (2015) Internet of Things (IoT): a literature review. J Comput Commun 3(3):164–173
17. Gubbi J, Buyya R, Marusic S, Palaniswami M (2013) Internet of Things (IoT): a vision, architectural elements, and future directions. Future Gener Comput Syst 29(7):1645–1660
18. https://old.4dsystems.com.au/downloads/4DGL-Display-Modules/uLCD-144-G2%28GFX%29/Docs/uLCD-144-G2GFX-DS-rev1.pdf [Online]. Accessed June 2017
19. Wang M, Zhang G, Zhang C, Zhang J, Li C (2013) An IoT-based appliance control system for smart homes. In: Fourth international conference on in intelligent control and information processing (ICICIP)
20. Parameswaran G, Sivaprasath K (2016) Arduino based smart drip irrigation system using internet of things. Int J Eng Sci 5518
21. Wu J, Zhang Y, Zukerman M, Yung EKN (2015) Energy-efficient base-stations sleep-mode techniques in green cellular networks: a survey. IEEE Commun Surv Tutor 17(2):803–826
22. RL B, Louis N. Electronics devices and circuits
23. Mano M (2012) Digital design. Pearson
24. http://www.ipofferings.com/IoT-patents-Internet-of-Things-Patents-for-sale.html, [Online]. Accessed 2017

Dynamic Routing in Software-Defined Networks

Mohammed Moin Mulla, Akshay Khot, Anusha Patil and D. G. Chandani

Abstract The Internet is definitely the greatest contributor to globalization which has brought together the whole world and has made every nook and corner attainable. The conventional IP networks have not been able to serve the purpose of a simplified infrastructure even after their extensive acquisition. Service provider networks are not fully fledged in providing (1) fast switching in the core network without any routing lookup, load balancing and retort to faults, (2) reorganize the network according to prevailing network policies and terms simultaneously. Software-defined network (SDN) which operates on OpenFlow protocol is a revolution in networking which aims to remodel the traditional network by disintegrating the data and control planes. It bifurcates the control logic from the various network devices like routers and switches, by providing a core supervisory control logic for the entire network and delivering aptness to code the network. In traditional routing, the information is flooded to the entire network which causes overutilization of resources, high bandwidth requirements, and many other drawbacks. Compared to the legacy routing, SDN is more effective in route computations and provides complete control for packet transmission. The paper proposes a method to find the shortest path routing between the source and destination using the Bellman–Ford routing algorithm.

M. M. Mulla (✉)
School of Computer Science & Enginering, KLE Technological University,
Hubli, Karnataka, India
e-mail: moinbvb@gmail.com

A. Khot · A. Patil · D. G. Chandani
Department of Electronics & Communication, B.V. Bhoomaraddi College
of Engineering & Technology, Hubli, Karnataka, India
e-mail: akshaykhot1000@gmail.com

A. Patil
e-mail: anush30896@gmail.com

D. G. Chandani
e-mail: chandanidevanand96@gmail.com

© Springer Nature Singapore Pte Ltd. 2019
V. Sridhar et al. (eds.), *Emerging Research in Electronics, Computer Science
and Technology*, Lecture Notes in Electrical Engineering 545,
https://doi.org/10.1007/978-981-13-5802-9_89

Secondly, the routing emulations for various network topologies are presented and compared using Mininet which implements routing for SDN. The comparative analysis of both the scenarios shows that the routing algorithm proposed in this paper contributes utmost QoS.

Keywords Networks · SDN · Mininet · POX controller · Routing

1 Introduction

The meteoric advent of diverse computer applications with networking substructure and variety of requirements pose many demands to network intellectuals. Though the traditional IP networks are widely implemented, they raise severe problems to handle. To adapt to evolving network paradigm, each networking device should be configured using distributor-specific and basic-level instructions. Automated restructuring and reaction mechanisms are practically not present in current IP networks [1]. To make things even more difficult in the prevailing networks, the data plane and the control plane are combined together. The control plane which makes decisions to route the traffic and data plane aka forwarding plane which forwards the data packets to destination, as logic is combined inside the networking devices which declines the workability and restricts the renovation of the networking infrastructure. Adopting an entirely new fully fledged protocol will take more than a decade for analyzing, designing, development, implementation verification, and refinement stages [1]. Eventually, the existing conditions have boosted the functional overhead and inflated the capital of regulating the IP networks.

SDN is a blanket term which includes various network technologies and focuses on building a versatile network, which gives a new dimension to existing network infrastructure. Firstly, it decentralizes the vertical combination of the control plane from the data-forwarding devices like routers and switches. Secondly, this implementation simplifies the functionality of routers and switches as there exists a centralized controller which enforces control over entire network, which thereby simplifies strategy imposition. The disassociation of control plane and data plane is achieved with the help of an unambiguous programming interface between the centralized controller and switches. SDN uses OpenFlow protocol, which is the first standard communication interface between the control and data planes of the SDN architecture. The internal flow table of the OpenFlow uses its controller to remotely control data transfer in both hardware- and software-based routers and switches.

The legacy routing protocols are posing high-performance setbacks and are not able to cope with high-speed developing internet [2]. Legacy infrastructure has unavailability of programmable interfaces which pose a great hindrance to application developers from developing a flexible network structure that can automatically handle any type of network spikes. Traditionally centralized protocols have good robustness, self-healing capacity, etc., but as the flooding mechanism is involved in forwarding link state updates affects greatly the convergence time or cost metric.

Taking all these drawbacks into consideration, SDN network has proved to provide compact set of policies and satisfy user requirements like QoS, resilience, and congestion control Kreutz et al. [1]. The paper aims to provide a comparative analysis of some of the network parameters like throughput and delay, defining the QoS of the network by considering two network scenarios. The first scenario is the conventional network which uses flooding to transmit data packets to destination, and the other scenario is the modern network implementing Bellman–Ford shortest path algorithm. The Bellman–Ford algorithm is an efficient algorithm that computes the shortest path with minimum convergence delay provides high bandwidth and helps in achieving large rate of fault tolerance in network.

The paper is organized as follows: Sect. 2 briefly describes emulation platform and the literature review of the paper. Section 3 explains the proposed work with the operation of Bellman–Ford routing algorithm. Section 4 of the paper contains the results and the performance estimation of traditional network and SDN with and without routing. Section 5 recapitulates proposed work and future scope of project.

2 Related Work

In this section, we describe the tools required for SDN emulation, literature survey and discuss the shortcomings of traditional networks.

2.1 Mininet Emulator

Mininet is the virtual network platform which is extensively used in SDN applications [3]. It has the capacity to employ large networks having network components like routers, layer 2 switches, layer 3 switches, hosts, and links [4]. The main purpose of Mininet is to pave the way for exploration in the field of SDN. It provides practicality and eases the work with low cost. Mininet also can be used by various application developers to work on the same network topology simultaneously.

2.2 POX Controller

POX is an open-source controller which renders a systematic way to execute the OpenFlow protocol. This Python-based controller supports different applications like firewall, switches, and hubs. The packet flow between the POX controller and the OpenFlow devices can be traced by various packet capture tools [4]. It is suitable for any operating environments, and it comes preinstalled in Mininet.

2.3 Drawbacks of the Conventional Network

In traditional networks, a hub may be used which acts as a general connecting point for all devices comprising a network. The networking devices in traditional networks do not have the capacity to filter data and therefore they flood data to all other devices in the network. All devices in a network have a single-collision domain when they are connected by a hub. They do not have the intelligence in them as compared to routers and therefore they are the main reasons for a disorganized network. In a hub, even though the packet received is unicast, it is flooded through every port of the hub; this causes inefficiency and adds more traffic in the network that leads to unsatisfactory response time of the network. In a hub-based transmission the bandwidth is shared between all the ports of the hub when multiple PCs are transmitting data, which leads to the degradation of the entire network performance.

2.4 Literature Survey

There are many researches carried out in the field of SDN. Kreutz et al. [1] provides a thorough analysis on SDN. It is a new approach in the succession of networking, providing a new rate of advancement in networking architecture. Following a bottom-up approach [1, 10] provides the inspiration of SDN, how it diverges from conventional networks, it analyzes the cross layer issues, standardization of SDN, industrial and academic support in shaping SDN, and so on. The paper synopsis provides the conceptualization of SDN, components of SDN, prevailing solutions and future scope of SDN [8].

The failure recovery mechanism provided by SDN is presented in [5] through algorithmic emulation of SDN architecture. The importance of shortest path algorithm in fault tolerance is provided by a relative study on Dijkstra's algorithm and Bellman–Ford algorithm. The paper concludes that Dijkstra's algorithm is resilient and processing time in new route estimation is least in case of link failure.

In [2], experiments are conducted using Floodlight controller to study the routing convergence time of conventional networks and SDN network. The paper [2] concludes that in a large-scale network, SDN with distributed routes provides scalability and self-recovery mechanism. The paper considers node-forwarding speed and convergence time under different link delays for comparison between traditional and SDN protocols.

Fig. 1 System model

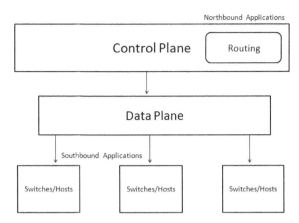

3 Proposed Work

The section describes the proposed work for dynamic routing in SDN using routing algorithm. Bellman–Ford algorithm and Pox controller is used for implementing routing mechanism for SDN [6, 9].

3.1 System Model

The architectural overview is presented through System Model (Fig. 1).

(a) Control Plane: It determines the most efficient path for data transmission and signals the data plane.
(b) Data Plane: It does the task of forwarding packets from input to output as determined by control plane.
(c) OpenFlow Switches: An OpenFlow switch is a device used to forward traffic in SDN environment; it could be a software program or a hardware component. If a packet's flow is unknown, the OpenFlow switch contacts the SDN controller to know about the flow of packets.
(d) OpenFlow Hosts: The end devices that receive or transmit data are called hosts.

3.2 Bellman–Ford Algorithm

In this work, Bellman–Ford shortest path algorithm is considered to test the network performance with routing. The Bellman–Ford is a graph-search distance-vector routing algorithm which computes the shortest path from the given source vertex to all other vertices in a directed graph [5]. The primary structure of Bellman–Ford algorithm is same as Dijkstra's algorithm. The algorithm primarily combines routing details (statistics) provided by various routers in an internetwork and learns about the prevalent conditions of the network to route packets to their destination. It uses the relaxation principle in which an estimation of the correct distance is successively replaced by more precise values up till optimal solution is obtained. It is more versatile than the Dijkstra's algorithm, as it can be applied to negative weights [5].

Algorithm 1: Bellman-Ford

Require: Cost Metric

Ensure: Shortest Path

1. *For each vertex v in G:*

   2. *d[v]->infinity ,previous[v]=null, d[src]=zero (1.1)*

   3. *While (Network .nodes) > zero*

   4. *For every iteration i from 1 to |v|-1*   *(1.2)*

   5. *For each edge (u,v) with weight w :*

   6. *if d[u] + w < d[v]:*

   7. *distance[v] := distance[u] + w*

   8. *predecessor[v] := u.*

Algorithm 1 describes the initialization. At the start, the distance from the source node to all other nodes is initialized to infinity and distance of source is set to zero. In (1.2), the edges are marked E1, E2, …, Em and this set of edges is relaxed $|v| - 1$ times where $|v|$ is the number of vertices in the graph.

4 Implementation

In this section, a scenario-based study of the SDN is presented. POX is used as SDN controller to implement dynamic routing. The proposed solution is tested with four different topologies, and performance of network is carried out for both routing and non-routing as shown in Table 1.

Table 1 Topology configuration

Topology no	No. of switches	No. of links	No. of hosts
1	5	7	2
2	5	7	2
3	4	7	2
4	6	9	2

4.1 Topologies Deployed

Figure 2 shows the Topology 1 which is the basic topology among all the other topologies considered. As shown in Table 1, it has 5 OpenFlow switches, 2 hosts, and 7 links connecting all the network devices.

As shown in Fig. 3, Topology 2 consists of 5 OpenFlow switches connecting to 2 hosts by 7 links as shown in Table 1.

Figure 4 shows the Topology 3 which is complex than Topology 1 and Topology 2. Topology 3 consists of 4 OpenFlow switches, 7 links, and 2 hosts as shown in Table 1.

Figure 5 shows Topology 4 which is the advanced topology of all topologies deployed for testing the network performance. From Table 1, we see that Topology 4 has 6 OpenFlow switches with 9 links, and 2 hosts.

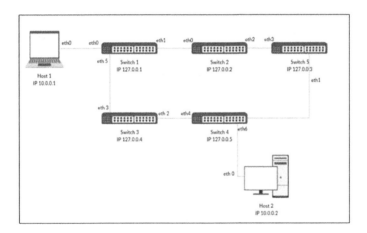

Fig. 2 Topology 1

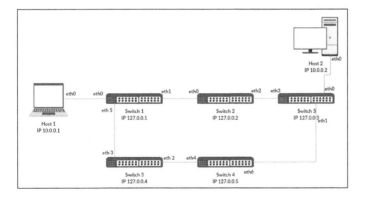

Fig. 3 Topology 2

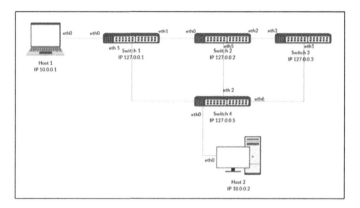

Fig. 4 Topology 3

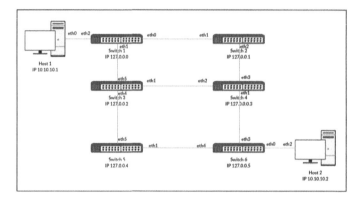

Fig. 5 Topology 4

The topologies that are considered here are based on the complexities. Proposed work also tries to address the problem of looping. Generally, when the switches are connected to each other (forming a ring structure), the control packets [7] start to move from one switch to other and the packets are never delivered to the destination. So, to handle this issue, Bellman–Ford algorithm is used.

5 Results and Performance Estimation

The results were obtained for all the topologies for both routing and non-routing scenarios. Comparative analysis on QoS parameters of both scenarios is obtained. The results state that the Bellman–Ford algorithm is the most efficient in terms providing high data throughput and minimizing the delay in any given topology compared to traditional network where no routing algorithm is employed.

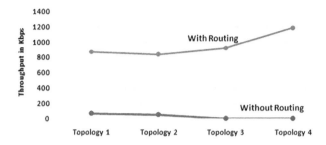

Fig. 6 Comparative analysis of bandwidth obtained with routing and without routing

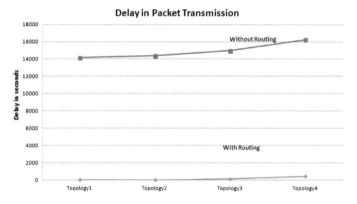

Fig. 7 Comparative analysis of delay in packet transmission with routing and without routing

Figure 6 shows bandwidth achieved for the topologies with routing and without routing scenarios. It is observed that bandwidth achieved is low with increasing network complexity in topologies with no routing. This is the main drawback of the traditional networks. Better bandwidth results are obtained after applying Bellman—Ford routing algorithm which uses distance as a parameter to find the best suitable path thus reducing the need to send the packets to all the switches which in turn increases the bandwidth.

Figure 7 shows the delay occurred in packet transmission. It is observed that delay occurred in packet transmission is minimum in topologies where Bellman—Ford routing algorithm is applied. This is due to the packets that are passed to particular switches thus reducing the traffic. Delay is high in conventional networks as the packets flood through all nodes in the network thus deteriorating the network performance.

Figure 8 shows that the packet loss occurred with routing are ignorable. There is high packet loss when data is transmitted with no routing mechanism. The reason

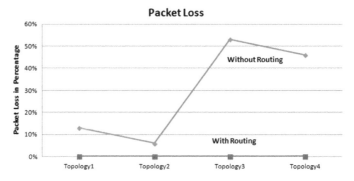

Fig. 8 Comparative analysis of packet loss occurred with routing and without routing

for negligible packet loss is because the looping is avoided by specifying a path for the packet to travel. Bellman–Ford algorithm being considered as the single-source shortest path algorithm can detect the negative cycles in the graph. But when it comes to efficiency, Dijkstra's algorithm is considered to be more efficient.

6 Conclusion

SDN helps organizations in advance application development and reduces IT costs in drastic way. In this paper, study conducted on the QoS achieved in case of traditional network and SDN network for routing and non-routing scenarios. When the packets are flooded, the bandwidth of the channel decreases as the complexity increases. By using Bellman–Ford algorithm, complex networks can be efficiently implemented with negligible packet loss. The problem of infinite looping is also addressed which leads to increased throughput. The results obtained emphasize the importance of routing in achieving better throughput with minimum delay and no packet loss as compared to traditional networks through network emulation.

7 Future Scope

SDN is an emerging technology which will help in revolution with the changing network trends. The existing Bellman–Ford algorithm-based approach can further be optimized for better QoS performance. This can also be applied further for combining traffic engineering and routing. Considering other networking parameters involved in a software-defined network for the performance analysis of network.

References

1. Kreutz D, Ramos FMV, Veríssimo PE, Rothenberg CE, Azodolmolky S, Uhlig S (Jan 2015) Software-defined networking: a comprehensive survey. In: Proceedings of IEEE, vol 103, no 1, pp 14–76. https://doi.org/10.1109/jproc.2014.2371999
2. Zhang H, Yan J (2015) Performance of SDN routing in comparison with legacy routing protocols. In: 2015 international conference on cyber-enabled distributed computing and knowledge discovery, Xi'an, pp 491–494. https://doi.org/10.1109/cyberc.2015.30
3. Home—Mininet. https://www.mininet.org/. Accessed 28 May 2018
4. Mulla MM, Narayan DG, Meena SM. Load balancing for software-defined networks
5. Waleed S, Faizan M, Iqbal M, Anis MI (2017) Demonstration of single link failure recovery using Bellman Ford and Dijikstra algorithm in SDN. In: 2017 international conference on innovations in electrical engineering and computational technologies (ICIEECT), Karachi, pp 1–4. https://doi.org/10.1109/icieect.2017.7916533
6. Open Networking Foundation. https://www.opennetworking.org. Accessed 28 May 2018
7. Home—Iperf. https://iperf.fr
8. Jarraya Y, Madi T, Debbabi M (Fourthquarter 2014) A survey and a layered taxonomy of software-defined networking. IEEE Commun Surv Tutor 16(4):1955–1980. https://doi.org/10.1109/comst.2014.2320094
9. Magzhan K, Jani HM (2013) A review and evaluations of shortest path algorithms. Int J Sci Technol Res 2(6)
10. Feamster N, Rexford J, Zegura E (2014) The road to SDN: an intellectual history of programmable networks. ACM SIGCOMM Comput Commun Rev 87–98

Design of an Energy-Efficient Routing Protocol Using Adaptive PSO Technique in Wireless Sensor Networks

R. Nagesh, Sarika Raga and Shakti Mishra

Abstract Demand of wireless sensor networks has increased dramatically due to their significant use in various real-time industrial, military, and medical field applications. Due to their vast applications, WSNs have become an attractive field of research. These sensor networks are easy to deploy and can efficiently monitor the area and environment, but due to limited resources, such as memory, battery capacity, and computation capacity, it becomes a challenging task. In this work, we focus on the network lifetime enhancement by developing particle swarm optimization (PSO)-based technique. In order to achieve the desired performance, the complete proposed model is divided into various stages where first of all, sensor nodes are deployed randomly. Later, cluster head selection is performed followed by the shortest path identification. In order to minimize the energy consumption, we apply multi-objective PSO scheme. However, fitness function computation suffers from the slow convergence which leads to the premature solution resulting in degraded communication performance. In order to address this issue, we present a new fitness function computation which considers residual energy parameter and formulates a new energy consumption model for each node which helps to optimize the power consumption during data transmission and reception by considering the sleeping phases of sensor nodes. An extensive simulation study is carried out using MATLAB simulation tool, and the performance of the proposed approach is compared with the state-of-the-art techniques. Results and discussion of this approach show that the proposed approach can achieve better performance in terms of QoS, packet delivery rate, and network lifetime enhancement.

Keywords Energy-aware routing · Wireless sensor network · Multi-objective PSO · QoS · Network lifetime

R. Nagesh (✉)
Centre for PG Studies Muddenahalli, VTU, Muddenahalli, India
e-mail: nagesh.rajudvg@gmail.com

S. Raga
Department of DECS, VTU, CPGS, Bangaluru Region, Muddenahalli, Chikkaballapur, India

S. Mishra
Department of ISE, NMIT, VTU, Bangalore, India

© Springer Nature Singapore Pte Ltd. 2019
V. Sridhar et al. (eds.), *Emerging Research in Electronics, Computer Science and Technology*, Lecture Notes in Electrical Engineering 545,
https://doi.org/10.1007/978-981-13-5802-9_90

1 Introduction

Demand of wireless sensor network-based communication has gained lot of attraction for daily life scenario, industries, military, health monitoring, security and surveillance, underground mines, and research applications [1] due to its significant nature of monitoring the indoor and outdoor environmental conditions [2]. Wireless sensor networks are self-organized in the nature and contain limited computing resources, communication requirements, storage, and limited power resources [3]. According to their demand, the aforementioned applications require prolonged network lifetime and efficient packet delivery rate to improve the quality of the service (QoS) of any sensor network-based application [4].

Moreover, these sensor networks are generally deployed in the hostile environments such as battlefield, forests, and flood-affected regions where these sensor nodes are not accessible and hence cannot be replaced or recharged their battery capacity [5]. In order to deal with these issues, energy consumption minimization can help to maximize the network lifetime in WSNs. Therefore, several techniques and researches have been presented in the field of energy consumption minimization which can help to improve the network lifetime.

During the communication phase of sensing applications, a packet which contains the required information is transmitted from the source node to the sink node via multi-hop communication. In this stage, route identification is a challenging task which can enhance the packet delivery performance and can observe other performance factors such as load balancing and energy-efficient communication. During last decade, this field has attracted the attention of researchers and several techniques have been introduced to improve the performance of the system by mitigating the issues of energy consumption, delay, load balancing, data aggregation, and packet routing schemes. However, efficient routing scheme can be helpful for improving the overall performance by means of improving the energy consumption, delay, and packet drop. These routing schemes are categorized into three main categories which are as follows: data-centric routing techniques, location-based routing, and hierarchal routing algorithms. According to the data-centric scheme, routing information is identified and updated during the message transmission phase. Semchedine et al. [6] presented data-centric routing protocol using directed diffusion data-centric algorithm which also performs the load balancing task in the network. SPIN [7] is a data-centric protocol for wireless sensor network which has a significant impact on the network performance. The intermediate sensor nodes can perform some form of aggregation on the data originating from multiple source sensor nodes and send the aggregated data toward the sink node. Therefore, these routing schemes can be deployed easily and strong self-organizing capability, but due to "flooding" effects, the unwanted overhead increases on the nodes; hence, these schemes are generally implemented for the small-scale sensor network development.

In the next type, location-based routing algorithms are discussed where positions of nodes are identified to establish the route from source node to sink node. These algorithms are always combined with the other techniques for any specific applications. The main advantages of these algorithms are that the path between sensor nodes can be found quickly as the communication initiates. Moreover, it provides accurate routing information but suffers from the efficiency issue due to the varying geographical environmental conditions. Some of the known techniques of location-based routing algorithms are GREES [8], HGMR [9], SPAN [10], and GEAR [11].

On the other hand, hierarchical routing algorithms are widely adopted in the field of WSN. According to these routing schemes, the complete sensor nodes would be divided into multiple parts by using some rules or similarity and each party is known as cluster. In every cluster, a superior node is selected which acts as the cluster head (CH) and other remaining nodes act as the cluster members. In these protocols, cluster members collect the required information which is later collected by the cluster head and forwarded to the sink node. These algorithms have several advantages such as efficient data delivery, balanced energy consumption, and robust performance. However, recently, large numbers of nodes are deployed where energy consumption and performance remain a challenging task which can affect the overall performance of the network [12]. In this field, evolutionary and intelligent computation-based schemes have also been introduced. Shokouhifar and Jalali [13] introduced application-specific low-power routing protocol (ASLPR) for optimal cluster head selection which further optimized using genetic algorithm-based scheme of optimization. Similarly, Gupta and Jana [14] also presented genetic algorithm-based clustering and routing scheme. This clustering scheme uses the information such as residual energy of gateways, distance from sensor to the cluster head.

Motivated by these researches, in this work the authors focus on the development of energy-aware routing scheme for WSN. According to the proposed approach, the authors formulate an optimization problem for improving the performance of WSN communication. Later, particle swarm optimization-based strategy is applied to further optimize the performance of WSN communication. This helps to improve the energy consumption performance. Moreover, the authors present a simple model for load balancing in WSN for increasing the network lifetime.

The rest of the paper is arranged as follows: Sect. 1 presents a brief discussion about recent studies in the field of energy-aware communication in WSN. In Sect. 2, we discuss the proposed approach for energy-aware routing and load balancing in WSN. Section 3 presents the discussion about experimental study, and the performance of the proposed approach is compared with the other state-of-the-art models. Finally, Sect. 4 provides concluding remarks and future directions of the work for improving the network performance.

2 Proposed Model

This section presents discussion about the proposed approach to improve the network performance by improving the network lifetime and quality of service. The complete model is divided into multiple sections as: network lifetime maximization problem formulation, cluster head selection, applying shortest path computation, developing energy-efficient routing using particle swarm optimization (PSO).

2.1 WSN System Model

The WSN system model comprises a number of sensor nodes N and sink node S in the sensor field. Sink node collects the desired information from the sensor nodes. Initially, these sensor nodes are deployed randomly for monitoring the environmental conditions, and then, the location of sensor nodes starts moving. Hence, required information is getting generated continuously at a constant data generation rate D_i, i.e., $D_i > 0$ for each sensor node i where $i \in N$. However, it is also considered that sink node is mobile and can vary the location during the processing of the task in the network. Let us consider that L numbers of locations are present in the sensor field where the sensor node can occupy the location $l \in L$ at the time $t_l \geq 0$. It shows the total time spend by the sink node at the location l. In this model, the authors make some necessary assumption in the underlying network model.

These assumptions are as follows:

1. A base station is present in the network which is located at the remote location from the sensing field. These sensor nodes occupy the coordinates in the sensor field.
2. Entire network has multiple nodes which are homogenous in nature and carry the similar configurations and capabilities. In this process, each node is given a unique id.
3. These sensors can operate in active mode and low-power node.
4. Deployed sensor nodes can use power control strategy to vary the power consumption performance based on the distance required for data transmission.
5. Sensed data is always highly correlated.

Author's main aim is to reduce the energy consumption and improve the network lifetime performance. Hence, the author presents a simplified model for energy dissipation. In this multi-path fading and free-space channel models have been used which depend on the distance between transmitter and receiver. The required amount of energy to transmit 1-bit packet over d distance is expressed as:

$$E_{Tx}(l,d) = lE_{elec} + l\epsilon d^{\gamma} = \begin{cases} lE_{elec} + \varepsilon_{fs}d^2 \, d < d_0 \\ lE_{elec} + \varepsilon_{mp}d^4, \, d \geq d_0 \end{cases} \tag{1}$$

E_{elec} denotes the electronics energy which depends on the several aspects such as modulation schemes, and amplifier energy ($\varepsilon_{fs}d^2 \, or \, \varepsilon_{mp}d^2$) depends on the distance between communicating nodes and bit error rate. Based on these assumptions, energy consumption to receive the packet is given as:

$$E_{Rx}(l) = lE_{elec} \tag{2}$$

Here, the authors consider fifth assumption where collected data is considered to be highly correlated; hence, cluster head can easily aggregate the data from neighboring nodes and formulates a single length-fixed packet for further process. However, some schemes show that relay nodes can be used for packet aggregation from other clusters with its own packet, but due to low degree of correlation among data, this relay-based scheme is discarded for data aggregation. Let E_{DA} (nj/bit/signal) denote the energy consumption for data aggregation by a cluster head.

2.2 Problem Formulation

Let us consider that a static wireless sensor network is modeled as undirected graph $G(V, L)$ where V denotes the nodes and L denotes the set of communication links between two nodes. In this model, two sensor nodes i and j are connected to each other if they can establish the communication without exceeding the maximum transmission power requirement for each node. Hence, these links are considered to be bidirectional. The sensor nodes which are connected to node i by a link are expressed as N_i. Moreover, it is also considered that the network graph is connected; hence, there exists a path between nodes i and j.

Moreover, it is assumed that the transmission rate between node i and node j is fixed as X_{ij} and maximum time duration for data transmission through a link is given as t_{ij}. Hence, the maximum supported data flow by a link between node i and node j can be computed as $R_{ij} = X_{ij}t_{ij}$. Later, with the help of path loss model, the minimum power of receiver can be used for estimating the required power for transmission (P_{ij}) at a data rate of R_{ij} between communicating nodes i and j. Based on this assumption, let us consider that data flow from node i to j is r_{ij}. The average power consumption for this data flow at node i can be given as:

$$P_{ij}\frac{r_{ij}}{E_{ij}} = r_{ij}E_{ij} \tag{3}$$

In this model, we assume that each node contains an initial energy of battery as B_i. Let us consider that D_i is the data generation rate at node i which need to be communicated to the sink node. For the considered network flow, r, r_{ij} denotes the data flow rate from node i to j whose energy dissipation is E_{ij}. Based on this, the lifetime of sensing node i can be given as

$$T_i(r) = \frac{B_i}{\sum_{i \in N} r_{ij}E_{ij}} \tag{4}$$

We express the network lifetime $T_{network}$ under the data flow r to be the time duration until the node runs out of the minimum required energy. This can be written as:

$$T_{network}(r) = \min_{i \in N} T_i(r) \tag{5}$$

Here, our main aim is to reduce the energy consumption which can improve the network lifetime.

2.3 Cluster Head Selection

In order to achieve the reduced energy consumption by any node for data transmission, the authors present a cluster head selection methodology. In this work, the authors aim at the cluster formulation without any centralized controlled scheme and the certain number of clusters can be formed in each communication round. Initially, each sensor node i considers itself as a cluster head during the first round as $(r + 1)$ with cluster head node probability $P_{ci}(t)$. Hence, if N numbers of nodes are present in the considered network then the function of each node to be the cluster head can be denoted as:

$$E[CH] = \sum_{i=1}^{N} P_i(t) * 1 = k \tag{6}$$

Let $l_i(t)$ denote the function which indicates whether the node is selected as cluster head in the recent communication rounds $(r(\text{mod } (N/K))$. According to this assumption, if the $l_i(t) = 0$ then the particular node has been assigned as cluster head previously; otherwise, $l_i(t) = 1$ denotes the node as a cluster member. The probability of any node becoming the cluster head can be given at round r as follows:

$$P_i(t) = \begin{cases} \frac{k}{N - k*(r \bmod \frac{N}{k})} : l_i(t) = 1 \\ 0 : l_i(t) = 0 \end{cases} \tag{7}$$

Once the cluster head selection is finished, we apply Dijkstra's algorithm for shortest path identification [15]. However, this gives us the path which has less cost from source node to destination node but the node alive states are not considered during this process.

2.4 PSO-Based Routing

In this section, we describe the proposed approach for routing using particle swarm optimization (PSO)-based scheme. Particle swarm optimization is a process which contains predefined number of particles which are capable to provide the solution for any given multi-dimensional optimization problem, and each particle has the same dimension. The particle is denoted by $P_i, 1 \leq i \leq Np$ and has initial position as

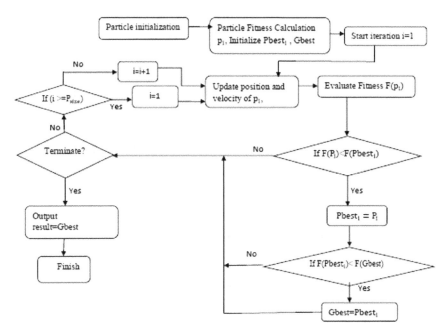

Fig. 1 Basic flowchart of PSO

X_{ij}, $1 \leq d \leq D$ and the velocity V_{id}. In this process, each particle is processed and the fitness of the particle is computed based on the fitness function. In order to achieve this, each particle tries to obtain the personal best and global best solution for updating the velocity. Figure 1 shows a basic flowchart of particle swarm optimization.

The velocity and position updates can be obtained by using the expression given as:

$$V_{i,d}(t) = \left(V_{i,d}(t-1) \times W\right) + c1 \times r1 \times \left(X_{pbest\,i,d} - X_{i,d}(t-1)\right)$$
$$+ c2 \times r2 \times \left(X_{gbest\,d} - X_{i,d}(t-1)\right) \tag{8}$$

Similarly, the position updates can be given as:

$$X_{i,d}(t) = X_{i,d}(t-1) + V_{i,d}(t) \tag{9}$$

where $c1$ and $c2$ are two nonnegative constants and $r1$ and $r2$ are the two random variables which are in the range of [0, 1]. Based on the PSO scheme, we present a routing algorithm as given in Fig. 2.

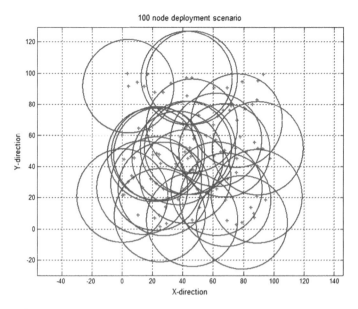

Fig. 2 Experiment scenario 1: 100 nodes

Input : set of generated cluster heads $\alpha = \{Ch_1, Ch_2, .. Ch_M\}$, PSO parameters, next hop and Hop count

Output: optimal route $R: \alpha \to \{\alpha + Ch_{M+1}\}$

Step 1: initialize the particles as $P_i, \forall_i, 1 \leq i \leq N_p$

Step 2: for $i = 1$ to N_p
(a) Compute the fitness as $F = Max\_Dist \times W_1 + Max\_Hops \times W_2$
(b) Find the personal best $P_{best} = P$
End
Step 3: find the global best (g_{best}) as
$\{P_{best_k} | Fitness(P_{best_k}) = \min\left(Fitness(P_{best_k})\right)$
Step 4: Until the optimal condition achieved *do*
    (a) *for* $i = 1: N_p$ do
    (b) Update the particle's velocity and positons.
    (c) Compute the fitness of current solution
    (d) Find the $P_{best_i} = P_i$, i.e. if $Fitness(P_i) < Fitness(P_{best})$ then
    (e) $P_{best_i} = P_i$
    (f) End
    (g) Find the $G_{best_i} = P_i$, i.e. if $Fitness(P_{best}) < Fitness(G_{best})$ then
    (h) $G_{best_i} = P_{best_i}$
    (i) end
    (j) end
Step 5: Compute Next Hop cluster using G_{best}
Step 6: Stop

Conventional PSO-based schemes suffer from the issue of slow convergence which may lead to premature solution identification. In order to deal with this issue, we present a new approach for fitness function computation by considering the node's residual energy estimation. This fitness function can be expressed as:

$$f(X_i) = \text{opt}(\gamma_1 \chi_1 + \gamma_2 \chi_2 + (1 - \gamma_1 - \gamma_2)\chi_2 \tag{10}$$

Subject to

$$\chi_1 = \sum_{n_j \in C_K} \left\{ \frac{\|n_j x_i\|}{|C_K|} \right\}$$

$$\chi_2 = \frac{\sum_{i=1}^{N} E(p_i)}{\sum_{j=1}^{|C_K|} E(n_j)} \quad E_{min} \leq E(n_j) \leq E_{max}$$

According to the proposed approach, γ_1 and γ_2 denote the weightage parameters. In this work, we have considered residual energy as the objective function which is associated with each particle P_i, and also, the sensor must contain a desired energy level in the range of $[E_{min}, E_{max}], C_k$ denotes the kth cluster, $|C_k|$ contains the total number of nodes available in the current cluster, X_1 denotes the cluster distance, and X_2 denotes the residual energy measurement.

As discussed before that two types of power losses can occur which are free-space and multi-path fading. In this model, we formulate small-sized clusters; hence, free-space power loss model is considered for analysis. Hence, the expected energy consumption for the data transmission for d distance can be given as:

$$E[d^2] = \int \int \varphi(x^2 + y^2)dxdy \tag{11}$$

where φ denotes the node deployment density which is considered based on the distance between the communicating cluster heads. Based on these assumptions, energy consumption for m-bit length data transmission over distance d can be expressed as given in (1). Hence, energy consumption used by a node to transmit/receive a packet can be given by considering the sleeping phases of the node. It can be given as:

$$\xi_{node} = (1 - S_p)[e_{tx} + e_{rx}] + S_p e_{sp} \tag{12}$$

where S_p denotes the sleeping phase and e_{sp} denotes the energy consumption during the sleeping phases.

3 Results and Discussion

This section deals with the experimental analysis using the proposed approach, and a comparative study is also presented by using state-of-the-art techniques. The complete experimental study is carried out using MATLAB simulation tool running of Windows platform with Intel i3 processor.

Experiment begins with by deploying the sensor network in a random manner where initially 100 sensor nodes are deployed. Each sensor is provided with initial energy as 0.5 J in the network area of 100×100 m. Each sensor node has some parameters related to the initial energy constraints such as amplification energy and power dissipation. Table 1 shows the complete simulation parameters used in this work.

The optimal path computation has been carried out using particle swarm optimization scheme. The considered simulation parameters for PSO are given in Table 2.

3.1 Performance Measurement Metrics

In this subsection, we briefly describe the performance measurement parameters which are applied in this work. These parameters are as follows: number of dead nodes where we find the total number of dead nodes during the communication phase, number of alive nodes where total number of alive nodes are identified during

Table 1 Simulation parameters

Parameter name	Parameter value
Network area	100 m $\times$ 100m
Number of nodes	100, 200, 300, 400 and 500
Tx amplifier energy dissipation	10 pJ/bit/m^2
E_{elec}	5 nJ/bit
ε_{mp}	0.0013 pJ/bit/m^2
E_0 (initial energy)	0.5 J
Data packet size	4000 KB

Table 2 Simulation parameters for PSO

Parameter name	Parameter value
Population size	1000
Number of iteration	1000
Social parameter c1	3
Cognitive parameter c2	1
Speed factor w	0.5

the complete simulation time, total packets transmitted to cluster head where total packets are transmitted to base station, packet delivered where we compute the total number of packet delivered successfully from source node to sink node and network throughput.

3.2 Experimental Scenario 1

According to the proposed model, the authors deploy 100 nodes randomly. Figure 2 shows a sample representation of sensor nodes in red color dots. Later, we apply a clustering scheme where similar residual energy nodes are clustered together for prolonged computation.

Once the network is deployed and sensor nodes are clustered, then we apply shortest path computation where source node is considered node 1 and destination node is 100. Figure 3 shows the shortest path computation phase where the shortest distance is computed between source node 1 and destination node 100 which shows a path cost of 34.83.

Dead Node Performance Comparisons

After identifying the shortest path, we initiate the communication, but due to frequent variations, the optimal path may vary. Therefore, we apply particle swam optimization scheme to obtain the optimal path in iterative process. Finally, we evaluate the performance of the proposed approach and compare with the state-of-the-art routing algorithms (Fig. 4).

Based on this study, we evaluate the average dead node performance. Conventional LEACH protocol has a node dead rate as 67.21%; modified LEACH, DEEC, SEP have node death rates as 59.82%, 77.77%, and 47.56%, respectively, whereas proposed

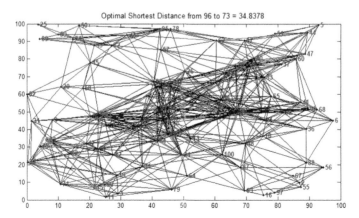

Fig. 3 Shortest path computation

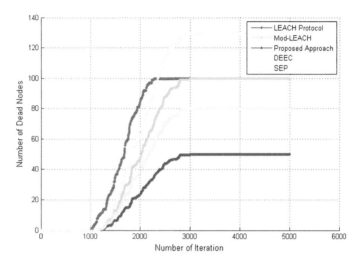

Fig. 4 Dead node performance comparisons

Table 3 Average dead node performance

	LEACH	Mod-LEACH	DEEC	SEP	Proposed
Avg. rate	67.21	59.82	77.77	47.86	29.91

Table 4 Average alive node performance

	LEACH	Mod-LEACH	DEEC	SEP	Proposed approach
Avg. rate	37.37	31.46	20.08	12.05	40.17

approach achieves node death rate as 29.91%. Table 3 shows average performance comparison.

Alive Node Performance Comparisons

In the next phase, we evaluate the performance of the proposed approach in terms of total alive nodes. Figure 5 shows a comparative performance in terms of total alive nodes in the network when the entire communication is completed.

From Fig. 5, it can be concluded that the proposed approach contains more number of alive nodes when compared with the other algorithms. Moreover, in the proposed system, node death starts after multiple iterations whereas conventional systems are not able to maintain the node alive state. According to this experiment, conventional LEACH, modified LEACH, DEEC, and SEP achieve node alive rates as 37.37%, 31.76%, 20.08%, and 12.05%, respectively, and the proposed approach achieves node alive rate as 40.17%. Table 4 shows average performance comparison.

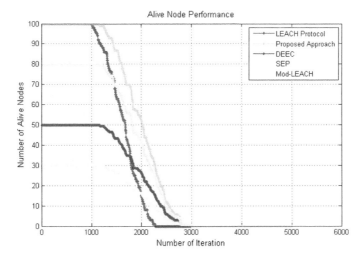

Fig. 5 Alive node performance

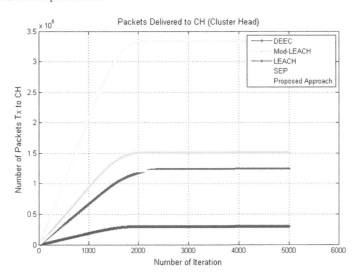

Fig. 6 Packets delivered to the cluster head performance

Packet Delivered to the Cluster Head Performance Comparisons

In this subsection, we evaluate the performance of successfully transmitted packets to the cluster head during communication. Figure 6 shows a comparative performance analysis where we show that the proposed approach achieves better performance in terms of packet delivery rate to the cluster head. Experimental analysis shows that the proposed approach is capable to deliver the packet to the cluster head efficiently. The performance of the proposed approach is compared with the conventional LEACH protocol, modified LEACH, DEEC, and SEP.

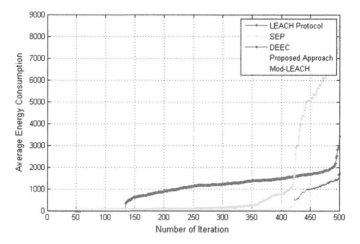

Fig. 7 Average energy consumption performance

Packet Delivered to the Cluster Head Performance Comparisons

This subsection presents the average energy consumption performance for 500 iteration scenarios. The performance of the proposed approach is compared with the state-of-the-art algorithms such as LEACH, modified LEACH, SEP, and DEEC whose average energy performance is obtained as 1010.67, 933.85, 212.24, and 202.13 J where average energy consumption using proposed model is 121.28 J (Fig. 7).

4   Conclusion

Demand of wireless sensor network is increasing rapidly for various real-time applications due to their several advantages such as easy deployment and efficient monitoring. However, these networks are efficient but due to limited resources such as battery capacity cause performance degradation. In order to deal with this issue, we present a novel approach for network lifetime enhancement using PSO technique. The performance of PSO is further improved by introducing a new fitness function which provides a new solution for data transmission by considering the sleeping phases of the sensor nodes. The proposed approach is implemented using MATLAB simulation tool as compared with the state-of-the-art techniques where it shows significant improvement in the network lifetime performance.

References

1. Akyildiz IF, Su W, Sankarasubramaniam Y, Cayirci E (2002) Wireless sensor networks: survey. Comput Netw 38:393–422
2. Amgoth T, Jana PK (2015) Energy-aware routing algorithm for wireless sensor networks. Comput Electr Eng 1(41):357–367
3. Yao, Cao Q, Vasilakos AV (2013) EDAL: an energy-efficient, delay-aware, and lifetime-balancing data collection protocol for wireless sensor networks. In: Proceedings of 10th IEEE MASS, 2013, pp 182–190
4. Aweya J (2013) Technique for differential timing transfer over packet networks. IEEE Trans Ind Inf 9(1):325–336
5. Thilagavathi S, Gnanasambandan Geetha B (2015) Energy aware swarm optimization with intercluster search for wireless sensor network. Sci World J 2015
6. Semchedine F, Bouallouche-Medjkoune L, Tamert M, Mahfoud F, Aïssani D (2015) Load balancing mechanism for data-centric routing in wireless sensor networks. Comput Electr Eng 1(41):395–406
7. Ehsan S, Hamdaoui B (2012) A survey on energy-efficient routing techniques with QoS assurances for wireless multimedia sensor networks. IEEE Commun Surv Tutor 14(2):265–278
8. Zeng K, Ren K, Lou WJ, Moran PJ (2009) Energy aware efficient geographic routing in lossy wireless sensor networks with environmental energy supply. Wireless Netw 15:39–51
9. Koutsonikolas D, Das SM, Hu YC, Stojmenovic I (2010) Hierarchical geographic multicast routing for wireless sensor networks. Wireless Netw 16:449–466
10. Chen B, Jamieson K, Balakrishnan H, Morris R (2002) SPAN: an energy-efficient coordination algorithm for topology maintenance in ad hoc wireless networks. Wireless Netw 8(5):481–494
11. Yu Y, Estrin D, Govindan R (2001) Geographical and energy-aware routing: a recursive data dissemination protocol for wireless sensor networks. UCLA Comp Sci Dept Tech Rep, UCLA-CSD TR-010023
12. Yetgin H, Cheung KT, El-Hajjar M, Hanzo LH (2017) A survey of network lifetime maximization techniques in wireless sensor networks. IEEE Commun Surv Tutor 19(2):828–854
13. Shokouhifar M, Jalali A (2015) A new evolutionary based application specific routing protocol for clustered wireless sensor networks. AEU-Int J Electron Commun 69(1):432–441
14. Gupta SK, Jana PK (2015) Energy efficient clustering and routing algorithms for wireless sensor networks: GA based approach. Wireless Pers Commun 83(3):2403–2423
15. Yao Y, Cao Q, Vasilakos AV (2015) EDAL: an energy-efficient, delay-aware, and lifetime-balancing data collection protocol for heterogeneous wireless sensor networks. IEEE/ACM Trans Netw (TON) 23(3):810–823
16. Narendra K, Varun VA (2014) Comparative analysis of energy-efficient routing protocols in wireless sensor networks. In: Emerging research in electronics, computer science and technology 2014. Springer, New Delhi, pp 399–405
17. Ho JH, Shih HC, Liao BY, Chu SC (2012) A ladder diffusion algorithm using ant colony optimization for wireless sensor networks. Inf Sci 193:204–212
18. Misra S, Thomasinous PD (2010) A simple, least-time and energy-efficient routing protocol with one-level data aggregation for wireless sensor networks. J Syst Softw 83:852–860
19. Ho JH, Shih HC, Liao BY, Chu SC (2012) A ladder diffusion algorithm using antcolony optimization for wireless sensor networks. Inf Sci 192:204–212

Detection of Retinal Disease Screening Using Local Binary Patterns

S. B. Manojkumar, U. Shama Firdose and H. S. Sheshadri

Abstract This work explores partial efficiency with effective structure based on fundus image to characterize among disease and normal images. The execution of LBP in the process of a surface description as retinal image had it investigated also contrasted and different description. The objective is to separate DR and typical fundus images investigating the surface of the retina foundation and keeping away from a past sore division. For each experiment, several classifiers were tested on an average sensitivity and specificity higher than 0.86 in all the cases, and almost of 1 and 0.99, respectively, for DR detection were achieved. These outcomes recommend that the strategy exhibited in this paper is a powerful calculation for portraying retina surface and can be valuable for the analysis which helps to framework for retinal disease screening.

Keywords Local binary patterns (LBPs) · Diabetic retinopathy (DR)

1 Introduction

Retinal disease may cause to any part of the retina. If it is untreated that may lead to visual blindness; among many retinal diseases like retinal tear, retinal detachment, macular hole, macular degeneration, retinitis pigmentosa, diabetic retinopathy also comes under retinal disease. This thesis focuses more on diabetic retinopathy. Diabetic retinopathy related to the retinal damage causes the blindness for diabetic

S. B. Manojkumar (✉)
PET Research Foundation, Mandya, India
e-mail: sbmanojkumar@gmail.com

U. Shama Firdose
Department of ECE, BGSIT, BG Nagar, Mandya, India
e-mail: shamafirdose2013@gmail.com

H. S. Sheshadri
Department of ECE, PES College of Engineering, Mandya 571401, India
e-mail: hssheshadri@gmail.com

© Springer Nature Singapore Pte Ltd. 2019   1055
V. Sridhar et al. (eds.), *Emerging Research in Electronics, Computer Science and Technology*, Lecture Notes in Electrical Engineering 545,
https://doi.org/10.1007/978-981-13-5802-9_91

patients. A few people are undergone screening regularly, while others not aware of it. The body cannot store the sugar from sustenance, and it courses through the circulatory system. This sugar responds with the dividers of the veins as it does as such, making them separate after some time. Diabetic retinopathy is the harm to the retina. As light beams come into the eye, through the viewpoint, it arrives on the retina to be transformed into electrical signs to be sent to the mind. Passages and veins take oxygen and supplement to your retina, and diabetes harms and pulverizes these veins.

The World Health Organization assesses that in 2010 there were 285 million individuals outwardly hamper nearby the globe. Despite the way that the quantity of visual deficiency cases has been essentially decreased as of late, nearly 80% of the instances of optical disability are avoidable or curable. Diabetic retinopathy and macular degeneration usually occur after mid-age which are the greatest continuous reasons for the visual deficiency and apparition problem. In addition, this disorder will encounter a high development later on because of diabetes occurrence increment and maturing populace in the present society. Their initial determination is very much necessary to identify this retinal disease through screening efforts.

Figure 1 shows the fundus images of healthy eye, diabetic retinopathy-affected eye, and age-related macular degeneration eye.

Diabetic retinopathy is divided into two types:

Non-proliferative diabetic retinopathy (NPDR) It is the primary phase of the infection in which manifestations will be mellow or nonexistent. In NPDR, the veins in the retina are weakening at the end. Little lumps in the veins, known as microaneurysm (MA), may release liquid into the retina. The spillage may prompt swelling to the macula.

Proliferative diabetic retinopathy (PDR) It is the main state of the malady. At this stage, flow issues deny the retina of the oxygen. Therefore, new frail vein can begin to emerge from the retina and into the vitreous, the gel-like liquid that fills the back of the eye.

2 Literature Survey

Morales et al.'s [1] paper researches segregation capacities in the surface of fundus to separate among neurotic and solid pictures. Specifically, the fundamental concentration lies in investigating the execution of local binary patterns (LBPs) as a surface descriptor for retinal pictures. It depends on looking at the local varieties around each and every pixel, and relegating marks to various nearby examples. From there on, the conveyance of the names is assessed and utilized as a part of the classification stage. There are numerous cases for the achievement of LBP used to depict and furthermore on account of medicinal imaging. Be that as it may, in regards to fundus image preparing, LBP have not been broadly utilized. Most state-of-the-art works

(a)　　　　　　　　　　　　**(b)**

(c)

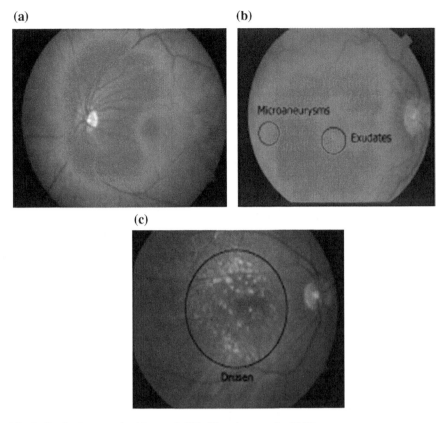

Fig. 1 Fundus images **a** healthy eye, **b** DR effected eye, and **c** AMD eye

that utilize the LBP system on fundus images locate center on the division of the retinal vessels rather than on a full determination framework, albeit a few cases can be found toward this path.

Ojala et al. [2] present a hypothetically exceptionally straightforward, yet effective, multi-determination way to deal with dark scale and revolution invariant surface grouping in light of neighborhood parallel examples and nonparametric separation of test and model dispersions. The technique depends on perceiving that specific nearby paired examples, named "uniform," are essential properties of neighborhood picture surface and their event histogram is turned out to be an effective surface component. We infer a summed up dark scale and pivot invariant administrator introduction that takes into account identifying the "uniform" examples for any quantization of the precise space and for any spatial determination and presents a technique for joining various administrators for multiresolution examination. The proposed approach is extremely hearty as far as dim scale varieties since the administrator is, by definition, invariant against any monotonic change of the dark scale. Another favorable position is computational straightforwardness as the administrator can be acknowledged with a couple of activities in a little neighborhood and a query table. Test comes about shows that great separation can be accomplished with the event measurements of basic turn invariant neighborhood parallel examples.

Ahonen et al.'s [3] paper exhibits a novel and proficient facial picture portrayal in view of neighborhood paired example (LBP) surface highlights. The face picture is separated into a few locales from which the LBP includes appropriations are removed and connected into an upgraded highlight vector to be utilized as a face descriptor. The execution of the proposed technique is surveyed in the face acknowledgment issue under various difficulties. Different applications and a few expansions are likewise examined.

Morales et al.'s [4] paper centers on investigating the execution of local binary pattern (LBP) as a surface descriptor for retinal pictures to separate among neurotic and sound pictures. In spite of the fact that LBP has been generally used to order surfaces, not much is accounted for on the investigation of the retina surface. Most works that utilized the LBP system on fundus pictures center on retinal vessel division and not on the analysis, albeit a few cases of analysis in light of LBP exist. Garnier et al. manage the AMD identification utilizing LBP. The surface data on a few scales is dissected through a wavelet deterioration of the fundus picture, and a LBP histogram is found from the wavelet coefficients. They do not consider DR arrangement. Mookiah et al. [8] separate irregular signs from fundus pictures to recognize ordinary fundus and two DR stages. The surface is found by LBP and laws vitality. A previous segmentation of the exudates include optic circle, veins are required for extraction. Shading data is not utilized; the RGB picture is changed over into dim scale. Krishnan and Laude consolidate LBP with entropies also, invariant minutes to produce a coordinated record for DR conclusion. Neither Mookiah et al. nor Krishnan and Laude think about AMD characterization.

Nanni et al.'s [5] work centers on the utilization of picture-based machine learning methods in therapeutic picture investigation. Variations of neighborhood paired examples (LBP) are introduced, which are broadly viewed as the cutting edge among surface descriptors, a point-by-point audit of the writing about existing LBP variations has been given, and the most remarkable methodologies are talked about alongside their advantages and disadvantages, new investigations are revealed utilizing a few LBP-based descriptors, and an arrangement of novel surface descriptors has been proposed for the portrayal of biomedical pictures. The standard LBP administrator is characterized as a grayscale invariant surface measure, got from a general definition of surface in a nearby neighborhood.

Gandhi and Dhanasekaran's [6] paper additionally centers on exudates for the reason that it gives data about prior diabetic retinopathy. The proteins and lipids getting spilled from the circulatory system into the retina through harmed veins are the main source of exudates. The screening procedure for diabetic retinopathy includes over the top expansion of student which influences the patients' eye. Along these lines, a mechanized strategy is exhibited in this paper for identification of exudates from the non-expanded shading fundus retinal pictures utilizing morphological process. In this paper, speedy and hearty strategy is acquainted with distinguishing the exudates by utilizing different morphological administrators on the low-quality non-expanded retinal fundus pictures. This method features the vague injuries in the retinal picture. This strategy is exceptionally compelling in portioning the exudates since it can perform rectify recognition and division of injuries. Our proposed technique additionally centers on surveying the seriousness level of the divided picture. SVM classifier is utilized for assessing the gravity of the diabetic retinopathy. This approach influences the screening to process simple without influencing the patient's eye and encourages ophthalmologists to distinguish the exudates rapidly.

3 Methods

3.1 Local Binary Patterns

LBP is an intense dark computation surface administrator utilized as a part of numerous PC vision applications in light of its calculation straightforwardness. The initial phase in LBP [7] is to create a name for every pixel in the picture where the mark is discovered in view of the nearby locality of the pixel which is characterized. Powerful neighboring dot stay threshold is used for the dark estimation of the focal pixel of the area producing a twofold string or, at the end of the day, a double example. The LBP is given as follow:

$$LBP_{P,R} = \sum_{p=0}^{P-1} s(g_p - g_c) \cdot 2^p, \quad s(x) = \begin{cases} 1 \text{ if } x \geq 0 \\ 0 \text{ if } x < 0. \end{cases}$$

where g_p and g_c are the dark estimations of the area and focal pixel, separately. P speaks to the quantity of tests going on the symmetric round neighborhood of sweep R. 2^p diverse double examples can be created in every area. LBP can have 36 different values (Fig. 2).

At the point when LBP are utilized for texture description, usually to incorporate a different quantity by characterizing the rotational invariant local variance is given in the below equation:

$$VAR_{P,R} = \frac{1}{P} \sum_{p=0}^{P-1} (g_p - \mu)^2, \quad \mu = \frac{1}{P} \sum_{p=0}^{P-1} g_p.$$

The LBP and VAR corresponding are consolidated toward upgrading the execution of the LBP administrator.

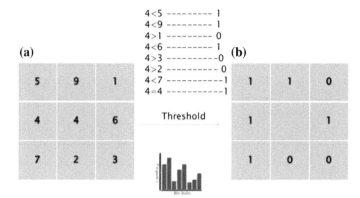

Fig. 2 LBP calculation: **a** estimations based on a roundabout area of range 1–8 bits. **b** Threshold of dim estimation focal pixel. The revolution invariant neighborhood parallel example produced is 11010011

3.2 Random Forest

One of the basic principles of random forest is it is the one of the modes of classifier and it can be used by machine learning to find out the classification and regression of the magnitude of the decision tree. The random forests equation is one in everything about least difficult among characterization calculations ready to group Goliath measures of data with precision. Arbitrary forests relate degree gathering learning system likewise thought of as a sort of closest neighbor indicator for grouping partner degreed relapse that build assortment of call trees at instructing time and yielding the class that is the method of the classifications yield by singular trees. Random forests might be a trademark of Leo Bremen and Adele monger for a troupe of call trees.

4   System Methodology

This paper researches separation capacities in the surface of fundus to separate among neurotic and sound pictures. Specifically, the primary concentration lies in investigating the execution of LBP as a surface descriptor for retinal pictures. The objective of this paper was to recognize DR and typical fundus pictures in the meantime and maintaining a strategic distance from any past division phase of retinal sores. The surface of the retina foundation is specifically broke down by methods for LBP [9].

The block diagram of detection of retinal disease using local binary patterns is as shown in Fig. 3 having the following functional units:

i. **Image Acquisition**: Images are procured from databases.

Fig. 3 Block diagram of detection of retinal disease using local binary patterns

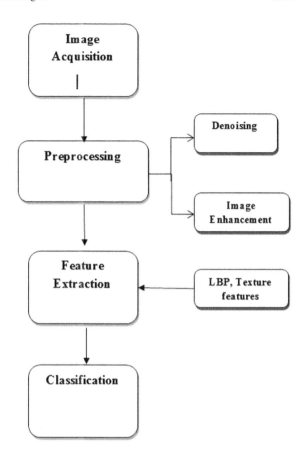

ii. **Preprocessing**: The aim of the preprocessing stage was to apply conceivable picture improvement procedures to get the required visual nature of the pictures. Picture upgrade methods.

- RGB channel extraction.
- Filtered image.
- Histogram equalization image.

- RGB channel separation: RGB channels are extracted from color image.
- Filtered image: An intermediate filter organizes a very good job at reducing the noise in image. This filter is applied in each channel of image for reducing the noise.
- Histogram equalization image: The complexity improvement of the picture can be seen by applying histeq (upgrade differentiates utilizing histogram balance).

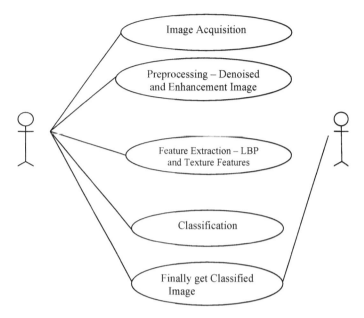

Fig. 4 Use case diagram

iii. **Feature Extraction**: In feature extraction stage, local binary pattern is used for extraction of features in each channel separately. Then extract the texture features for each channel of LBP image. After that, take average of all channel features for construct the final features. The final features are mean, standard deviation, entropy, kurtosis, and Skewness.

Figure 4 shows the use case diagram in the Unified Modeling Language (UML) which is a type of behavioral diagram defined by and created from a use case analysis. Its purpose is to present a graphical overview of the functionality provided by a system in terms of actors, their goals (represented as use cases), and any dependencies between those use cases. The main purpose of a use case diagram is to show what system functions are performed for which actor. Roles of the actors in the system can be depicted.

4.1 Preprocessing

The goal of the preprocessing stage is to apply conceivable picture improvement procedures to acquire the required visual nature of the pictures. Picture improvement strategies,

- RGB channel extraction
- Separated image

- Histogram equalization image

i. **RGB channel extraction**: In that R, G, and B channels are extricated from shading picture.

ii. **Filtered image**: A middle channel completes a great job at decreasing the commotion in picture. This channel is connected in each channel of picture for diminishing the clamor.

iii. **Histogram equalization image**: The difference improvement of the picture can be seen by applying histeq.

4.2 Feature Extraction

In feature extraction stage, local binary pattern is used for extraction of features in each channel separately. Then extract the texture features for each channel of LBP image. After that, take average of all channel features for construct the final features. The final features are mean, standard deviation, entropy, kurtosis, and skewness.

The feature extraction algorithm is as shown in Fig. 5 in which first the color image can be given to object cropping, the RGB channel can be extracted, and LBP computation can be performed to R G B extracted image finally the Features can be extracted with the help of LBP image.

4.3 Classification

The classification procedure is done from extraction of conclusive highlights. The primary algorithm used nowadays to classify the appropriate decision tree is a random forest (RF). RF classifier is connected over the highlights, and also the arrangement is finished. The random forest algorithm step is as shown in Fig. 6.

5 Results and Analysis

Figure 7 shows the process steps perform for the detection of retinal disease using LBP. The first step is to test an input image which is acquired from database. The second step is to preprocessing an image by using RGB channel extraction in which image has to be denoised and by using histogram equation image is enhanced. The third step is feature extraction by using RGB component in which mean, standard deviation, entropy, kurtosis, and skewness values can be obtained for each channel.

Figure 8 shows the final features and classification of test image having an average of RGB features and classification result: If the obtained class is 1 the output is disease eye and if it is 0 the output is normal eye (Table 1).

Fig. 5 Feature extraction using LBP images of RGB component

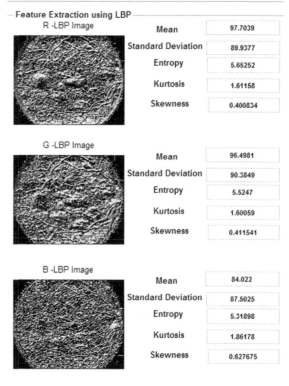

Fig. 6 Random forest algorithm steps

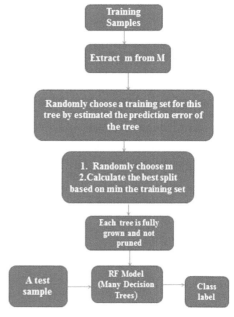

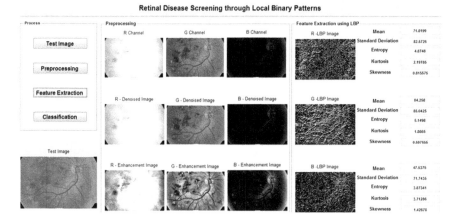

Fig. 7 Process perform for detection of retinal disease using LPB technique

Retinal Disease Screening through Local Binary Patterns

⊙ **Final Features**

Average of RGB Channel Texture Features

Mean	67.8718
Standard Deviation	79.7862
Entropy	4.63267
Kurtosis	2.5924
Skewness	0.94667

⊙ **Classification**

Classification Result

| Class | 1 |
| Output | Disease Eye |

Fig. 8 Final features and classification of test image

Table 1 Final average features of RGB channel

Class	Output	Mean	Standard deviation	Entropy	Kurtosis	Skewness
1	Disease eye	67.8718	79.7862	4.63267	2.5924	0.94667
0	Normal eye	47.9789	73.9333	3.87598	3.68939	1.43468

Fig. 9 Performance plot for age related macular degeneration and diabetic retinopathy

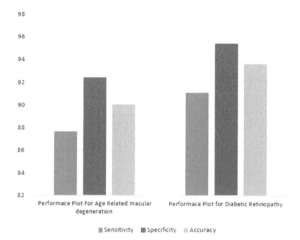

The performance plot for age-related degeneration and diabetic retinopathy is as shown in Fig. 9. The graph represents the comparison between performance for age-related degeneration and diabetic retinopathy. The blue shade shows the sensitivity, red shade shows the specificity, and green shade shows the accuracy.

6 Conclusion

In this paper, another approach for DR determination was obtained. It depends on dissecting surface separation abilities in fundus pictures to separate solid patients from DR pictures. The execution of LBP alongside various classifiers was tried and contrasted and other surface. The future technique is equipped for separating the modules in view of breaking down the surface of the retina foundation, evading past division of retinal injuries. Such sore division calculations may be tedious, along these lines maintaining a strategic distance from the division is helpful. The thesis shows that utilizing LBP as surface descriptor for fundus pictures gives helpful highlights to retinal infection screening.

Acknowledgements The authors would like to sincerely thank Dr. B. K. Narendra, Principal, BGSIT, BG Nagar, for providing the necessary facilities and support and Dr. M. B. Anandaraju, Professor and Head of the Department, Electronics and Communication Engineering BGSIT, BG Nagar, for their support and valuable suggestion to complete this paper.

References

1. Morales S, Engan K, Naranjo V, Colomer A (2017) Retinal disease screening through local binary patterns
2. Ojala T, Pietikinen M, Menp T (2001) A generalized local binary pattern operator for multiresolution gray scale and rotation invariant texture classification. In: 2nd international conference on advances in pattern recognition, 2001, pp 397–406
3. Ahonen T, Hadid A, Pietikainen M (2006) Face description with local binary patterns: application to face recognition
4. Morales S, Engan K, Naranjo V, Colomer A (2015) Detection of diabetic retinopathy and age-related macular degeneration from fundus images through local binary patterns and random forests
5. Nanni L, Lumini A, Brahnam S (2006) Face description with local binary patterns: application to face recognition. IEEE Trans Pattern Anal Mach Intell 28(12):2037–2041
6. Gandhi M, Dhanasekaran R (2013) Diagnosis of diabetic retinopathy using morphological process and SVM classifier
7. Yang Z, Ai H (2007) Demographic classification with local binary patterns. In: Lee SW, Li S (eds) Advances in biometrics. Lecture notes in computer science, vol 4642, pp 464–473
8. Mookiah M, Acharya UR, Martis RJ, Chua CK, Lim C, Ng E, Laude A (2013) Evolutionary algorithm based classifier parameter tuning for automatic diabetic retinopathy grading: a hybrid feature extraction approach. Int J Eng Adv Technol 6: 1–4
9. Oppedal K, Engan K, Aarsl D, Beyer M, Tysnes OB, Eftestol T (2012) Using local binary pattern to classify dementia in MRI. In: 9th IEEE international symposium on biomedical imaging (ISBI), May 2012, pp 594–597

Comparative Performance Analysis of Hybrid PAPR Reduction Techniques in OFDM Systems

A. V. Manjula and K. N. Muralidhara

Abstract Orthogonal Frequency Division Multiplexing (OFDM) is a promising multicarrier modulation technique used for high data rate communication. However, one of the major drawbacks is it suffers from high peak-to-average power ratio (PAPR). This paper is a study on different types of PAPR reduction techniques and proposes a new hybrid DCT with companding PAPR reduction technique. It is shown that proposed method is simple and provides better PAPR reduction compared to DCT, companding and conventional OFDM system.

Keywords Orthogonal frequency division multiplexing (OFDM) · Discrete cosine transform · PAPR · Companding · Complimentary cumulative distribution function (CCDF)

1 Introduction

Orthogonal frequency division multiplexing (OFDM) is the most widely used key technology in modern communication systems and provides high data rate with reasonable complexity and precision. OFDM is a special form of multicarrier transmission technique where the information is carried over narrow flat subcarriers to avoid intersymbol interference and provides spectral efficiency. OFDM is adopted for various wireless communication standards such as digital video broadcasting, digital audio broadcasting (DAB), and Worldwide Interoperability for Microwave Access (WiMAX). However, one of the major drawbacks of OFDM system is high peak-to-average ratio. High peak-to-average power ratio (PAPR), which seriously limits the

A. V. Manjula (✉)
Department of Electronics, PET Research Foundation, PES College of Engineering,
Mandya 571401, India
e-mail: manjularameshn@gmail.com

K. N. Muralidhara
Department of Electronics and Communication, PES College of Engineering,
Mandya 571401, India

© Springer Nature Singapore Pte Ltd. 2019   1069
V. Sridhar et al. (eds.), *Emerging Research in Electronics, Computer Science and Technology*, Lecture Notes in Electrical Engineering 545,
https://doi.org/10.1007/978-981-13-5802-9_92

power efficiency of the transmitter's high power amplifier (HPA), because the PAPR forces the HPA to operate in saturation region results in reduced efficiency. There are various methods to resolve this problem such as repeated clipping and filtering [1], Companding [2, 3], partial transmit sequence (PTS) [4], SLM [5], tone reservation and tone injection [6], and hybrid techniques. Among these, SLM is widely used method although it needs several IFFTs with high computational complexity. Further, there are numerous methods based on SLM with reduced computational complexity [7–11] which are discussed in the literature. Precoding methods [12–14] are more preferable to other technique as they do not require side information at the receiver to recover the original signal. This paper proposes a hybrid DCT with companding PAPR reduction technique, and here PAPR reduction is better when compared to companding-based PAPR reduction technique and DCT-precoding-based PAPR reduction technique. Section 2 provides an introduction to OFDM system PAPR and CCDF, Sect. 3 provides companding-based PAPR reduction technique and DCT-precoding-based PAPR reduction technique, Sect. 4 provides the proposed hybrid PAPR reduction technique, and Sect. 5 provides simulation results and conclusion.

2   OFDM System, PAPR, and CCDF

The block diagram of conventional OFDM is as shown in Fig. 1.

Let $Xk = [X(0), X(1) \ldots X(N-1)]$ denotes input symbol vector in the frequency domain, where Xk be the complex signal sequence transmitted on kth subcarrier.

The continuous time OFDM signal with N subcarriers is given by

$$x(t) = \frac{1}{\sqrt{N}} \sum_{k=0}^{N-1} X_k e^{j2\pi fkt}, 0 \le t \le NT \tag{1}$$

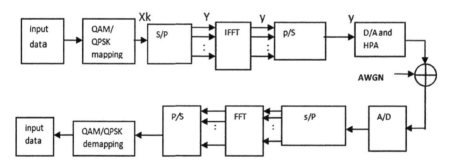

Fig. 1 Block diagram of conventional OFDM system

where fk be the kth subcarrier with $k = 0, 1 \ldots N - 1$ and subcarrier are chosen to be orthogonal with spacing between each subcarrier is $fk = \Delta fk = 1/(NT)$ and T is the symbol period. Discrete version of Nyquist-sampled OFDM signal is defined as

$$x[n] = \frac{1}{\sqrt{N}} \sum_{k=0}^{N-1} X_k e^{j\frac{2\pi nk}{N}}, \quad 0 \le n \le N - 1 \tag{2}$$

where N is the number of subcarriers.

PAPR of time domain OFDM signal is defined as the ratio of peak power to an average power of a signal and is given by

$$\text{PAPR}\{x(n)\} = \frac{\max_{0 \le n \le N-1} [|x(n)|^2]}{E[|x(n)|^2]} \tag{3}$$

where E[ ] is expectation operator.

Assume that the real and imaginary parts of time domain complex OFDM signal have Gaussian distribution for large number of subcarriers by the central limit theorem. However, amplitude of OFDM signal has Rayleigh distribution and power has chi-square distribution. The CCDF plots are the measure of performance; the cumulative distribution function of PAPR of OFDM signal with N subcarriers is given by

$$\text{CDF}(z_0) = \text{Pr}(\text{PAPR}(x(n)) \le z_0)$$
$$= (1 - \exp(-z_0))^N \tag{4}$$

where z_0 is the given threshold value of PAPR. Usually, CCDF is used as performance metric of PAPR reduction technique. Therefore, the complimentary cumulative distribution function of PAPR is given by

$$\text{CCDF}(z_0) = \text{Pr}(\text{PAPR}(x(n)) > z_0)$$
$$= 1 - (1 - \exp(-z_0))^N \tag{5}$$

3 Discrete Cosine Transform (DCT) and Companding-Based PAPR Reduction Technique

DCT is a Fourier-related transform similar to DFT but uses only real numbers. The main properties of DCT transform is de-correlation (i.e. minimizing or even removing the interdependencies between coefficients) and energy compaction property widely used as compression technique.

One-dimensional DCT of length N is defined as

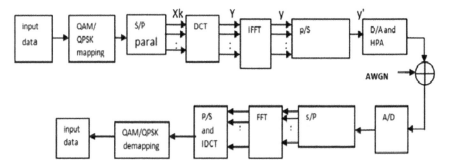

Fig. 2 Block diagram of DCT-precoding PAPR reduction technique

$$Y(k) = w(k) \sum_{k=0}^{N-1} y(n) \cos\left[\frac{\pi(2n+1)k}{2N}\right] \quad for\ k = 0, \ldots N-1 \qquad (6)$$

and inverse DCT is defined as

$$y(n) = \sum_{k=0}^{N-1} w(k)Y(k) \cos\left[\frac{\pi(2n+1)k}{2N}\right] \quad for\ n = 0, \ldots N-1 \qquad (7)$$

where w(k) is defined as

$$w(k) = \begin{cases} \frac{1}{\sqrt{N}}, & for\ k = 0 \\ \frac{2}{\sqrt{N}}, & for\ k \neq 0 \end{cases} \qquad (8)$$

The block diagram of DCT-precoding technique is as shown below in Fig. 2.

Here DCT transform is applied before IFFT operation. The resulting signal Y = CX where C is DCT matrix of order NXN.

The time domain OFDM signal is y = IFFT{Y} whose peak-to-average power ratio is measured and transmitted.

Evaluation of this method is explained in the next section.

4   Companding Technique

Companding-based PAPR reduction OFDM system is as shown below in Fig. 3. The time domain version of OFDM signal is passed through compander which employs a law/Mu law technique. This results in better performance than DCT and with slight degradation in BER.

The Mu law is defined as

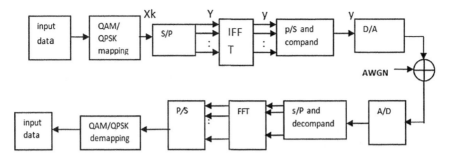

Fig. 3 Block diagram of companding-based PAPR reduction technique

$$y = \frac{V\log\left(1 + \frac{\mu|x|}{V}\right)}{\log(1 + \mu)}\, \text{sgn}(x) \qquad (9)$$

where V peak of the signal x, μ where log is natural logarithm and sgn is the sigmum function and μ is companding parameter usually set to 255. The average power low-amplitude signal is increased, high-amplitude signals are attenuated, and PAPR ratio is decreased. Since it is a nonlinear technique, there will be BER degradation at the receiver and expanding function is used at the receiver.

5 Proposed Hybrid PAPR Reduction Technique

This hybrid method uses both DCT function and companding function at the transmitter to reduce envelop variations. The input signal vector is modulated, and serial-to-parallel conversion is performed. Then DCT is applied, the transformed signal is passed through IFFT, and the time domain OFDM signal is passed through the compander. The signal is transmitted over AWGN channel expanding, and inverse DCT is applied at the receiver. This method is simple to implement, and better PAPR reduction ratio is achieved as shown in Fig. 4.

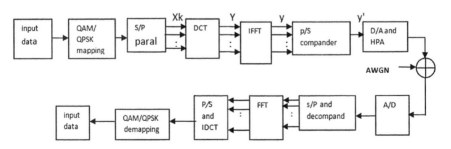

Fig. 4 Block diagram of proposed PAPR reduction technique

Y = CX, where C is a DCT matrix of order NXN and input signal vector X = $[X_0, X_1, \ldots X_{N-1}]^T$.

Therefore, modified time domain OFDM signal is

$$y = IFFT[Y] = [y_0, y_1, \ldots y_{N-1}]^T$$

6 Simulation Results

Simulation results have been carried out to evaluate the performance of OFDM, DCT, companding, and proposed method. This is evaluated for 10^6 bits of OFDM signal with N = 64, number of subcarriers. From the CCDF plots, it is shown that hybrid PAPR reduction methods provide better result compared to the other methods as shown in Figs. 5, 6, and 7.

In Fig. 5, CCDF performance of proposed method is compared with conventional OFDM and DCT methods. At 10^{-3}, PAPR is 2.1 dB, 8.2 dB, and 10.3 dB for proposed DCT and OFDM, respectively. BER performance of the proposed method is degraded due to companding function. However, the PAPR reduction is improved.

Figure 6 shows the CCDF performance of OFDM, DCT, and companding techniques. At 10^{-3} clip-level companding technique gives better PAPR reduction. Since it is a nonlinear technique, BER performance is reduced at the receiver.

Figure 7 shows the performance of proposed method with DCT, companding, and OFDM techniques. The hybrid technique uses both DCT and companding tech-

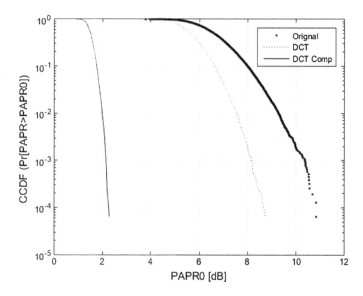

Fig. 5 Comparison of CCDF performance of OFDM, DCT, and proposed method

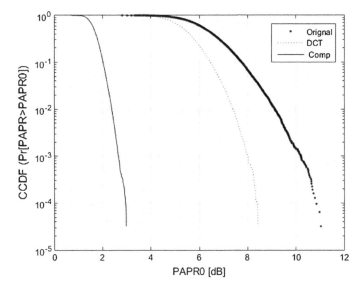

Fig. 6 Comparison of CCDF performance of OFDM, DCT, and companding method

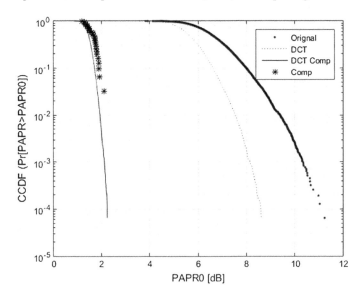

Fig. 7 Comparison of CCDF performance of OFDM, DCT, companding, and proposed method

Table 1 CCDF performance of proposed, DCT, companding, and OFDM techniques

No. of subcarriers	PAPR reduction technique	At 10^{-3} level (dB)
64	OFDM	10.5
64	DCT precoding	8.25
64	Companding-based	2.75
64	Hybrid DCT companding	2.1

niques; its CCDF performance at 10^{-3} is 2.1 dB. Therefore, the proposed hybrid PAPR reduction technique provides better performance than all the other three method discussed. The CCDF performance of all the methods is shown in Table 1.

7 Conclusion

The hybrid PAPR reduction technique uses two or more methods to reduce the PAPR ratio. The DCT, companding PAPR reduction techniques are studied and proposed hybrid DCT—Companding PAPR reduction technique and evaluated for better results compare to other methods. Further, BER analysis is to be carried out in the next paper.

References

1. Armstrong J (2002) Peak-to-average reduction for OFDM by repeated clipping and frequency domain filtering. IEEE Electron Lett 38(5):246–247
2. Huang X, Lu JH, Zheng JL, Letaief KB, Gu J (2004) Companding transform for reduction in peak-to-average power ratio of OFDM signals. IEEE Trans Wirel Commun 3(6):2030–2039
3. Jiang T, Yang Y, Song Y (2005) Exponential companding transformfor PAPR reduction in OFDM systems. IEEE Trans Broadcast 51(2):244–248
4. Muller SH, Huber JB (1997) OFDM with reduced peak-to-average power ratio by optimum combination of partial transmit sequences. IEEE Electron Lett 33(5):36–69
5. Jayalath DS, Tellambura C (2005) SLM and PTS peak-power reduction of OFDM signals without side information. IEEE Trans Wirel Commun 4(5):2006–2013
6. Krongold BS, Jones DL (2003) PAR reduction in OFDM via active constellation extension. IEEE Trans Broadcast 49(3):258–268
7. Yang L, Siu YM, Soo KK, Leung SW, Li SQ (2012) A low-complexity PAPR reduction technique for OFDM systems using modified widely linear SLM scheme. AEU Int J Electron Commun 66(12):1006–1010
8. Yang L, Soo KK, Siu YM, Li SQ (2008) A low complexity selected mapping scheme by use of time domain sequence superposition technique for PAPR reduction in OFDM system. IEEE Trans Broadcast 54(4)
9. Han SH, Lee JH (2004) A novel selected mapping technique for PAPR reduction in OFDM systems. IEEE Trans Broadcast 50(3)

10. Wang S-H, Sie J-C, Li C-P, Chen Y-F (2011) A low-complexity PAPR reduction scheme for OFDMA uplink systems. IEEE Trans Wirel Commun 10(4)
11. Hong E, Kim H, Yang K, Har D (2013) Pilot-aided side information detection in SLM-based OFDM systems. IEEE Trans Wirel Commun 12(7)
12. Wang ZP (2011) Combined DCT and companding for PAPR reduction in OFDM signals. J Signal Inf Process 2:100–104
13. Jiang Y (2010) New companding transform for PAPR reduction in OFDM. IEEE Commun Lett 14(4)
14. Virdi J (2013) PAPR reduction based on precoding techniques with companding in OFDM systems. Int J Sci Eng Res 4(5)

A Hardware Accelerator Based on Quantized Weights for Deep Neural Networks

R. Sreehari, Vijayasenan Deepu and M. R. Arulalan

Abstract The paper describes the implementation of systolic array-based hardware accelerator for multilayer perceptrons (MLP) on FPGA. Full precision hardware implementation of neural network increases resource utilization. Therefore, it is difficult to fit large neural networks on FPGA. Moreover, these implementations have high power consumption. Neural networks are implemented with numerous multiply and accumulate (MAC) units. The multipliers in these MAC units are expensive in terms of power. Algorithms have been proposed which quantize the weights and eliminate the need of multipliers in a neural network without compromising much on classification accuracy. The algorithms replace MAC units with simple accumulators. Quantized weights minimize the weight storage requirements. Quantizing inputs and constraining activations along with weights simplify the adder as well as further reduce the resource utilization. A systolic array-based architecture of neural network has been implemented on FPGA. The architecture has been modified according to Binary Connect and Ternary Connect algorithms which quantize the weights into two and three levels, respectively. The final variant of the architecture has been designed and implemented with quantized inputs, Ternary connect algorithm and activations constrained to +1 and −1. All the implementations have been verified with MNIST data set. Classification accuracy of hardware implementations has been found comparable with its software counterparts. The designed hardware accelerator has achieved reduction in flip-flop utilization by 7.5 times compared to the basic hardware implementation of neural network with high precision weights, inputs and normal MAC units. The power consumption also has got reduced by half and the delay of critical path decreased by three times. Thus, larger neural networks can be implemented on FPGA that can run at high frequencies with less power.

R. Sreehari (✉) · V. Deepu · M. R. Arulalan
Department of ECE, NITK, Surathkal, India
e-mail: sreehari234@gmail.com

V. Deepu
e-mail: deepu.senan@gmail.com

M. R. Arulalan
e-mail: perarulalan@gmail.com

© Springer Nature Singapore Pte Ltd. 2019
V. Sridhar et al. (eds.), *Emerging Research in Electronics, Computer Science and Technology*, Lecture Notes in Electrical Engineering 545,
https://doi.org/10.1007/978-981-13-5802-9_93

1 Introduction

Deep neural networks have been achieving state-of-the-art performance in various tasks such as image recognition, object recognition and speech recognition. Researchers have been designing new deep learning algorithms to fully exploit deep neural networks. They have been limited by the computational capability of general purpose systems. The demand for faster computation has led to the design of specialized hardware implementations of neural networks.

Researchers have come up with several FPGA implementations which provide high computational performance. But, numerous MAC units in neural network and weight storage requirements impose a limit on the size of the neural network that can be implemented on FPGA. Computationally, intensive deep neural networks have high power requirements. This makes them less feasible for power constrained applications. To make them more viable for commercial applications, designers had developed algorithms which eliminate multipliers from neural networks without affecting classification accuracy. Removing multipliers which are the most power-hungry components in neural networks improves power efficiency of hardware implementations. The algorithms use quantized weights which reduce weight storage requirements. Hardware implementation of neural network based on systolic array has been implemented on FPGA. Another variants of the architecture based on Binary Connect [1] and Ternary Connect [2] algorithms have also been tested on FPGA. Binary Connect algorithm constraints weight to +1 and −1 while the Ternary Connect algorithm quantizes weight to +1, 0 or −1. Ternary Connect version has given better classification accuracy than Binary Connect implementation without compromising much on performance. The architecture has also been modified with quantized inputs, ternary connect algorithm and activations constrained to +1 and −1 [3] which showed better performance. The paper is organized as follows: Sect. 2 discusses related literature in this field, Sect. 3 gives a detailed description about the architecture of the hardware accelerator and algorithms used to simplify the arithmetic, Sect. 4 explains how the algorithms have been integrated into the architecture, Sect. 5 analyses the results and Sect. 6 contains the conclusions.

2 Related Work

Recent developments in VLSI technology have made researchers look for both FPGA based and ASIC implementations of hardware accelerators for neural networks.

Out of the published literature on FPGA implementations, a popular architecture is the one that named as CNP [4]. It was then improved and renamed as NeuFlow [5]. Later on, with further improvements it was introduced as nn-X [6]. The architecture of CNP mainly contains a 32-bit soft processor and a vector arithmetic and logic unit (VALU). The VALU contains all the necessary operations for convolutional network layers. All the operations have been hardwired. The sequencing of operations has been done by the soft processor. It has been implemented on Spartan 3A DSP 3400 FPGA. 18-bit fixed point arithmetic has been used for multiplications. It has achieved a throughput of 12 giga operations per second (GOp/s) at 15 W. NeuFlow is a scaled up version of CNP. It consists of multiple coprocessing tiles. Each processing tile has been configurable. The data flow between the processing tiles has been routable at runtime. It has featured Virtex-6 VLX240T FPGA. 16-bit fixed point arithmetic has been used. It has given a throughput of 147 GOp/s at 11 W. NeuFlow has been ported to Zynq XC7Z045 to make use of the hardwired ARM processors and renamed as nn-X. The ARM processor acts as the host processor. Input data and configuration data have been transferred to the coprocessor, nn-X by the ARM processor. The coprocessor has been implemented in the programmable logic. It contains several processing blocks known as collections. Each collection comprises of a convolution engine, a pooling module, a nonlinear operator and a local memory router. It has achieved a throughput of 200 GOp/s at 4 W (FPGA, host and memory). Power efficiency of FPGA implementations has been low.

Recently, developed ASIC hardware accelerator is Origami [7] which does not use very large on-chip memories, thereby reducing the memory bandwidth. Image window SRAM always keeps a fixed portion of image in it. Image values are cached in such a way that they can be reused when moving to the next tile. Therefore, only one pixel value per clock cycle has to be loaded off-chip. It has obtained a throughput of 197 GOp/s and power efficiency of 803 GOp/s/W. YodaNN [8] is an efficiency improved version of Origami. It has employed Binary Connect approach which constrains real-valued weights to +1 and −1. It has achieved a throughput of 1510 GOp/s and power efficiency of 61.2 TOp/s/W.

3 System Model

A pipelined hardware accelerator for deep neural networks is designed. Various approaches available to simplify the arithmetic involved are examined.

3.1 Architecture

The design is targeted for a particular class of neural network called multilayer perceptron (MLP). Alternating orthogonal systolic array architecture [9, 10] is adopted for implementing MLPs.

3.1.1 Alternating Orthogonal Systolic Array

Alternating orthogonal systolic array is a pipeline plus systolic architecture. Two mapping schemes of systolic array are used in this architecture. In the first one,

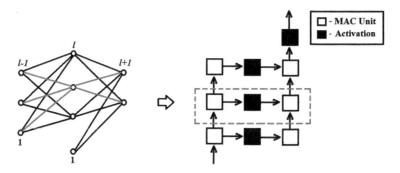

Fig. 1 Alternating orthogonal systolic array implementation of neural network

inputs are fed serially and outputs are produced parallely. In the other scheme, inputs are taken parallely and outputs are produced serially. These schemes are applied to alternate layers of the neural network. This allows the smooth interfacing of outputs of one layer within puts of adjacent layer. This also has enabled pipelining. Figure 1 shows the alternating orthogonal systolic array implementation of a neural network. A hidden neuron is implemented by the portion inside the dotted rectangle. A neural network implementation has as many such sections as the number of hidden neurons. The first MAC unit of the section is called as serial-in to parallel-out (SIPO) unit and the second as parallel-in to serial-out (PISO) unit. The weights of all the incoming connections to the hidden node are stored in SIPO unit. Weights of all outgoing connections from the hidden node are stacked in PISO unit. Activation function is implemented in the block between MAC units. The input vector is passed to the first systolic array serially. Accumulated value at each hidden node is calculated by the first MAC unit of each section. The accumulated values are fed to the second systolic array through activation function blocks. As soon as the computation of a SIPO unit is completed, the corresponding PISO unit is started. This has enabled the computation of second layer before the completion of first layer. The sum of number of input nodes and hidden nodes gives the number of clock cycles taken by the last input to reach the SIPO unit of the last section. By the time, computations of PISO unit of the preceding section are started. The accumulated values at the output nodes are streamed out serially by the PISO unit of the last section. It is passed through an activation function block to get the final results. Any N-layer neural network can be implemented by cascading several such set of arrays.

3.1.2 Basic Module of the Architecture

The basic building block of the architecture is formed by a combination of serial-in to parallel-out (SIPO) unit and parallel-in to serial-out (PISO) unit. Figure 2 shows the architecture of basic module.

Fig. 2 Block diagram of
basic module

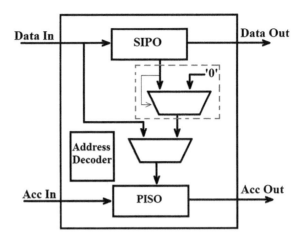

Weights of all the connections from layer $l - 1$ to a node in layer l are stored in the SIPO unit representing the same node. The weights of all the connections from the same node to layer $l + 1$ are contained in the PISO unit of the corresponding basic module. Accumulated value of the weighted inputs at the corresponding node is calculated by the SIPO unit. The accumulated result is fed to PISO unit through an activation function. The activation function used is rectified linear unit (ReLU). It is implemented using a multiplexer. The MSB of SIPO output is used as the select line of the multiplexer. The value itself is passed if the SIPO output is positive otherwise a zero. Various weighted values of its input are generated by PISO unit. Each weighted value contributes to the accumulated result of the corresponding nodes at layer $l + 1$. Weighted values generated by a PISO are added with corresponding weighted values from the preceding PISO unit.

The architecture of SIPO unit is shown in Fig. 3. Weights are stored in shift register. Incoming inputs are multiplied with its corresponding weights. Upon accumulating weighted inputs, the result is added with the bias value stored separately. The architecture of PISO unit is shown in Fig. 4. Shift register is loaded with weights of PISO unit. The weighted inputs from the preceding PISO unit are added with corresponding weighted values of its input. The new results are passed to the next PISO unit. Weights of both SIPO unit and PISO unit are fed through Data-In port. Address decoder selects either of the units for weight loading, depending on the address it receives. Data inputs are passed to next SIPO unit through Data-Out port.

Second multiplexer chooses between weights and input to the PISO unit. PISO unit begins its computation when it receives the start signal from SIPO unit. SIPO unit sends the start signal to PISO unit upon the completion of its accumulation. Any MLP can be implemented by replicating this basic block.

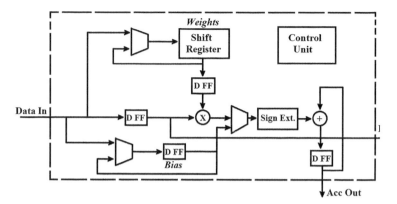

Fig. 3 Architecture of SIPO unit

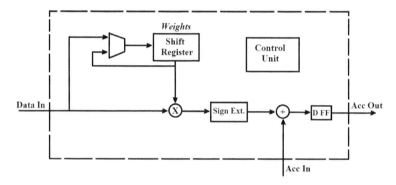

Fig. 4 Architecture of PISO unit

3.1.3 Neural Network Implementation

An MLP shown in Fig. 1 is the basic section of the architecture. It is implemented by cascading several basic modules. An example is shown in Fig. 5. The number of basic modules required is equal to the number of neurons in layer l. Data-Out and Acc-Out ports of every module are connected to the Data-In and Acc-In ports of next module, respectively. Acc-In port of first module is tied to ground. Weights and inputs are fed to the network through Data-In port of first module. Address decoder enables modules for loading weights into it depending on the address received. Every SIPO unit starts its operation upon the ready signal from the previous SIPO unit. A SIPO unit sends the ready signal to next SIPO unit when it starts passing inputs to it. The first SIPO unit gets its ready signal from outside the network, i.e. user. Outputs are available serially at the Acc-Out port of the last module. The bias module contains the bias values of layer $l + 1$. Outputs from last module are added with corresponding bias values. The results are then passed through ReLU activation function implemented using a multiplexer.

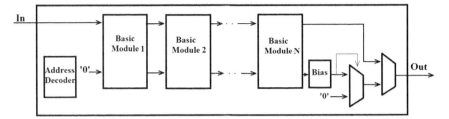

Fig. 5 Neural network implementation by cascading basic modules

Neural network with any number of layers can be implemented by cascading several basic sections. Out port of each section is connected to in port of next section. PISO unit of last module of every section generates the ready signal for the next section.

3.1.4   System Integration

The block diagram of the whole system is shown in Fig. 6. Weight memory holds the entire weights of the neural network, and biases memory contains the biases. Upon a load signal from user, the main control unit transfers all the weights to appropriate locations in the hardware implementation of neural network using address generator. Once weights are transferred, the biases are loaded into SIPO units and bias modules in the neural network implementation. SIPO unit stores its bias value separately from weights. Then the system waits for the start signal to begin the computations. The inputs are fed serially to the neural network from inputs memory. The weights, biases and inputs are transferred through the same bus using multiplexers. Final results are loaded into output memory. The main control unit ensures proper data flow between various modules.

3.2   Algorithm Optimization

MAC is the critical operation in neural network computations. Various methods to remove multipliers from the hardware implementation of the neural network are discussed below.

3.2.1   Binary Connect

Quantizing the weights to +1 and −1 will replace multiply–accumulate operations by simple accumulations [1].

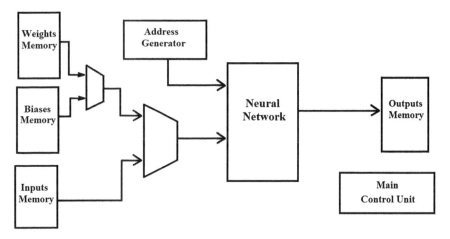

Fig. 6 Block diagram of the system

Deterministic Binarization

The weights can be binarized using the following function.

$$w = \begin{cases} +1, & if \ W \geq 0 \\ -1, & otherwise \end{cases} \tag{1}$$

where w is the binarized weight and W is the real-valued weight.

Stochastic Binarization

Another way is to binarize weights stochastically.

$$w = \begin{cases} +1, & with\ probability\ p = f(W) \\ -1, & with\ probability\ 1 - p \end{cases} \tag{2}$$

where w is the binarized weight and W is the real-valued weight and

$$f(x) = \max\left(0, \min\left(\frac{x+1}{2}\right)\right) \tag{3}$$

Using binary weights, the multiplication between inputs and weights is reduced to sign change in inputs. Multiplier in the hardware is replaced by a multiplexer which selects between the input and its negated value based on the weight. For a weight value of +1, the input itself is selected otherwise its negated value.

3.2.2 Ternary Connect

In the previous method, the weights were binarized to +1 and −1. However, in a trained neural network, many of the learned weights are 0 or close to 0. If we allow weights to be 0, the accuracy of the neural network will improve [2].

To allow weights to be 0, some modifications are required. The interval $[−1, 1]$ in which the entire real-valued weights lie is split into two subintervals: $[−1, 0]$ and $[0, 1]$. If a real-valued weight lies in one of the intervals, then it is stochastically sampled to one of the edge values of that interval.

Weights are quantized deterministically based on a threshold value.

$$w = \begin{cases} +1, & if \ W > \eta \\ 0, & \eta \geq W > -\eta \\ -1, & otherwise \end{cases} \tag{4}$$

where w is the quantized weight and W is the real-valued weight.

Multiplication between inputs and weights is converted into either sign change in inputs or nullification of inputs. A 3:1 multiplexer that selects input, complement of input or zero is used to replace the multiplier in hardware.

4 Experiments

A neural network with 784 input neurons, 32 hidden neurons and 10 output neurons is taken as the test case. MNIST data set is used for training and testing the neural network. As each image in the data set is of the size 28 × 28 pixels, we took the number of input neurons as 784 (28 * 28). According to the resources available in the Kintex-7(xc7k480tffv1156-1) FPGA, we constrained ourselves to one hidden layer with 32 hidden neurons. Since the data set contains 10 different classes of data (images of handwritten digits from 0 to 9), the number of output neurons is made 10. ReLU is used as the activation function for hidden neurons and softmax for output neurons. It is trained with MNIST data set on Tensor flow framework using Keras neural network library. Trained weights are quantized according to the adopted algorithms. The functionality and performance of the design in FPGA are evaluated with the trained weights from the software. In software, classification accuracy is calculated for both real-valued weights and quantized weights. The design is ported to Zynq(xc7z020clg484-1) SoC in zedboard to check classification accuracy in hardware. The classification accuracy of various algorithms is shown in Fig. 7.

The basic architecture of neural network is implemented for full precision weights and inputs. The inputs and weights are of 16 bits. Q3.13 format is used, with 3 bits representing the integer and 13 bits the fractional part. Classification accuracy, for MNIST data set, of 96.31% was obtained, which was almost equal to that of software implementation (96.56%). The difference in classification accuracy is due

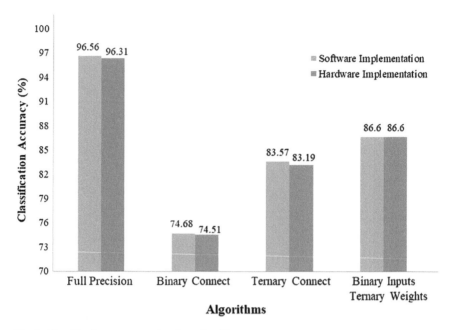

Fig. 7 Classification accuracy of various algorithms

to the difference in representation of numbers. Software has followed floating point representation while hardware has used fixed point.

Second variant of the architecture is designed based on Binary Connect algorithm. Neural network was trained in the software with weights constrained between +1 and −1. Deterministic binarization was used. Trained weights with values greater than or equal to zero were quantized to +1 and others to −1. 1 bit is used to represent binarized weights in hardware. Inputs and biases were 16 bits following the Q3.13 format. For MNIST data set, classification accuracy of software for real-valued weights was 93.01% and binarized weights were 74.68%. Classification accuracy of modified hardware for binarized weights was 74.51%.

The architecture of the third variant is based on Ternary Connect algorithm. Neural network was trained in the software with weights constrained between +1 and −1. Weights were quantized deterministically. The threshold for deterministic quantization was found to be 0.09 by trial and error method. Trained weights lying between 0.09 and −0.09 were quantized to 0. Weights greater than 0.09 were taken as 1 and others as −1. Quantized weights are then represented by 2 bits while inputs and biases by 16 bits following Q3.13 format. The same set of real-valued weights used in Binary Connect were quantized and used here. Software has a classification accuracy of 83.57% that of hardware implementation is 83.19%.

Ternary Connect is found to give better classification accuracy than Binary Connect without degrading the performance. Therefore, ternary connect algorithm is chosen for the final architecture. Inputs and biases are quantized. Activations are

Table 1 Resource utilization for various algorithms

Algorithm	LUT	FF	BRAM (Kb)	DSP slices
Full precision	6185	415,250	504	64
Binary connect	5199	32,900	90	0
Ternary connect	4790	58,693	126	0
Binary inputs, ternary weights	2730	54,745	126	0

Table 2 Delay of critical path for various algorithms

Algorithm	Max. delay (ns)
Full precision	6.547
Binary connect	2.675
Ternary connect	2.715
Binary inputs, ternary weights	2.170

Table 3 Power consumption for various algorithms

Algorithm	Static (W)	Dynamic (W)	Total (W)
Full precision	0.222	0.433	0.654
Binary connect	0.219	0.092	0.312
Ternary connect	0.219	0.126	0.346
Binary inputs, ternary weights	0.219	0.116	0.336

constrained to +1 and −1. These modifications have simplified the adder and further improved the performance. The same test case of one hidden layer with 32 neurons is used. The neural network has been trained in software with quantized inputs. Weights and biases are constrained between +1 and −1. Image values of MNIST data set were scaled down to the interval [0, 1]. Values less than 0.5 were quantized to 0 and others to +1. Sign function (gives +1 for zero and positive values while −1 for negative values) was used as activation function for hidden neurons. Inputs are represented in hardware with single bit while weights and biases with 2 bits. Software implementation resulted in a classification accuracy of 94.54% with real-valued weights and biases while a classification accuracy of 86.60% with quantized weights and biases. Hardware implementation also has the same classification accuracy as software (86.60%).

5   Results

The performance metrics of various implementations are shown in Tables 1, 2 and 3 have been obtained for an implementation on kintex-7(xc7k480tffv1156-1) FPGA.

The resource utilization of various designs is shown in Table 1. Multipliers in the basic design use DSP slices, at the rate of one per multiplier. Binary Connect and Ternary Connect algorithms eliminate the need of multipliers. Therefore, other designs require no DSP slices. Quantizing the weights has reduced the overhead of weight storage. As weights are stored in shift registers, the utilization of flip-flops has reduced accordingly across various designs. 2-bit ternary weight representation has reduced the usage of flip-flops in third and fourth architectures by more than 7 times compared to the full precision architecture. Flip-flop utilization of Binary Connect architecture which uses 1-bit weights is reduced by 12.6 times. 32-bit adder of full precision architecture has reduced to 23-bit adder (16 data bits + 7 guard bits) in Binary Connect and Ternary Connect architectures. This has decreased the LUT utilization. Final architecture has used 8-bit adder (2 data bits + 6 guard bits), and LUT usage has reduced by 56% in comparison with basic architecture. Before loading into the neural network, weights are received in block RAM. The size of BRAM has reduced according to the bit representation of weights for various designs.

Critical path of the design comprises of multiplier (combinational) and adder. The delay of critical path of various architectures is shown in Table 2. Multipliers are replaced by simple combinational logic in the architectures which have adopted Binary Connect and Ternary Connect. Therefore, the critical path delay is reduced by 59% for second and third architectures. With adders also getting simplified in the fourth architecture, the critical path has reduced further. Critical path has reduced by 67% of full precision architecture.

Table 3 gives the details of power consumption in various architectures. Power is calculated with a clock of 100 MHz. Removal of multipliers and reduction in other resources have considerably reduced the power consumption in the algorithm-based architectures. Power requirement of final architecture is reduced to half compared to basic architecture. Static power has been constant across all architectures. It is related to the targeted FPGA. Dynamic power which depends on the designs found to be reduced by 73% for the final architecture.

6 Conclusion

The hardware accelerator for deep neural networks is designed with quantized inputs and weights. As Ternary Connect algorithm has given better classification accuracy than Binary Connect, it is employed in the accelerator. Ternary Connect algorithm has eliminated multipliers. Activations of the neural network are constrained to +1 and −1. 2-bit quantized weights have reduced the overhead of weight storage while 1-bit quantized inputs and constrained activations have simplified the adder. The accelerator has achieved a reduction of 87% in the flip-flop usage and 56% in LUT usage compared to full precision implementation of neural network. Dynamic power consumption of the hardware accelerator has become one-fourth of the hardware implementation of neural network with full precision weights. The delay of the critical path of the accelerator has reduced to one-third.

In this work, training was done in software. Training is a time-consuming process. Implementing training phase with Binary Connect or Ternary Connect algorithms on hardware can accelerate the process.

References

1. Courbariaux M, Bengio Y, David JP (2015) Binaryconnect: training deep neural networks with binary weights during propagations. In: Proceedings of advances in neural information processing systems, pp 3123–3131
2. Lin Z, Courbariaux M, Memisevic R, Bengio Y (2015) Neural networks with few multiplications. arXiv:1510.03009
3. Hubara I, Courbariaux M, Soudry D, El-Yaniv R, Bengio Y (2016) Binarized neural networks. In: Proceedings of advances in neural information processing systems, pp 4107–4115
4. Farabet C, Poulet C, Han JY, LeCun Y (2009) CNP: an FPGA-based processor for convolutional networks. In: International conference on field programmable logic and applications, 2009, FPL 2009, pp 32–37. IEEE
5. Farabet C, LeCun Y, Culurciello E (2012) NeuFlow: a runtime reconfigurable dataflow architecture for vision. In: Proceedings of snowbird learning workshop, Apr 2012
6. Gokhale V, Jin J, Dundar A, Martini B, Culurciello E (2014) A 240 GOps/s mobile coprocessor for deep neural networks. In: Proceedings of the IEEE conference on computer vision and pattern recognition workshops, pp 682–687
7. Cavigelli L, Benini L (2017) Origami: a 803-GOp/s/w convolutional network accelerator. IEEE Trans Circuits Syst Video Technol 27(11):2461–2475
8. Andri R, Cavigelli L, Rossi D, Benini L (2016) YodaNN: an ultra-low power convolutional neural network accelerator based on binary weights. In: Proceedings of ISVLSI, pp 236–241
9. Murtagh P, Tsoi AC, Bergmann N (1993) Bit-serial systolic array implementation of a multilayer perceptron. IEE Proc E Comput Digit Tech 140(5):277–288
10. Gadea R, Cerdá J, Ballester F, Mocholí A (2000) Artificial neural network implementation on a single FPGA of a pipelined on-line backpropagation. In: Proceedings of the 13th international symposium on system synthesis, pp 225–230. IEEE Computer Society

Effective Protocols for Industrial Communication

G. Sridevi, Ananth Saligram and V. Nattarasu

Abstract The industry has undergone three revolutions mechanization, electrification, and informatization and now it is the era of fourth industrial revolution the Internet of things also called Industrial revolution 4.0 which is predicted its way into factory. The main vision of the fourth revolution is smart factory with globally networked and real-time capable industrial production. As a part of these, companies are aiming to create intelligent devices, storage systems, and supplies in industrial production. These intelligent devices in turn exchange data, perform action, control each other and also the products are aware of their current state. Furthermore, the challenge is to control of device in network with increase in their number and RT (real time) capability. The industrial communication network plays a vital role in automation industry. The industrial communication provides an effective means of data exchange, data controllability, and flexibility to connect other devices. The paper gives an introduction to industrial communication network and various industrial Ethernet protocols for real-time data exchange in automation industry. The paper mainly explains the effective role of EtherCAT protocol for the development of smart factory.

Keywords Fieldbus · Industrial Ethernet · IIOT · EtherCAT

1 Introduction

For the execution of any cyclic processes in automation industry without human interaction requires a lot of information to be shared between sensors, controllers, and actuators. The introduction of steam power relieved workers from hard manual

G. Sridevi (✉) · A. Saligram · V. Nattarasu
Department of ECE, JSS Science & Technology University, Mysuru, India
e-mail: sridevi_2017@yahoo.com

A. Saligram
e-mail: anathsaligram@hexmoto.com

V. Nattarasu
e-mail: nattarasu@sjce.ac.in

© Springer Nature Singapore Pte Ltd. 2019   1093
V. Sridhar et al. (eds.), *Emerging Research in Electronics, Computer Science and Technology*, Lecture Notes in Electrical Engineering 545,
https://doi.org/10.1007/978-981-13-5802-9_94

labor. The invention of mass production based on division of labor and machineries created a multitude of production. Then by digitization, the use of electronics and IT further lead to automate production. With the launch of IOT and Cyberphysical system (CPS) in industrial application not only the industrial production but also the whole industrial infrastructure shall be intelligently networked [1]. The industrial IOT is also termed Industry 4.0. The core of distributed automation system or smart factory is reliable exchange of information or industrial communication. Hence, communication plays a major role where it converges sensing and actuation. There should be some rules that define the method of communication called protocol. The communication protocol allows two devices to share information with each other using same language, so the protocol is restricted to one vendor. With the arrival of OSI concept, device from one vendor be able to communicate with other. In the early days of industrial communication evolved with the network called fieldbus system which was developed to overcome the limitations caused by parallel cabling between sensors, controllers, and actuators. Few fieldbuses include Profibus, Modbus, and Intranet. Real-time capable fieldbus solutions were used for device interconnection but the fieldbuses are subjected to the restriction of limited device. Hence, industrial Ethernet came to existence. Industrial Ethernet enables integration of all level of company with higher performance than traditional fieldbus. Few industrial Ethernet protocols include PROFINET, Sercos III, Power link, EtherCAT, etc. [2]. With the introduction of internet and wireless network in industry, the machine can be moved and connected with greater ease thereby bringing a tremendous change in industrial automation.

The paper consists of four sections including this Introduction section. Section 2 gives a brief introduction to industrial communication, Sect. 4 elaborates on various industrial communication technologies. Section 5 presents a case study based on the use of the EtherCAT protocol and discusses its relation to Industry 4.0. Finally, the paper concludes in Sect. 6.

2 Industrial Communication

Industrial communication is an essential part of automation system responsible for data transfer and data exchange between various devices. Industrial communication consists of some set of rules for communication called industrial communication protocols. The major control mechanisms used in industrial automation include programmable logic controller, supervisory control, and data acquisition and distributed control system. All these elements deal with supervisory controls, smart devices and HMI and many other field instruments.

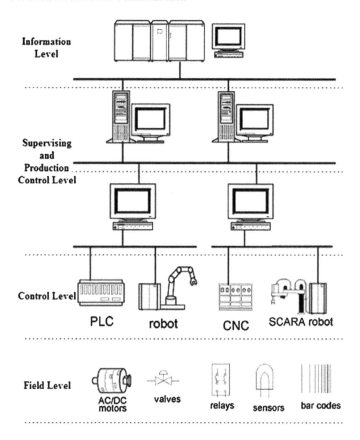

Fig. 1 Levels of industrial communication

2.1 Hierarchical Levels in Industrial Communication Network

The hierarchical levels in industrial communication are divided depending on the functionality of manufacturing or process industry, the data flows from field level to enterprise level. The main levels include device level, control level, and information level as shown in Fig. 1 [3]. Depending on the functionality sensors actuators and buses are at field level, control buses are at control level and information level is the topmost level.

- **Device level**: Device level consists of devices like sensors and actuators. The network consists of serial communication protocols like RS232, RS485 to transfer information to elements like PLC. Field level communication is characterized by factors such as response time and message size. The main task of devices at the field level is to exchange data between the manufactured product and technical process.

- **Control level**: Control level consists of computer system, distributed control units, and PLCs. The function performed at this level includes loading program and displaying variables on HMI. Control level communication is characterized by high speed, synchronization, and short data length.
- **Information level**: This is the topmost level of industrial automation which collects information from its lower level. Ethernet and WLAN are used at this level for factory planning and management. Ethernet networks can be used at this level as a gateway to connect to other industrial networks.

3 Design Principles of Industry 4.0

The main focus of Industry 4.0 is in process automation and data exchange, which bring IOT, cloud computing, and Cyberphysical systems together for fully automatic manufacturing and process control. The main key principles for the design of the smart factory include

- **Interoperability**: Interoperability indicates the ability of the system and humans to interact with each other.
- **Real-time capability**: Indicates the capability of the device to collect and produce the necessary data online in real time.
- **Decentralization**: Decentralization is the decision-making capability of the Cyberphysical System (CPS) on their own.
- **Service Orientation**: Offers data for sharing data through network.
- **Modularity**: Indicates the flexibility of the device in adapting the changes and expanding to the requirements of the new modules.

4 Industrial Communication Technologies

Three main industrial fieldbus technology are fieldbus technology, industrial Ethernet, and Industrial IOT. All these communication technologies are discussed in this section.

4.1 Traditional Fieldbus Technology

Fieldbus is a new digital communication network that is used for interconnection of field devices like sensors and actuators for data transfer or information exchange among them. The fieldbus has replaced 4–20 mA analog signal standard. Fieldbus is a two-way digital local area network communication dedicated to industrial automation. The fieldbuses are characterized on the basis of type of industry like discrete or manufacturing. The main intention of fieldbus is to replace the point to point connections between field devices with a single serial bus system. Different type includes Profibus, DeviceNet, Modbus, and CAN Bus. These are the common protocols which are responsible for acquiring the bus to manage synchronization between devices on the bus. Fieldbus is constructed with less cable which is simple and has digital technique, but yet there is no standardization for serial interface [3]. A set of rule are defined in order to establish data transfer between the devices along the bus. The main advantage of fieldbus is the savings associated with cable and maintenance. The disadvantage is different version of device due to different fieldbus standard.

4.2 Industrial Ethernet Technology

There are various fieldbus solutions capable of providing real-time environment, but fieldbuses are subjected to number of devices that can be networked and thereby limiting the scalability and interoperability between various solutions is not provided. Therefore, networking by means of industrial Ethernet prevails against fieldbus. The application of Ethernet to connect field devices offer many advantages compared to fieldbus [4]. The industrial Ethernet is defined as the use of Ethernet in industrial environment, designed to work in harsh environment. A RT capable industrial Ethernet is developed as remedy for deficiencies of standard Ethernet and TCP/IP- or UDP/IP-based communication. The industrial Ethernet has guaranteed delivery and has less jitter. Industrial Ethernet uses time division multiplexing method whereby each device is allowed to communicate in time slot. This provides synchronization among all devices. The above factors and the low cost of Ethernet have made Ethernet an attractive option for industrial communication application. There are three different classes of slave device implementations.

- Class A (Standard Ethernet Hardware and Software)
- Class B (Standard Ethernet Hardware, Modified Software)
- Class C (Modified Hardware and Software)

A. *PROFINET*

It is an industry technical standard designed for data communication, data collection, and controlling. PROFINET stands for Process Filed Net and maintained by PROFIBUS & PROFINET International. There are three PROFINET versions based on the three approach classes are:

- PROFINET CbA (Component-Based Automation) follows Class A approach
- PROFINET RT (Real Time) follows Class B approach
- PROFINET IRT (Isochronous Real Time) follows Class C approach

PROFINET CbA and RT are aimed at PLC applications while IRT is suitable for motion control. The cycle time and jitter for different versions are PROFINET CbA in the range of 100 ms, PROFINET RT up to 10 ms, PROFINET IRT less than 1 ms.

PROFINET CbA was the initial solution for industry Ethernet communication and is no longer supported. The PROFINET RT and IRT protocols are later renamed as PROFINET IO. PROFINET RT is based on the software tuning of stack which bypasses TCP and IP stacks. It has following limitations, delays in switches, delays in stacks, and TCP traffic. PROFINET IRT is based on time slicing concept. Its implementation is using both software and hardware changes. It requires special switches in all devices (master, slave, all infrastructure devices). It differentiates between real time and non-real traffic and routes accordingly. The bandwidth utilization is limited even though most applications only have TCP/IP communication and the bandwidth remains reserved for this kind of traffic. RT devices can be combined in IRT networks, if there is sufficient bandwidth and if the master supports this. The latest IRT v2.3 supports 31.25 µs cycle time.

B. *ETHERNET/IP*

Ethernet/IP is an industrial network protocol that adapts the Common Industrial Protocol (CIP) to standard Ethernet. It is based on approach Class A. CIP is the common object library for applications such as control, safety, synchronization, motion, configuration, and information. CIP is adapted by protocols such as Ethernet/IP, Device Net, CompoNet, and Control Net. Ethernet/IP is an efficient slave to slave communication.

Ethernet/IP requires broadcast communication and has large delay due to filtering in each device and has limited real-time capabilities. When tested with up to 80% bandwidth utilization, using both managed and unmanaged switches. Even though CIP Sync adds time synchronization, it does not reduce the cycle time or process data performance. The issues are as follows: limited number of connections; bus cycle time is typically 5–10 ms; reaction time is typically 15–30 ms; even though Ethernet/IP is aimed at the controller to controller level, it is more and more used for I/O communication as well.

C. *CC-LINK IE*

CC-Link is an RS485-based fieldbus technology introduced by Mitsubishi Electric and maintained by CLPA. CC-Link is promoted as an open-architecture technology and follows approach C. There are two main types, CC-Link IE Control and IE field used for controller and I/O communication. In Nov 2011, a Motion Control Profile was added for controller/controller communication and supports up to 119 slave stations. The information is transmitted using token passing method. If there is any problem in token passing or if the token frame is lost the entire token should be retransmitted and then, the real-time behavior is lost. The CC-Link IE Control frame is embedded directly in the Ethernet frame and the CC-Link IE Control needs a dedicated and separate network of its own. The cycle time is sensitive to no. of nodes and for 8 nodes, about 1.6 ms is observed.

D. *SERCOS III*

Sercos III is the third generation of the Sercos interface, standardized as an open digital interface for the communication between Ethernet nodes, IO devices, and motion control equipment. Working principle of the Sercos is similar to that of EtherCAT as the frames are processed "on the fly" mechanism. Sercos III follows master/slave arrangement and exchanging cyclic data between nodes. The master initiates all data transmission during a Sercos real-time cycle. All data transmissions begin and end at the master (circular). As the frame passes through each slave, the data is inserted (on the fly). Recovery time in case of cable failures <25 μs and cycle time of 31.25 μs.

E. *POWERLINK*

It is an open protocol introduced by Automation Company and managed by the Ethernet POWERLINK Standardization Group (EPSG). Previous versions are based on the approach B, while the new version support hard real time with approach C. The protocol uses hubs and replaces media access control by polling and uses time slicing mechanism. Guaranteed data transfer is achieved by time slicing mechanism in very short isochoric cycles. With configurable response time and synchronization of all nodes very high precision data transmission can be achieved.

F. *MODBUS/TCP*

Modbus is a serial communications protocol invented by Modicon. It follows approach A and is very simple to implement. Modbus/TCP client/master implementations are based on polling and can work on two ways wait for each response to return before the next request is issued and sends several requests at once in order to allow for parallel processing in the server/slave devices. Due to its operating principle, Modbus/TCP cannot guarantee delivery times or cycle times or provide precise synchronization.

G. *ETHERCAT*

The construction of the smart factory is based on the use of PLC controller motion control device, inverters connected through an intelligent industrial Ethernet. Industrial Ethernet is designed to work in extremely high temperatures, vibration and should be able to work for process control and automation with real time and reliable behavior. A firewall system is used for data exchange between individual network and office network. The office network is separated from IO network for better performance. MODBUS, Ethernet IP, and Profibus are the protocols used by PLC communication. EtherCAT is an Ethernet-based fieldbus system, invented by Beckhoff Automation suitable for both hard and soft real-time requirements in automation technology. The slave implementation of EtherCAT is a Class C approach. The key working principle of EtherCAT is "Frame processing on the fly" and thus requires dedicated slave controllers. EtherCAT uses a standard EtherCAT frame with Ether Type 0x88A4. Switches are not required if all devices present in the network use EtherCAT. Hence, there are no costs related to switches, their power supply, mounting, wiring, and configuration, and so on. The EtherCAT uses only standard Ethernet frames. Any number of drop lines or branches is possible, providing the most flexible topology [5]. Along with master/slave, it supports slave/slave communication. The adoption rate of EtherCAT is outstanding. Considering the design principles of Industry 4.0, EtherCAT has very less cycle time and has modularity. As EtherCAT communicates with different protocols hence provides interoperability. As EtherCAT technology satisfies most of the design principles of Industry 4.0, EtherCAT is a tailor made technology for the construction of smart factory.

4.3 Industrial IOT

In real-time Ethernet technologies, there is no solution without master component and special hardware. The industrial IOT is the use of IOT in manufacturing which is a part of larger concept called IOT. IOT is a network of intelligent devices, computer and objects that collect and share huge data [6]. The collected data is sent to the main cloud which is further shared at other end in a useful way. The main driving principle of IIOT is smart machine which provides accurate data capture and consistency, IIOT incorporate big data, machine to machine communication, machine learning, and automation technologies. The major focus of IIOT is on the interoperability between devices and machines that use different protocols and architecture. Industrial IOT (or industrial Internet or Industry 4.0) has created a new revolution in industry by enabling acquisition and accessibility of data at far place at higher speeds and greater efficiency than before. The main design principles for characterizing Industry 4.0 include interoperability, virtualization, decentralization, modularity, and real-time capability.

5 Case Study on EtherCAT

The case study is based on EtherCAT protocol to demonstrate the features of EtherCAT technology and its contribution for the development of a smart factory. Most of the available Variable Frequency Drives in the market are equipped with RS-485 MODBUS communication. By using MODBUS communication the Variable Frequency Drive cannot be added to industrial communication network. The unique features of EtherCAT make it best candidate for drive applications, hence the main focus is to replace the Variable Frequency Drive integrated with MODBUS communication by EtherCAT technology. In paper [7], the author has discussed the implementation of EtherCAT communication between Industrial PC and Variable Frequency Drive in detail. In this section, the main characteristics of the EtherCAT which aids the development of Industry 4.0 are discussed. The basic EtherCAT system architecture consists of one EtherCAT master and multiple EtherCAT slaves as shown in Fig. 2 [7] (Table 1).

Table 1 Comparison of various industrial ethernet protocols

Classifications	PROFINET	Ethernet/IP	CC-Link IE	SERCOS III	Powerlink	Modbus TCP	EtherCAT
Approach class	• CbA—Class A • RT—Class B • IRT—Class C	• Ethernet/IP—Class A • With CIP Sync—Class C	Class C	Class C	• V1&V2—Class B • V3&V4—Class C	Class A	Class C
Working principle	• CbA—TCP/IP on DCOM • RT—best effort by TCP layer bypassing • IRT—time slicing by ASICs	CIP adaption	Token passing	Extract and insert data on the fly	• V2: polling using hubs • V3: burst polling	Polling	Frame processing on the fly
Topology supported	Line, branch, tree	Line	• Control: ring • Field: line + star, ring	Line and ring	Line, star and daisy chain	Line	Most flexible topologies
Real-time capabilities	• CbA—Non real time • RT—soft realtime • IRT—hard real time	Limited real-time capabilities	Limited real-time capacities	Hard real-time capable	Soft real time	Non-realtime	Hard real time
Cycle time (Comparison not based on same nodes)	• CbA—in the range of 100 ms • RT—up to 10 ms • IRT—less than 1 ms (250 μs min)	5–10 ms	• Control: 1.6 ms • Field: 0.3 ms	31.25 μs	291 μs	10–20 μs	11 μs
Nodes supported	IRT—64	–	120	511	Limited	–	65535
Safety protocol	PROFIsafe	CIP safety	CC-Link safety	CIP safety	openSAFETY	openSAFETY	Safety over EtherCAT
Ease of use	No structuring concept—difficult to configure	Complex router configuration	No proper documents on usage	Average	Average	Very easy	Easy
Adaption rate (as on 2014)	614 entries	169 entries	No much of adoptions outside Mitsubishi	192 entries	95 entries	–	523

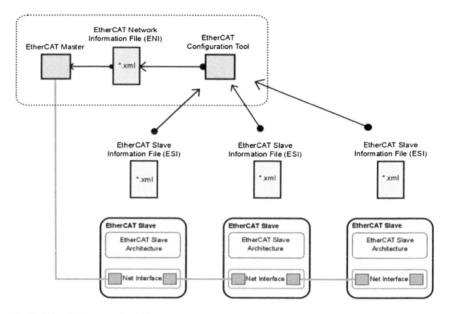

Fig. 2 EtherCAT network architecture

The main requirements of master are a standard Ethernet port, EtherCAT slave information (ESI) file and a real-time driver. The main requirements of EtherCAT slave are a standard Ethernet port, EtherCAT slave controller, EEPROM, and an Application controller. The complete setup for establishing communication between master and slave is as shown in Fig. 3 [7]. CX8090 is a control system with switched Ethernet port used as EtherCAT master, along with EK1110 coupler.

EK1110 extension is connected to the end of EtherCAT terminal block that offers an option for connecting EtherCAT cable with RJ45 connector. The master uses a standard Ethernet port and EtherCAT slave information (ESI) file. The ESI written in XML format is saved in TwinCAT master directory path. TwinCAT is a real-time environment driver embedded in the master PC that drives the slaves in the network. The Beckhoff Industrial PC CX8090 embedded with TwinCAT-2 reads the ESI files written in XML format and initializes the slave devices and the master prepares for establishing communication with slave device. The EtherCAT slave device will update the EEPROM with the slave information and prepare for communication and sends a frame to VFD. The VFD will respond for the frame sent by the application controller of slave device. When both master and slave device are ready for communication or information exchange, the master and slave devices will be in operational state the parameters received from the VFD is updated to the master and can be monitored in HMI as shown in Fig. 4 [7]. Mapping the variables in Twin-CAT IO devices to TwinCAT PLC is by using Structured Text Program. In master section, TwinCAT system manager and TwinCAT PLC control are the tools used for developing PLC code. By using Structured Text Language (STL), IO variables are

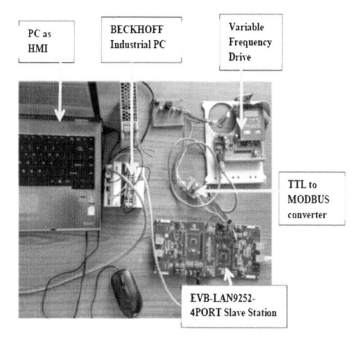

Fig. 3 Experimental setup for EtherCAT communication between industrial PC and variable frequency drive

created in TwinCAT PLC Control file, then the PLC IO variables are linked with the hardware IO in TwinCAT system manager and updated output can be monitored and controlled using master. EtherCAT has very less cycle time and jitter with efficient data communication due to which the data from the VFD is updated to TwinCAT master in real time. As EtherCAT is compatible with other industrial Ethernet protocols, it indicates modularity. With the use of TwinCAT, the EtherCAT technology is interoperable. With its service orientation nature, EtherCAT shares data among industrial communication. Comparing the above case study of EtherCAT with the design principles of Industry 4.0, EtherCAT is an effective industrial Ethernet for building of Smart factory.

6 Conclusion

Reliable communication is very essential for the development of smart factory. The three major milestones in field level networking: the fieldbus system, industrial Ethernet, and upcoming wireless field level network are discussed in this paper. Referring to Industry 4.0 discussed in the above section, EtherCAT fits with the many of its characteristics. EtherCAT satisfies interoperability, modularity, and real-time

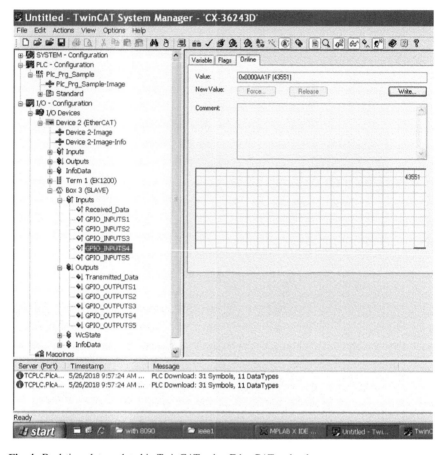

Fig. 4 Real-time data updated in TwinCAT using EtherCAT technology

capability. The adoptability rate of EtherCAT is increasing due to its excellent communication efficiency and networking. Most of the existing VFDs are available with RS-485 MODBUS communication. In order to add VFDs to EtherCAT network, VFDs should be implemented with EtherCAT technology. The drive parameters sent from the VFD can be monitored in TwinCAT master. EtherCAT meets the development trend of Variable Frequency Drive in real-time applications and industrial automation. Future work includes study on different communication profiles like SoE, FoE, and EOE, the application of EtherCAT for automation, EtherCAT-P, and study of TwinCAT master for various motion control applications.

Acknowledgements I would like to express my deepest gratitude and sincere respect to the Hexmoto team for their kind advice and assistance for the preparation of this thesis. Also I am thankful to Professor V Nattarasu and Professor B. A. Sujatha Kumari, Sri Jayachamarajendra College of Engineering, Mysuru, for their guidance and support.

References

1. Danielis P, Skodzik J, Altmann V (2014) Survey on real-time communication via Ethernet in industrial automation environments. IEEE
2. Langlois K, van der Hoeven T, Cianca DR, Verstratenb T (2018) EtherCAT tutorial. IEEE Robot Autom Mag. 1070-9932/18©2018 IEEE
3. Li S-C, Huang Y (2017) Using data mining methods to detect simulated intrusions on a Modbus network. In: 2017 IEEE 7th international symposium on cloud and service computing
4. Liu Z, Liu N, Zhang T, Cui L, Li H (2015) EtherCAT based robot modular joint controller. In: Proceeding of the 2015 IEEE international conference on information and automation
5. Wang L, Li M, Qi J, Zhang Q (2014) Design approach based on EtherCAT protocol for a networked motion control system. Int J Distrib Sens Netw. Article ID 750601
6. Farné S, Bassi E, Benzi F, Compagnoni F (2016) IIoT based efficiency monitoring of a Gantry robot. IEEE
7. Sridevi G, Saligram A, Nattarasu V (2018) Establishing EtherCAT communication between industrial PC and VFD. In: IEEE proceedings RTEICT-2018

Optimal Resource Allocation and Binding in High-Level Synthesis Using Nature-Inspired Computation

K. C. Shilpa, C. LakshmiNarayana and Manoj Kumar Singh

Abstract Allocation of resource and binding it to functional unit at high-level synthesis an optimal problem to minimize the area and performance in terms of resource sharing and binding is presented in this paper. The paper presents the comparative analysis of nature-inspired computation techniques for resource allocation and binding: 1. Evolutionary-based computation: genetic algorithm. 2. Swarm intelligence-based computation: particle swarm optimization. The comparative analysis of the results shows genetic algorithm surpasses particle swarm optimization in providing the precise mapping between the operation and functional unit sharing with zero errors in resource allocation.

Keywords Data flow graph · Genetic algorithm · High-level synthesis · Integer linear programming · Particle swarm optimization · Register-transfer level

1 Introduction

High-level synthesis means synthesizing register-transfer level (RTL) formation from the functional explanation. The two distinct tasks in high-level synthesis are scheduling and allocation [1]. Scheduling task describes the distinct start time for every process in the data flow graph (DFG). Scheduling gives the resource usage estimates. Allocation task ensures that sufficient numbers of resources are available for executing the operation.

K. C. Shilpa (✉)
Dr. Ambedkar Institute of Technology, Bangalore, India
e-mail: shilpa.kc2@gmail.com

C. LakshmiNarayana
Department of Electrical Engineering Science, BMSCE, Bangalore, India
e-mail: ln_gp@yahoo.co.in

M. K. Singh
Manuro Tech Research, Bangalore, India
e-mail: mksingh@manuroresearch.com

© Springer Nature Singapore Pte Ltd. 2019
V. Sridhar et al. (eds.), *Emerging Research in Electronics, Computer Science and Technology*, Lecture Notes in Electrical Engineering 545,
https://doi.org/10.1007/978-981-13-5802-9_95

The two steps in allocation are resource sharing and resource binding [2]. Resource sharing allows to control on the use of multiple hardware resources for implementing the operation. Resource binding maps between behavioral operations and the resources instances. Resource sharing and binding are NP (nondeterministic polynomial time) complete problem [3], which performs an exhaustive search in finding out the best answer.

2   Previous Work

Many novel techniques for resource binding and sharing are reported [4]. A clique partition algorithm for resource sharing and the coloring algorithm are the best method for resource sharing [5]. The ILP formulation [6, 7] for concurrent scheduling and binding provides successful solution of ILP problems for circuits of interesting size. Nature-inspired algorithms act as an optimized technique in solving the complex problem which is flexible in nature. Genetic algorithm is an optimization tool to solve high-complexity computation problems which are based on principles of Charles Darwin. Particle swarm optimization is swarm intelligence computation method-based stochastic algorithm.

Evolutionary-based search techniques are best to solve NP-Complete problem effectively.

3   Nature-Inspired Computations Method (Genetic Algorithm (GA), Particle Swarm Optimization (PSO))

Nature-inspired computations (NIC) are a method that is motivated by process focused from natural world. These computing methods led to the growth of working of algorithms so-called nature-inspired computation. The algorithms mainly focused toward the nature computational intelligence.

Nature-inspired computation algorithm is mainly categorized as follows:

Evolutionary Computation (EC): Evolutionary computation is a term used to illustrate an algorithm which was encouraged by 'survival of the fittest' or 'normal selection' principles proposed by Charles Darwin.

Swarm Intelligence (SI): Swarm intelligence is a phrase used to explain the algorithms and distributed problems-solvers mainly inspired by the cooperative cluster intelligence of swarm.

3.1 Genetic Algorithm (GA)

Genetic algorithm (GA) developed by John Holland [8]. The process of genetic algorithm is a search method used to compute to discover accurate or estimated solutions to optimization and search problems based on the rule of regular selection. Genetic algorithm is categorized as universal explore heuristics. Genetic algorithm [9] which is the group of evolutionary algorithms tools method motivated by evolutionary natural science such as inheritance, mutation, selection, and crossover.

3.2 Particle Swarm Optimization (PSO)

Eberhart and Shi [10] developed swarm intelligence method called particle swarm optimization, which emerges as a powerful stochastic optimization technique motivated by the communal activities of organisms such flocks of birds, schools of fish, or swarms of bees, and even human communal behavior, from which the behavior is emerged. Population-based search procedure in which individuals so called particles change their position (state) with time. The standard rule is particle swarm [11] move about toward the best position in explore space, identification based on each particle's best known position and global best known position.

4 Methodology

4.1 Problem Formulation

The objective of the allocation work aims to locate the resources in finding the appropriate correct number and type of resource sharing of the multiplier resources and ALU resources for each operation so that the design constraint is met.

4.2 Benchmark Problem for Resource Allocation

To illustrate the allocation problem, the scheduled sequencing time constraint graph displayed in Fig. 1, the problem based on hardware abstraction layer (HAL). Implementation by resource with type ALU is considered for the operation of type adders, subtractor, and comparator.

The scheduled graph from Fig. 1 indicates the operation for multiplier resources $\{(o_1), (o_2)\}$ is listed in the first time step, operation for multiplier resources $\{(o_3), (o_6)\}$ is listed in second time step, operation for multiplier resources $\{(o_7), (o_8)\}$ scheduled in third time step. Adders, subtractor, and comparator are generalized as the resource-type ALU. The operation for ALU resources (o_{10}) is scheduled in the initial control time step, operation for ALU resources (o_{11}) scheduled in second control time step, operation for ALU resources (o_4) scheduled in third time control step and operation for ALU resources $\{(o_5), (o_9)\}$ scheduled in fourth time control step. The obtained scheduled result under time constraint scheduling requires two multiplier operator units and two ALU operator units to fulfill the defined schedule graph.

4.3 Integer Linear Programming (ILP) Formulation for Allocation and Binding as a Constraint Optimization

To illustrate the allocation problem, the ILP formulation for operation binding as constraints optimization, for the scheduled data flow graph in Fig. 1 is as follows:

ILP model is a set of binary decision variables with two indices 'B' = { 'b_{ir}'; i = 0, 1, ... n; 'r' = 1, 2, ... a}, 'n' = number of operations, 'a' = number of resources. { 'b_{ir}' = 1} implies the operation 'o_i' in constraint graph bound to resource 'r', a ≤ n is an high bound on the numeral of resources to be set. Binary decision constants 'X' = 'x_{il}'; i = 0, 1, ... n; l = 1, 2, ... λ + 1, where { 'x_{il}' = 1} implies operation o_i start in the control step 'l' of the schedule, from the schedule 'l' = 't_i'.

The different ILP formulation constraints are:

- To obtain a binding, search a set of values of 'B', to allocate behavior operation to the resources such that the set of following constraints are met.

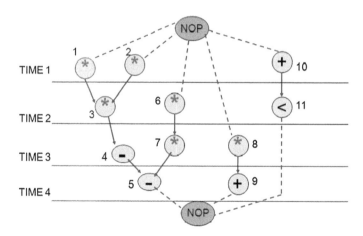

Fig. 1 Scheduled sequencing time constraint HAL benchmark problem

$$\sum_{r=1}^{a} b_{ir} = 1, \; i = 1, 2, \ldots, n \tag{1}$$

Equation (1) states every operation 'o_i' should assign to exactly one as well as only one resource of type 'a'.

- The resource allocation for Eq. (1) for 'resource 1' and 'resource 2' of the multiplier is summation of each operational units of multiplier by the 'resource 1' and 'resource 2' given below as follows:

$$b(1, 1) + b(1, 2) = 1$$
$$b(2, 1) + b(1, 2) = 1$$
$$b(3, 1) + b(3, 2) = 1$$
$$b(6, 1) + b(6, 2) = 1$$
$$b(7, 1) + b(7, 2) = 1$$
$$b(8, 1) + b(8, 2) = 1$$

- The resource allocation for Eq. (1) for 'resource 1' and 'resource 2' of the ALU is summation of each operational units of ALU by the 'resource 1' and 'resource 2' given below as follows:

$$b(10, 1) + b(10, 2) = 1$$
$$b(11, 1) + b(11, 2) = 1$$
$$b(4, 1) + b(4, 2) = 1$$
$$b(5, 1) + b(5, 2) = 1$$
$$b(9, 1) + b(9, 2) = 1$$

- Equation (2) states at each control step, one operation among resource r can be executed among those allocated.

$$\sum_{i=1}^{n} b_{ir} * \sum_{m=1-d_i+1}^{1} X_{im} \leq 1, \; 1 = 1, 2, \ldots \lambda + 1, r = 1, 2, \ldots a \tag{2}$$

$$b_{ir} \in \{0, 1\} \;, i = 0, 1 \ldots n; r = 1, 2, \ldots a \tag{3}$$

- Equation (3) constraint states decision variable 'B' are binate, either take (0, 1).

The resource allocation for Eq. (2) describes the summation of each multiplier operation by 'resource 1' with the product of each multiplier operation at scheduled time step is as follows:

$$b(1, 1) * x(1, 1) + b(2, 1) * x(2, 1) \leq 1$$

$$b(3, 1) * x(3, 2) + b(6, 1) * x(6, 1) \leq 1$$
$$b(7, 1) * x(7, 3) + b(8, 1) * x(8, 3) \leq 1$$

- The resource allocation for Eq. (2) by 'resource 2' of multiplier is as follows:

$$b(1, 2) * x(1, 1) + b(2, 2) * x(2, 1) \leq 1$$
$$b(3, 1) * x(3, 2) + b(6, 2) * x(6, 2) \leq 1$$
$$b(7, 1) * x(7, 3) + b(8, 2) * x(8, 3) \leq 1$$

- The resource allocation for Eq. (2) by 'resource 1' of ALU is as follows:

$$b(5, 1) * x(5, 4) + b(9, 1) * x(9, 4) \leq 1$$

- The resource allocation for Eq. (2) by 'resource 2' of ALU is as follows:

$$b(5, 2) * x(5, 4) + b(9, 2) * x(9, 4) \leq 1$$

5 Experimental Analysis and Data

To solve ILP formulation of operation binding as constraints optimization, the nature-inspired computations evolutionary computation genetic algorithm method, and swarm intelligence method are considered to work out the inequalities constraint value. There are '12' different variables for multiplier constraint equation, '10' different variables for ALU constraint equation. Thus, there are total '22' variables which have to be solved.

The allocation optimization specifications are as follows: Integer linear programming can be formulated for the objective function given in Eq. (4) as follows:

$$Minimize\ f;\ `f' = resources\ sharing \tag{4}$$

$$`f' = sum(abs(`rs')) \tag{5}$$

$$`rs' = [r\ \ r2];\ `r' = multiplier\ \ constraint\ equation,$$

$$`r2' = ALU\,constraint\,equation$$

- The algorithm is experienced with regular random numeral for population range (N) = 50.
- Dimension of the search space (D) = 22.

- Genetic Algorithm parameter setup: the crossover probability which is two-point factor = '1', mutation probability factor value = 0.01. Selection method tournament is used.
- Particle Swarm Optimization (PSO) parameter setup: Constriction factor (cf) value = 0.72, learning factor $(c1, c2)$ value of 2.5, inertia weight 'w' value is reducing from 1.2 to 0.1.

Allocation algorithm problem is solved using MATLAB.

6 Results and Discussion

6.1 Resource Binding Performance Analysis Using Genetic Algorithm

The 12 variables multiplier allocation results using GA are presented in Table 1. The 10 variables ALU allocation results are been listed as follows in Table 2.

Table 1 Results of genetic algorithms performance for multiplier allocation and binding

Allocation variables	Binding multiplier for resource type	Resource type
1	$b(1, 1)$	1
2	$b(1, 2)$	0
3	$b(2, 1)$	0
4	$b(2, 2)$	1
5	$b(3, 1)$	1
6	$b(3, 2)$	0
7	$b(6, 1)$	0
8	$b(6, 2)$	1
9	$b(7, 1)$	1
10	$b(7, 2)$	0
11	$b(8, 1)$	0
12	$b(8, 2)$	1

Table 2 Results of genetic algorithms performance for ALU allocation and binding

Allocation variables	Binding ALU resource type	Resource type
1	$b(10, 1)$	1
2	$b(10, 2)$	0
3	$b(11, 1)$	1
4	$b(11, 2)$	0
5	$b(4, 1)$	1
6	$b(4, 2)$	0
7	$b(5, 1)$	0
8	$b(5, 2)$	1
9	$b(9, 1)$	1
10	$b(9, 2)$	0

6.2 Discussion

In Table 1, $b(1, 1) = b(3, 1) = b(7, 1) = 1$; indicates operation for (o_1, o_3, o_7) done by 'resource 1' and results $b(2, 2) = b(6, 2) = b(8, 2) = 1$; indicates (o_2, o_6, o_8) operation done by 'resource 2'.

The ALU allocation result is tabulated in Table 2. The 10 variables results for ALU resources are presented in Table 2. In Table 2, $b(10, 1) = b(11, 1) = b(4, 1) = b(9, 1) = 1$; indicates operation for $(o_{10}, o_{11}, o_4, o_9)$ done by 'resource 1' of ALU and $b(5, 2) = 1$; indicate operation (o_5) done by 'resource 2' of ALU. In Fig. 2, the error in allocation using genetic algorithm is zero; the objective function given in Eq. (4) is minimized to zero which is the obtained optimal value.

The optimal scheduled and resource-bounded sequence graph obtained by solving the ILP constraint using genetic algorithm is shown in Fig. 3. Figure 3 describes multiplier 'resource 1' sharing is done for operation 'o_1', 'o_3', 'o' and indicated as $(1, 1)$. $((1, 1)$ indicate multiplier operations done by multiplier 'resource 1').

The multiplier 'resource 2' sharing is done for operation 'o', 'o_6', 'o_8' and is indicated as $(1, 2)$; $((1, 2)$ indicate multiplier operations done by multiplier 'resource 2').

ALU 'resource 1' sharing is done for operation 'o_{10}', 'o_{11}', 'o_4', 'o_9', and is indicated as $(2, 1)$; $((2, 1)$ indicate ALU operations done by ALU 'resource 1'). The ALU 'resource 2' sharing done for o_5 and is indicated as $(2, 2)$; $((2, 2)$ indicate ALU operations done by ALU 'resource 2'). Hence, the resource sharing and binding are done simultaneously for a solution under a larger set of constraints.

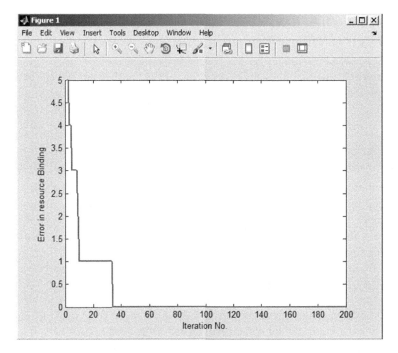

Fig. 2 Error in resource binding analysis for genetic algorithm

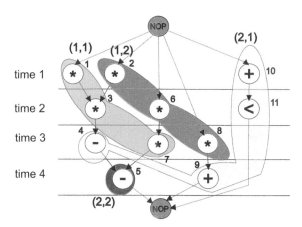

Fig. 3 Scheduled and resource-bounded graph obtained from GA

6.3 Resource Binding Performance Analysis Using Particle Swarm Optimization

The performances of multiplier allocation using PSO are shown in Table 3 and ALU allocation using particle swarm optimization is shown in Table 4.

6.4 Discussion

The multiplier allocation results are tabulated in Table 3. The 12 variables results allocating multiplier resources are presented in Table 3. Table 3 result $b(2, 1) = b(7, 1) = 1$; indicates (o_2, o_7) operation done by 'resource 1', and (o_6, o_8, o_1) operation have done by 'resource 2' and PSO fails to allocate resources sharing for operation (o_3).

The ALU allocation result using PSO is tabulated in Table 4. The 10 variables results for ALU resources are presented in Table 4. In Table 4, $b(10, 1) = b(4, 1) = 1$; indicates operation for (o_{10}, o_4) done by 'resource 1' of ALU and $b(5, 2) = b(11, 2) = 1$; indicates operation (o_5, o_{11}) done by 'resource 2' of ALU, but PSO fails to deliver the results for resources sharing for the operation (o_9).

The objective function is minimized to the value four as shown in Fig. 4. The error in allocation using particle swarm optimization is four; PSO fails to minimize the objective function to the optimal value of zero; and struck at local minima as shown in Fig. 4.

Table 3 Particle swarm performance for multiplier allocation	Allocation variables	Binding multiplier for resource type	Resource type
	1	b(1, 1)	0
	2	b(1, 2)	1
	3	b(2, 1)	1
	4	b(2, 2)	0
	5	b(3, 1)	0
	6	b(3, 2)	0
	7	b(6, 1)	0
	8	b(6, 2)	1
	9	b(7, 1)	1
	10	b(7, 2)	0
	11	b(8, 1)	0
	12	b(8, 2)	1

Table 4 Particle swarm performance for ALU allocation

Allocation variables	Binding ALU for resource type	Resource type
1	b(10, 1)	1
2	b(10, 2)	0
3	b(11, 1)	0
4	b(11, 2)	1
5	b(4, 1)	1
6	b(4, 2)	0
7	b(5, 1)	0
8	b(5, 2)	1
9	b(9, 1)	1
10	b(9, 2)	1

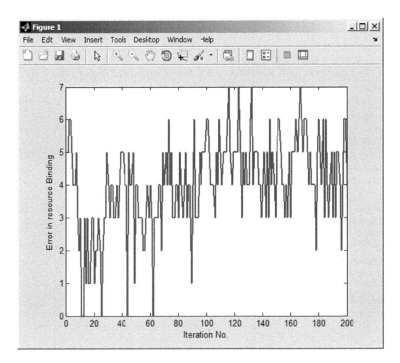

Fig. 4 Error in resource binding analysis for particle swarm optimization

7 Conclusion

Comparative analysis of resource allocation and binding of multiplier and ALU functional units is obtained by means of genetic algorithm which is one of the evolutionary computation methods and swarm intelligence method.

Genetic algorithm, an evolutionary method to find optimal solution for resource allocation and binding, achieves minimum objective function; i.e., 'f' = 0; is successfully with zero error in allocation. Particle swarm optimization, a swarm intelligence method, poorly gets struck at local minima and fails to obtain minimum objective function. Error in allocation exists in PSO method. The comparison results from GA and PSO show, GA is foremost in determining the binding of allocation problem in with zero errors.

References

1. Micheli GD (1994) Synthesis and optimization of digital circuits. McGraw-Hill, USA
2. Gajski D, Dutt ND, Wu A, Lin S (1992) High level synthesis: introduction to chip and system design. Kluwer Academic Publisher, USA
3. Ku D, DeMicheli G (1992) High level synthesis of ASICS under timing and synchronization constraints. Kluwer Academic Publishers, USA
4. Hafer L, Parker A (1992) Automated synthesis of digital hardware. IEEE Trans Comput Aided Des Integr Circuits Syst 31(2):365–370
5. Pangrle B, Gajski D (1987) A state synthesizer for intelligent silicon compilation. IEEE Trans Comput Aided Des 6(3):42–45
6. Devadas S, Newton AR (1989) Algorithms for allocation in data path synthesis. IEEE Trans Comput Aided Des Integr Circuits Syst 8(2):768–781
7. Thomas DE (1983) The automatic synthesis of digital systems. IEEE Trans Comput Aided Des Integr Circuits 69(10):1200–1211
8. Goldberg DE (1989) Genetic algorithms in search, optimization and machine learning. Addison-Wesley Publishing Co, Reading, MA
9. Mandal C, Chakrabarti PP, Ghose S (2000) GABIND: a GA approach to allocation and binding for the high-level synthesis of data paths. IEEE Trans Very Large Scale Integr (VLSI) Syst 8(6)
10. Eberhart RC, Shi Y (1998) Comparison between genetic algorithms and particle swarm optimization. In: Proceedings of seventh annual conference on evolutionary programming, pp 611–616
11. Kennedy J, Eberhart RC (1995) Particle swarm optimization. In: Proceedings IEEE international conference on neural networks (Perth, Australia), Piscataway, IEEE Service Center

Boundary Extraction and Tortuosity Calculation in Retinal Fundus Images

R. Manjunatha, Mahesh Koti and H. S. Sheshadri

Abstract Tortuosity and retina blood vessel dilation are important symptoms of plus disease in retinopathy of prematurity. This paper presents differential geometrical method for tortuosity measurement. The problem of tortuosity evaluation is formulated as one-dimensional differential geometrical curvature characterization. The vessel network extracted from retinal image is subjected to boundary extraction and individual vessel boundaries are extracted as planar curves, further these curves are segmented and differential curvature is computed at segment level and at vessel level for the individual vessels. The method is tested and validated on the available public data and local data set. Vessels with considerable tortuosity are found to be having significant curvature variation compared to the normal vessels.

Keywords ROP · OD · Vascular network · Tortuosity

1 Introduction

Recent clinical survey shows a number of premature infants being diagnosed with retinopathy of prematurity (ROP) a retinal disorder due to abnormal growth of blood vessels [1]. The potential risk of ROP and consequent threat of blindness can be dealt systematically by early screening and treatment [1, 2]. The plus disease of ROP is diagnosed by dilation and tortuosity of blood vessels. Severity of ROP is identified with stages based on visual characterization; ROP plus disease corresponds to one of these stages [1, 2]. The diagnosis of ROP can be made effective and simple by applying image processing techniques with the objective of identifying vascular changes in the offline retinal images. In this context, a number of algorithms and methods have been presented, like morphological and linear filtering, vessel tracking algorithms, based on arc length over chord length ratio [3], Recreantly, approaches like called the template disc method [4], mean curvature along condensed

R. Manjunatha (✉) · M. Koti · H. S. Sheshadri
PES College of Engineering, Mandya 571401, India
e-mail: rmanjunatha@gmail.com

© Springer Nature Singapore Pte Ltd. 2019
V. Sridhar et al. (eds.), *Emerging Research in Electronics, Computer Science and Technology*, Lecture Notes in Electrical Engineering 545,
https://doi.org/10.1007/978-981-13-5802-9_96

phase interfaces in two or three dimensions [5], estimation of the curvature along a condensed phase interface [6], are introduced.

This paper presents an extended differential geometrical curvature method for the measurement of tortuosity through the effective curvature analysis of the individual vessels. The method allows to compute the extent of tortuosity and helps in severity assessment. The paper is organized into four sections. Section 1 defines ROP and introduces different ROP measure approaches/algorithms.

In Sects. 2, 3, 4, a detailed view of the proposed method is presented with discussion of the model and algorithm. In Sect. 5, simulation results of the method are discussed, followed by conclusion in Sect. 6.

2 Tortuosity Measurement as Differential Geometrical Problem

Captured retinal image is multidimensional matrix, RI with RGB component pixel information. The matrix, RI contains optical disc and vessel network geometrical information in terms of pixel positions. RGB contrast and intensity information of RI are redundant for tortuosity and dilation analysis, as these can be interpreted and measured in terms vessel of twistedness and their width. The vessels can be interpreted as planar curves defined by large set of pixels having definite length and width. This representation allows identifying the twistedness of a vessel with curve differential curvature and dilation as the cross-sectional distance between boundary pixels of the vessel. With this, the problem of tortuosity analysis is formulated as geometrical curvature analysis problem.

One or the other way this formulation has been applied logically and doxastically. In this paper, an attempt is made to make this approach more realizable and epistemological.

Computing the curvature is computationally demanding task due to the definite width of the curves. To make the computational task, simpler curvature can be computed by taking the average projection of the curve or by computing the curvature for the boundary layer of the curve. Some of the earlier works computed tortuosity by former method which results in cumulative error. Here we propose and adopt the later method, i.e. curvature computation by considering curve boundary layers. This raises the question of which boundary layer to be considered as every planar curve has two boundaries, the method is equally applicable and gives almost the same results irrespective of the boundary being analysed. The geometrical computation is applied on retinal image through well-defined steps as illustrated in flow chart of Fig. 1. Section 3 presents details of that individual steps.

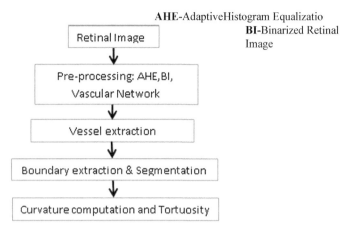

Fig. 1 Flow chart of tortuosity computation using curvature method

2.1 Pre-processing

Here the 8-bit greyscale image GI(x, y) is normalized to get better contrast of the image using AHE (adaptive histogram equalization), it is helpful to get the clear vasculature of the retinal fundus image and OD (Optic Disc) then it is subjected to binaries the greyscale image, i.e. BI(x, y) to reduce the computational complexity. The detection of OD is favourable for the analysis of retinal image; it can serve as a landmark for localizing and segmenting macula (fovea) and vessel structure [7]. The optic disc parameters of premature infants had no correlation with birth weight and gestational age [8].

Pre-problem formulation as presented mostly the prime objective is boundary extraction and tortuosity, extraction of vessels requires noise-free vascular network to accomplish this, the RI is pre-processed first. However, greyscale image can be employed for this, which results in calculation efficiency by eliminating three-channel processing. All the steps mentioned are carried on 8-bit greyscale image. The greyscale image is pre-processed with AHE, BI. The greyscale version of the RI will be affected by the luminous noise of the camera and artefacts due to the relative measurement of the eye's and camera. To make the greyscale image clear and free of noise, AHE is applied. Further to obtain vascular network, greyscale image is subjected to binarization.

In current work, fundus images from the Fire, Drive and Local database are used as input. The input image, RI(x, y) is normalized and converted into grey image, GI(x, y) followed by binarization, BI(x, y). The binarized images, BI(x, y) are subject to the vessel extraction, V(x, y) and characterization for tortuosity Tv_n.

2.2   Binary Image and Vascular Network

The greyscale intensity of the vessels is much prominent compared to the optic disc and retinal background intensity. This makes the vascular network extraction simpler. A vascular network, VN{x, y} is obtained by transforming the pre-processed greyscale image into binary image with dynamic threshold level D_{th}, corresponding to the vessel intensity.

$$VN\{x, y\} = 1 \, if \, GI\{x, y\} > \begin{Bmatrix} D_{th} \\ 0 \, else \end{Bmatrix} \tag{1}$$

Dynamic threshold is required as the grey scale intensity of the vessel varies depending on the image contrast. This approach is novel and distinct compared to the traditional thinning algorithms that have been frequently applied in blood vessel extraction [9]. The binary image contains skeleton of vascular network with geometrical information. Figure 3 shows the histogram information of Fig. 2b. Figure 2c shows vascular network for retinal image, where mv_n is minor vessels, M_{Vn} is major vessels and Bp_n are bifurcation points.

$$V_N = \begin{array}{l} 1\,0\,1\,1\,0\,1\,1\,0\,1\ \ 1\,0\,1\,1\,0\,1\,1\,0\,1 \\ 0\,1\,1\,0\,1\,1\,0\,1\,1\ \ 0\,1\,1\,0\,1\,1\,0\,1\,1 \\ 1\,0\,1\,1\,0\,1\,1\,0\,1\ \ 1\,0\,1\,1\,0\,1\,1\,0\,1 \\ 1\,0\,1\,1\,0\,1\,1\,0\,1\ \ 1\,0\,1\,1\,0\,1\,1\,0\,1 \\ 0\,1\,1\,0\,1\,1\,0\,1\,1\ \ 0\,1\,1\,0\,1\,1\,0\,1\,1 \\ 1\,0\,1\,1\,0\,1\,1\,0\,1\ \ 1\,0\,1\,1\,0\,1\,1\,0\,1 \end{array} \tag{2}$$

2.3   Major Vessel Extraction

Prime factor of ROP is associated with tortuosity and dilation of major vessels [1, 2]. This observation is considered in the current proposed method of tortuosity estimation by processing the vascular network for single major vessel isolation without bifurcation points. Figure 4 shows extracted single major vessels corresponding to the vascular network of Fig. 2c. The vessels extracted are two-dimensional curve patches with width (Wm) and length (Lm), as shown in Fig. 4. Single major vessels are extracted by applying RT (Radon Transformer) [10], Eq. 7

$$\text{No. of major vessels NV} \qquad V = \{V_1, V_2, V_3 \ldots V_n\} \tag{3}$$

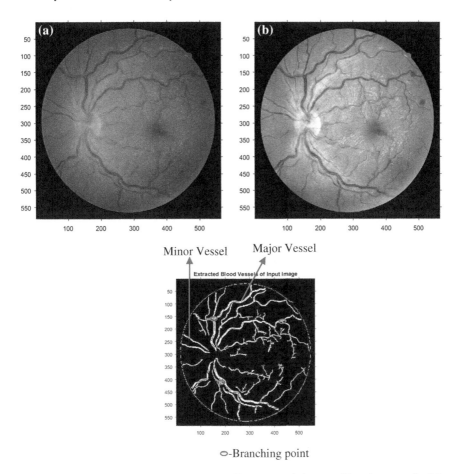

Fig. 2 **a** Original fundus retinal image. **b** Normalized greyscale image. **c** Vascular network of the binarized retinal image

Identify the major vessel length in the number of pixels and the corner pixel position.

$$V_l = \{V_{l1}, V_{l2}, V_{l3} \ldots V_{ln}\}$$
$$V_c = \{V_{c1}, V_{c2}, V_{c3} \ldots V_{cn}\} \tag{4}$$

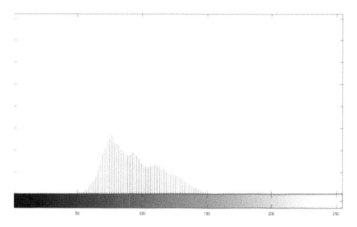

Fig. 3 Histogram of greyscale image of Fig. 2b

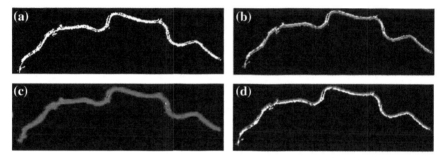

Fig. 4 a Single vessel extracted from the BI. **b** Single vessel traced on the lower edge. **c** Vessel traced on both edges. **d** Single vessel traced on upper edge

3 Boundary Extraction

Vessels in binarized retinal image $BI(x, y, \theta_n)$ are considered as polynomial functions, $f_{vn}(x, y, \theta_n)$. The functions correspond to curves of different shapes, lengths, Vnl and orientations with origin at optic disc.

$$BI(x, y, \theta_n) = \sum_{m=1}^{N} \cdot \sum_{n=1}^{N} f_{vn}(x, y, \theta_n) + ODx = \left\{ -\frac{X}{2}, \frac{X}{2} \right\}, y = \left\{ -\frac{y}{2}, \frac{y}{2} \right\} \quad (5)$$

$$f_{vn}(x, y, \theta_n) = (1 + \sum_{m=1}^{vn} x_m + x_m^2 + \cdots) a_m \cos \theta_n \theta_n = n * \theta \quad (6)$$

Equation (6) implies that individual vessel boundary can be extracted by masking the image, $BI(x, Y, \theta_n)$ with angular delta function $\delta(x - x') \delta(\theta - \theta_n)$ as

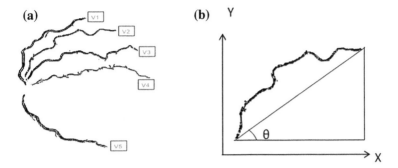

Fig. 5 **a** Major vessels extracted from binarized RI. **b** Theta calculation plot for the single vessel

$$f_{vn}(x, y, \theta_n) = \sum_{x=-\frac{X}{2}}^{\frac{X}{2}} BI(x, y, \theta_n)\delta(x\prime - x)\delta(\theta - \theta_n) \tag{7}$$

Figure 4 shows one extracted single vessel of boundary length LVn as per Eq. (7). This method of extracting boundaries is treating individual vessels as of single pixel width, this leads to loss of dilation information. Here the vessels are constructed to be continuous curves.

Boundary extraction of the individual vessel is done on the both edges/sides (upper and lower).

The geometrical pattern of the vessel network is random and this randomness makes boundary extraction challenging due to the arbitrary angular orientation of the vessels. As pointed out earlier, curvature is computed for the major vessels by considering either of their lateral boundaries. The lateral boundaries B1 and B2 of vessel Vn as shown in Fig. 4 are extracted by applying algorithm, i.e.

for m = 1 : length of vessel   theta = $COS^{-1}(X/hyp)$

B1(xm, y) = max(VNn(xm, y))

B2(xm, y) = min(VNn(xm, y))

end

By retaining the maximum and minimum Y-coordinate pixels at particular X-coordinate, this is repeated all along the length of the vessel. The maximum Y-coordinate pixels form a set corresponding to the boundary B1, where as the minimum corresponds to the boundary B2. In order to extract the boundaries in their intact shape, the vessels need to be rotated, i.e. to avoid abrupt transitions. Due to make the boundary extraction simpler, angular computation is applied to the individual vessels. The angle of rotation is found by computing orientation of the vessel with respect to x-axis of Cartesian coordinates at its origin, as shown in Fig. 5b.

Identify the angle subtended by the major vessels w.r.t the x-axis of the coordinate.

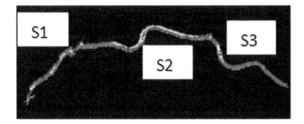

Fig. 6 Example of curve is divided into three segments

$$\theta = [\theta_1, \theta_2, \theta_3 \ldots \theta_n], \tag{8}$$

where θ the angle of vessels and n is the vessel number.

4   Segmentation and Average Curvature Computation

Each of the vessels exhibits running slope variation or curvature variation over length of the vessel. Tortuosity of the vessel also varies over length of the vessel, to measure the tortuosity statistical methods are adopted [4, 11, 12]. Curvature is rate of variation of a function with respect to the independent variable (Eq. 9), i.e pixel position.

$$c_{vn,sn} = \frac{df}{dx} \tag{9}$$

Each of the vessel exhibits running slope variation or curvature variation over length of the vessels, hence tortuosity of the vessel also varies over length of the vessel. Considering this statistical methods are adopted to measure the tortuosity [4, 9, 10]. These methods are focused on curvature computation at random sites of the pixels that are not part of the vessel boundaries, leading to temporal in accuracy. As stated earlier, in current method tortuosity of a major vessel is computed as average of the segment curvature (Eq. 11), by considering either the lower boundary or the upper. Depending on the length every vessel is divided into M number of segments, M = Vli/20 where factor 20 is arrived with iterative statistics. Curvature of the individual segments is average of the sample point curvature. Every segment consists of a number of pixels or sample points. Curvature at a sample point is computed by considering adjacent 4 points/pixels i.e m2 − m1, m3 − m2, m4 − m3, then sum of all differences i.e., d1 + d2 + d3 [11, 12] (Figs. 6 and 7).

$$C = \frac{Y2 - Y1}{X2 - X1} \tag{10}$$

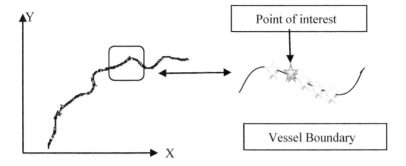

Fig. 7 Segment of curve shows adjacent pixels with point of interest

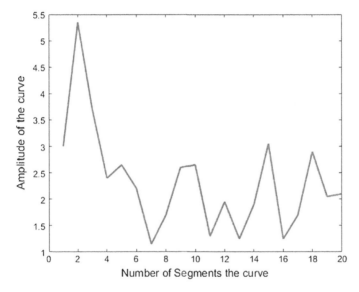

Fig. 8 Curvature variation of single vessel of (Fig. 4) considering 20 segments

The process results in segment curvature, for every vessel curvature is computed by taking average of segment curvatures represented by tortuosity index Z_i (Fig. 8).

$$Zi = \frac{1}{M} \sum_{i=1}^{M} Seg_c(i) \tag{11}$$

5   Results and Discussion

Figure 2C shows the vasculature of the test fundus retinal image for case 1, along with the one of the extracted vessel and its boundary extracted for both upper and

Table 1 Curvature calculations for different images

Sl no	Image name	Vessel name [Vn]	Theta (Vessel angle) [Θ]	Total curvature	Length of the vessel (No. of pixels) [LVn]	Angle (Auto selection)
1	P37_1 Case-1	V1	45	1.8125-ok	299	−45
		V2	59	2.3425-T	323	−31
		V3	73	2.37-T	343	−17
		V4	86	2.035-ok	353	−4
		V5	55	1.6275-T	275	7.5
2	S63_1 Case-2	V1	63	1.53-N	294	−27
		V2	59	2.32-F	340	−31
		V3	78.56	2.045-oK	361	−12
		V4	62.31	1.775-ok	297	−3
		V5	40	1.285-ok	248	30
		V6	32.75	0.965-ok	202	−58
3	M14 Case-3	V1	45	1.8625-N	219	21
		V3	36	1.6675-N	255	36
		V4	39	1.2175-N	227	−51
4	M13 Case-4	V2	66	3.9675-T	345	−9
5	11_test Case-5	V1	65.56	1.86-ok	350	−25
		V2	88.9	1.87-F	453	−2
		V3	52	2.057-ok	302	12
6	03_test Case-6	V3	71.73	3.6181-F	365	−18

T-True, N-Normal, Ok-Acceptable, F-False

Note In case 1, 6th column negative sign indicates the vessel rotates in clockwise direction and positive sign indicates vessel rotates in anticlockwise direction

lower part of the vessel is shown in Fig. 4. Table 1 shows the class demarcation for the extracted vessels.

The method is applied iteratively for every test retinal image (selected from Fire, Drive and local data set). Table 1, shows the details of computations for selective cases. The total curvature is calculated for major vessels, the vessel divided into randomly with number of segments for the table, and it is displayed 20 segments and eight segments. As discussed earlier to get better results it is necessary to rotate the vessel in horizontal direction, the method is calculating geometrically the angel theta and based on that it will rotate automatically in horizontal direction as it is displayed in the table. The angle of rotation is calculated by computing the θ angle formed by initial part of the curve w.r.t reference to horizontal line. Every vessel exhibits different orientations in Table 1 the column θ lists the orientation angle computed for major vessels of different retinal images. The negative angle sign indicates the vessel rotates in clockwise direction and positive sign indicates vessel rotates in anticlockwise direction.

The method can be further improvised with spectrum analyzer. The method can be tested for different segmented curves and the lengths appear to be intact irrespective of segment length. The method holds good in most of the curve excluding vessels with slow variations and symmetric curves. The method has been applied on a number of test images and found to be satisfactory or on par with the other methods in detection of ROP.

6 Conclusion

The paper introduces a novel geometrically characterized image processing method for the tortuosity detection in ROP cases with simple differential geometrical method for tortuosity measurement, although the method is simple and effective but it considers the vessels to be of single pixel leading to loss of dilation information hence resulting in loss of accuracy. The method can be improvised by updating the model considering curves in two dimensions.

Acknowledgements The authors are grateful to Dr. Satishkumar B V, Minto hospital, Bangalore for providing infant's images and also public database Drive, Fire data set. Thanks to the VGST of Karnataka for having funded this project under medical image analysis laboratory at our institution.

References

1. Mintz-Hittner HA, Kennedy KA, Chuang AZ (2011) Efficacy of intravitreal bevacizumab for stage 3+ retinopathy of prematurity. New England J Med 364(7)
2. Mannan MA, Moni SC, Shahidullah M (2014) Retinopathy of prematurity (ROP) current understanding of management. Bangladesh J Child Health 38(3):142–150
3. Grisan E, Foracchia M, Ruggeri A (2008) A novel method for the automatic grading of retinal vessel tortuosity. IEEE Trans Med Imaging 27(3)
4. Aghamohamadian-Sharbaf M, Pourreza HR, Banaee T (2016) A novel curvature-based algorithm for automatic grading of retinal blood vessel tortuosity. IEEE J Biomed Health Inform 20(2)
5. Bullard JW, Garboczi EJ, Carterb WC, Fuller Jr ER (1995) Numerical methods for computing interfacial mean curvature. Comput Mater Sci 103–116 (Elsevier)
6. Frette OI, Virnovsky G, Silin D (2009) Estimation of the curvature of an interface from a digital 2D image. Lawrence Berkeley National Laboratory-2009
7. Zhang D, Zhao Y (2016) Novel accurate and fast optic disc detection in retinal images with vessel distribution and directional characteristics. IEEE J Biomed Health Inform 20(1)
8. Park JW, Park SW, Heo H (2013) RetCam image analysis of the optic disc in premature infants. Eye 27:1137–1141 (Macmillan Publishers Limited)
9. Mustafa NBA et al (2016) A study of retinal vascular tortuosity in diabetic retinopathy. In: International conference on advances in electrical electronic and system engineering, 14–16 Nov 2016, Malaysia. IEEE

10. Pourreza R, Banaee T et al A radon transform based approach for extraction of blood vessels in conjunctival images, pp 948–956. ©Springer, Berlin, Heidelberg
11. Turior R, Uyyanonvara B (2012) Curvature-based tortuosity evaluation for infant retinal images. J Inf Eng Appl 2(8). ISSN 2224-5782
12. Turior R, Onkaew D, Uyyanonvara B, Chutinantvarodom P (2013) Quantification and classification of retinal vessel tortuosity. Sci Asia 39:265–277. https://doi.org/10.2306/scienceasia1513-1874.2013.39.265

Synthesis, Characterization of Hybrid Nanomaterials of Strontium, Yttrium, Copper Doped with Indole Schiff Base Derivatives Possessing Dielectric and Semiconductor Properties

Vinayak Adimule [ID], **P. Vageesha, Gangadhar Bagihalli** [ID], **Debdas Bowmik** [ID] **and H. J. Adarsha**

Abstract Objective: A set of different nanocomposite hybrid materials of $Sr_{0.5}$ $Y_{0.1}$ $Cu_{0.3}$ has been synthesized through co-precipitation synthetic method using Cetyl Trimethyl Ammonium Bromide (CTAB) and Tri ethyl amine (TEA) as surfactants. The different derivatives of indole Schiff base compounds (5a–5e) were doped to the nanocomposites in molar ratio of 1–2%. The entire hybrid material isolated by forming gelatinous network and calcinated. The hybrid nanomaterials were investigated for their semiconductor and dielectric properties. Method: Nanocompositional hybrid materials were prepared by co-precipitation method with the composition of $Sr_{0.5}$ $Y_{0.1}$ $Cu_{0.3}$ with doping of indole Schiff base derivative (ISB) of molar ratio 1–2%, and the reduction is done using surface reduction methods gelated precipitate of hybrid nanomaterials were calcinated, characterized by XRD, FT-IR, UV–Vis and SEM spectroscopic techniques. The semiconductor and dielectric properties of

V. Adimule (✉)
Department of Chemistry, Jain College of Engineering and Technology, Sainagar, Unkal, Hubli 580031, Karnataka, India
e-mail: adimulevinayak@yahoo.in

P. Vageesha
VTU Recognized Research Centre for Engineering Chemistry, Department of Chemistry, KLE Institute of Technology, Opposite Airport, Gokul Road, Hubballi 590030, Karnataka, India
e-mail: vageesha87@gmail.com

G. Bagihalli
Department of Chemistry, KLE Institute of Technology, Opposite Airport, Gokul Road, Hubballi 590030, Karnataka, India
e-mail: g.bagihalli@gmail.com

D. Bowmik
High Energy Materials Research Laboratory, Defence Research and Development Organization, Ministry of Defence, Government of India, Sutarwadi, Pune 411021, India
e-mail: voumik@yahoo.com

H. J. Adarsha
Centre for Research in Medical Devices, National University of Ireland (NUI), University Road, Galway H91TK33, Ireland
e-mail: a.hj1@nuigalway.ie

© Springer Nature Singapore Pte Ltd. 2019
V. Sridhar et al. (eds.), *Emerging Research in Electronics, Computer Science and Technology*, Lecture Notes in Electrical Engineering 545,
https://doi.org/10.1007/978-981-13-5802-9_97

pelletalized samples were measured with respect to various temperatures and frequency. The precursor material used for the synthesis is strontium carbonate, yttrium oxide and cuprous chloride which are reduced in presence of CTAB and urea. After isolating the hybrid materials ISB derivatives (5a–5e) were doped and the aqueous mixture of bluish-reddish precipitate was filtered, washed with ethyl alcohol and octanol mixture to remove any impurities present with the precipitate, dried at 50–120 °C, heat treated at 650–750 °C and obtained pure nanocomposite. Findings: Initial spectroscopic studies showed that grain size of copper was 20–30 nm in diameter. XRD pattern demonstrated the formation of trigonal copper and dopant addition considerably affects the crystal structure. The dielectric constant were measured and compared with undoped hybrid material. The band alignment and band gap obtained from the ISB material was further felicitating the fissile ejection of the electrons and ensuring the semiconductor properties of the materials.

Keywords Nanocomposite · Yttrium oxide · CTAB · Co-precipitation · Indole schiff base · Hybrid nanomaterials

1 Introduction

Novel hybrid pervoskite nanocomposites [1] of strontium and yttrium were reported for their transistor and dielectric related properties. Author envisaged that addition of copper to the extent of 0.3 mol could enhance the dielectric, semiconducting, transistor, photovoltaic, fluorescence and other electrical-related properties. We report here the addition of organic compounds doped to the metal oxide material, and literature reports for their dielectric and semiconductor properties. Earlier, organic polymer material used as a fabricating the pervoskite nanocomposite and thus imparting the material properties. The nanocomposites of $Sr_{0.5} Y_{0.1} Cu_{0.3}$ doped with organic material would enhance the dielectric and semiconductor properties. The pervoskite material has been prepared through co-precipitation methods [2, 3]. Yttrium oxide and strontium carbonate are used as precursor and by using ammonium hydroxide as gelation agent (pH > 12) during the precipitation, to the gel network copper was doped and isolated as hybrid pervoskite nanocomposite material [4]. The Sr-Y doped with Cu nanocomposites were further doped with hydrochloride salts of indole Schiff base derivatives [5–8] in 1–2 molar percentages and studied for their initial dielectric and semiconductor properties. It is envisaged that by doping appropriate amount of hydrochloride salts of ISB derivatives to the Sr-Y and Cu nanocomposites would enhance the electronic and electrical-related properties [9, 10]. The materials were obtained by using cetyl trimethyl ammonium bromide as surfactant as well as reducing agent in presence of urea and concentrated HCl at reflux condition in ethylene glycol as solvent. The hybrid pervoskite nanocomposites [11] were characterized by SEM and XRD analysis, and ISB compounds were characterized by ^{1}H-NMR, LCMS and IR spectroscopic analysis. The reddish-brown precipitate was dried, calcinated at different temperatures doped with copper and studied with their semiconductor characteristics [12].

2 Experimental

2.1 Synthesis of Sr-Y Nanocomposites

Strontium carbonate is added with CTAB, little amount of TEA (triethanol amine) in presence of concentrated HCl and refluxed for 8 h in an RB flask to this RM yttrium oxide is reduced in presence of urea and concentrated HCl was added and reflux was continued for 3 h The reduced Sr-Y nanocomposites were precipitated by adding NH$_4$OH solution drop-wise after the formation of gelation in 36 h the entire mass was concentrated and dried, calcinated at 650 °C and obtained Sr-Y hybrid nanocomposite. Yield 5.8 g; Colour of the compounds: Bluish white.

2.2 Purification and Isolation of Sr-Y Nanocomposites

The obtained Sr-Y nanocomposites were taken in a 25-ml RB flask added with 10% octanol water mixture and warmed in a water bath and re-precipitated by adding triethyl alcohol drop-wise, the precipitate was filtered, the filtered solid was further given with THF solvent wash and calcinated at 600 °C to get the pure Sr-Y pervoskite nanocomposite. Yield 4.8 g; Colour of the compounds: Off-white.

2.3 Doping of Copper to Sr-Y Nanocomposites

In a RB flask, cuprous chloride powder (appropriate amount) was added with concentrated HCl in presence of urea and TEA and refluxed for 2–3 h. The reaction mixture was cooled and added with isolated Sr-Y hybrid nanocomposite, and was made collapsing network with ammonium hydroxide and the precipitate was dried, the copper was doped to the mixture of Sr-Y hybrid pervoskite nanocomposites dissolved in TEA and processed to obtain the desired copper doped with yttrium and strontium hybrid oxide nanocomposites.

2.4 Synthesis of Substituted Derivatives of Carbohydrazide (2a–2e)

Substituted various derivatives of phenyl carboxylic acid (1 mol) are treated with ethylchloroformate (1.2 mol), hydrazine hydrazide (3 mol) in 100 ml of THF solvent at 0–5 °C and the reaction mixture was stirred overnight. Completion of the reaction is confirmed by TLC, RM is poured over crushed ice, solids that are separated and washed with water, washed with ethanol–water mixture and dried, and the dried solid is recrystallized from ethanol–water and obtained pure carbohydrazide. Yield 10.2 g; Colour of the compounds: white.

2.5 Synthesis of Various Analogues of Indole Schiff Base Derivatives (4a–4e)

Indole-3-carboxaldehyde (1.2 mol) treated with substituted derivatives of carbohy-drazide (4a–4e) (1.2 mol) in presence of catalytic amount of acetic acid and refluxed using ethanol as solvent for 1–2 h. TLC showed completion of the reaction, solvents are evaporated, the obtained solid was recrystallized from ethanol–water mixture. Yield 1.2–1.6 g (4a–4e); Colour of the compounds: Off-white.

2.6 Synthesis of Hydrochloride Salts of Indole Schiff Base Derivatives (5a–5e)

In a 100-ml RB flask fitted with nitrogen, the different derivatives of Schiff base compounds were treated with 1,4-dioxan HCl in presence of 1,4-dioxane as solvent, the RM was stirred overnight, salts that are separated was filtered, dried under nitro-gen atmosphere and obtained as hydrochloride salts of the corresponding Schiff base compounds. Yield = 3.2 g; Colour: Off-white; M.P- 145–150 °C (Figs. 1, 2 and 3).

2.7 Dielectric and Semiconductor Properties

The dielectric constant is almost 9×10^3 kV/mm at near-room temperature for the hybrid pervoskite nanocomposite (Fig. 4) doped with 1–2% of Schiff base deriva-tives as compared with $Sr_{0.5} Y_{0.1}$ undoped material which is almost 5×10^3 kV/mm (Fig. 4). The copper-doped material relatively shows less dielectric constant as com-pared with the doped hybrid material. At high temperature (250–550 °C) measured with different frequency range from 2 to 1000 kHz. $Sr_{0.5} Y_{0.1} Cu_{0.3}$ doped with indole Schiff base derivatives the dielectric constant increases from 20 to 80 kV/mm

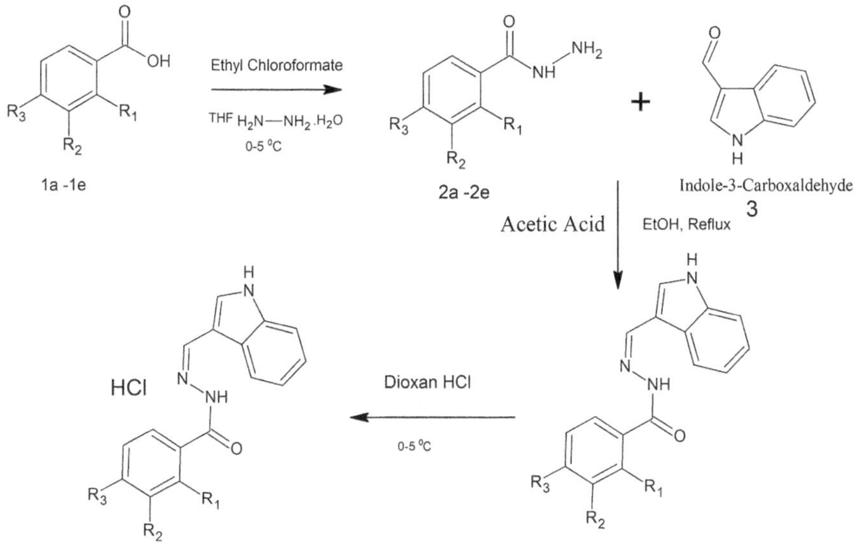

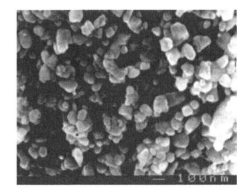

Fig. 1 Synthetic reaction scheme representing various steps involved in the preparation of hydrochloride salts of the indole Schiff base derivatives

Fig. 2 Scanning electron microscope image of Sr-Y nanocomposites doped with copper

(Fig. 5) as compared with the $Sr_{0.5} Y_{0.1} Cu_{0.3}$ and $Sr_{0.5} Y_{0.1} Cu_{0.2}$ undoped material. Critical current density is measured with respect to the doped and undoped hybrid nanocomposites at different elevated temperatures in the presence of magnetic field. The doped material shows considerable increase in the current density as compared with the undoped Sr, Y and Cu nanocomposites. Current gain is maximum for the doped nanocomposite (Fig. 4) as compared with the undoped Sr-Y nanocomposite. Presence of magnetic field current increases exponentially with the doped hybrid nanocomposite. The undoped Sr-Y nanocomposite shows differential distribution of the current as compared with the doped nanocomposites.

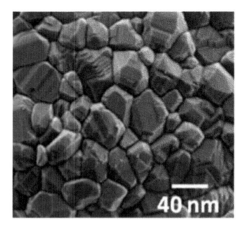

Fig. 3 Scanning electron microscope image of Sr-Y nanocomposites doped with copper the particle size distribution is 40 nm

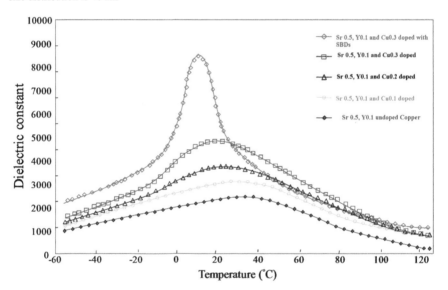

Fig. 4 Representing the variation of dielectric constant of the $Sr_{0.5}$ $Y_{0.1}$ and $Cu_{0.1-0.3}$ as well as doped Schiff base derivatives at various different temperatures

2.8 Synthetic Reaction Scheme

See Fig. 1.

1a: $R_1 = H$, $R_2 = H$, $R_3 = CH_3$; 1b: $R_1 = H$, $R_2 = H$, $R_3 = OCH_3$
1c: $R_1 = H$, $R_2 = H$, $R_3 = $ tert-butyl; 1d: $R_1 = H$, $R_2 = H$, $R_3 = Ph$
1e: $R_1 = H$, $R_2 = OCH_3$, $R_3 = OCH_3$

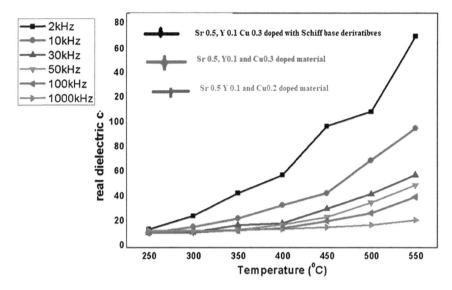

Fig. 5 Real-time curvatures of the different derivatives of $Sr_{0.5}$ $Y_{0.1}$ and $Cu_{0.1-0.3}$ and doped with Schiff base compounds to the nanocomposite at elevated temperatures

3 Materials and Methods

All the chemicals and solvents are purchased from SD-Fine and Spectrochem Ltd, and used without purification all the synthesized nanocomposites were characterized by UV–Vis, XRD in Poorna Prajna Scientific Industrial Research, Bangalore, SEM Images has been recorded in IISc, Bangalore, Karnataka, India. Co-precipitation method is employed for the synthesis of hybrid nanocomposites. All the dielectric constant measurements were done at KLE, Institute of Technology, Hubli, Karnataka, India (Table 1).

3.1 Spectral Analysis Data

3.1.1 1H-indole-3-carbaldehyde (**3**): ^{1}H NMR: δ 7.05 (1H, dd, $J = 8.2, 7.8, 1.5$ Hz), 7.22 (1H, ddd, $J = 8.2, 7.5, 1.5$ Hz), 7.55 (1H, ddt, $J = 8.0, 1.43, 0.4$ Hz), 7.68 (1H, ddt, $J = 8.4, 1.5, 0.5$ Hz), 7.87 (1H, t, $J = 0.5$ Hz), 10.15 (1H, s).; LCMS: [M+1]-147.

3.1.2 N'-[(Z)-(1H-indol-3-yl)methylidene]-4-methylbenzohydrazide (**4a**): ^{1}H NMR: δ 2.33 (3H, s), 7.05–7.23 (4H, 7.08 (ddd, $J = 8.0, 7.91, 1.3$ Hz), 7.20 (ddd, $J = 8.0, 7.81, 1.8$ Hz), 7.18 (ddd, $J = 8.5, 1.2, 0.6$ Hz)), 7.48 (1H, ddt, $J = 8.1, 1.3, 0.4$ Hz), 7.55 (1H, t, $J = 0.4$ Hz), 7.78 (1H, ddt, $J = 8.0, 1.8, 0.4$ Hz), 7.94 (2H, ddd, $J = 8.6, 1.7, 0.5$ Hz), 8.19 (1H, s); LCMS: [M+1]-279; M.P.-176 °C.

Table 1 Showing the dielectric constant of the various samples of doped with indole Schiff base derivatives (ISB) with respect to the undoped copper as well as doped with copper

Sample	W g (1×10^4 radius/s)	Rgb (ohm/kV/mm)	Dielectric constant ($\mathcal{E}$) (/ohm/kV/mm or/ohm/kV/cm)	Permittivity* (μ) (F/m × 10^{-12})
Sr-Y, $Cu_{0.1}$	1.23	1323.00	345.00	7.89
Sr-Y, $Cu_{0.2}$	2.34	986.00	456.00	8.02
Sr-Y, $Cu_{0.3}$	3.45	658.00	567.00	7.56
Sr-Y, $Cu_{0.3}$ ISB (1%)	0.97	567.00	1234.00*	8.12
Sr-Y, $Cu_{0.1}$ ISB (2%)	0.18	1453.00	1456.00*	8.01
Sr-Y, $Cu_{0.1}$ ISB (3%)	2.45	15678.00	1567.00*	8.34
Undoped Sr-Y	1.22	654.00	234.65	8.56

*Refers to relatively high permeability values

3.1.3 N'-[(Z)-(1H-indol-3-yl)methylidene]-4-methoxybenzohydrazide (**4b**): ^{1}H NMR: δ 3.9 (3H, s), 7.07–7.22 (4H, 7.12 (ddd, J = 8.0, 7.82, 1.3 Hz), 7.10 (ddd, J = 8.6, 1.2, 0.4 Hz), 7.17 (ddd, J = 8.0, 7.8, 1.6 Hz)), 7.48 (1H, ddt, J = 8.0, 1.3, 0.4 Hz), 7.65 (1H, t, J = 0.4 Hz), 7.79 (1H, ddt, J = 8.0, 1.7, 0.4 Hz), 8.06 (2H, ddd, J = 8.6, 1.8, 0.4 Hz), 8.19 (1H, s); LCMS: [M+1]-295; M.P.-127 °C.

3.1.4 4-*tert*-butoxy-N'-[(Z)-(1H-indol-3yl)methylidene]benzohydrazide(**4c**): ^{1}H NMR: δ 2.33 (3H, s), 7.09–7.24 (4H, 7.09 (ddd, J = 8.0, 7.8, 1.3 Hz), 7.18 (ddd, J = 8.0, 7.8, 1.7 Hz), 7.19 (ddd, J = 8.5, 1.2, 0.5 Hz)), 7.55 (1H, ddt, J = 8.0, 1.3, 0.5 Hz), 7.55 (1H, t, J = 0.4 Hz), 7.73 (1H, ddt, J = 8.0, 1.8, 0.4 Hz), 7.90 (2H, ddd, J = 8.5, 1.7, 0.5 Hz), 8.16 (1H, s); LCMS: [M+1]-321; M.P.-156 °C.

3.1.5 N'-[(Z)-(1H-indol-3-yl)methylidene][1,1'-biphenyl]-4 carbohydrazide (**4d**): ^{1}H NMR: δ 7.05–7.22 (2H, 7.09 (ddd, J = 8.0, 7.8, 1.3 Hz), 7.19 (ddd, J = 8.0, 7.8, 1.6 Hz)), 7.48 (2H, dddd, J = 8.1, 7.5, 1.8, 0.5 Hz), 7.41–7.51 (2H, 7.55 (ddt, J = 8.0, 1.4, 0.4 Hz), 7.78 (tdd, J = 7.2, 1.7, 1.2 Hz)), 7.55 (1H, t, J = 0.4 Hz), 7.87–7.93 (7H, 7.71 (ddd, J = 8.8, 1.91, 0.4 Hz), 7.85 (dddd, J = 7.9, 1.7, 1.7, 0.5 Hz), 7.73 (ddt, J = 8.0, 1.6, 0.4 Hz), 7.79 (ddd, J = 8.7, 1.8, 0.5 Hz)), 8.15 (1H, s) LCMS: [M+1]-341; M.P.-126 °C.

3.1.6 N'-[(Z)-(1H-indol-3-yl)methylidene]-3,4-dimethoxybenzohydrazide (**4e**): ^{1}H NMR: δ 3.89 (3H, s), 3.92 (3H, s), 6.66 (1H, dd, J = 1.7, 0.5 Hz), 6.92 (1H, dd, J = 7.6, 1.6 Hz), 7.04–7.20 (2H, 7.10 (ddd, J = 8.0, 7.8, 1.3 Hz), 7.25 (ddd, J = 8.0, 7.8, 1.6 Hz)), 7.45 (1H, ddt, J = 8.0, 1.3, 0.4 Hz), 7.65 (1H, t, J = 0.4 Hz), 7.83 (1H, ddt, J = 8.0, 1.6, 0.4 Hz), 7.82 (1H, dd, J = 7.6, 0.5 Hz), 8.14 (1H, s); LCMS: [M+1]-325; M.P.-134 °C.

4 Results and Discussion

In this research work, we have synthesized $Sr_{0.5}$ $Y_{0.1}$ and $Cu_{0.3}$ nanocomposites doped with different concentrations of indole Schiff base hydrochloride salts and studied for their dielectric constant measurements at room temperature range and real-time dielectric measurements at elevated temperature range was measured with respect to the undoped, partially doped and indole Schiff base doped materials. It is found that doped organic indole Schiff base compounds (ISB) shows higher dielectric susceptibility without much dielectric loss as compared with undoped oxide nanocomposite having constant of 9×10^3 kV/mm (Fig. 4) with related to undoped copper having dielectric constant of 5×10^3 kV/mm (Fig. 5). The hybrid pervoskite nanocomposites were synthesized by co-precipitation methods, isolated, purified and obtained the SEM images (Figs. 2 and 3) of the indole Schiff base (ISB) doped and undoped assembly of $Sr_{0.5}$ $Y_{0.1}$ oxide hybrid nanomaterials. XRD absorption intensity pattern elucidates the morphological arrangement of the crystal lattice. Studies were also carried out for the indole Schiff base doped, undoped nanocomposite as initial level in which it is found that the particle size is less than 50 nm. Real-time measurement of the dielectric constant of the indole Schiff base doped (ISB) nanocomposite at 2 kHz at much higher temperature shows 4–5 times increased constant as compared with partially, undoped mixture whose real-time dielectric constant measure at frequencies from 2 to 1000 kHz. The $Sr_{0.5}$ $Y_{0.1}$ and $Cu_{0.3}$ material shows 1.5–2 times higher dielectric constant as compared with the undoped copper material whose dielectric constant does not varies even at 1000 kHz frequency. Current gain is maximum for the indole Schiff base derivative and Cu doped nanocomposite as compared with the undoped Sr-Y nanocomposite. Presence of frequency field considerably affects the current gain characteristics which increase exponentially with the doped hybrid nanocomposite. Higher dielectric constants were obtained with larger grain size of the nanocomposites. Further studies are in progress.

5 Conclusion

In this research work, hybrid pervoskite nanocomposites of $Sr_{0.5}$ $Y_{0.1}$ $Cu_{0.3}$ have been synthesized by co-precipitation method and characterized by SEM and XRD analysis. ISB compounds are synthesised and characterized by 1H-NMR and LCMS spectroscopic methods. The hybrid material properties are effectively enhanced by doping 1–2 molar percentages of ISB compounds to the hybrid nanocomposites and studied for real-time dielectric constant with respect to temperature and varying the frequency from 2 to 1000 kHz. It is found that organic indole Schiff base compound (ISB) shows higher dielectric constant as compared with undoped oxide nanocomposite having constant of 9×10^3 kV/mm with related to undoped copper having dielectric constant of 5×10^3 kV/mm. Further the nanomaterial is studied for various organic photovoltaic characteristics.

Acknowledgements Authors are also thankful to IISc, for providing the spectral and analytical data. Authors are also thankful to DRDO, Ministry of Defence, Government of India for their support, encouragement for this research work.

References

1. Tiwari A, Snure M, Kumar D, Abiade JT (2008) Ferromagnetism in Cu-doped ZnO films: role of charge carriers. Appl Phys Lett 92(6). Article ID: 062509. https://doi.org/10.1063/1.2857481
2. Buchholz DB, Chang RPH, Song JY, Ketterson JB (2005) Room-temperature ferromagnetism in Cu-doped ZnO thin films. Appl Phys Lett 87(8). Article ID: 082504. https://doi.org/10.1063/1.2032588
3. Daisuke M, Yoshi N, Kazuyuki U, Ichiro T (2017) Improving the carrier mobility of pentacene thin film transistors by surface flattened polysilsesquioxane gate dielectric layers. J Soc Mater Sci Jpn 66(9):644
4. Miaomiao C, Lifang S, Yanan D, Zhiqiang S, Qingyun L (2017) N,N′-Di-carboxymethyl perylene diimide functionalized magnetic nanocomposites with enhanced peroxidase-like activity for colorimetric sensing of H2O2 and glucose. New J Chem 41(13):5853–5862
5. Jin WB, Hyung-Seok J, Won HP and Sang YK (2017) Triacetate cellulose gate dielectric organic thin-film transistors. Organ Electron 41:186–189
6. Samir M, Joanna RS, Albert MB (2017) Artificial miniaturized luminescent materials based on perylene-covered glass surfaces. New J Chem 41(14):6083–6088
7. Katariya SB, Dinesh P, Lydia R, Alswaidan IA, Ramasami P, Nagaiyan S (2017) Triphenylamine-based fluorescent NLO phores with ICT characteristics: solvatochromic and theoretical study. J Mol Struct 1150:493–506
8. Wu ZJ, Zhao XB, Tu J, Cao GS, Tu JP, Ahu TJ (2007) Synthesis of Li1+xV3O8 by citrate sol-gel route at low temperature. J Alloy Compd 403:345–348
9. Wu Y, He Y, Wu T, Chen T, Weng W, Wan H (2007) Influence of some parameters on the synthesis of nanosized NiO material by modified sol-gel method. Mater Lett 61:3174–3178. https://doi.org/10.1016/j.matlet.2006.11.018
10. Sahi S, Daud AR, Hashim M (2007) A comparative study of nickel-zinc ferrites by sol-gel route and solid-state reaction. Mater Chem Phys 106:452–456. https://doi.org/10.1016/j.matchemphys.2007.06.031
11. Mazen SA, Mansour SF, Zaki HM (2003) Some physical and magnetic properties of Mg-Zn ferrite. Cryst Res Technol 38:471–478. https://doi.org/10.1002/crat.200310059
12. Young SS, Moonjeong B, Eunju L (2017) Carrier transport of carbon nanotube embedded organic semiconductor composite. Mater Res Bull 90:232

Study of Clustering Approaches in Wireless Sensor Networks

M. Revanesh, V. Sridhar and John M. Acken

Abstract Ever since its introduction, wireless sensor networks have enabled us to do things which were previously unimaginable by simplifying more tasks and enhancing quality of life to millions of technology-dependent groups of people. Just like every other cutting edge technology, WSN also has its own needs and challenges with respect to that of the usage or transmission of data packets. This study paper is an attempt to introduce the research community to some of the clustering approaches followed in WSN along with the challenges that one should be familiar with before working on clustering approaches in WSN.

Keywords Wireless sensor networks · Clustering · Energy consumption · LEACH

1 Introduction

Wireless sensor networks (WSNs) are typically formed by combining large set of tiny sensor nodes which offer a powerful combination of distributed sensing, computing, and communication. These networks are more often deployed in cumbersome and unreachable area randomly to monitor or control conditions, such as agriculture, health monitoring, military base, home networks, and quality measurement at different industries [1].

These sensor nodes operate with limited battery power, which has turned out to be a major bottleneck problem for the constant advancement of technology. Most of the work [2–6] carried out in the field of WSN in one way or the other intends

M. Revanesh (✉) · V. Sridhar
Department of E&CE, PES College of Engineering, Mandya, Karnataka, India
e-mail: revaneshm@pesce.ac.in

V. Sridhar
e-mail: venusridhar@yahoo.com

J. M. Acken
Department of Electrical & Computer Engineering, Portland State University, Portland, USA
e-mail: acken@pdx.edu

© Springer Nature Singapore Pte Ltd. 2019
V. Sridhar et al. (eds.), *Emerging Research in Electronics, Computer Science and Technology*, Lecture Notes in Electrical Engineering 545,
https://doi.org/10.1007/978-981-13-5802-9_98

to enhance the lifetime of networks; also, the sensor nodes in these networks are usually designed with extensive constraints related to size and cost which results in extremely limited computational ability and memory. So every unit of energy present in this network must be carefully utilized.

Wireless sensor network energy utilization can be broadly classified into three categories: sensing, signal processing, and communication. More than 65% of energy in WSN is utilized for communicating the sensed data from one of sensor location to the base station, majority of which is wasted owing to the fact that these networks operate in an unattended hostile environment.

Consequently, any protocols or algorithms intended for enhancement of such systems must have self-sorting out capacities to guarantee precise and effective working of the system. Owing to the stringent challenges and environmental conditions in which these networks operate, different types of protocols have been proposed for enhancing the life of WSN and for directing the right information to the base station [4–10]. One of the most vital parameters to be considered for designing such algorithms is distance of transmission; as the distance of transmission increases and reliability of data over the network reduces, so researcher and industry experts consider multi-hop communication as one of the top preferred algorithms for extended lifetime of network.

The rest of the paper shares information to the readers in the following manner: Sect. 2 explains various clustering algorithms which are helpful for WSN. In Sect. 3, detailed analysis about the challenges and attributes designer must consider for designing efficient clustering methodology is described. Section 4 briefs some of the standard clustering algorithms which are proposed for WSN. Comparative results are plotted in Sect. 4, and finally, Sect. 5 summates the entire work in a systematic fashion.

2 Clustering Technique in WSN

The most vital piece of bunching strategies is that the whole system is separated into little gatherings called clusters. Every cluster has its own cluster head which handles the responsibility of transferring sensed data from the member node to the base station and also advocates and controls the member node as shown in Fig. 1. Usage of clustering topology plays a very significant role in reducing the energy consumption of WSN.

3 Challenges for Clustering in WSN

There are a few key qualities that designers should deliberately consider, which are of specific significance in remote sensor systems while designing clustering methodologies, for example:

Fig. 1 Typical cluster
structure of WSN

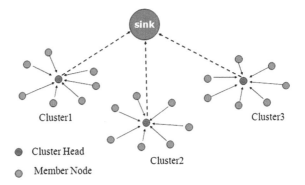

1. **Clustering Expenses**:

In spite of the fact that clustering plays a significant role in sorting sensor network topology, there are other numerous assets to be considered such as communication and tasks of preparing errands required in the creation and upkeep of the grouping topology. Such expenses are to be minimized as in such cases the required assets are not being utilized for information transmission or sensing tasks.

2. **Choice of Cluster heads and Clusters**:

The concept of grouping sensors into small groups offers enormous advantages for remote sensor systems. In any case, when planning for a specific application, designers and researchers should deliberately analyze the arrangement of clusters in the system. Contingent upon the application, certain prerequisites for the quantity of hubs in the cluster or its physical size may assume a vital part in its task. This essentially may affect how cluster heads are chosen in any required application.

3. **Synchronization**:

One of the essential confinements in wireless sensor networks is the restricted vitality limit of operating hubs called nodes. Selective and opportunistic transmission plans (such as TDMA) enable nodes to frequently plan rest interims to limit the usage of available restricted amount of energy. However, applying such plans to resource-constrained networks always demands synchronization principles to set up and keep up the transmission plan. Thus, while considering a clustering option, one must seriously look into synchronization and congestion control mechanisms to enhance the lifetime of the overall network.

4. **Information Aggregation**:

One noteworthy preferred standpoint of remote sensor systems is the capacity for information collection to happen within the network. In a thickly populated system, there is more than one node which detects comparable data. So usage of information aggregation permits the separation between repeated multiple detected information and helpful information. Inter- and intra-network clustering of sensor network makes this procedure easily conceivable even in a resource-constrained environment such as

WSN and it becomes an added advantage as the power required for handling and data processing tasks is substantially less than power required for communication. In that capacity, the measure of information moved in system ought to be limited. Numerous clustering algorithms give information conglomeration abilities, and in that capacity, the necessity for information collection ought to be painstakingly considered while choosing a bunching approach.

5. **Robustness and Scalability**:

Owing to the environment in which wireless sensor networks operate, they are frequently inclined to node versatility, node demise, and interference from other signals; these circumstances can bring about connection disappointment. Hence, it becomes an inevitable duty of researchers to address these issues when studying clustering algorithms, so that in case of harsh or undisciplined environmental conditions link recovery and reliable data communication can be possible.

4 Standard Clustering Algorithms

Clustering algorithms are classified into diversified manner and the most predominant among these are as follows:

- clustering in homogeneous and heterogeneous network;
- centralized clustering and distributed clustering.

Among the proposed clustering approaches, low-energy adaptive clustering hierarchy (LEACH) [11] is an extremely famous versatile clustering approach which upgrades energy proficiency of the framework by forming clusters in light of signal strength received. LEACH is an application-specific information dispersal approach that works on the principle of grouping and selection of random cluster head to extend the life span of resource-constrained sensor networks. Figure= 2 demonstrates the time line of LEACH, which generally works in two phases called to be set up stage and enduring state where it experiences these accompanying tasks:

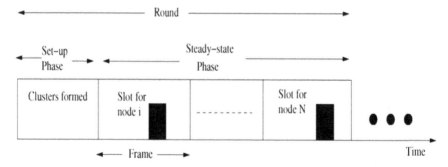

Fig. 2 Time line operation of LEACH

1. Every sensor chooses itself to be a cluster head with a particular likelihood, which is set to be 5% in the analyses.
2. After the cluster heads have been chosen, they will communicate their data to the remaining sensors in the system.
3. Based on the signal strength of the information received from different cluster heads, the sensors choose the cluster in which they continue their operation.
4. The cluster heads will make a transmission plan for the sensors in their own groups. Every sensor in the cluster speaks with their cluster head in a solitary bounce TDMA fashion.
5. The cluster heads gather and wire the information from the sensors and then send the amassed information to the BS utilizing code-division multiple access scheme.

LEACH always adopts random rotation principle for selection of local cluster heads to uniformly distribute the energy load among the sensors in the network. Each constituent node in the network conveys the information it has accrued to the cluster head which then transfers all the valuable part of amassed information to the rest of the network.

Some of the notable disadvantages of LEACH are that it does not ensure appropriate cluster head selection nor distribution, and also, it assumes uniform usage of energy throughout the network for CH selection. Hence, LEACH usage may lead to imbalanced selection of cluster heads which may often lead to reduced lifespan of the network. Also, LEACH does no longer perform well in heterogeneous conditions.

Power-Efficient Gathering in Sensor Information Systems (PEGASIS) [12] is another chain-based hierarchical protocol widely accepted by WSN research group. The nodes in this routing algorithm are arranged in the form of chain for transportation and aggregation; it is also considered to be a greedy chain-based protocol in which data communication takes place between the closest neighbors. PEGASIS exhibits an improvement in performance of LEACH by saving energy at different stages like usage of local gathering, thus reducing the distance of transmission of data compared to LEACH; also, the amount of data that a cluster head receives is almost 1/10th of size when measured against LEACH.

Hybrid Energy-Efficient Distributed (HEED) [10] algorithm is a multi-hop inter-clustering algorithm based on LEACH, while it also addresses issues related to inter-cluster data transfer by assuming some standard assumptions. CHs in this network are chosen based on two important parameters: unused energy and intra-cluster communication cost. A probabilistic model is used based on the value of unused energy to choose the CH initially. HEED provides opportunity for uniform cluster head selection throughout the system which leads to uniform distribution of energy usage. However, HEED strongly demands knowledge about the entire system to decide intra-cluster communication cost.

Stable Election Protocol (SEP) [13] is a bizarre clustering scheme proposed for more than one level heterogeneous type of network. SEP is a dynamic clustering approach which does not assume any prior distribution of the different levels of energy in the sensor nodes and also allows the nodes in the network to independently elect themselves as cluster heads without the knowledge of every node's energy in the network. SEP proves to be equally well efficient irrespective of size of network on which it is applied. However, SEP does not use to manage higher-level nodes efficiently.

This weakness in SEP was overcome in Distributed Energy-Efficient Clustering Protocol (DEEC) [14] where cluster head selection is more routinely based on enduring energy of node and overall energy of the network. The algorithm also offers fair chance for the high energy node to become cluster head than low-energy node; thus, it helps in balancing the average energy consumption of network.

In Threshold Sensitive Energy-Efficient Sensor Network Protocol (TEEN) [15], authors introduce a new network protocol, for reactive networks where transmission of data is event driven and no longer continuous. Every node in the network takes a turn to become cluster heads for a period of time called cluster period. The protocol outperforms many of the proposed protocols by sending both hard threshold for sensed data values and soft threshold values for reporting small change in the sensed attributes. TEEN works on the principle that message transmission consumes more energy than data sensing so the primary motive of the researchers [15] was to minimize the number of transmissions to save energy. TEEN proves to be very handy in applications which require fast transmission and save considerable amount of energy and response time.

Enhanced MODLEACH (E-MODLEACH) [16] proposes cluster head selection in the same manner as proposed in HEED [10] but based on different equations and energy hole removing mechanism to control the total count of cluster heads involved actively in the network. The nodes are usually pushed to sleep mode based on the count of number of active nodes in the cluster.

5   Simulation and Analysis

In this study, we have compared few standard algorithms such as LEACH, MOD-LEACH, E-MODLEACH, TEEN, SEP, DEEC which are described in Sect. 2 using MATLAB, and some important attributes in these algorithms are shown in Figs. 2 and 3 (Fig. 4).

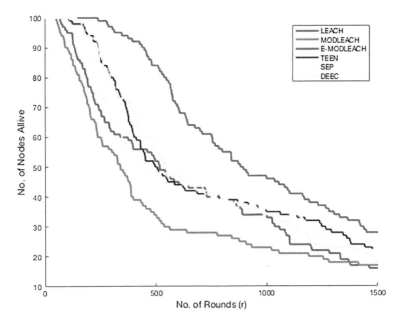

Fig. 3 Number of node alive versus number of rounds

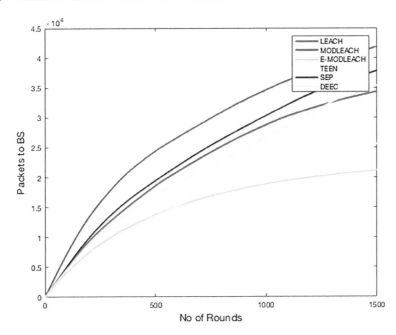

Fig. 4 Successful packets delivered to BS versus number of nodes

Table 1 Parameters used for simulation

Description	Value
Distance along x-axis	500 m
Distance along y-axis	500 m
Number of nodes installed	100 nodes
Cumulative energy of network	1 J
Possibility of being selected as cluster head	0.5
Total number of rounds	4000

6 Conclusion

The main objective of this research is to present a survey of existing standard clustering approaches and also to brief about the different challenges that one should consider before designing clustering algorithms for WSN.

In this paper, we presented a case study on standard clustering algorithms proposed for usage in WSNs and compared the number of nodes alive after few rounds of data transfer which clearly shows LEACH and its successors outperform other algorithms; also in terms of successful packet delivery to the base station, LEACH and MODLEACH show better results when compared to other standard algorithms (Table 1).

References

1. Akyildiz I, Su W, Sankarasubramaniam Y, Cayirci E (2002) Wireless sensor networks: a survey. Comput Netw 38(4):393–422
2. Enzinger M (2012) Energy-efficient communication in wireless sensor networks. Network Architectures and Services, Aug 2012. https://doi.org/10.2313/net-2012-08-2_04
3. Nagaraj S, Biradar RV (2017) Applications of wireless sensor networks in the real-time ambient air pollution monitoring and air quality in metropolitan cities—a survey. In: Proceedings of SmartTechCon Aug 2017, Bengaluru, India. https://doi.org/10.1109/smarttechcon.2017.8358594
4. Taruna S, Lata JK, Purohit GN (2011) Performance analysis of energy efficient routing protocol for homogeneous WSN. Trends in network and communications: WeST 2011, NeCoM 2011, WiMoN 2011. Communications in computer and information science, vol 197. Springer, Berlin, Heidelberg
5. Yan I, Zhou M, Ding Z (2016) Recent advances in energy-efficient routing protocols for wireless sensor networks: a review. Digit Object Identifier (IEEE). https://doi.org/10.1109/access.2016.2598719-2016
6. Hu Y et al (2017) An energy-efficient adaptive overlapping clustering method for dynamic continuous monitoring in WSNs. IEEE Sens J 17(3):834–847
7. Malik M, Arora A, Singh Y (2013) Analysis of LEACH protocol in wireless sensor networks. IJARCSSE 3(2). ISSN 2277 128X
8. Roy A, Kar P, Mishra S, Obaidat MS (2017) Distributed approach for the detection of dumb nodes in wireless sensor networks. Int J Comput Syst

9. Varshney S, Kumar C, Swaroop A (2015) A comparative study of hierarchical routing algorithms in wireless sensor networks. In: 2nd international conference on computing for sustainable global development (INDIACom), New Delhi, 2015, pp 1018–1023
10. Younis O, Sonia F (2004) HEED: a hybrid, energy-efficient, distributed clustering approach for ad hoc sensor networks. IEEE Trans Mob Comput 3(4):366–379
11. Heinzelman WR, Balakrishnan H, Chandrakasan A (2000) Energy-efficient communication protocol for wireless microsensor networks. In: International conference on system sciences, Jan 2000, Hawai
12. Lindsley S, Raghavendra CS (2003) PEGASIS: power-efficient gathering in sensor information systems. In: IEEE aerospace conference proceedings, Apr 2003
13. Smaragdakis G, Matta I, Bestavros A (2004) SEP: a stable election protocol for clustered heterogeneous wireless sensor networks. In: Proceedings of the international workshop on SANPA, 2004, pp 251–261
14. Chamam A, Samuel P (2010) A distributed energy-efficient clustering algorithm for wireless sensor networks. Comput Electr Eng 36:303–312
15. Manjeshwar A, Agrawal DP (2001) TEEN: a routing algorithm for enhanced efficiency in wireless sensor networks. In: Proceedings 15th international parallel and distributed processing symposium, IPDPS 2001, San Francisco, CA, USA, 2001, pp 2009–2015
16. Pandya NK, Kathiriya HJ, Kathiriya NH, Pandya AD (2015) Design and simulation of advance MODLEACH for wireless sensor network. In: International conference on computer, communication and control (IC4), Indore, 2015, pp 1–6

Novel Color Image Data Hiding Technique Based on DCT and Compressed Sensing Algorithm

M. K. Shyla and K. B. Shiva Kumar

Abstract Information security and its research are getting significant, and therefore, the steganographic technique is used in high level to send data secretly using a cover image such that its presence cannot be detected. In his paper, an improved RGB image steganographic technique which is a novel approach for hiding the secret image based on compressive sensing algorithm has been proposed. In the proposed approach, the RGB planes of payload image are extracted and compressed; then, the coefficients are reshaped and discrete cosine transform (DCT) is applied over 2 * 2 matrices. The compressed payload image is embedded with chaotically chosen random keys in the segmented RGB planes of cover image. The proposed method results in significant improvements with high PSNR value and payload capacity.

Keywords Compressive sensing algorithm · DCT · RGB image steganography

1 Introduction

Digital communication techniques on digital data or information play an important role nowadays, because of its fast access features. Large number of technologies are required for end-to-end protection to overcome the security threats in modern digital communication. In the present scenario, data hiding in digital multimedia is being applied in all security techniques and various applications vary from image steganography, secret communications, watermarking to digital signatures.

M. K. Shyla (✉)
SSAHE, Tumakuru, India
e-mail: shylamk@ssit.edu.in

K. B. Shiva Kumar
Department of TCE, SSAHE, Tumakuru, India
e-mail: kbsssit@gmail.com

© Springer Nature Singapore Pte Ltd. 2019
V. Sridhar et al. (eds.), *Emerging Research in Electronics, Computer Science and Technology*, Lecture Notes in Electrical Engineering 545,
https://doi.org/10.1007/978-981-13-5802-9_99

Image data hiding is a technique used to hide information in the form of text, audio, image, or video in a cover file. The data that is to be hidden itself is changed to some other form called cipher data in cryptography. This makes the hacker to easily suspect about the end-to-end transformation of data. To hide data secretly in such a way that any hacker should find it difficult to suspect is a big challenge in steganographic technique which is the advantage over cryptographic technique. Both encryption of data using key and data hiding are employed in some applications.

Security as well as embedding capacity is less in hiding text in a text. If we use audio or video files as cover files to hide secret data, for some small changes in an audio or video files lead to large changes because these two files consist of moving information. An Image file has a large number of unessential bits or pixels to embed payload data; hence, the image data hiding is the most commonly used technique.

2 Literature Review

Shivakumar et al. [1] proposed payload transformation-based technique where the cover image is divided into 2 × 2 blocks and the matrix for payload hiding is considered based on the threshold value fixed by calculating adjacent pixel intensity differences. The transformation matrix obtained is based on the identity matrix and the payload bit pair. And key is generated with first bit of payload matrix at the sending end and the same key is used to extract the payload from the stego-image. Masud Karim et al. [2] and AbdelQader and AlTamimi [3] introduced an approach to substitute LSB of RGB true color image and a concept of secret key encryption for the hidden information to protect it from unauthorized users.

Bhowmik and Bhowmik [4] proposed a method where the cover image is divided into 2 × 2 non-overlapping blocks; then, secret data is embedded using first bit of red, green, and blue layers and secured with hash values. Singh and Singh [5] proposed an LSB technique for 24-bit images by embedding the information into RGB planes of image in such a way that it enhances the quality of image and achieves high payload capacity. Jain et al. [6] explained that the text can be considered as secret information and is embedded in proportion to 2R, 2G, and 4B combinations of red, green, and blue layers of cover image. Sohag et al. [7] explained edge detecting techniques using an image as cover medium and considered text as secret image.

Gupta et al. [8] described balanced data hiding and proposed a least significant bit matching algorithm. This algorithm searches message bit that should not be same as least significant bit of cover image; if it finds such bits, it increments or decrements cover pixel by one and embedded data in that cover pixel. Patel and Patel [9] and Raja et al. [10] described and implemented different LSB and enhanced LSB hiding techniques for data hiding using discrete cosine transform and embedded using SVD method along with RSA algorithm and compression techniques to provide better security. Ghasemi et al. [11] and Shirali-Shahreza et al. [12] analyzed genetic algorithms which are based on optimization method. Mondal et al. [13] and Joshi et al. [14] proposed and combined different types of image data hiding in non-transform and transform domains. Charan et al. [15] and Jain et al. [16] explained cryptography techniques along with steganography to achieve better security. Orsdemir et al. [17] proposed LSB replacement data hiding which is a replacement method that modifies even pixel values and leaves odd values unchanged. Wang et al. [18] introduced data hiding algorithm which uses histogram statistical properties of an image. Patsakis and Aroukatos [19] proposed data hiding technique based on LSB or DCT features and compressive sensing domain. Donoho [20] proposed compressive sensing of payload data applied to SVD transform and then embedded. Devi and ShivaKumar [21] used SVM classifier to increase the data embedding rate.

III PROPOSED MODEL

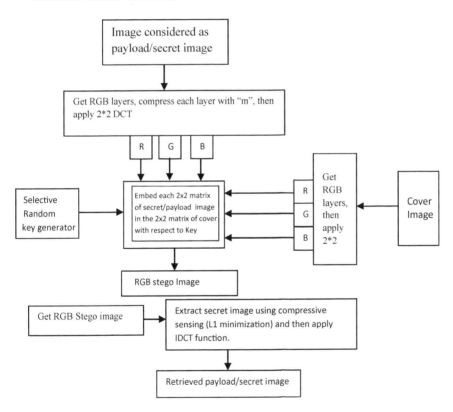

Fig. 1 Proposed model

Proposed Algorithm:

1. Load the secret image. Extract the red, green, and blue planes.
2. Compress each planes separately using compressive sensing algorithm, with the parameter "m." The value of "m" determines how much the information is being compressed; that is, the lesser the value of "m" the more is the compression attained.
3. Reshape the array of data obtained after compression into 2×2 matrix.
4. Apply DCT to the matrices (separately for RGB layers).
5. Load the cover image of size 256 * 256 and get R, G, B layers separately Apply DCT to these layers and subdivide them into blocks of size 2 * 2.
6. The secret image which is divided into 2 * 2 DCT is embedded into cover image with respect to key generated randomly.
7. The key generated is selective because it depends on compressive sensing parameter "m."
8. The above steps are repeated until all compressed secret information is embedded into cover image.
9. Decoding and reconstruction of secret message: The selective random key which is used at the transmitter side is used to locate the matrix that contains information in the stego-image. l_1 Minimization and IDCT functions are used to reconstruct Information as shown in Fig. 1.

3   Results and Discussions

We have simulated proposed approach in MATLAB R2017a version with different cover images of sizes 512 * 512 and 256 * 256 with different secret images of sizes

Table 1 Peak signal-to-noise ratio (PSNR) between different stego- and cover images

Cover image	Payload image	PSNR with [3]	PSNR with proposed method
Elephant	Aero	40.4571	63.117
Nature	Android	41.3426	65.456
Baboon	Lena	42.1507	66.3981

Table 2 Peak signal-to-noise ratio between payload image and retrieved payload image

Payload image	PSNR with [3]	PSNR with proposed method
Aero	43.9598	62.117
Android	37.2983	52.456
Lena	39.3217	53.3981

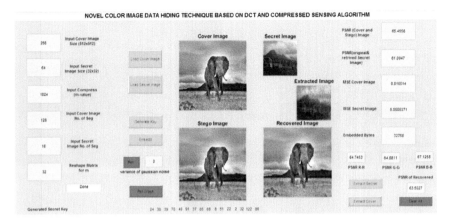

Fig. 2 GUI of proposed approach considering 256 * 256 cover image and 64 * 64 secret image

16×16, 32×32 and 64×64, 128×128. Peak signal-to-noise ratio, mean square error obtained for the proposed method are tabulated for different payload capacity and compressive sensing parameter "m" (Tables 1 and 2). Figure 2 shows GUI of proposed approach considering 256 * 256 cover image and 64 * 64 secret/payload image.

4 Conclusions

The proposed approach is based on compressive sensing domain with the use of the three-layer color image over DCT features, to enhance the security, secrecy, and payload capacity. The compressed information is reshaped and embedded in chaotically chosen matrices of cover image. The information is reconstructed at the receiver side using compressed sensing reconstruction algorithm based on l_1 minimization and inverse DCT functions. The results show that the proposed technique has better PSNR with regard to the stego-image as well as the extracted payload with good embedding capacity (Fig. 3).

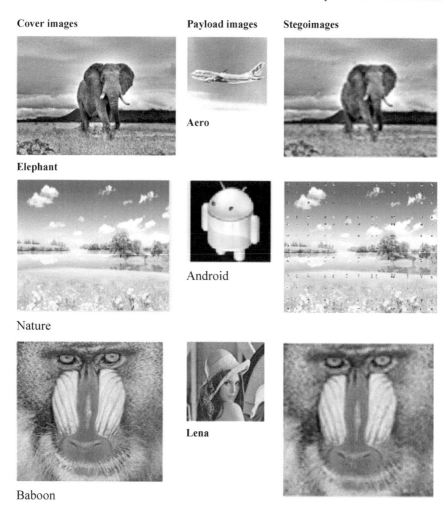

Fig. 3 Different cover, payload, and corresponding stego-images

References

1. Shiva Kumar KB et al (2011) Steganography based on payload transformation. IJCSI Int J Comput Sci Issues 8(2)
2. Masud Karim SM, Saifur Rahman Md, Ismail Hossain Md (2011) A new approach for LSB based image steganography using secret key. In: 14th international conference on computer and information technology (ICCIT 2011), 22–24 Dec 2011, Dhaka, Bangladesh
3. AbdelQader A, AlTamimi F (2017) A novel image steganography approach using multi-layers DCT features based on support vector machine classifier. Int J Multimed Appl (IJMA) 9(1)
4. Bhowmik S, Bhaumik AK (2016) A new approach in color image steganography with high level of perceptibility and security. In: International conference on intelligent control power and instrumentation (ICICPI)

5. Singh A, Singh H (2015) An improved LSB based image steganography technique for RGB images. In: IEEE international conference on electrical, computer and communication technologies (ICECCT), pp 1–4
6. Jain N, Meshram S, Dubey S (2012) Image steganography using LSB and edge detection technique. Int J Soft Comput Eng (IJSCE) 2(3)
7. Sohag SA, Kabirul Islam Md, Baharul Islam Md (2013) A novel approach for image steganography using dynamic substitution and secret key. Am J Eng Res (AJER) 2(9):118–126
8. Gupta S, Gujral G, Aggarwal N (2012) Enhanced least significant bit algorithm for image steganography. Int J Comput Eng Manag (IJCEM) 15(4)
9. Patel P, Patel Y (2015) Secure and authentic DCT image steganography through DWT–SVD based digital watermarking with RSA encryption. In: IEEE 5th international conference on communication systems and network technologies (CSNT), pp 736–739
10. Raja KB, Chowdary CR, Venugopal KR, Patnaik LM (2005) A secure image steganography using LSB, DCT and compression techniques on raw images. In: IEEE international conference on intelligent sensing and information processing (ICISP), pp 170–176, Dec 2005
11. Ghasemi E, Shanbehzadeh J, Fassihi N (2011) High capacity image steganography using wavelet transform and genetic algorithm. In: International multiconference of engineers and computer scientists, vol 1
12. Shirali-Shahreza M (2006) Stealth steganography in SMS. In: Proceedings of IFIP international conference on wireless and optical communication network, pp 316–321
13. Mondal S, Debnath R, Mondal BK (2016) Color image steganography technique in spatial domain. In: Proceedings of 9th international conference on electrical and computer engineering, Dhaka, Bangladesh, pp 582–586, 20–22 Dec 2016
14. Joshi SV, Bokil AA, Jain NA, Koshti D (2012) Image steganography combination of spatial and frequency domain. Int J Comput Appl 53
15. Charan GS, Nithin Kumar SSV, Karthikeyan B, Vaithiyanathan V, Divya Lakshmi K (2015) A novel LSB based image steganography with multi-level encryption. In: 2015 international conference on innovations in information, embedded and communication systems (ICIIECS), pp 1–5. IEEE
16. Jain M, Lenka SK (2015) Secret data transmission using vital image steganography over transposition cipher. In: 2015 international conference on green computing and internet of things (ICGCIoT), pp 1026–1029. IEEE
17. Orsdemir A, Altun HO, Sharma G, Bocko MF (2008) On the security and robustness of encryption via compressed sensing. In: IEEE military communications conference, pp 1040–1046
18. Wang Q, Zeng W, Tian J (2013) Integrated secure watermark detection and privacy preserving storage in the compressive sensing domain. In: IEEE international workshop on information forensics and security, Guangzhou, China, pp 67–72
19. Patsakis C, Aroukatos NG (2014) LSB an DCT steganographic detection using compressive sensing. J Inf Hiding Multimed Signal Process 5(1):20–32
20. Donoho DL (2006) Compressed sensing. IEEE Trans Inf Theory 52(4):1289–1306
21. Devi A, ShivaKumar KB (2017) Novel secured reversible covert communication over encrypted domain using SVM classifier. In: 2017 international conference on advances in computing, communications and informatics (ICACCI)

GSM-Based Advanced Multi-switching DTMF Controller for Remotely Monitoring of Electrical Appliances

Sumit Kumar, Aman Ranjan Verma and C. H. Nagesh

Abstract This paper presents the design and implementation of a GSM-based dual-tone multi-frequency (DTMF) controller for remotely monitoring of electrical appliances. The present system provides an added feature like the secure connection with a passcode and reliable control of various devices without perturbation. The device can be controlled from any location using a mobile phone. For this, one has to make a call from a cell phone to control the electrical appliances. Since mobile phones are available with everyone, it will be much easier to employ this technology in practical life. In this paper, the main focus is on the controlling of more devices without ambiguity. The developed system is cost effective and can be used to control up to 128 devices with a secured connection unlike the 8–12 devices in the conventional systems.

Keywords DTMF · Mobile phone · Transmitter · Receiver · Microcontroller · Encoder · Decoder

1 Introduction

The world is getting digitalized in every aspect especially in terms of communication and automation with the advancement of technology. Smart devices are increasingly popular for controlling electrical and electronic devices from remote locations. Remote control technologies are being used in fields like industrial automation and space exploration for years, in places where human access is difficult [1]. The DTMF technology was initially developed for the telephone signaling to and from the local

S. Kumar (✉) · A. R. Verma · C. H. Nagesh
IIIT Manipur, Imphal 795002, India
e-mail: sumit@iiitmanipur.ac.in

A. R. Verma
e-mail: v.aman@iiitmanipur.ac.in

C. H. Nagesh
e-mail: nagesh@iiitmanipur.ac.in

© Springer Nature Singapore Pte Ltd. 2019
V. Sridhar et al. (eds.), *Emerging Research in Electronics, Computer Science and Technology*, Lecture Notes in Electrical Engineering 545,
https://doi.org/10.1007/978-981-13-5802-9_100

exchange, though today it finds several applications in the field of telecommunications and industrial automation. GSM-based DTMF controller as an agriculture device for monitoring and controlling from a remote location through mobile phone has been studied [2].

GSM-based DTMF controller can control electrical appliances such as cooler fans, bulbs, refrigerator, air conditioner, and heating units from a remote location through a mobile phone before/after arriving home or industry. The usage of electronic, electrical, and mechanical devices is increasing exponentially. It will be challenging to manage and control so many appliances as the conventional DTMF are restricted to controlling of only 8–12 devices [3]. In this paper, GSM-based DTMF controller uses a mobile phone as a remote to control up to 128 home/industry electrical, electronic, or mechanical devices. The adaptability of this DTMF controller is accomplishable for any community because of the readily available technology implied on it.

The system is operated by a mobile phone. It generates different signal frequencies corresponding to the pressed keys. The proposed DTMF controller consists of a DTMF decoder that decodes 4-bit binary data from those signal frequencies. These 4-bit binary data is used in relay switching and controlling the appliances. The system is proficient in providing a secure connection by using a passcode. In order to operate the device, the user needs to be logged in by placing a call to multi-switching DTMF controller system. The system verifies the caller user id with the successful entry of a passcode. Each appliance is coded to work on a unique combination of frequency. This paper is further organized as follows. The basic principles of DTMF decoder are presented in Sect. 2. The details of the proposed DTMF controller are explained in Sect. 3. The results and discussion are discussed in Sect. 4, and finally, the paper is concluded.

2 Basic Principles of DTMF Decoder

DTMF is the technical term for the sound frequencies produced when a key is pressed on the mobile phone keypad. DTMF generates a sequence of two different frequencies (one low frequency and another high frequency) corresponding to the key pressed and the convolution of these two frequencies gives the resultant unique frequency [4]. A different frequency is assigned to each key in the mobile phone. DTMF keypad is in the form of a 4×4 matrix. Rows represent the lower frequency, and columns represent the higher frequency components. The four rows of DTMF keypad are assigned to a low-frequency group, and the three columns are assigned to a high-frequency group. The fourth column of key named as A, B, C, and D is an optional, and it is mostly used in military networks. For example, the number 3 is pressed, it will generate the combination of two frequencies that consist of 697 Hz for the low group and 1477 Hz for the high group. Similarly, the DTMF generated a wave with a unique frequency can be expressed mathematically as shown in Eq. (1):

Table 1 DTMF decoder output binary codes

Keys	Low DTMF frequency (Hz)	High DTMF frequency (Hz)	Q4	Q3	Q2	Q1
1	697	1209	0	0	0	1
2	697	1336	0	0	1	0
3	697	1477	0	0	1	1
4	770	1209	0	1	0	0
5	770	1336	0	1	0	1
6	770	1477	0	1	1	0
7	852	1209	0	1	1	1
8	852	1336	1	0	0	0
9	852	1477	1	0	0	1
0	941	1336	1	0	1	0
*	941	1209	1	0	1	1
#	941	1477	1	1	0	0

$$F(t) = A_H \sin 2\pi f_H t + A_L \sin 2\pi f_L t \qquad (1)$$

where A_H is the amplitude of higher frequency wave, A_L is the amplitude of lower frequency wave, f_L and f_H are lower frequency and higher frequency of the wave, respectively [5]. Further, frequency sequences and specifications of DTMF [6] are given in Table 1.

3   Proposed DTMF Controller

Figure 1 represents a block diagram of the proposed system. The system consists of two types of receivers, and these are labeled with numeric starting from 0 to 15 for addressing. The block diagram and complete schematic diagram of the receiver 0 are shown in Fig. 2a and Fig. 3, respectively. Further, the operation and working principle of the proposed DTMF controller are described. For controlling and monitoring of electrical appliances, one has to establish the connection with the DTMF system through mobile phone by placing a call as shown in Fig. 2a. After making a call to a DTMF system, it will ask for the secure passcode to establish a connection. After the successful interfacing, the user can give the command to the system for controlling appliances. The unique frequency generated corresponding to the key pressed in mobile phone comes to receiver 0 through GSM. Simultaneously, a mobile phone gives this signal to the DTMF decoder through the 3.5 mm earphone jack as shown in Fig. 3. The DTMF decoder decodes the frequency and generates equivalent binary 4-bit data. The respective frequencies of the corresponding keys and their 4-bit output data array (Q4–MSB to Q1–LSB) are given in Table 1.

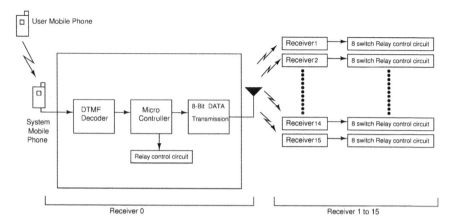

Fig. 1 System block diagram

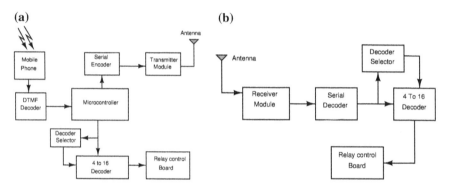

Fig. 2 Block diagram of **a** receiver 0 **b** receiver 1

The receiver 0 holds dual nature which acts as both transmitter and receiver as shown in Fig. 2a. The 4-bit data from Q4 to Q1 is decoded from the input, and it is passed through the microcontroller [7] which generates 8-bit parallel binary code (D5–D12) as shown in Fig. 3. Microcontroller converts this 4-bit binary code into decimal number and stores in its memory and further waits for next input. If the next input is a number, once again repeat the same process called the store and wait. In the other case, if the next input is '*', then microcontroller resets the stored decimal numbers and waits for the new input; in case the next input is '#', the microcontroller converts the stored decimal number into 8-bit binary code. Table 2 shows a proposed 8-bit binary code with respect to key codes. First four bits of data decide the address of the receiver and rest of four bits decide the position of the appliances according to Table 3.

The processed 8-bit code from the microcontroller is given to serial encoder. Serial encoder converts this 8-bit parallel code into an 8-bit serial code and transmits the same over a radio frequency by an antenna to receiver 1–15.

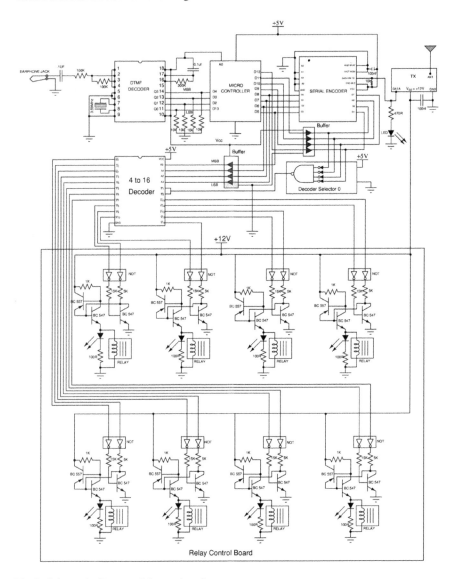

Fig. 3 Schematic diagram of the receiver 0

Table 2 8-bit binary code generated by microcontroller and respected appliance activity

Key code entered by user	8-bit binary output of microcontroller	Appliances activity
1#	00000001	Appliance 1 will ON
2#	00000010	Appliance 1 will OFF
–	–	–
–	–	–
62#	01111110	Appliance 31 will ON
63#	01111111	Appliance 31 will OFF
–	–	–
–	–	–
254#	11111110	Appliance 127 will ON
255#	11111111	Appliance 127 will OFF

Table 3 Address of the receiver according to the first four-bit data

First four-bit of 8-bit data	Address of receiver	Appliances control
0001	Receiver 1 will be active	Appliance 9–16
0010	Receiver 2 will be active	Appliance 17–24
–	–	–
–	–	–
1110	Receiver 14 will be active	Appliance 112–119
1111	Receiver 15 will be active	Appliance 119–126

The receiver 1 block diagram and the complete schematic diagram are shown in Fig. 2b and Fig. 4, respectively. Similarly, the receiver 2–15 can be depicted. At the receiver side 1–15, the decoder selector decides which decoder [8] to be enabled or disabled depending on the address of the receiver. If the decoder is in enable state, then it decodes the last 4-bit code and gives to the relay control board. The relay control board controls the relays according to the decoder output [9]. Relay control board has eight transistor switches, and transistor switch has two inputs for ON and OFF states, respectively.

Similarly, remaining receivers such as a 2–15 can be used for the same application like receiver 1 with the help of different decoder selectors. The decoder selectors are used to create a unique address to each receiver as shown in Fig. 5. With this method, a total of 128 electrical appliances, 8 by receiver 0, and 120 by receiver 1–15 can be controlled.

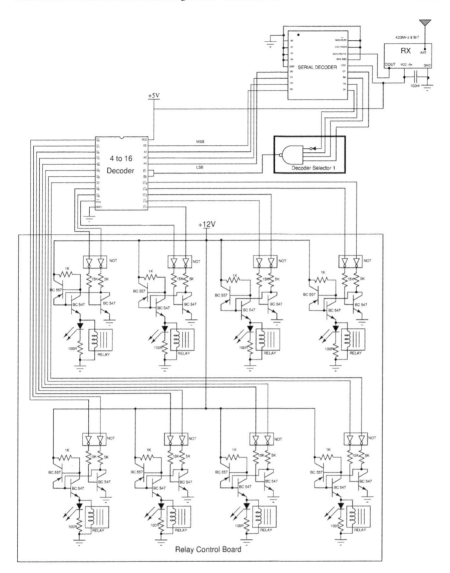

Fig. 4 Schematic diagram of receiver 1

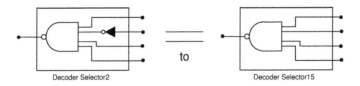

Fig. 5 Decoder selectors

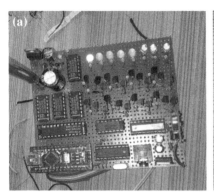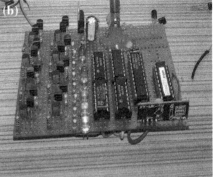

Fig. 6 Practical demonstration of DTMF controller **a** receiver 0 **b** receiver 1

4 Results and Discussion

This system enables switching of electrical appliances from a remote location through a mobile phone. Overcoming the limited range of IR and radio remote controls the system works through GSM globally where a network is accessible.

The system working principle and the proposed method have been successfully demonstrated by controlling the working of fans and bulbs as well as other home appliances. The user was kept at a distance of 5 km from the location. First, the user placed the call to the mobile phone which is attached to receiver 0. The next, user needs to enter the passcode for establishing a secure connection between the system and user mobile phone. All other possible combinations of controlling of 128 appliances have been tested using LED. The working model using LEDs is shown in Fig. 6a and b, respectively.

The designed system can be used to open doors, control DC motors, electrical appliances, and heavy-duty motors. Overcoming the barriers to achieving to control up to 128 devices will prove huge gain in preexisting DTMF technology.

5 Conclusion

An advanced multi-switching DTMF control system has been designed and demonstrated successfully. The present system is designed to control up to 128 electrical appliances including electronic devices from a remote location through GSM. The DTMF decoder was designed to increase the effective utilization of power by reducing the wastage of electricity. The designed system is affordable having ease of installation and comes with an economical price compared to other technologies like IOT. Finally, the system provides a solution for the uncertainty in the switch position with the added advantage of a secure connection. In future, the aim is to make an android interface to control the system with the call that transmits the code over GSM.

Acknowledgements The design and implementation were carried out at IIIT Manipur with the support of TEQIP-III, NPIU, and Government of India. Finally, authors would like to thank Department of ECE as well as others who have helped in the demonstration of DTMF controller for the said practical application.

References

1. Islam MM, Chowdhury MH. DTMF Based home appliances control using cell phone
2. Getu BN, Hamad NA, Attia HA (2015) Remote controlling of an agricultural pump system based on the dual tone multi frequency (DTMF) technique. J Eng Sci Technol 10(10):1261–1274
3. Sharma R, Kumar K, Vig S (2006) DTMF based remote control system. In: IEEE international conference on industrial technology, 2006, ICIT 2006, pp 2380–2383. IEEE
4. Lee KM, Lai J (2005) Speech versus touch: a comparative study of the use of speech and DTMF keypad for navigation. Int J Hum Comput Interact 19(3):343–360 (Taylor & Francis)
5. Ghosh R (2012) DTMF based controller for efficiency improvement of a PV cell & relay operation control. Int J Eng Res Appl (IJERA) 2(3):2903–2911
6. Popović M (2003) Efficient decoding of digital DTMF and R2 tone signalization. Facta Universitatis Ser Electron Energ 16(3):389–399
7. Denysyuk P, Teslyuk T (2013) Main algorithm of mobile robot system based on the microcontroller arduino. In: 2013 XVIIIth international seminar/workshop on direct and inverse problems of electromagnetic and acoustic wave theory (DIPED), 2013, pp 209–212. IEEE
8. Gajski DD (1997) Principles of digital design
9. www.sierraic.info

Design and Development of 15-Level Asymmetrical Cascaded Multilevel Inverter

J. Madhusudhana, Mohamed Rafiq A. Chapparband and P. S. Puttaswamy

Abstract In this paper, a photovoltaic model is designed and developed for generating 110 V (RMS) is presented. The voltage obtained out of the photovoltaic (PV) module is comparatively less and variable in nature. The model presented in this paper consists of three voltage fed-back boost converters that are designed and modeled using state-space averaging technique (SSA) in order to obtain a higher and stabilized constant DC output voltage. This boosted output is fed to an asymmetrical 15-level multilevel inverter to convert DC to AC. The switching angles for the 15-level H-bridge multilevel inverter are designed using equal area criteria. The designed circuit is developed using IRFP250N and IRF840 MOSFETs. The simulation and hardware results compared in the result section convey that the proposed design is able to produce 110 V (RMS) for variable loads.

Keywords DC/DC boost converter · Photovoltaic module · Equal area criteria · Cascaded H-bridge inverter · Multilevel inverter

J. Madhusudhana (✉) · M. R. A. Chapparband
Department of Electrical Engineering, UVCE, Bangalore, India
e-mail: madhutmkr@yahoo.com

M. R. A. Chapparband
e-mail: mrafiqkid@gmail.com

P. S. Puttaswamy
Department of Electrical Engineering, PES College of Engineering, Mandya 571401, Karnataka, India
e-mail: psputtaswamy_ee@yahoo.com

© Springer Nature Singapore Pte Ltd. 2019
V. Sridhar et al. (eds.), *Emerging Research in Electronics, Computer Science and Technology*, Lecture Notes in Electrical Engineering 545,
https://doi.org/10.1007/978-981-13-5802-9_101

1   Introduction

In the near future, the need for electric energy is expected to increase more rapidly due to the global population growth and industrialization. Currently, a large share of electricity is generated from fossil fuels, especially coal due to its low prices. As the demand for the electricity increases, consequently the usage of the fossil fuels also increases which are perishable. To overcome the drawbacks associated with generation of electricity from fossil fuels, renewable energy sources come into picture for generation of electrical energy. One of the renewable energy sources that can be used for this purpose is the light received from the sun (solar). This light can be converted to clean electricity through the photovoltaic process. The photovoltaic (PV) panels are manufactured from a semiconductor material. The semiconductor material is selected based on its ability to gather high concentration of electrons. Silicon is the most widely used semiconductor material in PV panels. When a photovoltaic cell is exposed to sunlight, the solar radiation increases the energy levels of the electrons in the semiconductor resulting in generation of electricity; this phenomenon is called photovoltaic effect. The converters and inverters play a very important role in transferring the power from the PV panels to the load.

Nowadays, various DC–DC converter topologies such as buck, boost, buck—boost, and Cuk converter are widely used in switched mode power supplies. These converters are used to convert a dc voltage to a desired dc voltage level, often providing a regulated output. The buck and boost are the basic converter topologies, and other converters are derived from these two basic converter topologies. Among all the available converters, boost converter is widely used to step up the unregulated dc output of the photovoltaic module to desired higher constant output voltage.

But most of the loads available are operated with AC source. The inverters are used to convert DC to AC source. An **inverter** is a circuit that changes direct current (DC) to alternating current (AC). There are various types of inverters available, among all of them multilevel inverters are most widely used for its various merits.

2   Proposed Model

Here in this work, an asymmetrical three-stage cascaded H-bridge inverter is considered for generating 15-level AC output. The three-stage cascaded H-bridge inverter requires three separate DC sources. Hence, three batteries of 12 V each are considered and the output of the batteries is fed to three closed-loop boost converters which convert 12 V to constant output of 27, 54, and 108 V. The schematic diagram of closed-loop boost converter is as shown in Fig. 2, and the specifications and designed values of boost converters are shown in Tables 1 and 2. These voltages are fed to

Table 1 Specification of the proposed boost converter (BC) and its designed values

Mode	BC1	BC2	BC 3
Output voltage (V_o)	27	54	108
Switching frequency	100 kHz		
Input voltage (V_{in})	12 V		
R_L load	20 Ω		
Voltage ripple	1%		

Table 2 Designed values proposed boost converter (BC)

Circuit	V_{in} (V)	V_o (V)	D	L_{min} (μH)	L (μH)	C_{min} (μF)	I_L (A)
BC1	12	27	0.55	11.13	13.92	27.5	2.96
BC2	12	54	0.77	4.07	5.019	38.5	11.34
BC3	12	108	0.88	7.28	9.1	42	23.43

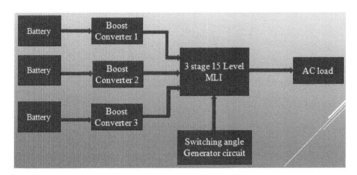

Fig. 1 Block diagram of the proposed model

three-stage inverter for converting this DC to AC form at the load side in stepped form to generate 110 V (RMS). This output can be converted into 220 V RMS by passing this through a 1:2 step-up transformer. The step-up transformer acts like an isolator and also as an inductive filter which helps in smoothing the output signal which results in reduced THD (Fig. 1).

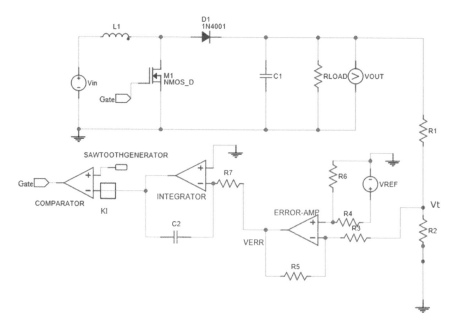

Fig. 2 Closed-loop boost converter

The input of boost converters is 12 V DC battery. The outputs of the boost converters are selected in such a way so as to achieve 110 V RMS at the inverter output, i.e., in the ratio 1:2:4.

$V_{out1} = 27$ V, $V_{out2} = 54$ V, $V_{out3} = 108$ V. These outputs of the boost converters are fed as inputs to 3 H-bridges. The output of the inverter will be $Vout$ of

$$\text{Inverter} = \frac{V_{out}1 + V_{out2} + V_{out3}}{\sqrt{2}}$$

$$= \frac{27 + 54 + 108}{\sqrt{2}} = 133.6 \text{ V (RMS)}$$

3 Multilevel Inverters

A multilevel inverter is a power electronic system that synthesizes a desired output voltage waveform from several DC source as input MLI has stepped output and with an increase in no. of levels, the output waveform approaches near to sinusoidal signal and the quality of the output waveform enhances with considerable reduction in THD (Fig. 3).

In comparison with the hard-switched two-level inverter, multilevel inverter can operate at high voltage with lower dv/dt. There are three basic MLI topologies and are classified based on the number of input DC sources used in the circuitry. The neutral-

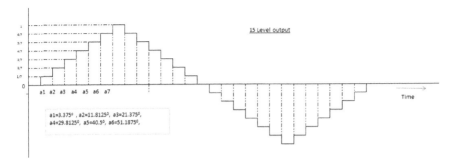

Fig. 3 Typical output of a multilevel inverter

point-clamped, flying-capacitor MLIs, consists one dc source, and cascaded H-bridge MLI (CHB-MLI), requiring separate dc sources. The latter becomes a very attractive feature in the case of PV systems, because solar cells can be assembled in a number of separate generators. Since their output voltage is a modulated staircase, they outperform two-level PWM inverters in terms of total harmonic distortion (THD), without the use of bulky expensive and dissipative passive filters. Further cascaded H-bridge MLI is classified as: (1) symmetrical H-bridge MLI: The input voltage levels of the cascaded inverter cells are equal. (2) Asymmetrical H-bridge MLI: The input voltage levels of the cascaded inverter cells are not equal.

Advantages of Asymmetrical Over Symmetrical MLI, Flying Capacitor MLI, Diode-Clamped MLI

The number of power devices required is reduced. More number of output levels can be obtained with less number of H-bridges. Hence, better quality of output voltage and less THD with less components. Losses will be reduced, and hence, efficiency will be more. For 15 level symmetric needs 28 switches. whereas asymmetric needs only 12 switches.

4   Simulation Results

The proposed design is simulated using MATLAB/Simulink software. The performance of the boost converter is tested with different values of input voltage and duty cycle, and the simulation results are captured for both without feedback and with feedback. From the simulation results, the proposed converter is able to give a constant DC output voltage. Below figure gives boost converter circuit and simulation results (Figs. 4, 5, 6, and 7).

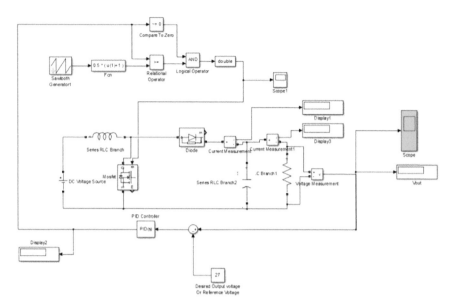

Fig. 4 Boost converter with feedback

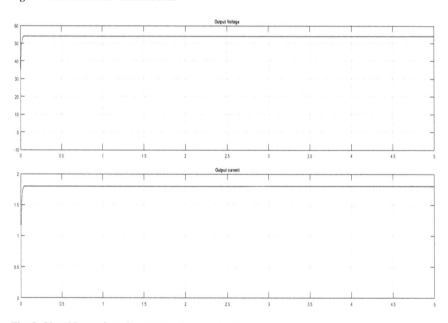

Fig. 5 V and I waveform for output voltage (27 V)

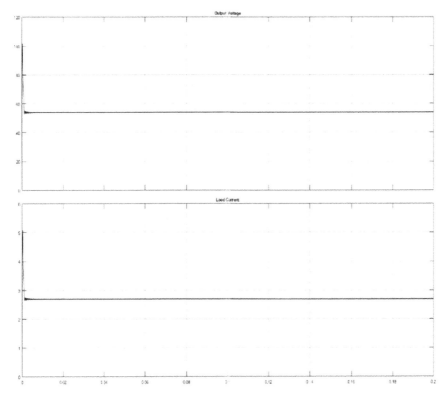

Fig. 6 V and I waveform for output voltage (54 V)

4.1 15-Level H-Bridge Symmetrical Multilevel Inverter

This circuit uses seven equal DC voltage sources which are taken in the ratio of 1:1:1:1:1:1:1 (i.e., $V_1 = V_2 = V_3 = V_4 = V_5 = V_6 = V_7 = V_{dc}$). The circuit is analyzed to obtain 28 switching states, i.e., V, 2 V, 3 V, 4 V, 5 V, 6 V, 7 V, 0, $-V$, -2 V, -3 V, -4 V, -5 V, -6 V, and -7 V (Figs. 8 and 9).

4.2 15-Level H-Bridge Asymmetrical Multilevel Inverter

This circuit uses three unequal DC voltage sources which are taken in the ratio of 1:2:4 (i.e., V1 = Vdc, V2 = 2 Vdc, and V3 = 4 Vdc). The circuit is analyzed to obtain 15 switching states, i.e., V, 2V, 3 V, 4 V, 5 V, 6 V, 7 V, 0, $-V$, -2 V, -3 V, -4 V, -5 V, -6 V, and -7 V.

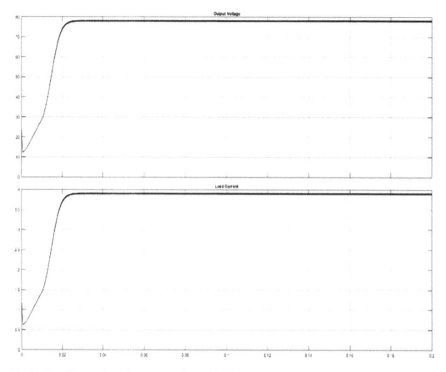

Fig. 7 V and I waveform for output voltage (78 V)

4.3 Equal Area Criteria Method

Equal Area Criterion:

- EAC is a simple technique executed to get minimum THD for any number of levels. This technique is used mainly to obtain initial switching angles; these angles are obtained with reference to the fundamental sine wave. The fundamental sine wave is divided into horizontally and vertically with step voltage and time (ms), respectively.
  The A1 and A2 areas shown in Fig. 10 should be equal in order to get minimum THD. The fundamental switching frequency is 50 Hz. The a_1, a_2, a_3, ... a_n are the switching angles for N-level MLI and should vary between 0° and 90°.
- Mathematical formula for angle calculation:
  Nth switching angle in (deg.) = [[Time at which the Nth-level vertical line touches the time axis (x-axis)] * [2 * fundamental frequency]] * 180°.

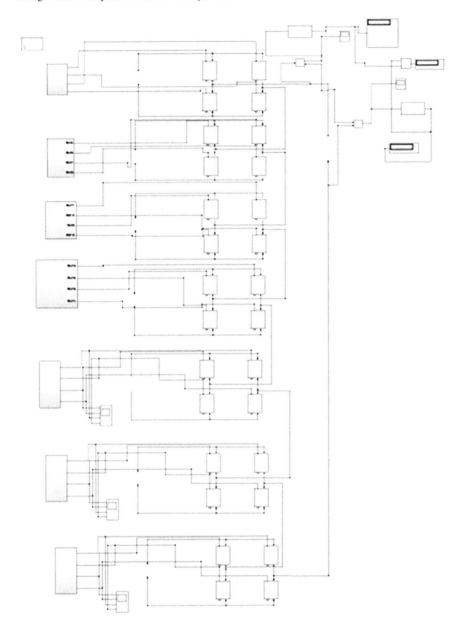

Fig. 8 15 H-bridge symmetrical inverter

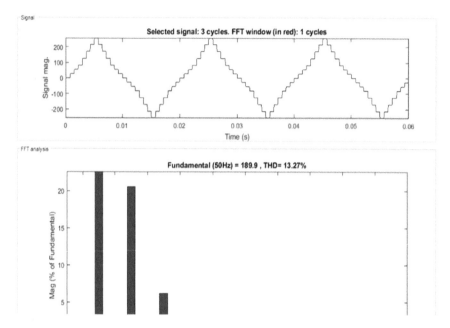

Fig. 9 15 H-bridge symmetrical inverter simulation output

Fig. 10 Equal area
calculation for 15 levels

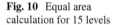
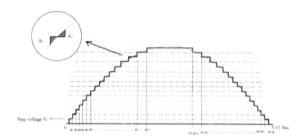

The number of switching angles required for N number of levels is obtained using
[(Number of levels-1)/2].

- The switching angles obtained for 15 levels are: $a_1 = 3.375°$, $a_2 = 11.8125°$, $a_3 = 21.375°$, $a_4 = 29.8125°$, $a_5 = 40.5°$, $a_6 = 51.1875°$, and $a_7 = 66.375°$. These switching angles are converted into time (ms), and in these time intervals, the power switches are turned ON.

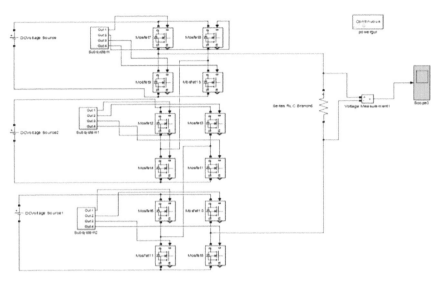

Fig. 11 15 H-bridge symmetrical inverter

4.4   Simulink Model of a New 15-Level Asymmetrical Multilevel Inverter Topology with DC Source

See (Figs. 11 and 12).

5   Hardware Implementation

The hardware model is designed by using MOSFETs as switches for both boost converters and H-bridge inverter circuits. The module is designed to have two PCBs, one for boost converter and other for inverter circuit. Boost converter output can be varied by varying the duty cycle of the switch. The gate signals are generated as per the value of the angles obtained by equal area criterion using an Arduino board. The Arduino board has the flexibility of simple coding for the required levels of output. The board is tested to obtain output for 11, 13, 15 levels by varying the duty cycle of the boost converters to obtain desired voltage levels (Fig. 13).

25ohm + 100mH

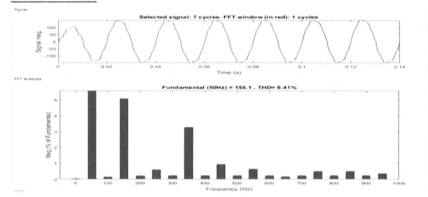

Fig. 12 15 H-bridge symmetrical inverter simulation output

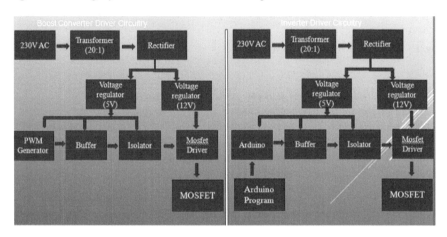

Fig. 13 Hardware implementation block diagram

The input voltage required for the controllers was 5 and 12 V in order to drive them by using a step-down transformer and rectifier 12 V DC is obtained. By using LM7805 and LM7812 regulator, regulated voltage is obtained. The MOSFET component is selected based on the criteria that the Vgs > 10 V, i.e., IRFP250N. The IRFP250N is a HEXFET power MOSFET with model no. TO-247AC. A power diode MUR1560G is used for power circuit. The controllers used for generating the pulses of required amplitude in the required sequential manner in order to drive the MOSFETs are TL494. The drivers are selected in order to drive the MOSFETs, is IR2101.

5.1 Controller: Arduino

The Atmel AVR® core combines a rich instruction set with 32 general-purpose working registers. All the 32 registers are directly connected to arithmetic logic unit (ALU), allowing two independent registers to be accessed in a single instruction executed in one clock cycle. The resulting architecture is more code efficient while achieving throughputs up to ten times faster than conventional CISC microcontrollers. An optocoupler-based driver circuit TLP250 is employed to trigger the MOSFETS (Figs. 14 and 15).

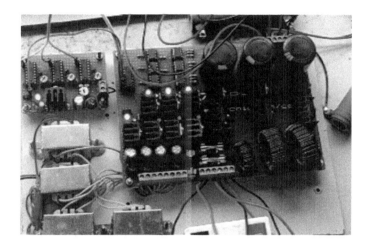

Fig. 14 Boost converter

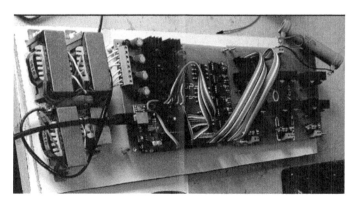

Fig. 15 15-level multilevel inverter

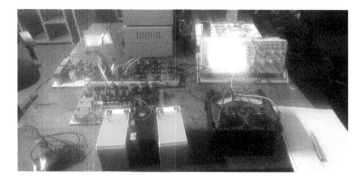

Fig. 16 Boost converter and inverter together

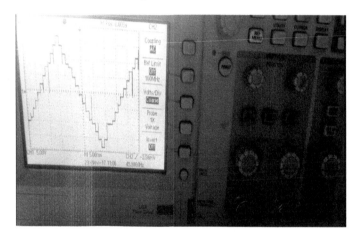

Fig. 17 Practical 15-level output

5.2 Boost Converter Integrated with 15-Level MLI

The hardware model designed is tested to obtain output for 11, 13, 15 levels by varying the duty cycle of the boost converters to obtain desired voltage levels (Figs. 16 and 17).

6 Conclusion

Here in this paper, simulation studies made on 15-level symmetrical and asymmetrical 15-level cascaded multilevel inverter with equal area criteria switching technique has been presented. The results show that asymmetrical circuit gives more output with less loss. Also, asymmetrical circuit uses less number of switches, hence able to produce more output, and has more efficiency which has less cost compared to symmetrical circuit. The circuits are simulated using MATLAB/Simulink. To validate the simulated results, the 15-level asymmetrical circuit has been developed using a hardware model, and the hardware circuit is also tested with different loads. The simulated and hardware results obtained are tabulated in the table. The topology gives a total harmonic distortion maximum of 6.5% for a load of $R = 25 \ \Omega$, $L = 100$ mH. The output from 15-level asymmetrical hardware model has been obtained satisfactorily.

This work is done on 15-level cascaded multilevel inverter. This work may be carried out for any higher levels by varying the number of H-bridges and by varying the ratios of the DC input voltage values. Also, the same circuit can be tested for different advanced control techniques (like soft switching techniques) which may result in lesser THD and a quality output signal.

Comparative Study of 31-Level Symmetrical and Asymmetrical Cascaded H-Bridge Multilevel Inverter

Rakshitha R. Prabhu, J. Madhusudhana and P. S. Puttaswamy

Abstract Multilevel inverters (MLI) are suitable for high power and medium voltage applications. Number of topologies has been introduced among which the cascaded H-bridge (CHB) inverter is widely used because of its simplicity. It consists of number of power semiconductor switches and DC voltage sources to generate step voltage waveform. The use of separate DC voltage source for each H-bridge allows the CHB inverter to be easily integrated with photovoltaic systems. Depending upon DC voltage source, the CHB inverter has two types: symmetrical CHB inverter which consists of equal DC voltage sources and asymmetrical CHB inverter with unequal DC voltage sources. Symmetrical inverter topology suffers from increased number of power devices, complexity and losses with the increase in number of output levels, whereas asymmetrical topology uses less number of power devices for producing higher level output voltage waveform. In this paper, analysis and simulation results for 31-level symmetrical and asymmetrical CHB MLI are presented.

Keywords Multilevel inverter (MLI) · Cascaded H-bridge inverter (CHB) · Total harmonic distortion (THD)

1 Introduction

MLI technology is a useful solution for reducing switching loss in high power application. There have been immense growth of technology and advancement of this type of inverters leading to its increased industrial application.

R. R. Prabhu (✉) · J. Madhusudhana
Department of Electrical Engineering, UVCE, Bangalore, India
e-mail: rakshithaprabhu10@gmail.com

J. Madhusudhana
e-mail: madhutmkr@yahoo.com

P. S. Puttaswamy
Department of Electrical Engineering, PES College of Engineering, Mandya 571401, Karnataka, India
e-mail: psputtaswamy_ee@yahoo.com

© Springer Nature Singapore Pte Ltd. 2019
V. Sridhar et al. (eds.), *Emerging Research in Electronics, Computer Science and Technology*, Lecture Notes in Electrical Engineering 545,
https://doi.org/10.1007/978-981-13-5802-9_102

MLI has many advantages over conventional 2-level inverters such as higher power quality, better electromagnetic interface, less harmonic content, lower switching losses, lower harmonic distortion and higher efficiency [1]. In addition to this, the electromagnetic interference and size are reduced [2]. It is noted that the above advantages have a direct relation with the number of levels of the output voltage produced by the inverter. Higher the number of levels, closer the waveform to sine wave, thereby decreases the THD [3, 4].

There are three kinds of basic MLI topologies: neutral point clamped (NPC), flying capacitor (FC) and cascaded H-bridge (CHB) MLI. NPC topology uses diodes and gives different voltage levels to the capacitor banks connected in series. FC topology uses capacitors to transfer voltage to electrical devices. In CHB inverters, H-bridges containing separate DC sources and switches are cascaded. Among these, CHB is preferable because of its simple structure, easy expandability to higher voltage levels, reliability, modularity and interfacing capability with the renewable energy resources (RER).

2 Symmetrical Cascaded H-Bridge Inverter

For a MLI, several H-bridges are connected in cascade and each of the H-bridges consists of a separate DC source. In case of symmetrical CHB inverters, the values of the DC voltage sources are equal. As the number of output voltage level increases, the number of H-bridges increases, thereby increasing the number of switching devices in the structure. This contributes to more switching losses, thus reducing the overall efficiency of the inverter.

Figure 1 shows the general circuit for 'm' level symmetrical CHB inverter having 'N' H-bridges in cascade. Table 1 shows the switching states for the same.

In order to generate 'm' level output voltage in symmetrical configuration:

$$\text{The number of H-bridges to be cascaded} = N = (m-1)/2 \tag{1}$$
$$\text{The number of separate DC sources required} = (m-1)/2 \tag{2}$$
$$\text{The number of switching devices in the circuit} = 2(m-1) \tag{3}$$

The equation to obtain 'm' level output voltage:

$$V_0 = V_1 + V_2 + \cdots + V_N = \sum_{n=0}^{(m-1)/2} V_n \tag{4}$$

where $V_1, V_2, \ldots, V_k$ are the voltage output of each H-bridge. And V_0 is the sum of the voltages of 'N' such H-bridge to obtain multilevel output voltage.

Similarly to obtain m = 31-level output voltage, the number of H-bridges is N = 15 and the number of switching devices required is 60.

Fig. 1 Circuit for 'm' level symmetrical CHB inverter having N H-bridges

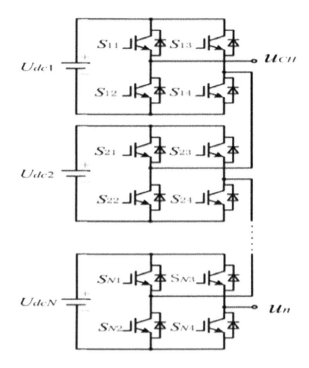

Table 1 Switching table for Nth H-bridge inverter

Switches in ON state	Output voltage (Vo)
S_{N1}, S_{N4}	VDC
S_{N1}	0
S_{N3}	0
S_{N2}, S_{N3}	−VDC

3 Asymmetrical Cascaded H-Bridge Inverter

In asymmetrical CHB inverters, the values of the DC voltage sources are unequal. The values are in specific ratios such as 1:2:3:4 or 1:2:4:8. These ratios should be given in such a way that all output voltage levels can be generated.

By implementing asymmetrical topology, more levels in the output voltage can be obtained with less number of H-bridges. This makes it cost-effective, compact and efficient.

Figure 2 shows circuit for 31-level asymmetrical CHB inverter having DC voltage sources in the ratio 1:2:4:8. Table 2 shows the switching states to generate 31-level output voltage. The pulses are given to switches by connecting pulse generator to the gate terminal of each switch. Equal phase angle technique is used to generate these pulses.

The number of levels can be increased to get lower values of THD by cascading more H-bridges to the below circuit.

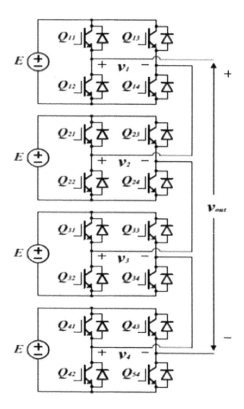

Fig. 2 Circuit for 31-level asymmetrical CHB inverter with DC voltage sources in ratio 1:2:4:8

Table 2 Switching table for 31-level asymmetrical CHB inverter for source ratio 1:2:4:8

E	Q_{11}	Q_{12}	Q_{13}	Q_{14}	Q_{21}	Q_{22}	Q_{23}	Q_{24}	Q_{31}	Q_{32}	Q_{33}	Q_{34}	Q_{41}	Q_{42}	Q_{43}	Q_{54}
15	1	0	0	1	1	0	0	1	1	0	0	1	1	0	0	1
14	1	0	0	0	1	0	0	1	1	0	0	1	1	0	0	1
13	1	0	0	1	1	0	0	0	1	0	0	1	1	0	0	1
12	1	0	0	0	1	0	0	0	1	0	0	1	1	0	0	1
11	1	0	0	1	1	0	0	1	1	0	0	0	1	0	0	1
10	1	0	0	0	1	0	0	1	1	0	0	0	1	0	0	1
9	1	0	0	1	1	0	0	0	1	0	0	0	1	0	0	1
8	1	0	0	0	1	0	0	0	1	0	0	0	1	0	0	1
7	1	0	0	1	1	0	0	1	1	0	0	1	1	0	0	0
6	1	0	0	0	1	0	0	1	1	0	0	1	1	0	0	0
5	1	0	0	1	1	0	0	0	1	0	0	1	1	0	0	0
4	1	0	0	0	1	0	0	0	1	0	0	1	1	0	0	0
3	1	0	0	1	1	0	0	1	1	0	0	0	1	0	0	0

(continued)

Table 2 (continued)

E	Q_{11}	Q_{12}	Q_{13}	Q_{14}	Q_{21}	Q_{22}	Q_{23}	Q_{24}	Q_{31}	Q_{32}	Q_{33}	Q_{34}	Q_{41}	Q_{42}	Q_{43}	Q_{54}
2	1	0	0	0	1	0	0	1	1	0	0	0	1	0	0	0
1	1	0	0	1	1	0	0	0	1	0	0	0	1	0	0	0
0	1	0	0	0	1	0	0	0	1	0	0	0	1	0	0	0

4 Analysis and Simulation Results

The proposed 31-level symmetrical and asymmetrical CHB inverter is simulated using MATLAB/Simulink. The voltage rating of the output voltage of inverter is fixed to be:

$$V_{orms} = 230 \text{ V}$$

Therefore, the peak voltage is given by:

$$V_m = \sqrt{2} * V_{orms} = \sqrt{2} * 230 = 324 \text{ V}$$

Output voltage waveform is obtained, and harmonic analysis is done for different RL loads. These results are then compared for symmetrical and asymmetrical topologies.

4.1 Symmetrical Cascaded H-Bridge 31-Level Inverter

Figure 3 shows the MATLAB/Simulink circuit for symmetrical CHB 31-level inverter in which 15 H-bridges and 60 switching devices (MOSFETs) are used.

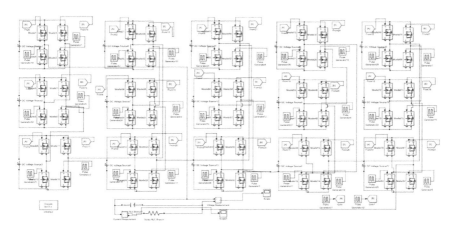

Fig. 3 MATLAB/Simulink circuit for 31-level symmetrical CHB inverter

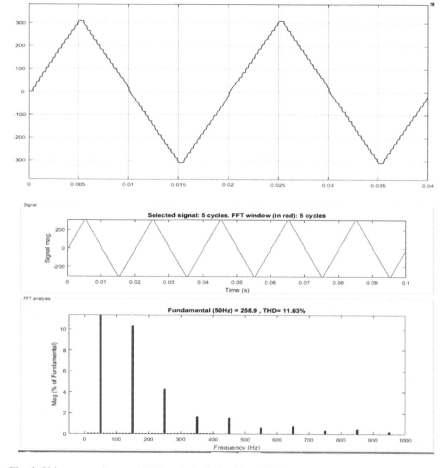

Fig. 4 Voltage waveform and FFT analysis for load R = 50 Ω and L = 50 mH

Therefore, 15 separate DC sources are required with equal values:

$$V_m/31 = 324/31 = 21.6 \text{ V}$$

Thus to generate higher level output voltage, more H-bridges are cascaded in this case. Therefore, large number of switches and DC voltages sources are needed which makes the inverter bulky, expensive and complicated. The voltage waveform is obtained, and FFT analysis for symmetrical CHB 31-level inverter is done and presented as shown in Figs. 4, 5 and 6.

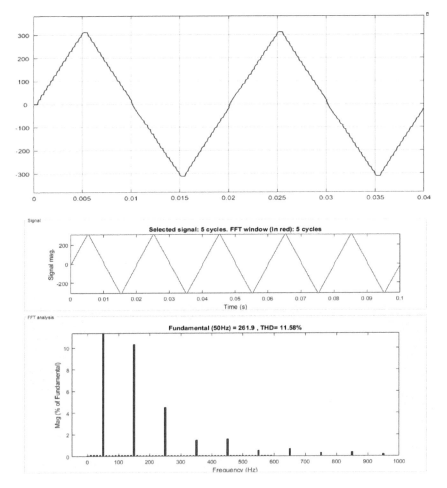

Fig. 5 Voltage waveform and FFT analysis for load R = 50 Ω and L = 100 mH

4.2 Asymmetrical Cascaded H-Bridge 31-Level Inverter

Figure 7 shows the MATLAB/Simulink circuit for asymmetrical CHB 31-level inverter in which 4 H-bridges and 16 switching devices (MOSFETs) are used. The DC voltage sources are in ratio 1:2:4:8 having values are:

$$V_{DC1} = 21.6 \text{ V}, \ V_{DC2} = 43.2 \text{ V}, \ V_{DC3} = 86.4 \text{ V}, \ V_{DC4} = 172.8 \text{ V}$$

$$\text{Sum gives}: \quad V_{DC1} + V_{DC2} + V_{DC3} + V_{DC4} = V_m = 324$$

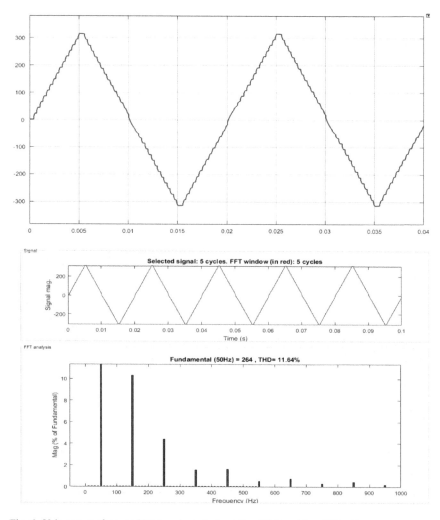

Fig. 6 Voltage waveform and FFT analysis for load R = 75 Ω and L = 100 mH

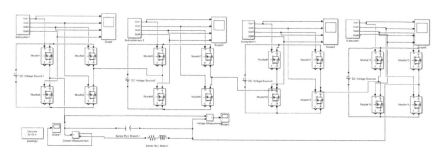

Fig. 7 MATLAB/Simulink circuit for 31-level asymmetrical CHB inverter

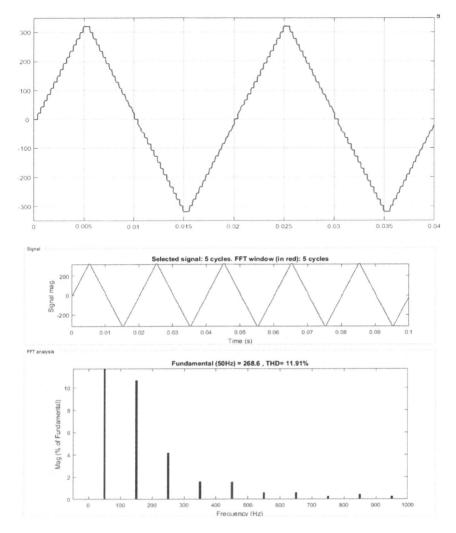

Fig. 8 Voltage waveform and FFT analysis for load R = 50 Ω and L = 50 mH

This topology is more efficient, compact and cost-effective compared to the symmetrical topology. But the main drawback is that the voltage stress on each switch is different and also the gate pulse given to each of the switches is complex. The voltage waveform is obtained, and FFT analysis is done for asymmetrical CHB 31-level inverter and presented as shown in Figs. 8, 9 and 10.

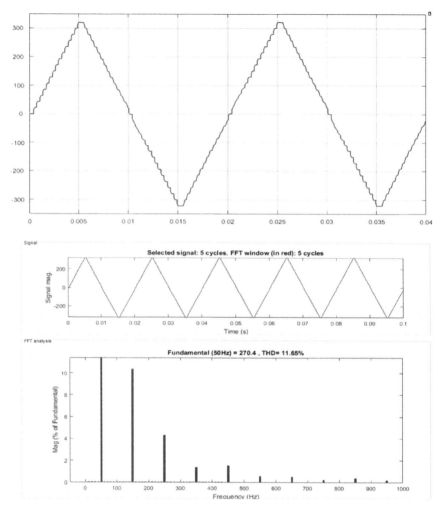

Fig. 9 Voltage waveform and FFT analysis for load R = 50 Ω and L = 100 m

4.3   Simulation Results

The results are tabulated for 31-level symmetrical and asymmetrical CHB inverter in Tables 3 and 4, respectively, for different loads. From the table, it is observed that the value of the output RMS voltage (V_{orms}) is more in asymmetrical topology for the same load. This is because the number of switching device (16) in this topology is less compared to that of symmetrical topology (60), contributing to less voltage drop across each switch, thereby increasing the power delivered to the load.

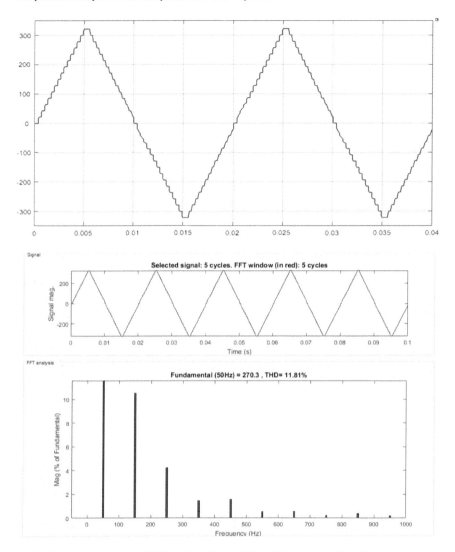

Fig. 10 Voltage waveform and FFT analysis for load R = 75 Ω and L = 100 mH

Table 3 Tabulated results of various parameters for 31-level symmetrical CHB inverter for different loads

R (Ω)	L (mH)	Vorms (V)	Iorms (A)	Porms (W)	THD (%)	No of switches	nth Harmonic component			
							3rd	5th	7th	9th
50	50	184	3.5	646	11.63	60	10.3	4.3	1.6	1.6
50	100	186	3.15	586	11.58	60	10.3	4.5	1.5	1.6
75	100	187	2.3	432	11.64	60	10.3	4.4	1.6	1.6

Table 4 Tabulated results of various parameters for 31-level asymmetrical CHB inverter for different loads

R (Ω)	L (mH)	Vorms (V)	Iorms (A)	Porms (W)	THD (%)	No of switches	nth Harmonic component			
							3rd	5th	7th	9th
50	50	191	3.64	695	11.91	16	10.6	4.1	1.5	1.5
50	100	192	3.25	624	11.65	16	10.4	4.3	1.4	1.5
75	100	192	2.36	453	11.81	16	10.5	4.2	1.5	1.6

The total harmonic distortion (THD) in both the topologies is observed to be same. Because the value of THD solely depends on the number of levels of output voltage and is independent from the type of topology used.

5 Conclusion

From the above analysis, the asymmetrical CHB inverter has higher output voltage and power, making it more efficient. Also, to generate same level output voltage, the number DC sources and switches in asymmetrical topology is significantly reduced making it more compact and cost-effective.

The THD value is observed to be independent of the type of topology used. To get lesser values of THD, more levels must be present in the output voltage.

6 Future Scope

Rather than using equal phase angle switching technique as above, other optimized switching techniques such as genetic algorithm, neural network can be used to control switching action of the switches. This can reduce the harmonic contents in the output voltage.

Furthermore, closed-loop control can be incorporated to regulate the output voltage of required value.

Also, a photovoltaic array can be given as an input to each H-bridge inverter instead of constant DC voltage supply.

References

1. Fallah M, Imani M, Abarzadeh M, Kojabadi HM, Hejri M (2016) Load compensation n based on frame considering low-order dominant harmonics and distorted power system. Control Eng Pract 51:1–12

2. Ali US, Kamaraj V (2013) Bipolar multicarrier pwm techniques for cascaded quasi-z-source multilevel inverter. In: International conference on circuits, power and computing technologies (ICCPCT), pp 236–240
3. Kangarlu MF, Babaei E (2013) Cross-switched multilevel inverter: an innovative topology. IET Power Electron 6(4):642—651
4. Salam Z, Majed A, Amjad AM (2015) Design and implementation of 15-level cascaded multi-level voltage source inverter with harmonics elimination pulse-width modulation using differential evolution method. IET Power Electron 8(9):1740–1748

Three-Phase Shunt Active Filter for Cuk-Sepic Fused Converter with Solar–Wind Hybrid Sources

M. R. Harshith Gowda and K. U. Vinayaka

Abstract At the present time, the use of nonconventional energy resources is having a huge demand as the conventional energy sources are depleting in nature and causing more pollution which ensures the need of renewable energy resources. This paper deals with the design of a cuk-sepic converter with a three-phase inverter feeding a nonlinear load. Harmonics will be introduced to the system due to the use of nonlinear load which will affect the equipment in both source and load end, so there is a need of filter to mitigate the harmonics. Here, a shunt active filter is used which will reduce the harmonics introduced in the circuit. The desired low harmonic three-phase voltage is obtained as per the IEEE standard of below 5% as the filter results in 1.33% total harmonic distortion (THD). The simulations are carried out and analyzed by using PSIM software.

Keywords Cuk-sepic converter · Three-phase inverter · Dqo conversion · Active filter · Rectifier load

1 Introduction

Due to inadequate nonrenewable energy sources like fossil fuels as the power demand has been augmented, the renewable energy source has become a greater benefit. Pollutions are caused by the recourses based on fossil fuels. This will formulate us to think about the renewable energy resources which are abundant in nature and causes less pollution to the environment. The installation cost and space is more for the renewable energy systems, but the operating cost will be less as they use their principal sources by nature which are complimentary. As the different readily

M. R. H. Gowda · K. U. Vinayaka (✉)
Department of Electrical and Electronics Engineering, Siddaganga Institute of Technology, Tumakuru, India
e-mail: vinay.ene@gmail.com

M. R. H. Gowda
e-mail: appuarjun009@gmail.com

© Springer Nature Singapore Pte Ltd. 2019
V. Sridhar et al. (eds.), *Emerging Research in Electronics, Computer Science and Technology*, Lecture Notes in Electrical Engineering 545,
https://doi.org/10.1007/978-981-13-5802-9_103

available renewable energy resources are in nature, wind and solar energy sources have potential to meet the power demand.

Since the renewable energy sources have their application in microgrid (MG) systems, distributed grid (DG) systems, Green Offices and Apartments (GOA), etc. The lone negative aspect of these resources is they are unpredictable, as the weather changes and they are intermittent in nature. So there is a need of hybrid systems which will work with two or more resources (usually wind and solar) as per their existence in nature, and thus, the efficiency and lifetime of these systems are improved and also reduce the requirement of storage to an extent. As these systems will use numerous sources, the installing amount is high and becomes tangled which needs controlled supervision. There is a necessity of three-phase power for the industrial applications with low THD.

The cuk-sepic fused converter is used to generate the power by the renewable energy sources (solar and wind) which is fed to a three-phase inverter to generate the three-phase voltages. The load contains the nonlinear load which introduces the harmonics to the system which will be mitigated by the active filter.

2 Objective

The paper implements a single fused converter for the wind and solar hybrid system. This work proposes a dual-input, single-output DC–DC converter for a hybrid wind–solar energy system. The proposed topology allows both the sources to meet the load demand either individually or simultaneously depending on their availability. A three-phase inverter is proposed to generate the three-phase power, so by using the output of the proposed converter and a three-legged rectifier is used as the nonlinear load. The closed-loop mechanism of this circuit is simulated by using a simulation tool PSIM 9.1.1 (Fig. 1).

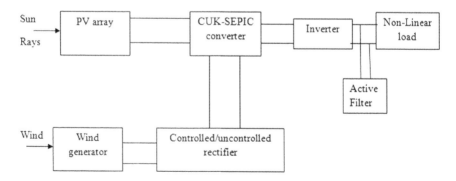

Fig. 1 Proposed block diagram

For stand-alone system, the proposed CUK-SEPIC converter operates as CUK converter when only PV source is available. It acts as a SEPIC converter when only wind source is available. When both the sources are available, the switches will turn ON. When both sources are unavailable, the switches will turn OFF. The output of this converter is fed to a three-phase inverter which consists of six MOSFET switches in a three-leg arrangement fed by a SPWM switching pulse generator; the output of this three-phase inverter is fed to a nonlinear load (a three-leg rectifier).

3 Proposed System

The proposed system has a Cuk-Sepic converter, a three-phase inverter, load, and an active filter. But as for here we have took the Photo voltaic array module is represented as the dc voltage source and the wind generator with the controlled rectifier is also represented as the dc source for simulation purpose (Fig. 2).

A Cuk-Sepic converter is a high-efficient DC–DC boost converter which will act as boost converter which has dual inputs, i.e., solar and wind. This converter works either both or any one of the sources is present. The converter boosts the voltage to feed a three-phase inverter (Fig. 3).

A three-phase inverter converts the dc source to the three-phase ac source. The power inverter is a device which produces stepped sine wave; the inverter output is more clearly a three-step wave (modified sine wave). The inverter will produce the three-phase sinusoidal waveform, and the RMS value of the line–line voltage should be more than 410 v (Fig. 4).

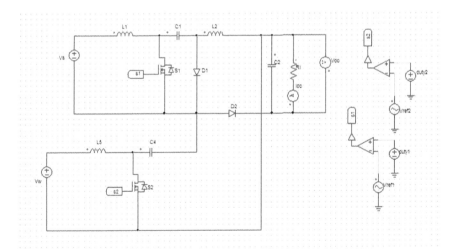

Fig. 2 Cuk-Sepic converter

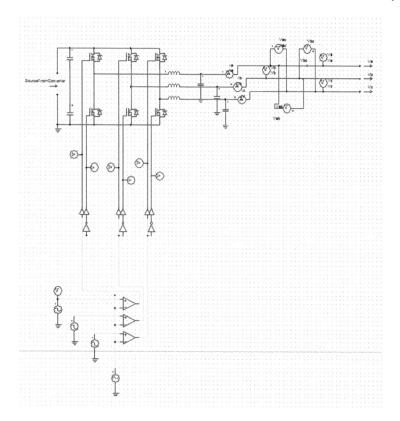

Fig. 3 Three-phase inverter

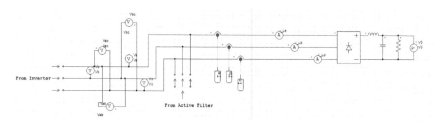

Fig. 4 Load (three-phase rectifier/nonlinear)

The output of the inverter is fed to the load which is a three-phase rectifier. The nonlinear load introduces the harmonics which will affect the source 5, 7, 11, and 13th harmonics which will highly affect the source. So, we have to use a filter which mitigates the harmonics. There are two types of harmonic filters, i.e., active filter and passive filters. The passive filter is a LC or LCL arranged to mitigate the harmonics (Fig. 5).

A passive filter is an arrangement of LC (inductor–capacitor) in series and parallel. Here, inductor is arranged in series and capacitor is placed in parallel to the inductor; the passive filter arrangement will reduce the some order of harmonics but not as per the requirement. The active filter is used to mitigate the harmonics (Fig. 6).

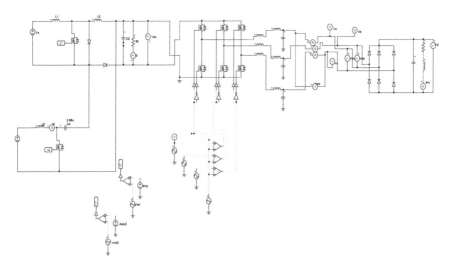

Fig. 5 Cuk-Sepic converter with only passive filter

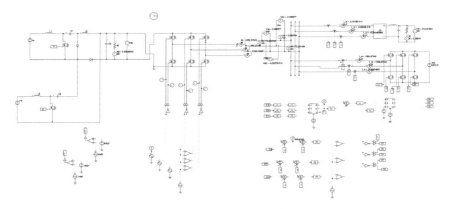

Fig. 6 Cuk-Sepic converter with only active filter

As we all know that the active filter is a very efficient type of harmonics filter as the active filter senses the harmonics in the source side and generates the reference current harmonics so that the reference current harmonics are equal to the source harmonics, so that the harmonics can be mitigated (Fig. 7).

Here, a shunt active filter which is a three-phase active will produce the source which is equal and opposite to the source power, so this will use the we have used this for this circuit. Here, the active filter will produce the reference waveform by using dqo compensation which is as shown in the above figure. In the dqo compensation, the source current is compared with the reference current; the resultant current is obtained and fed to the circuit. The reference current is so important in SAF. For eliminating harmonics of source current, SAF must inject a current that source current be sinuous form.

4   Calculation for the DQO Compensation

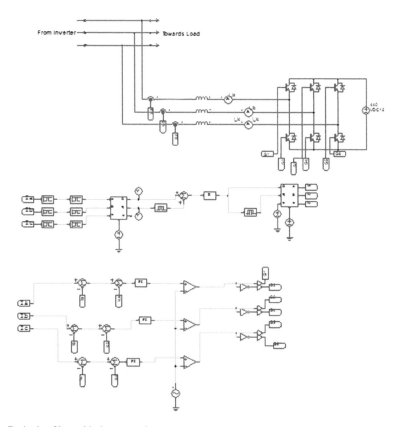

Fig. 7 Active filter with dqo control

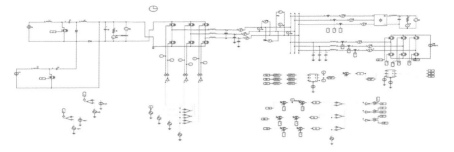

Fig. 8 Cuk-Sepic converter with combination of active and LC passive filters

$$i^*_{(1)ca} = i_{la} - i^+_{(1)la} \tag{1}$$

$$i^*_{(1)cc} = i_{lb} - i^+_{(1)lb} \tag{2}$$

$$i^*_{(1)cc} = i_{lc} - i^+_{(1)lc} \tag{3}$$

The relation between the above signals and positive, negative, and zero sequence is shown below (Fig. 8).

$$\begin{bmatrix} i_d \\ i_q \\ i_0 \end{bmatrix} = \frac{2}{3} \begin{bmatrix} 1 & -\frac{1}{2} & -\frac{1}{2} \\ 0 & -\frac{\sqrt{3}}{2} & -\frac{\sqrt{3}}{2} \\ \frac{1}{2} & \frac{1}{2} & \frac{1}{2} \end{bmatrix} \begin{bmatrix} 1 & 1 & 1 \\ 1 & \alpha^2 & \alpha \\ 1 & \alpha & \alpha^2 \end{bmatrix} \begin{bmatrix} i^+ \\ i^- \\ i^0 \end{bmatrix} \tag{4}$$

where $\alpha = 1 \llcorner 120°$

$$i^+ = \frac{1}{2} (i_d + j.i_q) \tag{5}$$

$$i^- = \frac{1}{2} (i_d - j.i_q) \tag{6}$$

5   Simulation Results

In Fig. 9, the wave shows the output voltage of the Cuk-Sepic fused converter which will use the solar and wind sources.

Figure 10 shows the waveform which is the output of the inverter without any filter; this will have more distortion, and the THD will be more so that the harmonics will be more (32.67, 45.88, and 33.32%, respectively), so we have to design a filter to mitigate the harmonics.

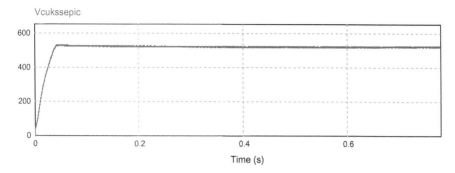

Fig. 9 Output voltage of cuk-sepic converter

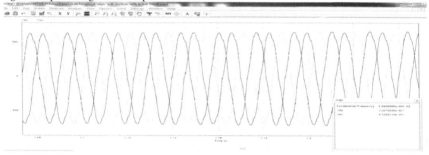

Fig. 10 Output voltage of inverter before adding filter

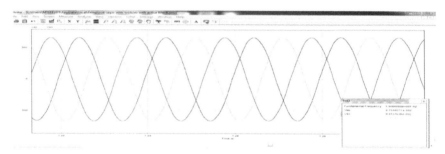

Fig. 11 Output voltage of inverter after adding LC filter

Figure 11 waveform will show the output waveform of the inverter with the passive (LC) filter which will be mitigate the harmonics will be at the passive filter which is an arrangement of L & C to eradicate the harmonics; due to this arrangement, the harmonic will be mitigated to some extent as the passive filter will mitigate the harmonics up to some extent (9.753, 9.913, and 9.842%, respectively).

Figure 12 shows the waveform which represents the output of the inverter with only active filter where the active filter will mitigate the harmonics of the circuit to a greater extent as the harmonics will be of extent 6.873, 7.110, and 4.822%,

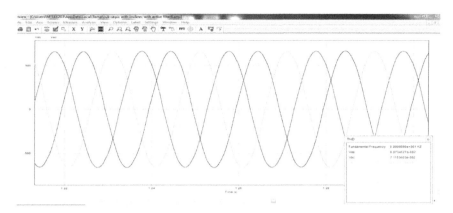

Fig. 12 Output voltage of inverter with active filter

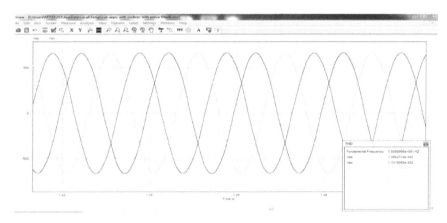

Fig. 13 Output voltage of inverter an active and passive filters

respectively, as this will be having the very low THD, but this THD is not satisfactory; so we have used the combination of the active and passive filters.

Figure 13 shows the output of the inverter with the combination of the active and passive filters where this combination of the filter will mitigate the harmonics to a greater extent so that the THD will be very much lower than the standard THD value, i.e., below 5% (1.2607, 1.323, and 1.2788%, respectively) so that this is an effective filter to mitigate the harmonics.

Figure 14 shows the source harmonics and reference current waveforms as the reference current is generated to mitigate the harmonics which are introduced in the system which will be equal to the source harmonics current.

Figure 15 shows the inverter current waveforms after the addition of the filter, where the harmonics are mitigated and a pure sine wave is obtained.

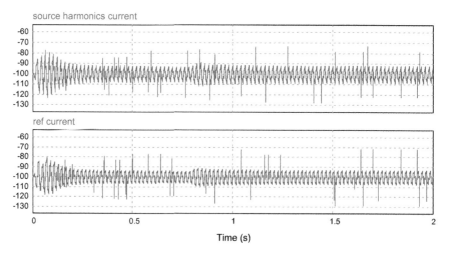

Fig. 14 Waveforms of the source and reference current

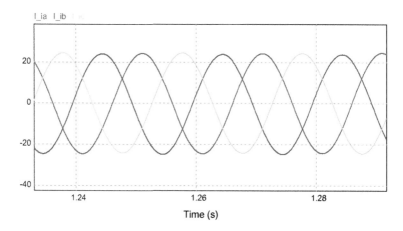

Fig. 15 Output current waveforms

6 Results

As we have got the waveforms and results by simulating the circuit, we have obtained the results using PSIM software.

i. Output of the cuk-sepic converter

$$V_{cuk-sepic} = 530v$$

ii. Output voltage of the load/circuit

$$V_0 = 650\,v$$

iii. Output power of the circuit

$$P_0 = 3.125\,KW$$

7 THD with Various Filters

Table 1 shows the work which contains the comparison of various filters which are used for this circuit, and the result is obtained from them. The filter which we have come to conclusion is a combination of an active and passive filter which will give the harmonics desired in the IEEE standards.

8 Conclusion

The paper discusses the fused cuk-sepic converter with a three-phase inverter for the industrial applications.

The output of the inverter obtained is having 410 v AC voltage with a minimum harmonics which is in permissible level.

The harmonics in the system is mitigated so that the damage of the loads by the harmonics; this ensures the safety of the equipment at the load side.

The Cuk-Sepic converter is an efficient converter to produce the energy by the solar and wind sources.

According to the IEEE standards 519–2014 is 5% but this converter circuit operates at 1.33% maximum, so this system has more benefit.

Table 1 THD comparison of various filters

THD using various filters

Filters	Vab (%)	Vac (%)	Vbc (%)
Without filter	32.67	45.88	33.32
With LC (passive) filter	9.753	9.913	9.842
With active filter	6.873	7.110	4.822
With combination of active and passive filters	1.2788	1.323	1.2607

References

1. Vinayaka KU, Krishnan V (2016) Applications of fused DC-DC converters using hybrid wind-solar sysetms. In: 1st IEEE International conference on power electronics, intelligent control and energy systems (ICPEICES-2016)
2. Asadi M, Jalian A, Farahani HF (2010) Compensation of unbalanced non linear load and neutral currents using stationary reference frame in shunt active filter. In: 14th international conference on harmonics and quality of power (ICIIQP)
3. Ahuja RKR, Verma S, Dhull B Simulation of three phase active filter for harmonics reduction and reactive power compensation. Int J Adv Res Electr Electron Instrum Eng
4. Viji AJ, Sudhakaran M Three phase active shunt power filter with simple control in psim simulation. J Inf Eng Appl
5. Kothuru S, Kotturu J, Kumar CH (2014) Reduction of harmonics in 3-phase, 3-wiresystem by the use of shunt active filter. In: International conference on circuit, power and computing technologies (ICCPCT)
6. Rahman T, Motakabber SMA, Ibrahimy MI (2016) Design of a switching mode three phase inverter. In: International conference on computer & communication engineering
7. Nayeripour M, Niknam T Design of a three phase active power filter with sliding mode control and energy feedback. World Acad Sci Eng Technol
8. Leonardo B, Camphol G, Sérgio A, Silva O, Goedtel A Application of shunt active power filter for harmonicreduction and reactive power compensation in three phase four-wire systems. IET Power Electron

Study of Different Modelling Techniques of SMA Actuator and Their Validation Through Simulation

Prakruthi Vasanth, G. M. Kamalakannan and C. S. Shivaraj

Abstract With the increased emphasis on both reliability and functionality, shape memory alloys (SMAs) are fast becoming an enabling technology capturing the attention of engineers and scientists worldwide. The thermal-electrical-mechanical dynamics of SMA are nonlinear and hysteretic in nature, possessing a problem for the researchers to model the actuator. The increased range of applications and better realisation of SMA actuators have led to the research on modelling of SMA's thermo-mechanical response. The paper discusses various SMA actuator modelling approaches such as Preisach model, Fermi–Dirac statistics, Duhem hysteresis model and Brinson model and attempts to elucidate their advantages and limitations through Simulink-based models and simulation results.

Keywords Shape memory alloy · Phase transformation · Dynamics · Martensite · Austenite · Modelling · Simulation

1 Introduction

The shape memory alloy (SMA) is a smart actuator, which has the ability to memorise the trained shape or form and return to it after deformation when subjected to certain stimulus. The core advantages of SMA actuator include high strength to weight ratio, lightweight and noiseless. But the SMA suffers from hysteresis, and the actuator is nonlinear in nature.

The SMA exhibits unique property of remembering its previous crystalline structures when transformed from martensite to austenite phase. When the SMA actuators are subjected to Joule heating, the SMA wire is subjected to thermal-electrical-

P. Vasanth (✉) · C. S. Shivaraj
Department of Electrical and Electronics Engineering,
The National Institute of Engineering, Mysuru, Mysuru, India
e-mail: prakruthivasantha@gmail.com

G. M. Kamalakannan
CSMST, CSIR-NAL, Bangalore, India

© Springer Nature Singapore Pte Ltd. 2019 1211
V. Sridhar et al. (eds.), *Emerging Research in Electronics, Computer Science and Technology*, Lecture Notes in Electrical Engineering 545,
https://doi.org/10.1007/978-981-13-5802-9_104

mechanical dynamics. These dynamics also include nonlinearity and hysteretic behaviour that are difficult to be modelled accurately. Also, due to the fatigue behaviour of SMA along with its initial thermal mechanical conditioning. The direct design and implementation of SMA model would pose a difficulty to the designers.

Khandelwal and Buravalla [1] classified the SMA modelling techniques into microscopic and macroscopic levels. The microscopic study of the SMA deals with the crystal and the lattice dynamics, whereas the macroscopic study is used to understand the phase field, hysteresis and the propagation from one phase to another, which is more relevant for actuator applications.

In general, for the macroscopic analysis of SMA, a three-prong method is applied [2]. They are:

1. Thermodynamic model
2. Phase transformation model
3. Kinematic model.

The thermodynamics is mainly used to correlate the supply voltage or current as a function of time with the temperature rise in the SMA actuator under heat loss condition. The phase transformation is the relation between the martensite/austenite fraction and temperature rise. Since the SMA simultaneously possess both martensite and austenite phases at varying degrees as a nonlinear function of temperature and other parameters, accurate modelling becomes difficult. The phase transformation phenomenon is the core contributor of hysteresis, and many different research approaches are found in the literature. The main approaches are discussed in this paper. The kinematic model is mainly used to calculate the stress or strain along with the displacement that could be linear or rotational. The kinematic model mainly depends on the shape of the actuator, the type of motion and the stress–strain relationship.

Many researchers have investigated the use of different modelling techniques for the implementation of shape memory alloy using Simulink or LabVIEW. Tanaka et al. [3] used the stress–strain–temperature behaviour of SMA in thermo-mechanics perspective to explain the kinetics of transformation. But the major drawback of Tanaka et al. model [3] is that the model does not explain the stress-induced detwinning of the martensite phase and also the martensite fraction is assumed as a function of temperature only.

Muller and Xu [4] and Falk [5] proposed a model based on a polynomial that describes the thermo-mechanical behaviour of SMA. Though the model was simple and provided good description about the system dynamics, it failed to represent the hysteresis of the material. Also, Aurichhio and Lubliner [6] generalised the SMA model based on only two internal variables: single variant martensite fraction and multiple variant martensite fraction, but in practical cases, the phase transformation also depends on the stress loading and unloading.

Bekker and Brinson [7] derived the model of SMA based on the phase diagram approach. The phase diagrams of SMA did not have defined procedure for tracking the actual behaviour of the alloy. In the paper [8], the Brinson model was used to obtain the phenomenological model under antagonistic configuration, but the theoretical and empirical results of strain and temperature did not match. Using the Brinson's [2] and dimensional model of Liang and Rogers [9], Abiri et al. [10] have constructed a state-space model, but since the equations are nonlinear, the state-space representation could not clearly model the state of the SMA actuator.

Furst et al. [11, 12] developed the SMA model based on the Gibbs free energy landscape and the probability of constitutive grain of SMA material switching phases. But the model in [11] holds good as long as SMA's behaviour is repeatable. Huo [13] initially uses Landau–Devonshire free energy to realise the thermodynamic properties of individual crystallites, resulting in the four-dimensional Preisach space which could not be practically analysed.

Sayyadi et al. [14] explain the theoretical aspects of Tanaka, Liang and Brinson model. He compared the theoretical models with the experimental test results of differential scanning calorimeter (DSC) test and loading tests [1, 14]. Based on the comparison, the corrected evolution kinetics was proposed for the Brinson model. However, the corrected evolution kinetics is very complex for analysis and simulation. In paper [15], the modelling and simulation of advanced shape memory alloy effects such as reorientation of martensite under multiaxial loading, training of two-way shape memory alloy and thermo-mechanical coupling were discussed. But in practicality, these advanced effects are rarely used as these make the modelling even more complex.

The paper [16] summarises the list of researchers who modelled the SMA along with their approach details. The paper [16] did not provide exact details about the constitutive modelling approaches. Paiva and Savi [17] validated five phenomenological theories such as to explain the general thermo-mechanical behaviour of SMA. The authors have also tried to explain the phase transformation due to temperature variations and internal subloops due to incomplete phase transformation. But from the results, the Brinson model proved to be better than the other phenomenological models. Khandelwal and Buravalla [1] classified the modelling techniques based on their own discretion for better understanding. The paper was only able to provide theoretical aspects of modelling and did not provide evolution equations for obtaining the models through MATLAB/Simulink.

In the following sections, the most commonly used models are constructed using MATLAB/Simulink and the modelling approaches are analysed using the parameters given in the literature. In the addition, the thermodynamics of SMA, advantages and drawbacks of the modelling techniques are discussed.

2 Thermodynamics of SMA

The thermodynamics of SMA mainly is used to relate the physical parameter (temperature) with the electrical parameter (power). From the law of conservation of energy, the rate of temperature rise is proportional to the difference between the supplied power and heat losses [2, 18–24]. The equation of thermodynamics is provided in Eq. (1) with L_0 and d_0 which are the length and the diameter of the SMA wire.

$$\rho c \frac{\pi d_0^2 L_0}{4} \frac{dT}{dt} = RI^2 - \pi d_0 L_0 h(T - T_0) \tag{1}$$

where t is the time-independent variable, c is specific heat constant, ρ is wire density, R is electrical wire resistance, h is the convective heat coefficient, T_a is ambient temperature, i(t) is the input current, and T(t) is the temperature. The Simulink representation of the thermodynamics is presented in Fig. 1. In Fig. 2, for the initial temperature of 25 °C, the SMA wire requires a finite time for the temperature to rise.

Also, in the paper [25, 26], the temperature dynamics is based on the first law of thermodynamics and Fourier's law as in (2).

$$\rho c \frac{dT}{dt} = \nabla \cdot (k \nabla T) - h(T - T_0) + P_e \tag{2}$$

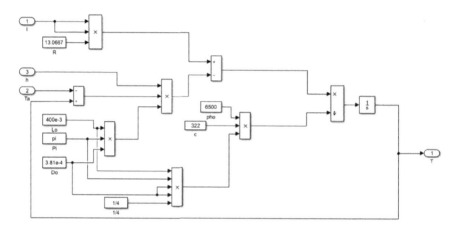

Fig. 1 Simulink diagram for thermal model of SMA

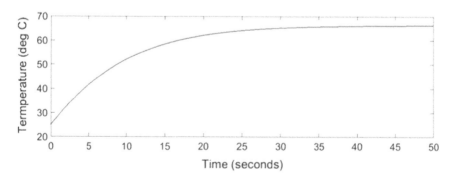

Fig. 2 Thermal response of SMA

ρ, ∇, P_e and c are material density, gradient vector, electrical power and specific heat coefficient. In comparison with Eq. (1), the equation consists of the additional term for gradient vector to include the geometry of the temperature vector. In the Eq. (2), the partial derivatives of the vector along y and z-axis are negligible as the SMA is assumed to be circular. Also, the response of the heat conduction in the x-axis is at a much faster rate than the heat convection. So, Eq. (2) can be simplified as Eq. (1) itself. But this simplification does not hold when the designer needs to model the SMA strip instead of wire.

The convective heat coefficient 'h' can be obtained from many methods such as trial and error method, as a second-order polynomial [27], as a nonlinear function of T [22, 23] and by the use of Nusselt number [28, 29].

In the paper [22, 23], the specific heat constant c and the convective heat transfer coefficient h are given as the nonlinear functions of temperature with a_1, $a_2, a_3, a_4, b_1, b_2, m_1, m_2, n_1$ and n_2 as the constant parameters that need to be assumed leading to the ambiguity in the obtained value.

$$h = \begin{cases} a_1 - a_2 T; & \dot{T} \geq 0 \\ a_3 + a_4 \, \mathrm{erf}\left(\frac{T - m_1}{n_1}\right); & \dot{T} \leq 0 \end{cases} \tag{3}$$

$$c = b_1 + b_2 \mathrm{erf}\left(\frac{T - m_2}{n_2}\right) \tag{4}$$

In the paper [27], the second-order polynomial is used to calculate the h value with h_o, h_1 are the curve fitting parameters.

$$h = h_o + h_1 T^2 \tag{5}$$

From the papers [28, 29], the heat convection coefficients can be calculated by the following equations:

$$h = \frac{N_u k}{L} \tag{6}$$

where N_u is the Nusselt number, K is thermal conductivity of air $= 1/T$ for air, L is characteristic length $= V/S$, and V and S are the volume and surface area of the wire. The Nusselt number is obtained from Eq. (7) with Gr (Grashof number) and Pr (Prandtl number).

$$N_u = \left(0.6 + \frac{0.387(G_r P_r)^{\frac{1}{6}}}{\left[1 + (0.559/P_r)^{\frac{9}{16}}\right]^{\frac{8}{27}}}\right)^2 \tag{7}$$

The simulation results of temperature profile with the use of different convective heat transfer coefficient formulae are given in Fig. 3. All the curves follow the same profile despite the changes in the h parameter. There is overall of $\pm 5\%$ changes in the

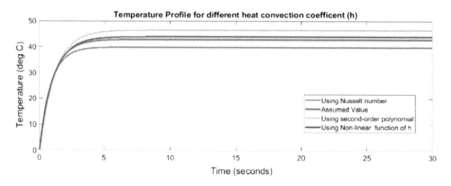

Fig. 3 Temperature profile for different convective heat coefficients

curve. Also, the Nusselt number method can be considered as the optimum method for h calculation as it does not have any curve fitting/assumed parameters like the second-order polynomial and the nonlinear function method.

3 Phase Transformation of SMA

The phase transformation in SMA is due to its inherent property of being able to remember its previously deformed shape. The phase transformation is mainly used to correlate the temperature rise of the SMA with the martensite/austenite fraction. Different prominent approaches for modelling the phase transformation in SMA are discussed in the following subsections.

3.1 Preisach Model

The Preisach model [30] is generally used to derive the hysteretic relationship between magnetic field and magnetisation of a material. The similar principle is used to estimate the hysteresis relation between the martensite fraction, strain and temperature of the shape memory alloy.

Instead of fixed mathematical equations, Preisach model makes use of experimental results to develop the model for the shape memory alloy. Separate tests are conducted for both major hysteresis loop and minor hysteresis loops. The plots of strain versus current and strain versus time are obtained to understand the behaviour of the alloy under different loading conditions. The Preisach model uses the information from each minor loop and then on integration obtains the overall hysteresis (8).

$$w(t) = \int_0^\infty \int_{-\infty}^\infty w(r, s)\Re_{s-r,s+r}[v](t)dsdr \tag{8}$$

Though Preisach model is widely used for SMA hysteresis model, it is unable to represent the dead zones of transformation or the drift of hysteresis loops with cyclic loading during partial transformation [1, 23, 30]. Also, the computation of the weighing functions in the hysteresis region is very tedious as the experimental results may change due to any external disturbances.

3.2   Duhem Hysteresis Model

The Duhem model provides an analytical description of hysteresis, so it is widely applied in structural, electrical and mechanical systems [31]. This model makes use of black box approach. Tai and Ahn [22] and Dutta and Ghorbel [23] tried to model the SMA based on the similar black box approach.

In the paper [22, 23], the author uses Duhem differential hysteresis model to explain the hysteresis with R_m as martensite fraction and temperature T. The R_m-T model is represented in Eq. (9) with $R_m(0) = 0$. The hysteresis model signifies the parameter values during increasing and decreasing curves.

$$\frac{dR_m}{dT} = \begin{cases} \frac{h_-(T)+R_m-1}{h_+(T)-h_-(T)}g_+(T); \dot{T} > 0 \\ \frac{h_+(T)+R_m-1}{h_-(T)-h_+(T)}g_-(T); \dot{T} > 0 \end{cases} \tag{9}$$

where the $g_{+/-}$ and $h_{+/-}$ are given in Eqs. (10) and (11). The function *erf* is the error encountered in integrating the normal distribution with μ and σ^2 are the mean and the covariance which are physically not significant.

$$g_{+/-}(u) = \frac{1}{\sigma_{+/-}\sqrt{2\pi}}exp\left(-\frac{\left(u - \mu_{+/-}\right)^2}{2\sigma_{+/-}^2}\right) \tag{10}$$

$$h_{+/-}(u) = \int_{-\infty}^u g_{+/-}(u')du' = \frac{1}{2}\left[1 + erf\left(\frac{u - \mu_{+/-}}{\sqrt{2}\sigma_{+/-}}\right)\right] \tag{11}$$

Using the martensite fraction, the strain incurred on the SMA wire is calculated using the approximated polynomial Eq. (12). The values k_1, k_2 and k_3 are the constant parameters. Using the strain value, Eq. (13) can be used to find the electrical resistance of the SMA.

$$\varepsilon = \varepsilon_0 + k_1 R_m + k_2 R_m^2 + k_3 R_m^{50} \tag{12}$$

$$\frac{1}{R} = \frac{\pi d_0^2}{4L_0(1 + 2\varepsilon)}\left\{\frac{1 - R_m}{\rho_a(T)} + \frac{R_m}{\rho_m(T)}\right\} \tag{13}$$

The $\rho_a(T)$ and $\rho_m(T)$ are the electrical resistivity of austenite and martensite, respectively, obtained using nonlinear expressions (14) and (15) with the p_1, p_2, p_3, q_1, q_2 and α_i ($i = 1$ to 9) as the constant parameters.

$$\rho_a(T) = p_1 + p_2\exp(-p_3(T - T_0)) \tag{14}$$

$$\rho_m(T) = (q_1 - q_2T)\left[1 + erf\left(\frac{T - m_3}{n_3}\right)\right] + \sum_{i=1}^{9}\alpha_i(T - T_0)^2 \tag{15}$$

The parameter values used in the Duhem model are represented in Table 1. The Simulink representation of Duhem differential model of SMA is in Fig. 4.

Table 1 SMA Simulink parameters for Duhem model

Parameter	Value	Parameter	Value
R	55 Ω	μ_+	78.9 °C
d_0	3.81×10^{-4} m	μ_-	34 °C
l_0	400 mm	σ_+	11.2 °C
ρ	6500 kg m^{-3}	σ_-	5.8 °C
T_a	25 °C	ε_0	0.5
a_1	165 Wm^{-2}°C^{-1}	k_1	0.0204
a_2	0.5 Wm^{-2}°C^{-1}	k_2	0.01293
b_1	140J/kg°C	k_3	0.0027
b_2	1J/kg°C	p_1	9.2×10^{-7} Ωm
m_2	65 °C	p_2	8.4×10^{-7} Ωm
m_3	70 °C	q_1	3.4×10^{-8} Ωm
n_2	0.5 °C	q_2	5.7×10^{-10} Ωm
α_0	8.7×10^{-7}	α_5	1.2×10^{-12}
α_1	4.8×10^{-8}	α_6	-2.5×10^{-14}
α_2	-7.8×10^{-8}	α_7	3.2×10^{-16}
α_3	7×10^{-10}	α_8	-2.2×10^{-18}
α_4	-3.7×10^{-11}	α_9	6.7×10^{-21}

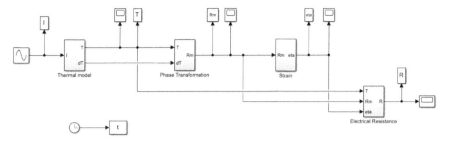

Fig. 4 Duhem differential model of SMA

The plots of martensite fraction, strain and electrical resistance w.r.t to time are indicated in Figs. 5, 6 and 7. There exists a linear relationship between the strain and the martensite fraction of the SMA as in Fig. 8. The parameter utilised in the strain equation was obtained empirically. Also, most of the parameters were obtained through nonlinear least square optimisation method.

The Duhem model [22] has time-consuming execution with the inaccurate results. The model handles the complex equations with the parameters obtained empirically

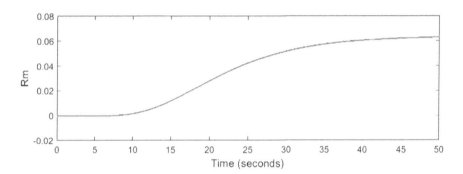

Fig. 5 Martensite fraction

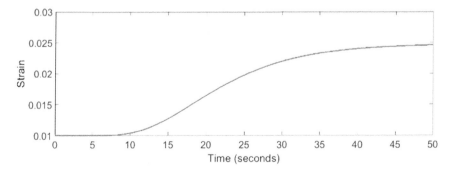

Fig. 6 Strain on SMA

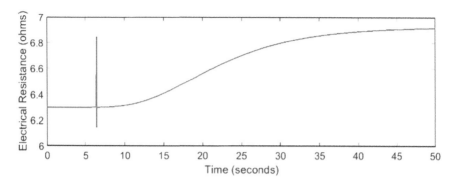

Fig. 7 Electrical resistance

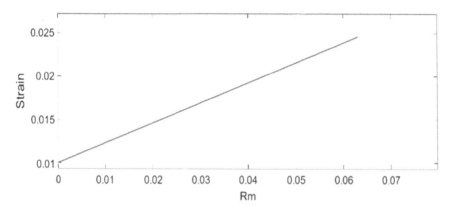

Fig. 8 Relation between martensite fraction and strain

or through nonlinear least square optimisation method making it difficult for the designers to model accurately.

Both the Preisach and Duhem model predict the inner loop response of the SMA, but both the methods are complex and tedious when antagonistic configuration and multiple variants of SMA are considered. Also, these models do not provide much insight about the phase transformation process of SMA [1].

3.3 Fermi–Dirac Statistics

Basically, Fermi–Dirac statistics [27] explains the distribution of electrons in normal and excited state. The similar analogy can be used to explain the SMA phase transformation during heating and cooling.

According to the Fermi–Dirac statistics, the austenite fraction (ξ) during heating phase is given as:

$$\xi = \frac{\xi_m}{1 + \exp\left(\frac{T_{fa} - T}{\sigma_a} + K_a \sigma\right)} \tag{16}$$

where ξ_m is the fraction of the martensite phase prior to the present transformation, T_{fa} is the transition temperature, σ_a is an indication of the range of temperature around the transition temperature, and K_a is the stress curve fitting parameter which is obtained from the loading plateau of the stress–strain characteristic with zero temperature change. During the cooling phase, the same Eq. (16) holds well except that the martensite fraction ξ is found out with all the other parameters referring to the austenite state. It should be considered that the sum of mole fraction of austenite and martensite should be equal to unity.

Under all cases, the behaviour of the SMA cannot be equated to that of an electron. Also, the speed of electron movement from normal to excited state is very high as compared with the transformation under heating and cooling phases. Also, the statistics holds good for a single electron, which cannot be practically equated to the entire crystalline structure of the SMA.

3.4 Ikuta Model

Dutta and Ghorbel [23] gave a unique approach for the modelling of SMA. The model used Ikuta theory [25, 26] for dividing the SMA into two parallel layers and then uses Duhem differential hysteresis theory [22] to explain the relation between martensite fraction and the temperature change.

In order to explain the martensite or austenite ratio, Ikuta [23, 25, 26] establishes variable sublayer model. The SMA is considered as a composition of two parallel layers of martensite and austenite that are normally randomly distributed. As the ratio of martensite/austenite changes, the corresponding cross-sectional areas and volumes of the two phase changes. Equation (17) provides the phase fraction during heating and the similar equation can be framed under the cooling phase (Fig. 9).

$$\xi_a = \begin{cases} 0, T \le A_s \\ \dfrac{T - A_s}{A_f - A_s}, A_s \le T \le A_f \\ 1, T \ge A_f \end{cases} \tag{17}$$

The stress and strain are related by the use of generalised Hooke's law [32]. Hooke's law makes use of Young's modulus in martensite (E^M) and austenite (E^A) with ε^e being the elastic strain given by Eq. (18).

$$\sigma = E\varepsilon^e = \left(E^M \xi_m + E^A \xi_a\right)\varepsilon^e \tag{18}$$

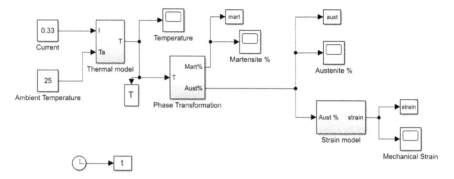

Fig. 9 Ikuta model of SMA actuator

The temperature dynamics and phase transformation can be modelled in MATLAB/Simulink providing results as shown in Figs. 10, 11 and 12 with the Simulink diagram in Fig. 9. From the graph, it is clear that the strain profile follows the austenite profile that is not true for the cases of transformation.

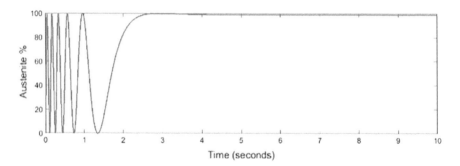

Fig. 10 Phase transformation during heating

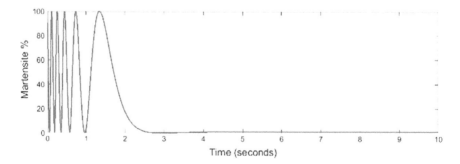

Fig. 11 Phase transformation during cooling

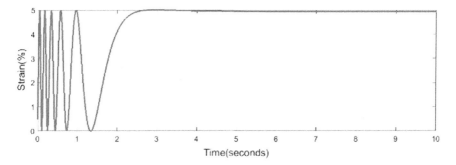

Fig. 12 Mechanical strain

3.5 Liang Constitutive Model

Liang proposed a strain-based modelling approach for SMA. The basic principle is Liang's solution of the actuator dynamics which is the integration of Newton's second law to obtain the position (strain) from the force (stress). Hence, stress obtained by the SMA is the output of the strain-driven model which is also the input to the actuator dynamics model. For calculating the stress value, the martensite phase fraction $(0 \leq \xi \leq 1)$ is required [8, 17, 18, 21, 24]. For martensite fraction calculation, the cosine function is used.

$$\xi = \frac{\xi_M}{2}\{\cos[a_A(T - A_s) + b_A\sigma] + 1\} \tag{19}$$

$$\xi = \frac{1 - \xi_A}{2}\left\{\cos\left[a_M(T - M_f) + b_M\sigma\right] + \frac{1 + \xi_A}{2}\right\} \tag{20}$$

where $a_A = \frac{\pi}{A_f - A_s}$, $a_M = \frac{\pi}{M_s - M_f}$, $b_A = -\frac{a_A}{C_A}$, $b_M = -\frac{a_M}{C_M}$ are the curve fitting parameters, ξ is martensite phase fraction, ξ_M is maximum martensite fraction during cooling, ξ_A is maximum austenite fraction during heating, σ is stress, A_s, A_f are austenite start and finish temperatures and M_s, M_f are martensite start and finish temperatures.

The constitutive equation relating the stress and the strain [8, 9, 14] is given as:

$$\sigma - \sigma_0 = E(\varepsilon - \varepsilon_0) + \Omega(\xi - \xi_0) + \theta_T(T - T_a) \tag{21}$$

The simulation parameters for the SMA model are given in Table 2 using the manufacturer datasheet of the SMA. The simulation is carried out for 30s with 0.0001s as the sampling time. The Simulink model of the SMA actuator wire is given in Fig. 13. The plots of temperature, stress, strain and displacement w.r.t to time are given in Figs. 14, 15 and 16.

Table 2 SMA Simulink parameters for strain-driven model

Parameter	Value	Parameter	Value
d	150 μm	M_s	72 °C
R	55 Ω/m	M_f	62 °C
T_a	25 °C	C_A	10 MPa/°C
h	150 Wm^{-2} °C^{-1}	C_M	10 MPa/°C
A_w	0.477 mm^2	ξ_M	0.1
ρ	6.45 × 10^{-3} kgm^{-3}	E	51.5 GPa
V_w	0.02 × 10^{-3} m^{-3}	ϵ_0	0
C_w	322 J kg^{-1} °C^{-1}	θ_T	−0.055
l_0	0.75 m	ϵ_{max}	4%
A_s	68 °C	m, b, k	0.1
A_f	78 °C	I_{max}	440 mA

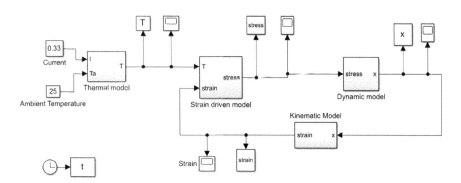

Fig. 13 Liang model of SMA wire actuator

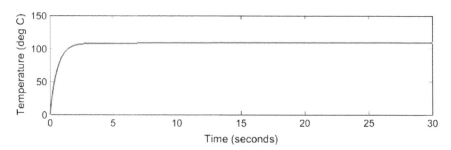

Fig. 14 SMA temperature versus time

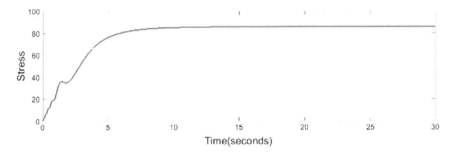

Fig. 15 Output stress profile of strain-driven model

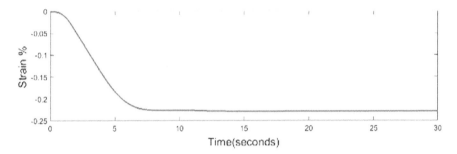

Fig. 16 Strain profile of strain-driven model

The results of the Liang model are corresponding to the practical behaviour of the SMA. Also, the provision of stress–strain relation enables the designer to understand and correlate their functionality.

3.6 Brinson Model

The Brinson model [2, 7, 14, 33, 34] is used to address the special cases of SMA such as the detwinning effect of the SMA. Firstly, the martensite fraction (ξ) is divided into stress-induced (detwinned martensite, ξ_s) and temperature-induced (twinned martensite, ξ_t) martensite fractions. Using the detwinned fractions, Eq. (21) is altered as:

$$\sigma - \sigma_0 = E(\xi)\varepsilon - E(\xi_0)\varepsilon_0 + \Omega(\xi)\xi_s - \Omega(\xi_0)\xi_{s0}$$
$$+ \theta(T - T_0) \tag{22}$$

Based on the initial conditions [35], the equation can be rewritten as:

$$\sigma = E(\xi)(\varepsilon - \varepsilon_L\xi_s) + \theta(T - T_0) \tag{23}$$

The equations evolved for conversion from martensite to detwinned martensite are as follows:

For $T > M_s$ and $\sigma_s^{cr} + C_M(T - M_s) < \sigma < \sigma_f^{cr} + C_M(T - M_s)$,

$$\xi_s = \frac{1 - \xi_{s0}}{2} \cos\left\{\frac{\pi}{\sigma_s^{cr} - \sigma_f^{cr}}\left[\sigma - \sigma_f^{cr} - C_M(T - M_s)\right]\right\} + \frac{1 + \xi_{s0}}{2}$$

$$\xi_T = \xi_{T0} - \frac{\xi_{T0}}{1 - \xi_{s0}}(\xi_s - \xi_{s0}) \tag{24}$$

For $T < M_s$ and $\sigma_s^{cr} < \sigma < \sigma_f^{cr}$,

$$\xi_s = \frac{1 - \xi_{s0}}{2} \cos\left\{\frac{\pi}{\sigma_s^{cr} - \sigma_f^{cr}}\left(\sigma - \sigma_f^{cr}\right)\right\} + \frac{1 + \xi_{s0}}{2}$$

$$\xi_T = \xi_{T0} - \frac{\xi_{T0}}{1 - \xi_{s0}}(\xi_s - \xi_{s0}) + \Delta_{T\varepsilon} \tag{25}$$

But the drawback of the Brinson model is that for certain thermo-mechanical loading ($T < M_s$) and stress–temperature histories, the value of ξ becomes greater than unity which is in-acceptable. Also, when $\sigma = \sigma_f^{cr}$, the transformation should be complete, and only stress-induced martensite should be present. But, the Brinson model structure could not achieve this result.

3.7 Kinematic Model for SMA

The kinematics of the SMA actuator mainly depends on the type of load such as antagonistic load, spring load, wire load and so on. This design mainly depends on the designer's discretion and the type of SMA application. Also, the kinematics can be designed with or without considering the strain of the actuator.

4 Conclusion

The important modelling techniques for SMA with corresponding Simulink models and their simulation results were presented with more stress on the implementation aspects. Also, the pros and cons of the different macroscopic modelling approaches of phase transformation were presented. Though a number of modelling approaches for SMA are proposed, there is no single approach that meets all the aspirations of the SMA actuator designer.

The Fermi–Dirac statistics fails to provide the exact analogy of the SMA with the electron as the rate of electron energy transformation is much higher than that of the phase transformation in the SMA. Also, the Duhem hysteresis model had many curve fitting parameters that are to be obtained by the optimisation techniques making it difficult for the designers to handle all the unknown parameters. Also, Ikuta model being the simplest method could not provide satisfactory results. The Fermi–Dirac statistics, Duhem hysteresis and the Ikuta model are not applicable to practical implementations.

The Preisach model is preferred for modelling where the experimental results under different loading conditions are available. The Liang constitutive model could be selected for modelling when the controller needs to be designed using MAT-LAB/Simulink, embedded system and LabVIEW platforms. The Brinson model is selected for complex and accurate modelling for SMA such as the implementation using artificial intelligence (genetic algorithm, particle swarm optimisation and neural networks).

Acknowledgements This work was carried out at CSMST division, CSIR-NAL, Bengaluru. The authors would like to thank Jitendra J Jadhav, Director, CSIR-NAL, for providing us the platform to carry out the research. The authors also thank Dr. Dayananda G N, Chief Scientist, CSMST, CSIR-NAL, for reviewing the paper, valuable discussions and advice.

References

1. Khandelwal A, Buravalla V (2009) Models for shape memory alloy behaviour: an overview of modelling approaches. Int J Struct Chang Solids-Mech Appl 1(1):111–148
2. Brinson LC (1993) One-dimensional constitutive behaviour of shape memory alloys: thermo-mechanical derivation with non-constant material functions and redefined martensite internal variable. J Int Mater Syst Struct 4
3. Tanaka K, Kobayashi S, Sato Y (1986) Thermomechanics of transformation pseudoelasticity and shape memory effect in alloys. Int J Plast
4. Muller I, Xu H (1991) On the pseudo-elastic hysteresis. Actuator Metall Mater 39(3):263–271
5. Falk F. Model free energy mechanics and thermodynamics of shape memory alloys. Actuator Metall 28(12):1773–1780
6. Aurichhio F, Lubliner J (1997) A uniaxial model for shape memory alloys. Int J Solid Struct
7. Bekker A, Brinson LC (1998) Phase diagram based description of the hysteresis behaviour of shape memory alloy. Published by Elsevier Science Ltd
8. Ho M, Desai JP (2013) Modelling, characterisation and control of antagonistic SMA springs for use in a neurosurgical robot. In: IEEE international conference on robotics and automation (ICRA), 2013
9. Liang C, Rogers CA (1990) One-dimensional thermomechanical constitutive relations for shape memory materials. J Intell Mater Syst Struct 1(2):207–234
10. Abiri R, Kardan I, Nadafi R, Kabganian M (2016) Nonlinear state space modelling and control of shape memory alloy spring actuator. Int J Eng Sci (IJES)
11. Furst SJ, Crews JH, Seelecke S (2013) Stress, strain and resistance behaviour of two opposing shape memory alloy actuator wires for resistance based self-sending applications. J Intell Mater Syst Struct
12. Furst SJ, Seelecke S (2012) Modelling and experimental characterization of the stress, strain and resistance of shape memory alloy actuator wires with controlled power input. J Intell Mater Syst Struct
13. Huo Y (1989) A mathematical model for the hysteresis in shape memory alloys. Contin Mech Thermodyn. Springer-Verlag

14. Sayyaadi H, Zakerzadeh MR, Salehi H (2012) A comparative analysis of some one-dimensional shape memory alloy constitutive models based on experimental tests. Sci Iran B 19(2):249–257

15. Cisse C, Zaki W, Zineb TB (2016) A review of modelling techniques for advanced effects in shape memory alloy behaviour. Smart Mater Struct. https://doi.org/10.1088/0964-1726/25/10/103001. IOP Publishing

16. A review on phenomenological shape memory alloy constitutive modelling approaches. Appendix: SMA modelling

17. Paiva A, Savi MA (2006) An overview of constitutive models for shape memory alloys. In: Mathematical problems in engineering, Hindawi Publishing Corporation, 2006. ArticleID: 56876

18. Quintanar-Guzman S, Kannan S, Aguilera-González A, Olivares-Mendez MA, Voos H. Operational space control of a lightweight robotic arm actuated by shape memory alloy wires: a comparative study. J Int Mater Syst Struct

19. Abdelaal WGA, Nagib G. Modelling and simulation of SMA actuator wire. 978-1-4799-6594-6/14/ ©2014 IEEE

20. Elahinia MH, Siegler TM, Leo DJ, Ahmadian M. Sliding mode control of a shape memory alloy actuated manipulator. In: International conference on intelligent materials (5th) (Smart Systems & Nanotechnology)

21. Alsayed YM, Abouelsoud AA, El Bab AMRF (2016) Hybrid sliding mode fuzzy logic-based PI controller design and implementation of shape memory alloy actuator. In: 2016 8th international congress on ultra-modern telecommunications and control systems and workshops (ICUMT). IEEE

22. Tai NT, Ahn KK (2011) Adaptive proportional-integral-derivative tuning sliding mode control for a shape memory alloy actuator. Smart Mater Struct. https://doi.org/10.1088/0964/1726/20/5/055010

23. Dutta SM, Ghorbel FH (2005) Differential hysteresis modelling of a shape memory alloy wire actuator. IEEE/ASME Trans Mechatron

24. Elahinia M, Koo J, Ahmadian M, Woolsey C (2005) Backstepping control of a shape memory alloy actuated robotic arm. J Vib Control

25. Ikuta K, Tsukamoto M, Hirose S (1991) Mathematical model and experimental verification of shape memory alloy for designing micro actuator. In: Proceedings-IEEE micro electro mechanical systems, Nara, Japan, 1991

26. Lee CJ, Mavroidis C (2002) Analytical dynamic model and experimental robust and optimal control of shape memory alloy bundle actuators, ASME, 2002

27. Jayender J, Patel RV, Nikumb S Ostojic M (2008) Modelling and control of shape memory alloy actuators. IEEE Trans Control Syst Technol 16(2)

28. Eisakham A, Ma W, Gao J, Culham JR, Gorbet R (2011) Natural convection heat transfer modelling of shape memory alloy. In: Smart materials, structures and NDT in aerospace, conference NDT, Canada

29. Favelukis JE, Lavine AS, Carman GP (1999) Experimentally validated thermal model of thin film NiTi. In: Symposium on smart structures and materials, CA, US

30. Ahn KK, Kha NB (2008) Modelling and control of shape memory alloy actuators using Presaich model, genetic algorithm and fuzzy logic. Mechatron 18:141–152

31. Fuad MFM, Ikhouane F (2013) Characterisation of hysteresis Duhem model. In: 5th IFAC (The international federation of automatic control) international workshop on periodic control systems, France, July 2013

32. Shu SG, Lagoudas DC, Hughes D, Wen JT (1997) Modelling of a flexible beam actuated by shape memory alloy wire. Smart Mater Struct

33. Brinson LC, Lammering R (1993) Finite element analysis of the behaviour of shape memory alloys and their applications. Int J Solids Struct 30(23):3261–3280

34. Chung JH, Heo JS, Lee JJ (2007) Implementation strategy for the dual transformation region in the Brinson SMA constitutive model. Smart Mater Struct 16:N1–N5

35. Brinson LC, Huang MS (1996) Simplifications and comparisons of shape memory alloy constitutive models. J Intell Mater Syst Struct 7:108–114

Maximum Power Point Tracking for an Isolated Wind Energy Conversion System

D. Lakshmi and M. R. Rashmi

Abstract Isolated energy systems are gaining popularity for supplying power to remote and rural areas. Wind energy conversion systems (WECS) are a good choice among various options. For efficient operation, hill climbing search (HCS) maximum power point tracking (MPPT) algorithm is applied to extract maximum power from wind turbine. This paper presents the simulation study and harmonic analysis of self-excited induction generator-based WECS for a nonlinear load by adapting the maximum power point tracking mechanism.

Keywords Harmonics · Maximum power point tracking · Hill climbing search (HCS) algorithm · Excitation capacitors

1 Introduction

Power generation using conventional technologies introduces atmospheric pollution, climate change, emission of poisonous and harmful gases, depletion of fossil fuels, etc. Hence, these conventional methods are being replaced with various renewable energy technologies. These include solar, wind, tidal, geothermal, hydro, biomass. These energy sources are either used in conjunction with conventional technologies or as separate stand-alone systems. For power supply to remote and rural areas, conventional transmission lines will not be feasible because of both technical and economic reasons. In such cases, either any one of renewable energy sources or their combinations as hybrid systems are popular. The generation of power using wind is gaining importance because of less space occupancy, zero carbon emission operation, and low cost of electricity production. In these wind energy systems, energy contained

D. Lakshmi (✉) · M. R. Rashmi
Department of Electrical and Electronics Engineering, Amrita School of Engineering,
Bangalore, Amrita Vishwa Vidyapeetham, Bangalore, India
e-mail: lakshmidevdas@gmail.com

M. R. Rashmi
e-mail: rashmi.power@gmail.com

© Springer Nature Singapore Pte Ltd. 2019
V. Sridhar et al. (eds.), *Emerging Research in Electronics, Computer Science and Technology*, Lecture Notes in Electrical Engineering 545,
https://doi.org/10.1007/978-981-13-5802-9_105

in wind at varying velocities is converted into electrical power. The output power varies with respect to wind speed. Hence to determine the optimal generator speed that will guarantee the maximum power, various MPPT algorithms have to be used. Basically, three MPPT control algorithms are applied for WECS, namely tip-speed ratio (TSR) control, hill climbing search (HCS) control and optimum relationship-based (ORB) control.

For such isolated systems, power quality (PQ) issues will be much more intense than that for conventional grid. These PQ issues include voltage sag, swell, unbalance, distortion, interruption, notching, flickering, harmonics. Among these issues, harmonics is one among a major issue that needs attention. The increased use of various nonlinear and power electronic devices injects significant amount of harmonic components to network. These harmonic components adversely affect functioning of sensitive electronic equipment connected at the point of common coupling (PCC). A harmonic analysis has to be carried out in the design of various passive and active filtering devices. Harmonic analysis is the process of calculating magnitude and phase angle of both fundamental and its harmonic components of system. The simulations circuits are also provided.

2   Wind Energy Conversion System

The basic components of a WECS include wind turbine (WT) coupled to a generator, three-phase diode bridge rectifier, DC–DC converter, battery, inverter, and loads as shown in Fig. 1. The turbine extracts energy content in wind and transfers it to the shaft. Generator then converts this energy into electrical energy. Various types of generators can be used depending on applications namely permanent magnet synchronous generators (PMSG), squirrel-cage induction generators (SCIG), doubly fed induction generators (DFIG). SCIGs are the most widely used generator type for WECS due to its simple construction, robustness, less maintenance, etc. These types

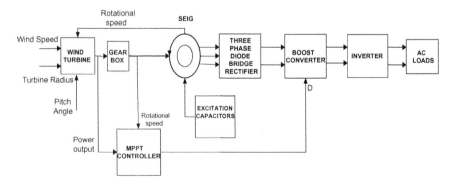

Fig. 1 Block diagram of an isolated WECS

of generator require a reactive power source for its operation. Based on techniques used to provide reactive power support, these are two types, namely self-excited induction generator (SEIG) and grid-connected (doubly fed) induction generator (GCIG/DFIG). For remote area applications, SEIG is preferred over its counterpart. The output from generator is then fed directly to three-phase diode bridge rectifier followed by a DC–DC converter. This output can then be connected directly to DC loads or to AC loads through an inverter.

3 Wind Turbine Modeling

The mechanical power P_m extracted from the wind by a turbine can be expressed as:

$$Pm = \frac{1}{2}C_p(\lambda, \beta)\rho A V_w^3 \tag{1}$$

where

$$Cp(\lambda, \beta) = 0.5176\left(\frac{116}{\lambda_i} - 0.4\beta - 5\right)e^{\frac{-21}{\lambda_i}} + 0.0068\,\lambda \tag{2}$$

$$\frac{1}{\lambda_i} = \frac{1}{\lambda + 0.08\beta} - \frac{0.035}{\beta^3 + 1} \tag{3}$$

$$\lambda = \frac{\omega R}{V_w} \tag{4}$$

where

C_p Power coefficient
P   Density of air (1.225 kg/m^3)
A   Swept area of rotor disk (m^2)
V_w Wind velocity (m/s)
λ Tip speed
B   Pitch angle
ω Turbine rotational speed (rad/s)
R   Turbine radius (m).

Simulation circuits of WT are given in Figs. 2, 3, 4, and 5.

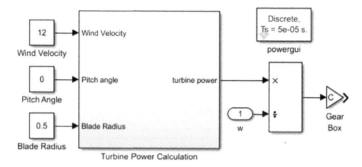

Fig. 2 Model of WT in MATLAB

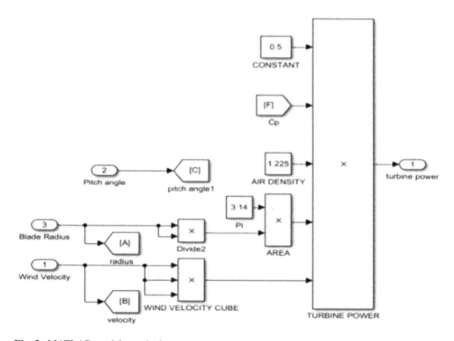

Fig. 3 MATLAB model to calculate power

4 Excitation Capacitor Design for SEIG

The induction generator needs a reactive power source for operation. In remote area applications, this requirement is provided by capacitor banks connected across its stator terminals. The selection of capacitance is very crucial. For self-excitation to occur, the value of selected capacitance should be more than the minimum value. The equations used for calculating the minimum value for excitation capacitors needed for self-excitation to occur are given as

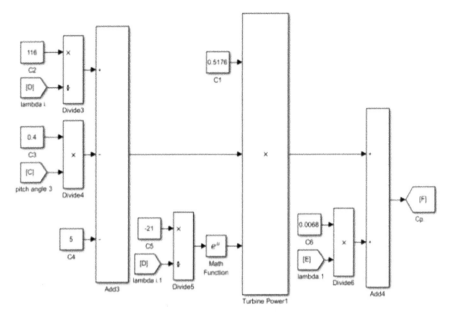

Fig. 4 MATAB model to calculate C_p

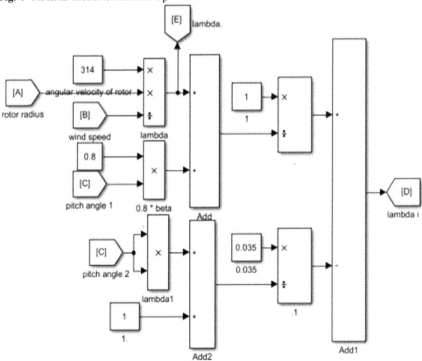

Fig. 5 MATLAB model to calculate λ_i

$$Q = \frac{V^2}{X_L} = V^2 X_C \qquad (5)$$

where

$$X_L = 2\Pi f L_m \qquad (6)$$

$$X_C = 2\Pi f C \qquad (7)$$

The value of excitation capacitors needed for the operation of induction generator is calculated as:

$$C = \frac{Q}{V^2 2\Pi f} \qquad (8)$$

5 Hill Climbing Search MPPT Algorithm

In order to extract the maximum energy available in wind, an MPPT tracking algorithm has to be used. Basically, three MPPT tracking methods are used for WECS, namely hill climbing search (HCS) algorithm, optimum relationship-based (ORB) control, and tip-speed ratio (TSR) control algorithm.

A typical power v/s rotational speed characteristics of a WT for different wind speed will be as shown in Fig. 6. Corresponding to each wind speed, there will be a unique MPP. Here A, B, C, D, and E correspond to MPP at wind speeds of V_1 m/s, V_2 m/s, V_3 m/s, V_4 m/s, and V_5 m/s, respectively, where $V_5 > V_4 > V_3 > V_2 > V_1$. MPPT algorithms do the function of searching this optimum value at which power generated is maximum for given wind speed.

Among the three, HCS algorithm is the simplest MPPT technique. This algorithm is based on the fact that, at MPP, $\frac{dP}{d\omega} = 0$. The steps of HCS MPPT algorithm are indicated in Fig. 7.

6 Simulation Results

The simulation model of SEIG driving RL load is given in Fig. 8.

The specifications of induction machine used for simulation are given below:
Power rating (P): 5.4 HP (4 kW)
Voltage (V): 415 V

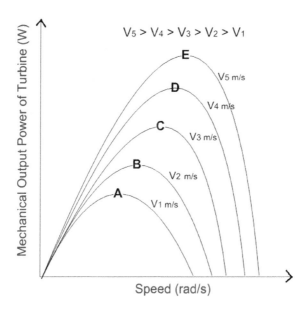

Fig. 6 Power versus speed characteristics of wind turbine

Frequency (f): 50 Hz
Speed (N): 1430 rpm
Mutual inductance (L_m): 0.1722 H
No. of poles: 4

The maximum mechanical power extracted by the wind turbine at a wind speed of 12 m/s is shown in Fig. 9.

The minimum capacitance value required for excitation of SEIG is obtained as 59 μF. Also, when an induction machine operates as a generator, it runs at a speed greater than synchronous speed (N_s). The N_s of machine used for simulation work is 1500 rpm (Ns = 120 * f/P). The speed of induction generator is shown in Fig. 10.

The voltage generated by SEIG without connecting to load and the THD is shown in Figs. 11 and 12, respectively.

The voltage buildup by SEIG connected to load and the THD is shown in Figs. 13 and 14, respectively.

The output of induction generator is connected to a three-phase diode bridge rectifier. The output of diode bridge rectifier is given as

$$Vout = 1.65 * V_m \tag{9}$$

where

V_m Peak value of input voltage

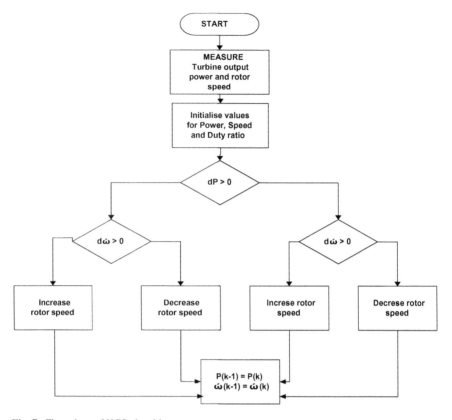

Fig. 7 Flow chart of HCS algorithm

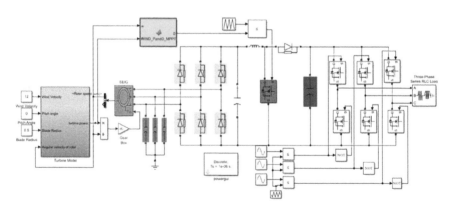

Fig. 8 MATLAB model of SEIG driven by wind turbine connected to AC loads

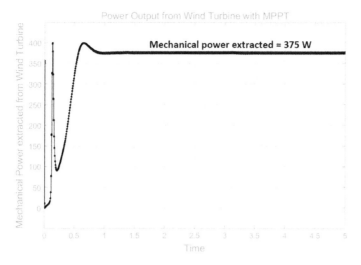

Fig. 9 Mechanical power extracted by wind turbine

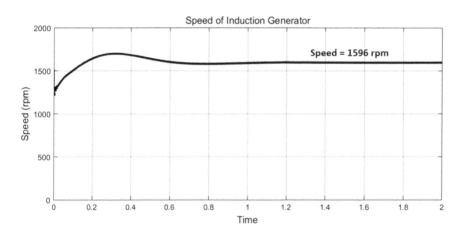

Fig. 10 Speed of induction generator

The output of three-phase diode bridge rectifier is given in Fig. 15.

The output of three-phase diode bridge rectifier is fed to a DC–DC boost converter. The gate pulse to this converter is provided by the MPPT controller. The DC link voltage is given in Fig. 16.

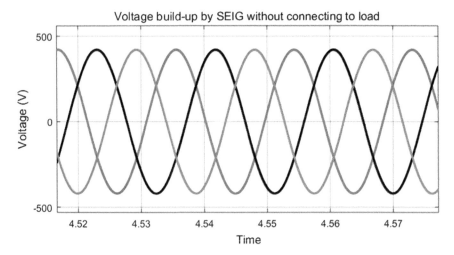

Fig. 11 Output voltage of SEIG without load

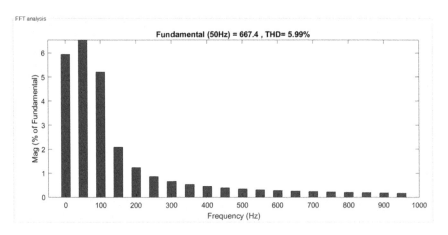

Fig. 12 THD of SEIG output voltage without connecting to load

7 Conclusions

An isolated WECS feeding an AC load has been simulated in the paper. Mathematical modeling of wind turbine has been done. Hill climbing search MPPT algorithm is used to track maximum mechanical output power from the wind turbine. Design of excitation capacitors, which acts as a source of reactive power, has been done. The

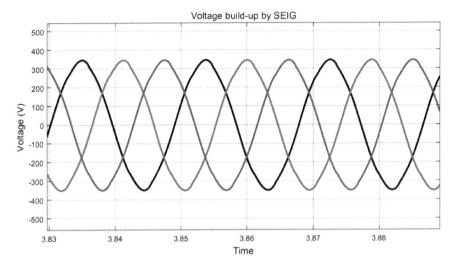

Fig. 13 Output voltage of three-phase SEIG

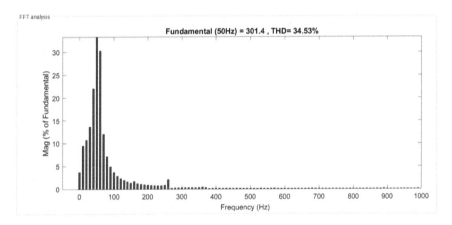

Fig. 14 FFT analysis of output voltage of SEIG

FFT analysis of SEIG voltage with and without connecting to load has been found out. From the simulation result, it has been found that the THD increases from 5.99 to 34.53%, by connecting to loads. Further, a control algorithm can be developed to bring down the THD value to an acceptable range.

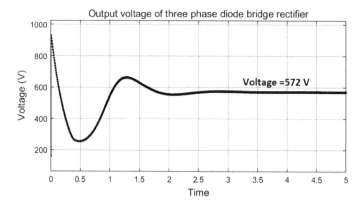

Fig. 15 Output of three-phase diode bridge rectifier

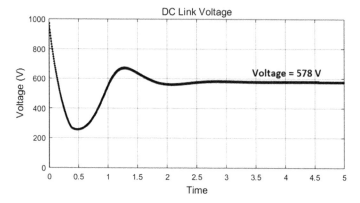

Fig. 16 DC link voltage

References

1. Solangi KH, Islam MR, Saidur R, Rahim NA, Fayaz H (2011) A review on global solar energy policy. Renew Sustain Energy Rev 5(4):2149–2163
2. Mekhilef S, Saidur R, Safari A (2011) A review on solar energy use in industries. Renew Sustain Energy Rev 15(4):1777–1790
3. Samith MV, Rashmi MR (2016) Controller for integrating small scale power generation to hybrid AC/DC grid. In: IEEE international conference on inventive computation technologies ICICT
4. Sivakumar K, Ramprabhakar J, Shankar S (2017) Coordination of wind-hydro energy conversion system with sliding mode control. In:1st IEEE international conference on power electronics. Intelligence Control Energy System, Delhi, pp 1–5
5. Hussain J, Mahesh K, Mishra (2016) Adaptive maximum power point tracking control algorithm for wind energy conversion systems. IEEE Trans Energy Convers 31(2):697–705
6. Le HT, Santoso S, Nguyen TQ (2012) Augmenting wind power penetration and grid voltage stability limits using ESS: application design, sizing, and a case study. IEEE Trans Power Syst 161–171

7. Zhao H, Wu Q, Hu S, Xu H (2014) Rasmussen CN review of energy storage system for wind power integration support. Elsevier J 137:545–553
8. Dalala ZM, Zahid ZU, Yu W, Cho Y, Lai JS (2013) Design and analysis of an mppt technique for small-scale wind energy conversion systems IEEE Trans Energy Convers 28(3)
9. Xia Y, Ahmed KH, Williams BW (2011) A new maximum power point tracking technique for permanent magnet synchronous generator based wind energy conversion system. IEEE Trans Power Electron 26(12):3609–3620
10. RazaKazmi SM, Goto H, Guo HJ, Ichinokura O (2011) A novel algorithm for fast and efficient speed-sensorless maximum power point tracking in wind energy conversion systems. IEEE Trans Ind Electron 58(1):29–36
11. Koutroulis E, Kalaitzakis K (2006) Design of a maximum power tracking system for wind-energy-conversion applications. IEEE Trans Ind Electron 53(2):486–494
12. Satpathy AS, Kishore NK, Kastha D, Sahoo NC (2014) Control scheme for a stand-alone wind energy conversion system. IEEE Trans. Energy Convers 29(2):418–425
13. Datta R, Ranganathan VT (2003) A method of tracking the peak power points for a variable speed wind energy conversion system. IEEE Trans Ener Convers 18(1):163–168
14. Narayana M, Putrus GA, Jovanovic M, Leung PS, McDonald S (2012) Generic maximum power point tracking controller for small-scale wind turbines. Renew Energy 44:72–79
15. Hidalgo RM, Fernandez JG, Rivera RR, Larrondo HA (2002) A simple adjustable window algorithm to improve fft measurements. IEEE Trans Instrum Meas 51(1):31–36
16. Simon J, Ramprabhakar J (2015) Wind-Photovoltaic systems for isolated load condition. In: Proceedings. of IEEE International. conference on computation of power, energy, information and communication, Chennai, pp 200–204

Phase Shift Control Scheme of Modular Multilevel DC/DC Converters for HVDC-Based Systems

H. U. Shruthi and K. C. Rupesh

Abstract Among the different multilevel topologies, the modular multilevel converter (MMC) has now become a subject of intense research, where it offers some interesting and useful features. In this project, DC/DC converters are proposed for the HVDC-based systems to reduce the transmission losses. The full-bridge converters and three-level flying capacitor circuits are combined and integrated by employing the phase shift control scheme which can be easily applied to achieve 0-voltage and proposed for the high step-down and HVDC-based systems, and also which has a capability to generate the high-quality power under various conditions. Importantly, in this project the voltage auto-balance ability among the cascaded modules is achieved by the flying capacitor which removes the additional components or control loops, and it also allows the operation at higher frequencies and at higher input voltages without scarifying the efficiency. The neutral point clamped (NPC) converters and flying capacitor-based converters are the major multilevel topologies for the high-power and high-voltage applications. Zero-voltage switching (ZVS) performance for both the leading and lagging switches can be provided to reduce the switching losses by adopting the phase-shift control scheme. The time sequence of the leading leg in the phase-shift-controlled full-bridge converters is kept constant, and only the phase of the lagging leg is shifted to regulate the output voltage. A high DC voltage is required for the DC-based distribution and micro-grid systems to improve the delivery power capability which reduces the transmission losses. The switch voltage stress is reduced, and thus, the circuit reliability is enhanced in this project. The MMC concept can be easily extended to N-stage converter to satisfy the high-voltage applications with low-rated voltage switches. The circuit operation and converter performance are analyzed by simulations. The result of input voltage sharing across the capacitors is of 300 V. Thus, the input voltage auto-balance is achieved excellently. The input voltage is stepped down to 53 V. The modes of operations and

H. U. Shruthi (✉) · K. C. Rupesh
Department of Electrical and Electronics Engineering,
Siddaganga Institute of Technology, Tumakuru, India
e-mail: pintu.shruthi@gmail.com

K. C. Rupesh
e-mail: rupeshkc.sit@gmail.com

© Springer Nature Singapore Pte Ltd. 2019   1243
V. Sridhar et al. (eds.), *Emerging Research in Electronics, Computer Science and Technology*, Lecture Notes in Electrical Engineering 545,
https://doi.org/10.1007/978-981-13-5802-9_106

converter performance are analyzed and simulated by using P-Sim software. The three-stage converter is designed to increase the step-down ratio when compared to two-stage converter. This operation is similar to the two-stage converter.

Keywords Neutral point clamping · TLC multilevel DC-to-DC converter · ZVS performance · Phase shift control scheme

1 Introduction

Modular multilevel converters (MMCs) usually come from essential of two different kinds of converters—high-power converters and high-output frequency converters with low-switching frequencies. For the high-power converters which are needed, the design should be found on conventional circuits, paralleling of power switches which are also considered. But, this option represents a few essential drawbacks—basically paralleling switching devices are highly difficult to apply. As current or voltages shares among the devices which is not an easy assignment. The major purpose for high-power converters is mostly centered on power machine drives which are in high and also for grid applications, for example, high voltage-based systems.

With the dissimilar multilevel topology, the modular multilevel converter has now become a focus of extreme investigation. Even it shares the interesting property of additional multilevel designs, it may offer some remarkable and valuable elements. Thus, nowadays the modular multilevel converter has become a research subjects. Although it is of advantage, the controlling of MMC has became a tough task. Therefore of its facts, it is not a matured technology and also there is no universal contract about this classification, control strategies. By the systematization of the MMC with the capacitor, filters will be the main target of this proposal.

DC/DC Converters
DC–to-DC converters are an electronic circuitry device which converts direct current to another. It is one of the power converters whose power varies as of low to high.

Uses of DC-To-DC Converter
DC/DC converters are used in portable devices such as cellular phones and laptops, the power supplies which is powered by batteries. Electronic device comprises the various sub-circuits where each circuit has its own requirement in terms of voltage level which is either supplied by external supply or battery.

DC/DC converter is mainly used for the regulation of output voltage with their certain exceptions such as high efficiency. LED source converter regulates the current through the LEDs, and easy charge pumps where output voltage is twice or thrice.

DC to DC converters are able to improvise the energy produce for photovoltaic system and also the wind turbines which are usually termed as power optimizers.

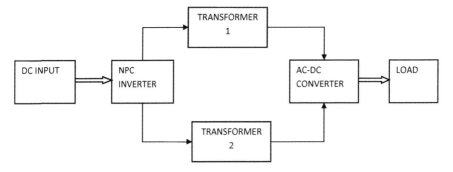

Fig. 1 Proposed diagram

Transformers are designed for the purpose of transfer of voltage to the supply frequency maybe 50 or 60 Hz.

This is more expensive, when eddy current in their core energy starts losses in their windings. Dc to dc converter uses transformers or inductors with its higher frequencies, along with some wound components which are cheaper, smaller, and lighter.

2 Proposed System

Figure 1 shows the proposed system of two-stage converter; in this, there are normally three scopes. From the scope 1, the output of the current and voltage can be shown. From the scope 2, the switching sequence of all the switches, primary voltage and primary current of the transformer 1 and transformer 2 can be shown. In the scope 3, the voltage across the input capacitors C1 and C2 can be shown.

3 System Design

The three-stage converter is designed to increase the step-down ratio, compared to two-stage converter here one more stage is increased, this means that three FB converters are connected in series and also one more flying capacitor is added. For example, for the purpose of simplicity, consider the input voltage as 600 V, in two-stage converters the input voltage is stepped down to 53 V. In three-stage converter, the input voltage is stepped down to 26 V (Fig. 2).

Here, the stepped ratio is increased. The operation of the three-stage converter is similar to two-stage converter to 26 V. Here, the stepped ratio is increased. The operation of the three-stage converter is similar to two-stage converter.

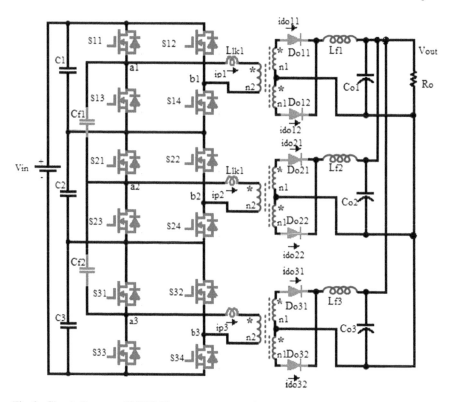

Fig. 2 Circuit diagram of MMC (three-stage converter)

In the secondary side of the derived MMC, the full-wave rectifier, full-bridge rectifier, current doublers rectifier, and, on the other side, the higher current-type rectifier are to be implemented. Here, it is greatly adapted to the full-wave rectifier. It is an symbolic to explore the circuit presentation of the projected modular level topology which is shown in the above Fig. 1.

3.1 Operation Analysis

MODE 1: The switches S_{11}, S_{14}, S_{21}, S_{24}, S_{31}, and S_{34} are turned ON. The flying capacitor C_1 is connected in parallel with C_f. The capacitor discharges the switch and flows through the transformer and continues the loop through the switch. But in stage 3, the switch S_{31} is turned on after some delay ($0.06T_S$). The primary voltage of the transformers is $V_{in}/2$, and the primary current of the transformers is increases linearly. The switch diodes D_{o11}, D_{o21}, and D_{o31} are forward biased.

MODE 2: Here, the switches S_{11}, S_{21}, and S_{31} are turned OFF. The capacitors C_1, C_2, and C_3 are disconnected from the circuit. The stored energy in the inductor flows to the transformer. The primary current starts to decay and the primary voltage starts to decrease gradually.

MODE 3: In this mode, the switches S_{13}, S_{23}, and S_{33} are switched ON. There is no path for the current to flow. Hence, both the primary voltage and current will be zero.

MODE 4: In mode 4, the switch S_{14} is turned off. Here, the switch diode of the switch S_{14} conducts, but it becomes reverse biased and also there is no energy in the inductance of the transformer L_{lk1}. In this mode also, both primary current and voltage will be zero.

MODE 5: Mode 5 is similar to the mode 4, and in this mode, the switches S_{24} and S_{34} are turned off when after some delay of S_{24} gets turned off. Here also, the primary voltage and current of both the transformers is zero.

MODE 6: Here, switch S_{12-} is turned ON. In this mode, C_2 is connected in parallel with C_f. The C_1 discharges through switch S_{12} and flows through the transformer in reverse direction and continues the switch S_{13-} through the loop. The primary voltage across the transformer 1 is $-V_{in}/2$, and the primary current of T_1 starts to flow in the negative half cycle. The other two bottom converters continue with the previous mode of operation. This means that the primary voltage and current will be zero.

MODE 7: In this mode, switch S_{22} is turned ON. Here also, C_2 is connected in parallel with C_f. The capacitor C_1 is discharged with the switch S_{12} and flows through the transformer T_1 in reverse direction and continuous the loop through the switch S_{13}. The primary voltage of T_1 is $-V_{in}/2$. For second stage, the capacitor C_2 is discharged with the switch S_{22} and flows through the transformer T_2 in reverse direction and continues the loop through the switch S_{23}. The primary voltage of T_2 is $-V_{in}/2$. For bottom stage, the capacitor C_3 is discharged with the switch S_{32} and flows through the transformer T_3 in reverse direction and continues the loop through the switch S_{33}. The primary voltage of T_3 is $-V_{in}/2$.

MODE 8: In mode 8, the switches S_{13}, S_{23}, and S_{33} are turned OFF. In this mode, there is no path for current. But both primary voltage and the current of the transformers will be zero.

4 Voltage Auto-Balance Mechanism

The input voltages of the auto-balance mechanism are used to propose modular multilevel DC-to-DC converter which is used to display the output and is shown in the above figure. The steady operation is future interested in the converter for the leading-leg switches S_{11} and S_{12} which is having the same time sequence, and the switches S_{13} and S_{23} are operated synchronously (Fig. 3).

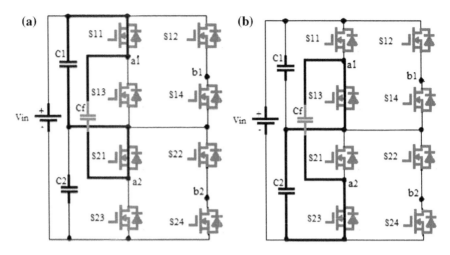

Fig. 3 **a** C_1 is parallel with C_f **b** C_2 is parallel with C_f

$$V_{cf} = V_{c1}$$

where switches S_{11} and S_{21} are turned to the ON; S_{13} and S_{23} switches to the OFF. The flying capacitor C_f is connected in parallel with the input capacitor C_{-1}. The flying capacitor is used to connect with the lagging-leg switches directly with it. The result of the operation on the flying capacitor is hardly affected to the state of the lagging-leg switches. The two phase switches angles can be ϕ_1 and ϕ_2 which take the control of the output voltage.

Effect of Different Factors:

The input voltage imbalance is one of the major drawbacks for most multilevel converters, which is mainly caused by the asymmetry of the component. It has been carried out that the transformer turns ratio difference (N), leakage inductance (L_{lk}), and phase shift angle (Ø). which are the main reasons for the input voltage imbalance in the steady state for the phase shift-controlled converter (Table 1).

Table 1 Effect of different factors

Cases	Results of unbalanced voltage
$N_1 > N_2$	$V_{c1} > V_{c2}$
$L_{lk1} > L_{lk2}$	$V_{c1} > V_{c2}$
$Ø_1 > Ø_2$	$V_{c1} > V_{c2}$

5   Operation Analysis of Proposed System

Design Analysis
To simplify the analysis, the following assumptions are made:

- All the power switches and diodes are ideal.
- The parasitic capacitors of the switches have the same value as C_S.
- The voltage ripples on the divided input capacitors, C_1 and C_2, and flying capacitors, C_f, are small due to their large capacitance.
- The turns ratio of both transformers is $N = n_2 : n_1$.
- The input voltage is balanced, and the auto-balance mechanism will be studied later.

Due to the symmetrical circuit structure and operation, only the first eight stages are analyzed as follows.

- The primary currents, i_{p1} and i_{p2}, are expressed as follows, which is increased to the peak value at the end of the **mode 1**

$$i_{p1}(t) = i_{p1}(t_0) + \frac{v_{in}/2 - NV_{out}}{L_{lk1} + N^2 L_{f1}}(t - t_0) \tag{1}$$

$$i_{p2}(t) = i_{p2}(t_0) + \frac{v_{in}/2 - NV_{out}}{L_{lk2} + N^2 L_{f2}}(t - t_0) \tag{2}$$

- The primary currents are derived at stage/**mode 3**

$$i_{p1}(t) = \frac{is1(t)}{N} \tag{3}$$

$$i_{p2}(t) = \frac{is2(t)}{N} \tag{4}$$

- At **mode 4**, the primary current is regulated by the formula:

$$i_{p1}(t) = i_{p1}(t_{03}) + \cos\omega(t - t_0) \tag{5}$$

where,

$$\omega = \frac{1}{\sqrt{2L_{lk2}C_s}} \tag{6}$$

- At **mode 5**, primary current i_{p2} is regulated by,

$$i_{p2}(t) = i_{p2}(t_4) + \cos\omega(t - t_4) \tag{7}$$

where

$$\omega = \frac{1}{\sqrt{2L_{lk2}C_s}} \tag{8}$$

- At **mode 6**, during the time interval t_5, i_{p1} declines steeply due to half-input voltage across the leakage inductor Llk1, ip1 is given by,

$$i_{p1}(t) = i_{p1}(t_5) - \frac{v_{in}/2}{L_{lk2}}(t - t_5) \tag{9}$$

- At **mode 7**, i_{p2} declines rapidly due to half-input voltage across the leakage inductor L_{lk2}, i_{p2} is given by,

$$i_{p2}(t) = i_{p2}(t_6) - \frac{v_{in}/2}{L_{lk2}}(t - t_6) \tag{10}$$

The output diode Do21 turns OFF after t8, and then a similar operation works in the rest stages.

5.1 Switching Sequence of the Three-Stage Converter

See (Table 2).

5.2 Parameters for Design

Table 3 shows the components list to design. Components are selected based on the requirements. Transformer, diodes, and MOSFETs are taken based on the

Table 2 Switching sequence of three-stage converter

Transformer 1	S_{11}	S_{13}	S_{14}	S_{12}
	0.75	0.25	0.95	0.45
Transformer 2	S_{21}	S_{23}	S_{24}	S_{22}
	0.75	0.25	0.978	0.478
Transformer 3	S_{31}	S_{33}	S_{34}	S_{32}
	0.75	0.25	0.006	0.506

Components	Parameters
Table 3 List of simulation parameters	
Input voltage	600 V
Output voltage	48 V
Switching frequency	100 kHz
Max output power	2000 W

requirements. The transformer turns ratio of primary, secondary, and tertiary windings is selected.

5.3 Simulation Diagram of DC-to-DC Converter with Filter and Without Filter

The three-stage converter is designed to increase the step-down ratio compared to two-stage converter here one more stage is increased, this means that three FB converters are connected in series and also one more flying capacitor is added. For example, for the purpose of simplicity, considered the input voltage as 600 V, in two-stage converters the input voltage is stepped down to 53 V. In three-stage converter, the input voltage is stepped down to 26 V. Here, the stepped ratio is increased. The operation of the three-stage converter is similar to two-stage converter (Fig. 4).

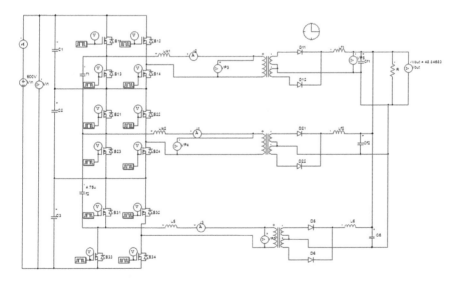

Fig. 4 Circuit diagram with and without C_f

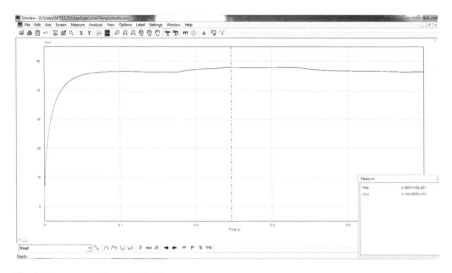

Fig. 5 Output waveform of circuit

5.4 Output Waveform

See (Fig. 5).

5.5 Output Waveforms of Switches, Voltages, Current

See (Fig. 6).

6 Comparison Analysis of Base Converter (Three-Stage Converter) and Proposed Converter (Two-Stage Converter)

See (Table 4).

7 Conclusion and Future Work

In this work, the MMC-based DC-to DC-converters are proposed for the HVDC systems. Because of the flying capacitor, it connects among the input capacitors alternatively. This leads to the sharing of voltage automatically and balancing without

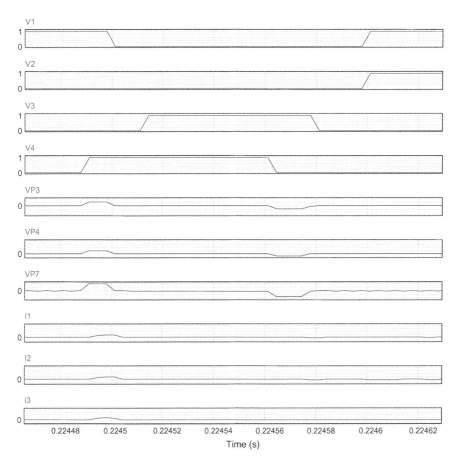

Fig. 6 Output waveforms of switches, voltages, and current

Table 4 Comparison between the converters

Two-stage converter	Three-stage converter
Step-down ratio is not considered	Designed to increase the step-down ratio
Two flyback converters are connected in series	Three FB converters are connected in series and also one more flying capacitor is added
The input voltage is stepped down to 53 V	Here, the input voltage is considered as 300 V. The input voltage is stepped down to 26 V
Stepped ratio is decreased	Here, the stepped ratio is increased

any additional power components and control loops. As a result, the voltage stress across the switches is reduced and also the reliability of circuit is improved.

In addition to this, high step-down ratio is achieved by increasing one more stage. Compared to the two-stage converter, step-down ratio is increased in three-stage converter. This system is suitable for high-power DC-based applications and also used for high step-down applications. The MMC-based DC-to-DC converter technique would be further extended to N number of stages with a load. The full-bridge modules are maintained with the dreadfully high-voltage applications.

References

1. Kakigano H, Miura Y, Ise T (2010) Low-voltage bipolar-type dc micro-grid for super high quality distribution. IEEE Trans Power Electron
2. Anand S, Fernandes BG (2013) Reduced-order model and stability analysis of low-voltage dc micro-grid. IEEE Trans Ind Electron
3. Anand S, Fernandes BG (2010) Optimal voltage level for DC microgrids. IEEE Conf Ind Electron (IECON)
4. Salomonsson D, Soder L, Sannino A (2008) An adaptive control system for a dc microgrid fordata centers. IEEE Trans Ind Appl
5. Park KB, Moon GW, Youn MJ (2011) Series-Input Series-Rectifier interleaved forward converter with a common transformer reset circuit for High-Input-Voltage applications. IEEE Trans Power Electron
6. Qain T, Lehman B (2008) Coupled input-series and output-parallel dual interleaved flyback converter for high input voltage application. IEEE Trans Power Electron
7. Chien CH, Wang YH, Lin BR, Liu CH (2012) Implementation of an interleaved resonant converter for high-voltage applications. In: Proceedings of IET power electron

Improvement of Power Quality in an Electric Arc Furnace Using Shunt Active Filter

K. U. Vinayaka and P. S. Puttaswamy

Abstract Stochastic performance of an electric arc furnace (EAF) and its associated power quality constraints has drawn the attention of the researcher's. In this paper, the power quality disturbances are investigated by characteristic modeling of an electric arc furnace and shunt active filter is incorporated with the system to suppress the effect of these disturbances. The nonlinearity of an EAF load results in distortion of the fundamental component leading to the occurrence of voltage flicker, harmonics, and inter-harmonics. The simulation studies are carried out in MATLAB (Simulink).

Keywords Electric arc furnace (EAF) · Power quality · Voltage flicker · Active filter

1 Introduction

Present-day steel manufacturing is carried using EAF due to its advantageous features, but the prominent benefits of an EAF are masked by the negative impacts of the arc furnace which introduces voltage flicker, harmonics, low power factor, thereby degrading the quality of power system. It is stated that a small voltage fluctuation of less than 0.5% in the range of frequency 5–10 Hz can cause visible flicker.

To probe the harmonic and voltage flicker introduced by an EAF in the electrical network, modeling of an EAF is carried based on the various stages of EAF operation and its associated characteristics.

K. U. Vinayaka (✉)
Department of Electrical and Electronics Engineering,
Siddaganga Institute of Technology, Tumakuru, India
e-mail: vinay.ene@gmail.com

P. S. Puttaswamy
Department of Electrical and Electronics Engineering, PES College of Engineering, Mandya
571401, Karnataka, India
e-mail: psputtaswamy_ee@yahoo.com

© Springer Nature Singapore Pte Ltd. 2019
V. Sridhar et al. (eds.), *Emerging Research in Electronics, Computer Science and Technology*, Lecture Notes in Electrical Engineering 545,
https://doi.org/10.1007/978-981-13-5802-9_107

Figure 1 puts forward the typical line-voltage fluctuations generated during the operation of a furnace. The voltage fluctuation altogether introduces a typical phenomenon termed as "flicker".

Due to the nonlinear variations in current of an EAF, the voltage gets deviated from its purest form, since the same potential is utilized by other loads of a common grid, it poses a severe threat to other devices. The variation of arc current is observed to be very large during the initiation of melting stage, but the severity in magnitudes of current is comparatively lower during other stages of steel making. A typical amplitude spectrum of the current—during melting is as demonstrated by Fig. 2.

Figure 3 exhibits the non-characteristics and characteristic distortions from the fundamental component under various stages of EAF operation.

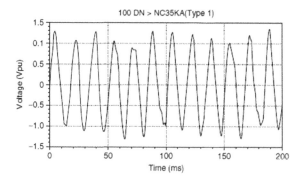

Fig. 1 Voltage flicker curve

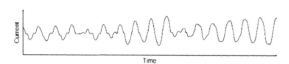

Fig. 2 Arc furnace current

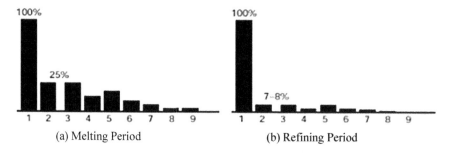

Fig. 3 Harmonic spectrum of arc furnace current

2   Electric Arc Furnace

In the recent years, manufacturing of steel by the aid of an electric arc furnace is widely accepted methodology. Here an electric arc is produced between the electrodes resulting in dissipation of excessive heat in temperature ranging between 3000 and 3500 °C.

The arc furnace has subsequent operations:

- Furnace charging
- Melting
- Refining
- De-slagging.

The process of steel making using an EAF is highly vulnerable in behavior. The rapid variations of an arc resistance make the V-I characteristic of an EAF be non-linear.

3   Modeling of Electric Arc Furnace

Definite electrical activities of an EAF have been sketched out as mentioned in the previous sections. As evident, high nonlinearity, unbalanced, and periodically varying are the characteristics of an EAF load. Such a random nature is hard to realize on a simulator.

The behavior of a working arc furnace is defined by solution of nonlinear differential equations, these equations are utilized to model the operation of an EAF [1].

Here, the characteristic model of an EAF is achieved based on V-I characteristics of the EAF (Fig. 4).

Fig. 4   Actual and approximated (linear piece wise) V-I characteristics of EAF

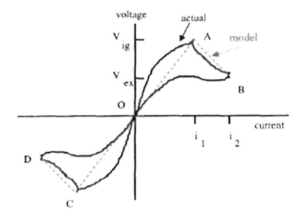

Fig. 5 Actual VI
characteristics of hyperbolic
model in static state

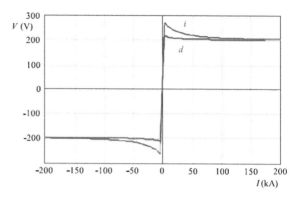

3.1 Hyperbolic Model

In a hyperbolic model, the parameters such as arc current and arc voltage are equated
as per the relationship (Fig. 5).

$$V = \left\{ VT + \frac{Ci, d}{Di, d} \right\} sign(I) \tag{1}$$

VT   Arc voltage threshold value, under the increasing arc current conditions (VT =
      200)
I   Arc current
V   Voltage.

3.2 Exponential Model

Here, the voltage-current attributes of an arc are articulated as an exponential function. The voltage and current relationship for this model are communicated as per
the underneath condition 2 (Fig. 6).

$$V = Vat\left(1 - e^{\frac{-|I|}{Io}}\right) sign(I) \tag{2}$$

VAT   Arc voltage threshold value, under the increasing arc current conditions.
Vat   200
I   Arc current
V   Voltage
Io   Constant value of current to model the sheerness of negative and positive
       currents.

The above tended to models (hyperbolic and exponential) can be consolidated to shape a solitary model by relevant evolution function,

For the case of consolidated model, hyperbolic model characteristic is observed in the voltage during low arc currents and follows exponential model characteristic during high arc currents.

3.3 Exponential-Hyperbolic Model

The voltage-current characteristic of the above-proposed model is given by Eq. 3 (Fig. 6).

The above-proposed model portrays the characteristics of an EAF behavior in time domain. Voltage flicker is introduced under the melting stage of furnace operation and refining stage presents characteristic and non-characteristic harmonic current and voltage at PCC (Fig. 7).

Fig. 6 Actual VI characteristic of exponential model in the static state

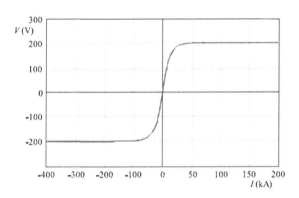

Fig. 7 Actual VI characteristic of proposed model

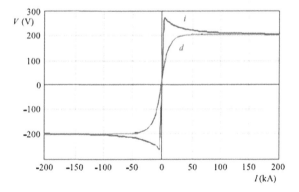

$$V = \begin{Bmatrix} VT + \frac{c}{D+I} & \frac{dI}{dt} \geq 0, I > 0 \\ VT * \left(1 - e^{\frac{-|I|}{I_0}}\right) & \frac{dI}{dt} < 0, I > 0 \end{Bmatrix} \tag{3}$$

4 Harmonic Suppression Techniques

Harmonics existing in the power system network can be effectively suppressed/mitigated by incorporating the various filters.

Out of the different methodologies of harmonic suppression, passive filter is simplest. As the approach is simple, the implementation becomes easier, but it suffers from several drawbacks like tuning requirements, bulkiness of system components for high-power requirements, and occurrence of resonance, thereby influencing stability aspects of power system.

Considering the significant improvement in semiconductor technology for power applications makes the use of active power filters (APF) as the effective solution for harmonic reduction, APF makes utilization of power semiconductor switches that produces signal with phase opposition to the line, thereby cancel out the harmonics to nullify the negative impacts on the source side.

In hybrid APF, the burden of harmonics suppression is carried by two filters. Where lower order dominant harmonics are canceled out by an APF and removal of less predominant higher order harmonics are taken care by passive filter. The objective of hybrid APF is to extract the functionalities of active and passive in providing an effective solution for harmonic reduction [2].

4.1 Active Power Filtering

Active filters are extensively in medium and low voltage distribution level. Figure 8 demonstrates the outline of active filter operation.

The estimation of the harmonic current existing in the system as a result of nonlinear load is achieved by reference signal estimator combined with various influencing parameters of the system. The estimated reference signal drives the system controller as well as another signal. PWM generator along with reference signal determines the pattern of switching.

4.2 Shunt Active Power Filter

Shunt active power filter is the widely accepted topology in the industrial sector. Figure 9 represents the system configuration shunt design.

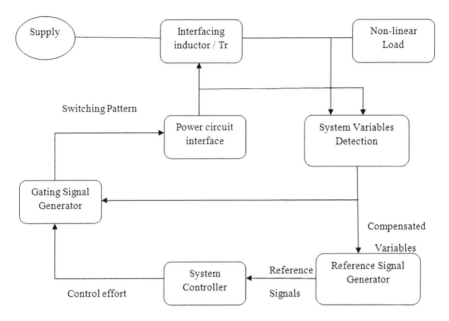

Fig. 8 Block diagram of APF

Fig. 9 Block diagram of VSI-based SAPF

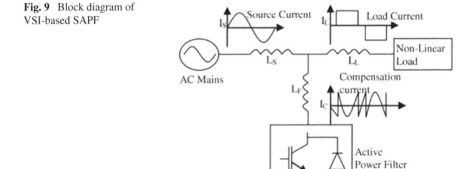

SAPF injects the current harmonic that is in phase opposition with the line currents at the PCC to mitigate the harmonics raised due to the nonlinear loads. As a result, cancelation of the harmonics occurs resulting in reduced distortion of source current. The SAPF also serves as reactive power compensation. Power filter includes of a DC link capacitor, power semiconductor switches, and a coupling inductor (Lf). SAPF effectively compensates the harmonic currents by behaving as a current source.

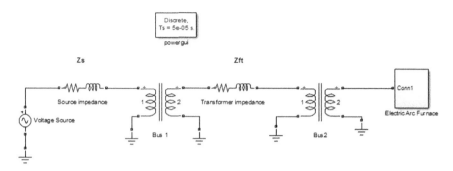

Fig. 10 Single phase test circuit of EAF

Items	Parameters
Table 1 System specifications	
System	V = 566 V, f = 50 Hz
	Zs = 0.0568 + j0.468 mΩ
	Zt = 0.3366 + j3.22 mΩ
Hyperbolic model	Melting stage
	Ci = 190 kW
	Di = 5000 A
	Refining stage
	Cd = 39 KW
	Dd = 5000 A

Desired results of an SAPF is obtained by "shaping" the compensation current waveform (ic), using the current controlled-VSI.

5   Results and Discussion

Attributes of different time-domain arc models are analyzed by an EAF in single-phase circuit. The EAF system arrangement is as shown in Fig. 10. The term Zs refers to the system impedance and PCC is visualized by the transformer on source side and the EAF bus is toward the secondary side of transformer having impedance as Zt. The EAF model is realized with MATLAB function block.

The specifications of the source, system impedance, and parameters of EAF are mentioned in Table 1.

The nonlinear behavior of the hyperbolic model, exponential model, and exponential-hyperbolic model in static state is as represented in the above Figs. 11, 12 and 13 respectively.

Fig. 11 **a** Hyperbolic model **b** exponential model and **c** exponential-hyperbolic model in static state

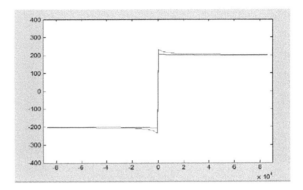

Fig. 12 Exponential model in static state

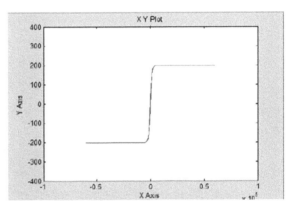

Fig. 13 Exponential-Hyperbolic model in static state

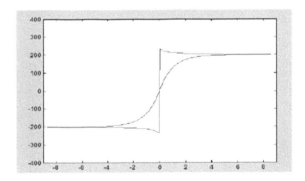

6 Harmonic Behavior of EAF System

Figure 14 demonstrates the test circuit of an EAF fed by three-phase source. A three-phase voltage source with suitable line impedance is used to couple the EAF to power system (Figs. 15, 16, 17, 18, 19 and 20).

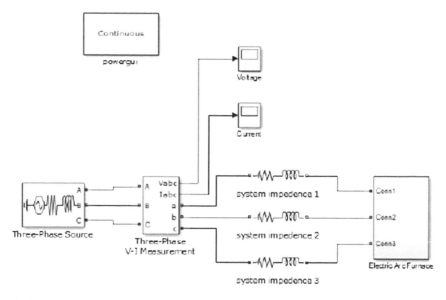

Fig. 14   Three-phase test circuit of EAF connect supply system

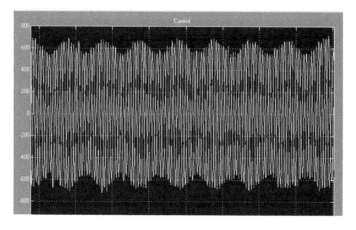

Fig. 15   Three phase Arc current Waveform during Melting stage

Table 2 presents the order of harmonic distortion in an arc furnace current of the above time domain models. It is observed that, due to the unstable arcing phenomenon in melting stage, the non-linearity is found to be high under this condition, indicating the existence of lower order harmonics contributing to the increased distortions in hyperbolic model, the melting stage is characterized by the gradual stabilization of the arc the nonlinear variations gradually reduces significantly, thereby resulting in reduced THD under refining stage of furnace operation.

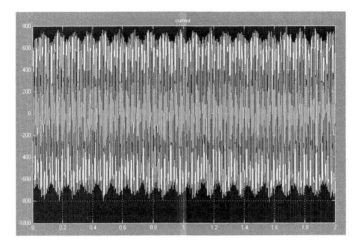

Fig. 16 Three phase Arc current Waveform during refining stage

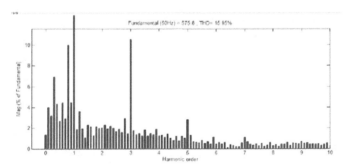

Fig. 17 Arc furnace current harmonic spectrum during melting

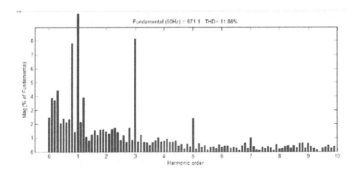

Fig. 18 Arc furnace current harmonic spectrum during refining

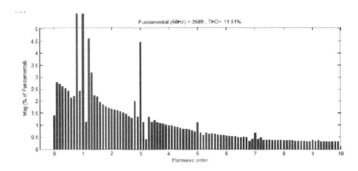

Fig. 19 Arc furnace current harmonic spectrum in exponential model

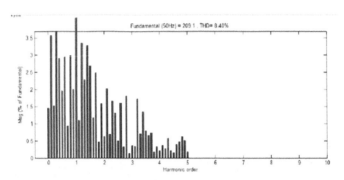

Fig. 20 Arc furnace current harmonic spectrum in exponential-hyperbolic model

Table 2 Harmonic component comparison of different stages of operation

Harmonic order	Hyperbolic		Exponential model	Exponential-hyperbolic model
	Melting stage	Refining stage		
3rd (%)	10.53	8.15	4.47	0.35
5th (%)	2.81	2.40	1.10	0.18
7th (%)	1.10	1.01	0.66	–
9th (%)	0.69	0.60	0.40	–
THD (%)	15.95	11.86	11.81	8.40

Exponential and Exponential-Hyperbolic model of an EAF signifies that, the characteristics move towards the linear zone, hence Exponential-Hyperbolic model comprises reduced order harmonics in comparison with hyperbolic model.

The harmonic spectrum of arc current of various characteristic models shows the noteworthy existence of inter harmonics—which inside and out adds to the expanded total of distortion levels of the system.

Table 3 Voltage flicker of different time domain models

Model	% voltage flicker
Hyperbolic-melting stage	1.54
Exponential-refining stage	2.01
Exponential	10.85
Exponential-hyperbolic	23.45

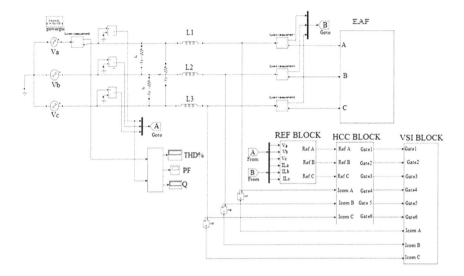

Fig. 21 Electric Arc Furnace simulated with SAPF

Table 3 infers the insight on the voltage flicker levels of different time domain models of an EAF, it is observed that the voltage flicker is high is case of hyperbolic-exponential model than the others.

The system configuration of an EAF with SAPF is realized as shown below in Fig. 21; the source voltage parameter is considered as 440 V at 50 Hz with an EAF as load, the harmonics and flicker introduced by a nonlinear and unbalanced operation of EAF.

SAPF is introduced in parallel to reduce the impact of harmonics and voltage flicker on supply side.

The EAF Simulink block is developed using MATLAB. Exponential model of an EAF is modeled to investigate the performance of the system. And the system specifications of the SAPF are as listed in Table 4.

From Tables 5 and 6, it can be interpret that, the voltage flicker and the harmonic levels in system feeding an EAF are dropped down measurably due to the insertion of Shunt active power filter. The harmonic spectrum of Arc furnace current with and without Shunt Active Power Filter is shown in Figs. 22 and 23, respectively.

Table 4 System specifications of SAPF

Parameters	Values
System	V = 440, f = 50 Hz
Line inductance	0.1 mH
DC capacitor	100 μF
Filter inductance	0.45 mH

Table 5 Voltage flicker simulation results with and without SAPF

Model	% voltage flicker without SAPF	% voltage flicker with SAPF
Exponential	10.85	7.2

Table 6 THD simulation results with and without SAPF

Model	% THD without SAPF	% THD with SAPF
Exponential	11.81	4.38

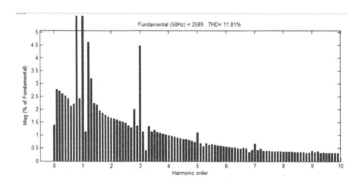

Fig. 22 The harmonic spectrum of Arc furnace current without shunt active power filter

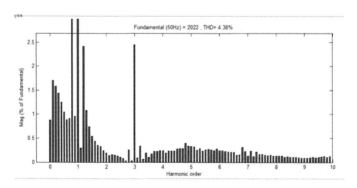

Fig. 23 The harmonic spectrum of Arc furnace current with shunt active power filter

7 Conclusion

EAF is an exceptionally nonlinear, timely varying load with clamorous conduct acquainting a few power quality unsettling influences with the system.

The static conducts of different kinds of electric arc furnace models are examined and the outcomes got show the presence of voltage flicker in the system. Hyperbolic and exponential model is contemplated in detail and another model is inferred. The new model displays attributes for both expanding and diminishing currents. This model clearly indicates unbalanced and flickering voltage behavior.

From the simulated results, the harmonic distortions and the voltage flicker of the arc models are exceeding the IEEE standards. These power quality problems cause disturbances to in the system. Hence, these issues with respect to arc furnace must be mitigated.

As indicated by IEEE 519-1992 STD, the current harmonics in the framework ought to be inside ±7% yet from the simulated results, the harmonic content in the framework is surpassing the IEEE guidelines. IEEE P1453 STD for the voltage flicker in the framework ought not to surpass ±5%, but rather from the reenacted comes about, the voltage flicker in the framework is surpassing the IEEE guidelines.

Henceforth to smother these vital issues investigated in the framework a hysteresis based SAPF innovation has been inculcated to serve the needs of power quality improvement. It is learnt that THD of the Arc current has been lowered significantly as per the Standards, proving the effectiveness of the Filter.

References

1. Golkar MA, Meschi S (2008) MATLAB modeling of arc furnace for flicker study. In: IEEE international conference on industrial technology, 2008. ICIT, 21–24 April 2008, pp 1–6
2. Singh B, Al-Haddad K, Chandra A (1999) A review of active filters for power quality improvements. IEEE Trans Ind Electron 46(5):960–971

Wireless Power Transfer for LED Display System Using Class-DE Inverter

A. Vamsi Krishna and M. R. Rashmi

Abstract In the present era, electricity is one of the essential needs of human society. Transmission lines are used in conventional power system which is expensive and less efficient. Transmission line losses account for the major reduction in transmission efficiency due to long transmission lines spanning several kilometres. One best solution for this old-age problem is to have wireless power transmission (WPT). Not only in transmission, can any application module can be made compact and energy efficient using WPT concept. In WPT, AC voltage is rectified, converted to high-frequency AC, and transmitted using inductive power transfer or capacitive power transfer approach. Inductive power transfer system contains transmitter and receiver coils designed for high-frequency AC voltage. Therefore, the coils' size is reduced and they can be made compact. In this paper, a WPT scheme is proposed for LED lighting which can be used in public information display system. The system is designed to drive 100 W LED display unit. Class-DE inverter is considered and series–parallel resonance is used in transmitter and receiver coil sides, respectively. The simulation results are presented.

Keywords LED display · Class-DE converter · Wireless power transfer · Series–parallel resonance

1 Introduction

To eliminate the losses in the transmission system, wireless power transfer is the best choice [1]. The WPT can use inductive power transfer or magnetic coupling or resonant coupling to transfer power between two coils. There are several

A. V. Krishna (✉) · M. R. Rashmi
Department of Electrical and Electronics Engineering, Amrita School
of Engineering, Bengaluru, Amrita Vishwa Vidyapeetham, Bengaluru, India
e-mail: vamsikrishna2950@gmail.com

M. R. Rashmi
e-mail: mr_rashmi@blr.amrita.edu

© Springer Nature Singapore Pte Ltd. 2019
V. Sridhar et al. (eds.), *Emerging Research in Electronics, Computer Science
and Technology*, Lecture Notes in Electrical Engineering 545,
https://doi.org/10.1007/978-981-13-5802-9_108

resonant topologies listed in the literature [2, 3] such as series–series (SS) topology and series–parallel (SP) topology of the magnetically coupled receiver and transmitter and their characteristics were elucidated in the paper. Various characteristics of electrical resonance coupling in wireless power transfer are discussed in [4]. The advantage of Class-D inverter for WPT, its design and operation was given in [5]. To alleviate the switching losses, zero-voltage switching was adapted. Class-E converter is a better choice over Class-D for WPT applications [6, 7] in terms of efficiency and low sensitivity to noise signals, and Class-E converter efficiency is good for high-frequency applications. Class-DE converter combines the better features of Class-D and Class-E converters. Class-DE inverter with fixed modulation index using series–parallel resonant circuit was proposed in [8, 9] for WPT applications. Zero voltage and zero current were introduced in this inverter to reduce high switching losses at high switching frequencies. In Class-DE converter, there will be capacitors across all the active switches. These capacitors' value depends on the type of resonance used in transmitter coil side of WPT system. A detailed design approach for these capacitors was provided in [10] and the design is based on the resonant frequency. Class-DE inverter may be of half bridge or full bridge. At a known coupling coefficient, power transfer gain is high when Class-DE inverters are used instead of Class-D/Class-E inverters. In Class-DE, all the switches of rectifier and inverter are operated in zero-voltage and zero-current switching. Hence, the switching losses are also minimized. It suggests the use of soft switching in Class-DE converter to curtail the switching losses further. The authors in [11] also discussed in detail design of Class-DE inverter and stated that Class-DE is the blend of best characteristics of both Class-D and Class-E amplifiers, leaving out their disadvantages are listed in the literature. A full-bridge Class-DE inverter was designed in [12] for WPT and was used in open loop. Author(s) in [9] also gave the method for the transition from series–parallel resonant network for 100 kHz to series resonant network for Class-DE inverter-based WPT system. The benefits of contactless energy transfer systems (CETSs) for various applications were given [13]. The various types of ferrites cores for transmitter and receiver coils with different geometries and their design aspects were also presented in [13].

A Class-DE full-bridge inverter with series–parallel resonance is presented in this paper. The circuit operation is discussed in Sect. 2. Design considerations are provided in Sect. 3. Simulation results and analysis are given in Sect. 4 and conclusion in the last Sect. 5

2   Circuit Description

A typical block diagram of WPT system is given in Fig. 1. Input taken from the AC source is fed to the rectifier which converts it to the DC and is further given to the inverter circuit to alter the frequency and ensuring that the frequency falls in the chosen range. The output of the inverter, an alternating signal with high frequency, is fed to the transmitting coil which produces the magnetic field. The receiving coil,

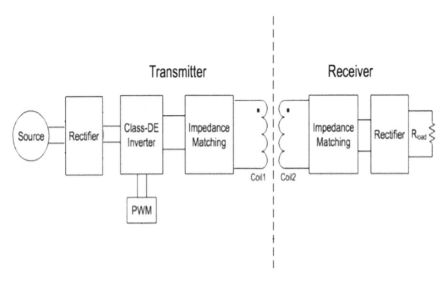

Fig. 1 Wireless power transfer system diagram

which is coupled with the transmitting coil with a certain coupling factor, is in the vicinity of the magnetic field engendered by the transmitting coil. Hence, an EMF is induced in the receiving coil which is converted into DC by the single-phase full-bridge rectifier with necessary filters to minimise the ripple content and is supplied to the load. The circuit diagram is shown in Fig. 2. Class-DE inverter with series resonance is used.

A Class-DE power amplifier can be modelled by two half bridges with a common DC source, a series inductor–capacitor pair that is connected from the mid-point of the four transistors, and in series to that a load is connected as shown in Fig. 3. Class-DE inverter operates in four modes based on the switching sequence indicated in Table 1.

2.1 Operating Mode During Interval 1 ($0 \leq \theta \leq \pi/2$)

During this mode, switches S1 and S2 are ON. The equivalent circuit during this mode is shown in Fig. 4a. During this inverter, output current $I_o > 0$ and I_o is positive. Positive terminal is connected to A and negative terminal is connected to B. Therefore, $V_o > 0$, V_o is positive. Therefore, the output voltage is given by Eq. (1)

$$V_o = V_{in} - V_l - V_c - V_{s1} - V_{s2} \tag{1}$$

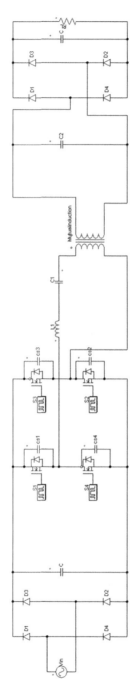

Fig. 2 Class-DE inverter with inductive coils, rectifier, and load

Fig. 3 Class-DE power
amplifier circuit schematics

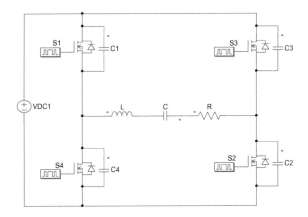

Table 1 Switching states of the inverter switches

	$0 \leq \theta \leq \pi/2$	$\pi/2 \leq \theta \leq \pi$	$\pi \leq \theta \leq 3\pi/2$	$3\pi/2 \leq \theta \leq 2\pi$
S1 and S2	ON	OFF	OFF	OFF
D1 and D2	OFF	ON	OFF	OFF
S3 and S4	OFF	OFF	ON	OFF
D3 and D4	OFF	OFF	OFF	ON

2.2 Operating Mode During Interval 2 ($\pi/2 \leq \theta \leq \pi$)

During this, none of the switches are given pulses. Diodes D1 and D2 will be forward
biased. The energy from inductors will be freewheeled during this mode. The equivalent circuit of this mode is shown in Fig. 4b. During this inverter, output current
$I_o < 0$ and $V_o > 0$. Diodes conduct till the energy stored in inductor becomes zero.
The output voltage during this interval is given by the expression (2)

$$V_o = V_{in} + V_{d1} + V_l - V_c + V_{d2} \tag{2}$$

2.3 Operating Mode During Interval 3 ($\pi \leq \theta \leq 3\pi/2$)

During this mode, switches S1 and S2 are ON. The equivalent circuit during this mode
is shown in Fig. 4a. Therefore, the inverter output current is in reverse direction that
is $I_o < 0$. The output voltage is negative $V_o < 0$. The output voltage is given by
Eq. (3).

$$V_o = -V_{in} + V_l - V_c + V_{s3} + V_{s4} \tag{3}$$

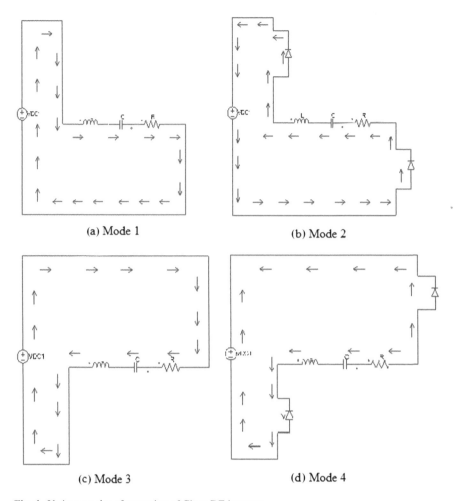

Fig. 4 Various modes of operation of Class-DE inverter

2.4 Operating Mode During Interval 4 ($3\pi/2 \leq \theta \leq 2\pi$)

During this, none of the switches are given pulses. Diodes D3 and D4 will be forward biased. The equivalent circuit of this mode is shown in Fig. 4d. Whenever anti parallel are diodes conduct, current direction will reverse that is $I_o > 0$. Voltage is of the same polarity that is $V_o < 0$. The output voltage during this interval is given by the expression (4)

$$V_o = -V_{in} + V_{d3} - V_l - V_c + V_{d4} = 0 \tag{4}$$

3 Design Considerations

The system is designed for 100 W output. The rectified output in the receiver should drive a LED display of 100 W at 12 V. The switching frequency is 100 kHz.

$\omega = 2\pi f$ where $f = 100 * 10^3$ Hz

The coupling coefficient $K = 0.2$ for air cored mutually inductive coils.

At the receiver side, output is 12 V with 100 W; therefore, the equivalent resistance is given by (5)

$$R_{load} = V^2/P = \frac{12^2}{100} = 1.44\,\Omega \tag{5}$$

At the receiver side's output, 1.44 Ω with 100 W is obtained which results in output current $I_{load} = 8.33$ A.

3.1 Receiver-side Rectifier Specifications

$$V_o = 2Vm/\pi \tag{6}$$

Therefore, $vm = 18.84$ V

$$Vm = Vrms * \sqrt{2} \tag{7}$$

Hence, $Vrms = 13.32$ V

3.2 Transmitter-side Class-DE Inverter Design

Series capacitor on the primary side is chosen as $C = 2 * e^{-6}$ F.

Resonant frequency is given by

$$f = 1/2\pi\sqrt{LC} \tag{8}$$

Using (8), series inductor L value is found to be $L = 3.97 * e^{-6}$ H.

Reviver's output voltage $vm = 18.84$ V by taking coupling factor $K = 0.2$, we get transmitter-side output voltage is $V_o = 133.21$ V.

3.3 Supply-side Rectifier Design

Using (6), the peak input voltage to the rectifier is $vm = 133.21 * \pi/2 \approx 210$ V
Therefore, the supply voltage $Vrms = 147.88$ V.

3.4 Transmitter Coil Design

Power $(pt) = 100$ W
Voltage $(Vt) = 134$ V
Current $(It) = \frac{Pt}{Vt} = \frac{100}{134} = 0.746$ A
Resistance $(Rt) = \frac{Vt}{It} = \frac{134}{0.746} = 179.62\,\Omega$
Inductance value

$$(Lt) = \frac{Qt * Rt}{w} \tag{9}$$

For series–parallel topology quality factor $Qt = 1098$

Therefore, $Lt = \frac{1098*179.64}{2*3.14*100*10^3} = 314 * 10^{-3}$ H

Spherical coils are used.

$$L(\text{mH}) = \frac{Di^2 * A^2}{(30 * A - 11 * Di)} = 314\,\text{mH} \tag{10}$$

Area of cross section of the coil is given by

$$A = \frac{Di + N * (w + s)}{2} \tag{11}$$

$$w = \frac{Wl}{N} \tag{12}$$

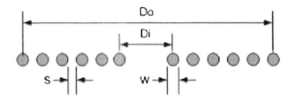

where

Di = inner diameter of coil = 2 cm;
Do = outer diameter of coil = 15 cm;
S = distance between coils = 0.25 cm;
N = number of turns = 26;
w = wire diameter;
Wl = wire length.

Using (11), wire diameter $w = 0.552$ mm and using (12), wire length Wl is found to be 14.375 m.

3.5 Receiver Coil Design

Receiver is designed for 100 W output.
Power $(pr) = 100$ W
Voltage $(Vr) = 18.84$ V
Current $(Ir) = \frac{Pr}{Vr} = \frac{100}{19} = 5.26$ A
Resistance $(Rr) = \frac{Vr}{Ir} = \frac{19}{5.26} = 3.61 \, \Omega$

$$RL = \frac{8}{\pi^2} * Rr = 2.929 \, \Omega$$

Inductance value

$$(Lr) = \frac{Qr * Rr}{w} \tag{13}$$

For series–parallel topology $Qr = 1031$

$$Lr = \frac{1031 * 2.929}{2 * 3.14 * 100 * 10^{\wedge}3} = 4.8 * 10^{-3} \text{ H6}$$

Receiver wire diameter = 0.536 mm and receiver $Wl = 13.95$ m.

4 Simulation Results

Simulation is carried out in MATLAB/Simulink environment. The simulation circuit is shown in Fig. 5. The AC input supply is shown in Fig. 6. The supply peak voltage is 210 V. Source-side rectifier output is shown in Fig. 7. The ripples in rectifier output are removed by using capacitor filter, and then, this output is given to high switching frequency inverter.

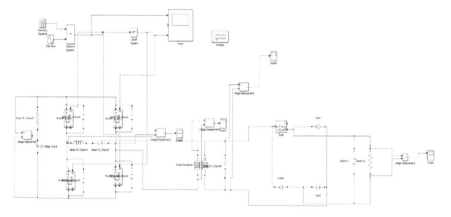

Fig. 5 Simulation circuit

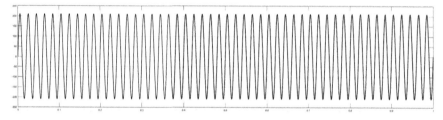

Fig. 6 Supply voltage

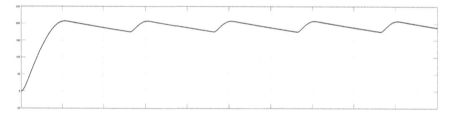

Fig. 7 Supply-side rectifier output voltage

The output voltage of Class-DE inverter at 100 kHz switching frequency is shown in Fig. 8. This is the voltage appearing at transmitting coil. The power in transmitter coil is transferred inductively to the receiver coil. An air-cored coupled coils are used in the simulation. The output voltage at the receiver side is shown in Fig. 9. The rectified voltage to drive 100 W load is shown in Fig. 10.

From Fig. 8, it is observed that the inverter output is not sinusoidal. The inverter output is passed.

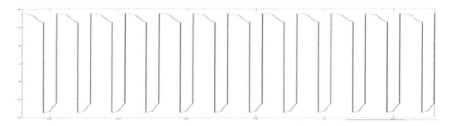

Fig. 8 Class-DE inverter output voltage

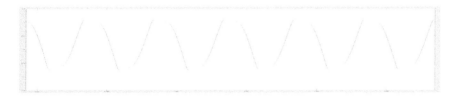

Fig. 9 Voltage at receiver terminals

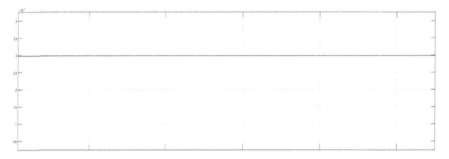

Fig. 10 Receiver-side rectifier output voltage

5 Conclusion

A wireless power transfer system was designed to drive LED unit of 100 W. Class-DE inverter was designed for this application for efficient energy transfer. The output of receiver was smoothened by proper resonant circuit design, and this AC voltage was rectified and fed to 100 W load. The required voltage level was obtained at the receiver side with stringent design considerations. The work can be further focused on regulating load terminal voltage under variable supply conditions due to the intermittency of renewable energy sources. This can be achieved by closed loop control of either Class-DE inverter or by controlling the receiver-side rectifier.

References

1. Khan, Qureshi MI, Rehman MU, Khan WT (2017) Long range wireless power transfer via magnetic resonance. In: 2017 Progress in Electromagnetics Research Symposium—Fall (PIERS-FALL). Singapore, pp 3079–3085
2. Ishihara M, Umetani K, Umegami H, Hiraki E, Yamamoto M (2016) Quasi-duality between SS and SP topologies of basic electric-field coupling wireless power transfer system. Electron Lett 52(25):2057–2059
3. Buja G, Bertoluzzo M, Mude KN (2015) Design and experimentation of WPT charger for electric city car. IEEE Trans Industr Electron 62(12):7436–7447
4. Umegami H, Ishihara M, Hattori F, Masuda M, Yamamoto M (2015) Basic experiment study on misalignment characteristic of electrical resonance coupling wireless power transfer. In: 2015 IEEE international telecommunications energy conference (INTELEC). Osaka
5. Bilsalam A, Haema J (2015) A high frequency isolated asymmetrical Class-D resonant inverter for induction heating saw blades application. 2015 12th international conference on electrical engineering/electronics, computer, telecommunications and information technology (ECTI-CON). HuaHin
6. Sokal NO, Sokal AD (1975) Class E-A new class of high-efficiency tuned single-ended switching power amplifiers. IEEE J Solid-State Circuits 10(3):168–176
7. Rohith T, Samhitha VS, Mamatha I (2016) Wireless transmission of solar power using inductive resonant principle. In: IEEE biennial international conference on power and energy systems: towards sustainable energy (PESTSE 2016)
8. Albertoni et al L (2016) Analysis and design of full-bridge Class-DE inverter at fixed duty cycle. In: IECON 2016—42nd annual conference of the IEEE industrial electronics society. Florence, pp 5609–5614
9. Udhayakumar G, Rashmi MR, Suresh A (2016) Interleaved boost converters with active clamping as power supply for artificial ozonator. Int J Control Theory Appl 9(36):601–617
10. Naik MK, Bertoluzzo M, Buja (2013) Design of a contactless battery charging system. In: 2013 Africon. Pointe-Aux-Piments, pp 1–6
11. Inaba T, Koizumi H, Sekiya H (2017) Design of wireless power transfer system with Class E inverter and half-bridge Class DE rectifier at any fixed coupling coefficient. In: 2017 IEEE 3rd international future energy electronics conference and ECCE Asia (IFEEC 2017—ECCE Asia). Kaohsiung, pp 185–189
12. Biten AB (2016) Wireless power transfer using Class-DE converter via strongly coupled two planar coils. Thesis and Dissertations, 1340
13. Albertoni L, Grasso F, Matteucci J (2016) Analysis and design of full-bridge Class-DE inverter at fixed duty cycle. In: IECON 2016—42nd annual conference of the IEEE industrial electronics society, 23–26 October 2016

Bidirectional Power Conversion by DC–AC Converter with Active Clamp Circuit

H. Anusha and S. B. Naveen Kumar

Abstract Solar is one of the most widely used energy sources due to its ease of availability and preferred for the generation of electricity. This paper presents a bidirectional power conversion from DC to AC by using non-complementary active clamp circuits. It consists of the bidirectional flyback converter. In order to interface the grid with low-voltage energy storage through single-stage power conversion, the bidirectional converter is used to convert low voltage directly into the grid voltage and regulates the grid current. By using the non-complementary operation approach, the flyback converter avoids the sudden increase in voltage and also decreases the energy loss. And hence by using single-stage power conversion approach and non-complementary active clamp circuits, the flyback converter attains high power efficiency and low total harmonic distortion. A control algorithm is developed to facilitate the bidirectional single power conversion. The flyback converter assures high voltage quality by this control algorithm. The simulation is done by using the PSIM software and analyzed in detail.

Keywords Energy storage system (ESS) · Powersim (PSIM) · Total harmonic distortion (THD)

1 Introduction

Environmental problems, such as fossil fuel reduction, global warming, and discharge of carbon dioxide, have stimulated the progress of renewable energy sources. However, the discontinuous nature of renewable energy sources affects a negative effect on the quality of the grid power. Because of these reasons, energy storage system (ESS) is becoming more and more important. ESS plays a major role to lessen the problem of intermittency of renewable energy sources. To connect the

H. Anusha (✉) · S. B. Naveen Kumar
Department of Electrical and Electronics Engineering,
Siddaganga Institute of Technology, Tumakuru, India
e-mail: anushaa382@gmail.com

© Springer Nature Singapore Pte Ltd. 2019
V. Sridhar et al. (eds.), *Emerging Research in Electronics, Computer Science and Technology*, Lecture Notes in Electrical Engineering 545,
https://doi.org/10.1007/978-981-13-5802-9_109

Fig. 1 Conventional
two-stage bidirectional
DC-to-AC converter

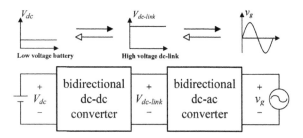

high-voltage grid to a low-voltage 48-V battery, a bidirectional DC–AC converter is needed. The value of the bidirectional DC-to-AC converter is estimated by power efficiency, battery power regulation, and grid power quality such as power factor and total harmonic distortion (THD). To meet these desires, numerous bidirectional DC-to-AC converters have been introduced. Figure 1 represents the two-stage typical bidirectional conversion of direct current to alternating current.

The charging or discharging function is achieved by the bidirectional DC–DC converter by converting the low voltage into high voltage. To interface the grid with the high-voltage DC link, a bidirectional DC-to-AC converter is used. Due to the two power processing stages, drawback of circuit complexity, high cost, and low power efficiency arises. To get the better way for the processing of power, the single-stage bidirectional DC–AC converters are introduced.

To enhance the efficiency of the power by single stage, the processing of the power is done by single-stage power conversion using DC–AC converter. The main disadvantage of the typical two-way DC-to-AC converter is that it has only step-down phenomena, and hence, the source voltage must be greater than the maximum value of the line voltage, that is why the number of batteries has to be series connected. This type of arrangement of battery not only decreases the reliability and lifetime of the energy storage system but also increases dimension and mass of the system.

The input supply to the bidirectional DC-to-AC converter is taken from two sources. One is the constant DC supply, and the other one is the variable solar supply. The control circuit is designed such that if the sun rays can be readily available then the solar PV is used as the input power supply. If it is too rainy or if the solar supply could not reach the desired value, then instead of solar supply the battery can be used as the source.

2   Block Diagram

The above block diagram shows the entire process of the DC-to-AC power conversion with non-complementary active clamp circuits. The supply voltage is taken from the 48-V DC and is given as the input to the bidirectional flyback converter. The main advantage of this converter is that it has high ratio of voltage conversion and evades the number of batteries connected in series. The above strategy avoids the sudden

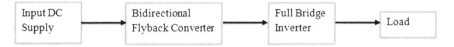

Fig. 2 Block diagram of the bidirectional flyback converter

increase in voltage and decreases energy losses by propagating energy to achieve the maximum power efficiency (Fig. 2).

3 Operation Principle

The circuit diagram of the closed-loop bidirectional flyback converter is as shown in Fig. 3. The main switches of the bidirectional flyback converter, i.e., S_{P1} and S_{S1}, will operate corresponding to each other. The duty cycle of these switches will be varied according to the grid voltage v_g. The two-way flyback converter controls the line current to get the maximum pf and decreased THD. Clamp capacitors C_P and C_S are meant to absorb the leakage energy of the transformer T. The body diodes of the switches S_{P2} and S_{S2} are turned on when the main switches are off; thus, the leakage current has to flow across these switches. So as to recycle outflow energy, switches S_{P2} and S_{S2} have to be turned on for a short time before S_{P1} and S_{S1} are switched on. The energy losses by the propagating energy need to be minimized through decreasing the function of active clamp circuits. During positive half cycle, switches S_1 and S_2 are turned on, and during negative half cycle, S_3 and S_4 are turned on of the grid voltage v_g.

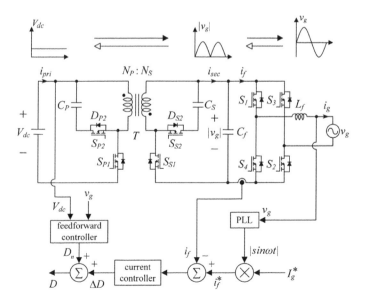

Fig. 3 Diagram of bidirectional DC–AC converter with control circuit

The bidirectional flyback converter has the symmetrical structure as shown in Fig. 3. And hence, the steady-state operation can be discussed either for the charging/discharging mode. The switching period is represented as T_S; in the steady-state operation, it is alienated into six operating modes.

4 Basic Operations of Converter

Mode 1 operation (t_0–t_1): At time t_0, the main switch S_{P1} is turned on. The energy of the battery is transferred to the magnetizing inductor L_m of the transformer T. At the secondary side, the voltage stress V_{S1} of the switch S_{S1} rises. When the voltage stress V_{S1} reaches to $|V_g| + V_{CS}$, the body diode of the active clamp switch S_{S2} is turned on. Hence, the leakage energy in L_{lk2} is transferred to the secondary clamp capacitor C_S and V_{S1} is clamped to the value $|V_g| + V_{CS}$. When L_{lk2} is totally discharged, the body diode D_{S2} is turned off and this interval finishes (Fig. 4).

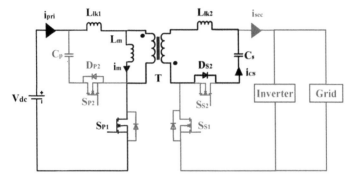

Fig. 4 Circuit diagram of mode 1 operation

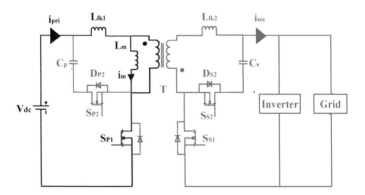

Fig. 5 Circuit diagram of mode 2 operation

Mode 2 operation (t_1–t_2): Only S_{P1} is turned on in this interval. At this time, the energy of the battery is still transferred to L_m and the primary side current i_{pri} increases linearly. The voltage stress of S_{S1} is the sum of reflected voltage and the folded grid voltage, e.g., $nV_{dc} + |V_g|$ where the turns ratio n is given by n_S/n_P. This period ends at t_2 when S_{S2} is turned on (Fig. 5).

Mode 3 operation (t_2–t_3): At time t_2, the active clamp switch S_{S2} is turned on for a short time. The absorbed leakage energy in mode 1 is transferred to the battery side in this interval. The voltage stress V_{S1} is changed to the value $|V_g| + V_{CS}$. This period ends at t_3 when S_{P1} and S_{S2} are turned off (Fig. 6).

Mode 4 operation (t_3–t_4): The main switch S_{S1} is turned on at time t_3. The magnetizing inductor L_m starts discharging, and the stored energy is delivered to the grid. At the primary side, the voltage stress V_{P1} of the main switch S_{P1} increases. When V_{P1} reaches $V_{dc} + V_{CP}$, the body diode of the active clamp switch S_{P2} is turned on. Consequently, the leakage energy in L_{lk1} is absorbed by the primary clamp capacitor C_P and the voltage stress V_{P1} is clamped to the value $V_{dc} + V_{CP}$. The body diode D_{P2} is turned off when the leakage inductor is fully discharged and this interval finishes (Fig. 7).

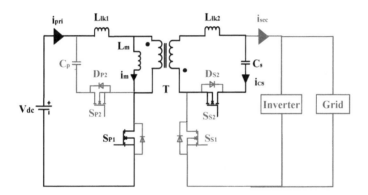

Fig. 6 Circuit diagram of mode 3 operation

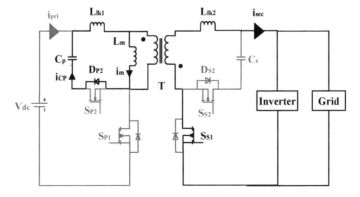

Fig. 7 Circuit diagram of mode 4 operation

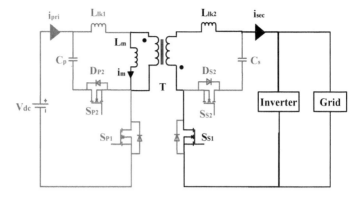

Fig. 8 Circuit diagram of mode 5 operation

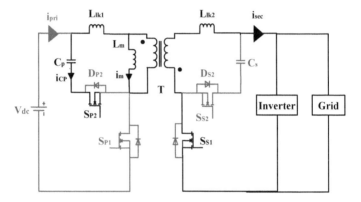

Fig. 9 Circuit diagram of mode 6 operation

Mode 5 operation (t_4–t_5): Only S_{S1} is turned on in this interval. The stored energy of L_m is still transferred to the grid, and the secondary side current i_{sec} decreases linearly. The voltage stress V_{P1} of the main switch S_{P1} is the sum of the dc storage voltage and reflected voltage, e.g., $V_{dc} + |V_g|/n$. This period ends at t_5 when S_{P2} is turned on (Fig. 8).

Mode 6 operation (t_5–t_6): At time t_5, the active clamp switch S_{P2} is turned on for a short time. In this interval, the absorbed leakage energy in mode 4 is transferred to the grid side. The voltage stress V_{P1} is changed to the value $V_{dc} + V_{CP}$. This period ends at t_6 when S_{S1} and S_{P2} are turned off (Fig. 9).

5 Control Algorithm for the Bidirectional Converter

Feasibility of the conversion of the power through single stage is attained by regulating the line current i_f. The line current comprises power flow direction, pf and THD.

The bidirectional DC–AC converter will operate in quasi-steady state at every single instant because the DC–AC converter operates slowly in the grid period when compared to single switching instant. Duty ratio of the switch S_{P1} is D, and magnetizing current deviation is Δim during the discharging mode. And the average voltage for Lm for the one switching period T_S can be attained as

$$V \mathrm{dc}\, D - \frac{|vg|}{n}(1 - D) = Lm \frac{\Delta im}{TS} \tag{1}$$

Duty ratio D can be considered as

$$D = \frac{|vg|}{n V \mathrm{dc} + |vg|} + \frac{n}{n V \mathrm{dc} + |vg|}(Lm \frac{\Delta im}{TS}) \tag{2}$$

The magnetizing current and line current depending on the duty ratio D can be given as

$$if = \frac{(1 - D)im}{n} \tag{3}$$

By using Eq. (3), the duty cycle in (2) can be re-expressed by means of the line current as

$$\begin{aligned} D &= \frac{|vg|}{n V \mathrm{dc} + |vg|} + \frac{n}{n V \mathrm{dc} + |vg|}\left(\frac{Lm}{TS}\right)\left(\frac{n \Delta if}{1 - D}\right) \\ &= \frac{|vg|}{n V \mathrm{dc} + |vg|} + \frac{n Lm}{TS\,V \mathrm{dc}}\Delta if = Dn + \Delta D \end{aligned} \tag{4}$$

The nominal duty cycle Dn and control duty cycle ΔD can be given by

$$Dn = \frac{|vg|}{n V \mathrm{dc} + |vg|}, \Delta D = \frac{n Lm}{TS\,V \mathrm{dc}}\Delta if \tag{5}$$

There is no need to calculate the duty cycle for the discharging mode because for both the modes it will remain same but the direction of the current is changed because of the corresponding switching operation of S_{P1} and S_{S1}. And hence, duty ratio of the switch S_{P1} in charging mode is equal to Eq. (4).

6 Simulation Results

Closed loop simulation of bi-directional DC-to-AC converter with single input:

The circuit shown in Fig. 10 is the bidirectional flyback DC-to-AC closed-loop converter which is simulated using the software PSIM. Here, the 48-V DC battery is taken as the input voltage source. Then, it is taken as the input to the flyback converter

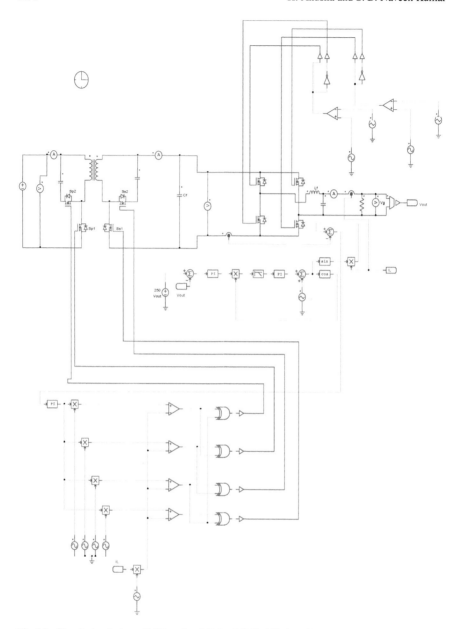

Fig. 10 Circuit simulation of bidirectional flyback DC–AC closed-loop converter

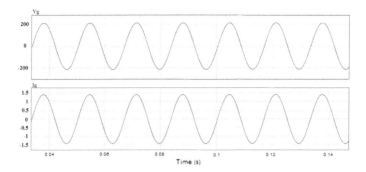

Fig. 11 Waveforms of grid voltage and current

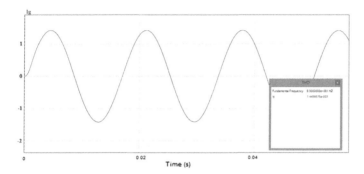

Fig. 12 THD of the grid current

which boosts the voltage. The output of this converter is given as input to the inverter which converts DC to AC. The output of the inverter is given to the 220-V grid.

The output voltage and current waveform of the single input converter are 213.05 V and 1.42 A, respectively as shown in the Fig. 11.

And the THD of the grid current is as shown in Fig. 12.

Closed loop simulation of bi-directional DC-to-AC converter with dual input:

The circuit shown in Fig. 13 is the bidirectional flyback DC-to-AC converter with dual input. One is the constant DC supply, and the other one is the variable solar supply. If the sun rays can be readily available, then the solar PV is used as the input power supply. If it is too rainy or if the solar supply could not reach the desired value, then instead of solar supply the battery can be used as the source. The solar PV panel is given as input to the converter. The output of the converter is taken as input to the single-phase inverter. The output of the inverter is given to the 220-V grid.

The output voltage and current waveform of the dual input converter are 211.9 V and 1.41 A respectively as shown in the Fig. 14.

And the THD of the grid current is as shown in Fig. 15.

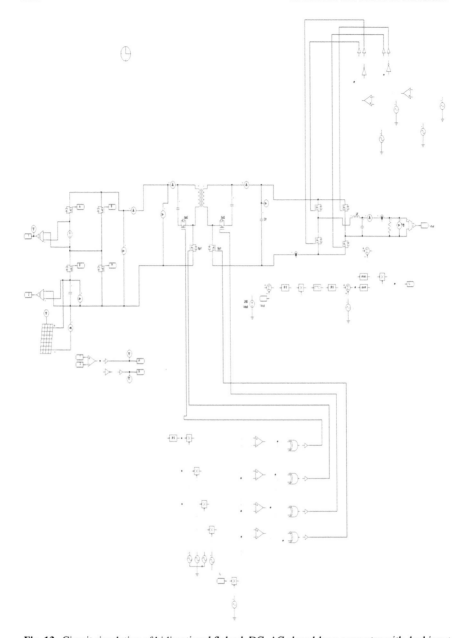

Fig. 13 Circuit simulation of bidirectional flyback DC–AC closed-loop converter with dual input

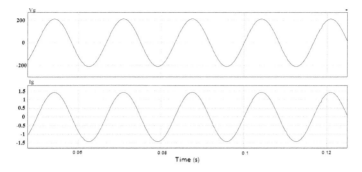

Fig. 14 Waveforms of grid voltage and current

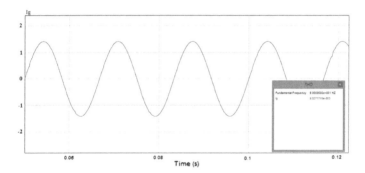

Fig. 15 THD of the grid current

7 Conclusion

The bidirectional single-stage power conversion using the flyback direct current to alternating current converter along with the non-complementary active clamp circuit is verified by the analysis and simulation results. Here, the bidirectional flyback converter uses the non-complementary active clamp circuit topology. This active clamp circuit prevents the sudden increase in the voltage and also decreases energy losses by propagating energy. By the use of controlling procedure, the realization of the single-stage power conversion has been done. The controlling procedure will remain same in both charging and discharging modes to attain the single-stage power conversion by the same controlling procedure. The converter is designed for 48 V input and 220 V output. Simulation results show that by the use of this converter THD of the output current is reduced. The simulation is done by using the PSIM software and analyzed in detail.

References

1. Lee SH, Kim KS, Cha WJ, Kwon JM (2016) Bidirectional single power conversion dc–ac converter with non-complementary active-clamp circuits. IEEE Trans Ind Elect
2. Wang H, Chen F, Qiao W, Qu L (2018) A grid-tied reconfigurable battery storage system. IEEE applied power electronics conference and exposition (APEC)
3. Kwon O, Kim JS, Kwon JM, Kwon BH (2018) Bidirectional grid-connected single-power-conversion converter with low-input battery voltage. IEEE Trans Ind Electron
4. Ogata K (2010) Modern control theory. Pearson Education, Inc, Publishing as Prentice Hall, One Lake Street, Upper Saddle River, NJ 07458
5. Shang YL, Xia B, Zhang C, Cui N, Yang J, Mi CC (2017) An automatic equalizer based on forward–flyback converter for series-connected battery strings. IEEE Trans Ind Electron
6. Hart DW (2011) Power electronics. McGraw Hill Education (India) Private Limited

Performance Study of DC–DC Resonant Converter Topologies for Solar PV Applications

Pattar Gayatri Kallappa and B. R. Rajeev

Abstract This paper proposes performance study of series, parallel and series—parallel resonant converter topologies for solar PV application. The performance studies are carried out considering the switching losses and power factor improvement, ZVS and ZCS switching techniques are implemented in each simulation model of DC–DC resonant converter topologies. The solar PV panel is introduced, and its simulation model is connected to DC–DC resonant converter input terminals, and complete system is simulated for the performance study under different topologies. The simulation tool PSIM 9.1.1 is used.

Keywords Solar PV panel · ZVS · ZCS · Boost converter · DC–DC resonant converter · Rectifier

1 Introduction

In the recent years, solar energy has become a common and a major source of electrical power generation. Many power industries are installing high capacity solar PV system to meet the increasing demand of electrical power. In this view, many works on solar PV system for better efficiency and better performance have evolved. One such work on solar PV converter is to minimize the switching losses and to improve the power factor at the inverted output of solar PV panel. This paper mainly deals on the improvement of power factor at the inverted solar PV output and to minimize the switching losses at the converter circuit. Here, in this paper, DC–DC resonant converter topologies are used in the solar PV conversion for minimizing the

P. G. Kallappa (✉) · B. R. Rajeev
Department of Electrical and Electronics Engineering, Siddaganga Institute of Technology, Tumakuru, India
e-mail: pattargayatri001@gmail.com

B. R. Rajeev
e-mail: rajeevbr@sit.ac.in

© Springer Nature Singapore Pte Ltd. 2019
V. Sridhar et al. (eds.), *Emerging Research in Electronics, Computer Science and Technology*, Lecture Notes in Electrical Engineering 545, https://doi.org/10.1007/978-981-13-5802-9_110

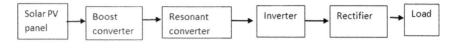

Fig. 1 Block diagram

switching losses and to improve the power factor at the inverted output. The simple block diagram which represents the complete system is shown in Fig. 1.

The computer simulation model of solar PV panel is introduced as an input to the DC–DC resonant converter circuit for the performance analysis, and the simulation tool is PSIM 9.1.1.

2 Computer Simulation Model of PV System

Figure 2 shows the details of the solar panel being employed in the simulation. The solar panel manufacture data sheet has number of cells, maximum power, open circuit voltage, short circuit voltage and the standard test condition including intensity and temperature. The intensity and temperature have standard values, where the intensity is 1000 W/mm^2 and the temperature is 25 °C. Output power graphs are also shown.

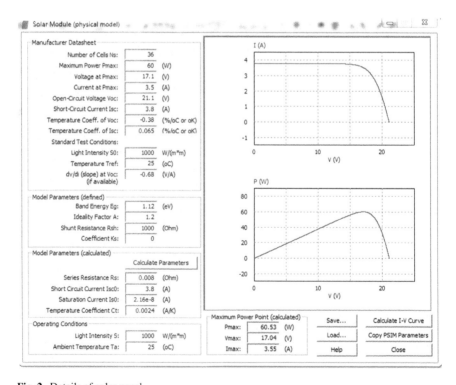

Fig. 2 Details of solar panel

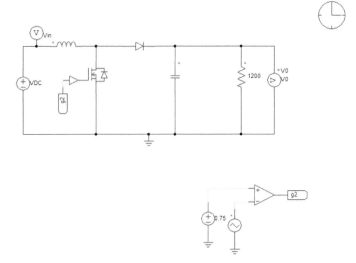

Fig. 3 Boost converter

3 Boost Converter

The boost converter to boost up the DC voltage from the PV Panel is used and it is nothing but a step-up converter. ON and OFF states of boost converter are shown below with simulation circuits (Figs. 3, 4 and 5).

4 Inverter

The inverter employing MOSFET is used here with high-frequency switching to invert the DC output and then the resonant converter is introduced in the simulation model. Inverter has two types of sources usually either current source or voltage source. If the inverter has current source, it is known as current source inverter. If the inverter has a voltage source, it is known as voltage source inverter. Figure 6 shows a single-phase inverter. And switching conditions are follows:

(1) From $0°$ to $180°$, switches Q_1 and Q_2 are closed and Q_3 and Q_4 are open.
(2) From $180°$ to $360°$ switches, Q_3 and Q_4 are closed and Q_1 and Q_2 are open.
(3) Here the switches Q_1 and Q_4 are in first leg and switches Q_2 and Q_3 are in second leg. The same leg switches should not conduct at a time because it becomes a short circuit.

The simulation model and output waveforms of 1-Φ full-bridge inverter are shown below in Figs. 7, 8 and 9.

The simulation circuit and output waveforms of SPWM inverter are shown in Fig. 10, reference signals and carrier signal waveforms are shown in Fig. 11, the output voltage, input voltage and current waveforms are shown in Fig. 12.

ON STATE

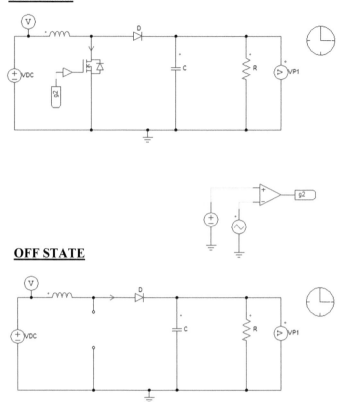

OFF STATE

Fig. 4 ON state and OFF state of boost converter

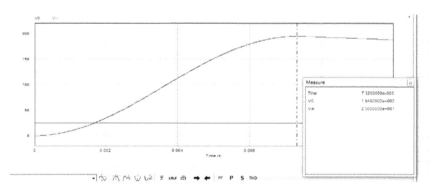

Fig. 5 Waveforms of boost converter

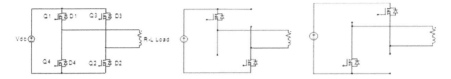

Fig. 6 1-Φ full-bridge inverter and conduction mode from, 0° to 180° and 180° to 360°

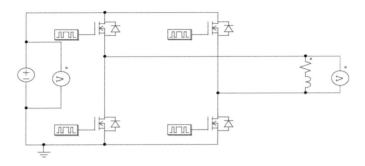

Fig. 7 Circuit simulation of 1-Φ full-bridge inverter

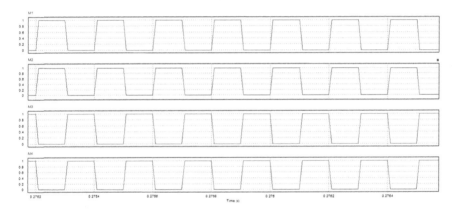

Fig. 8 Switching waveforms of inverter

5 DC–DC Resonant Converter

5.1 Operating Modes of DC–DC Resonant Circuit

Above figure shows the complete simulation model of the system, where solar PV variable DC output is boosted and made a constant output (Fig. 13). Boost converter output is given to SPWM inverter further to improve the performance, ZVS and ZCS resonant converters are connected. Via an isolation transformer, the output is analyzed across a load. Finally, the output is rectified to give it to a DC load.

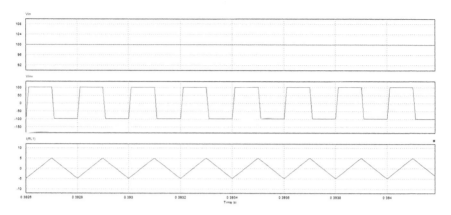

Fig. 9 Waveforms of input voltage, output voltage and current

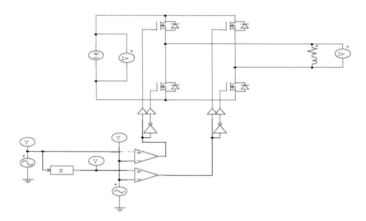

Fig. 10 Simulation circuit of SPWM inverter

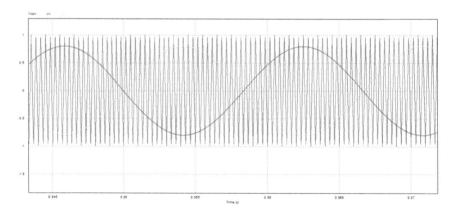

Fig. 11 Waveforms of reference and carrier signals

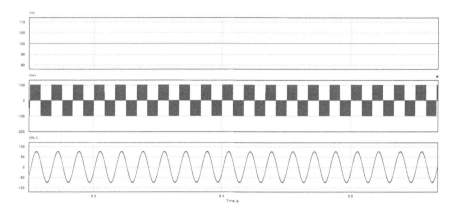

Fig. 12 Waveforms of input voltage, output voltage and current

6 Simulation, Results and Discussion

6.1 DC–DC Series Resonant Circuit

See Figs. 14, 15, 16 and 17.

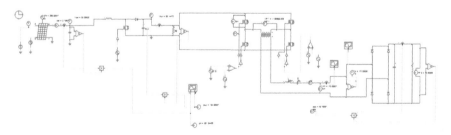

Fig. 13 DC–DC resonant circuit

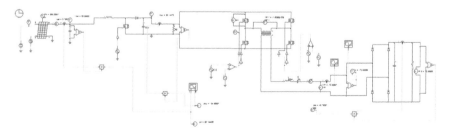

Fig. 14 DC–DC series resonant circuit

Table 1 Simulation results of DC–DC resonant circuit

Configuration	With resonant circuit (power factor)	Without resonant circuit (power factor)
Series	0.99	0.76
Parallel	0.99	0.76
Series parallel	0.99	0.76

6.2 DC–DC Parallel Resonant Circuit

See Figs. 18, 19, 20 and 21.

6.3 DC–DC Series–Parallel Resonant Circuit

See Figs. 22, 23, 24 and 25

6.4 DC–DC Without Resonant Circuit

See Figs. 26, 27, 28, 29 and Table 1.

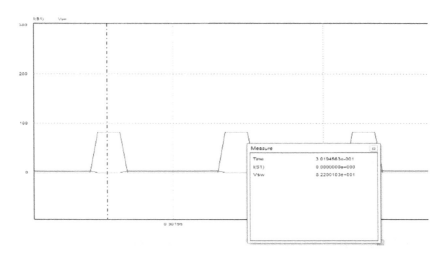

Fig. 15 Switching losses waveforms of DC–DC series resonant circuit

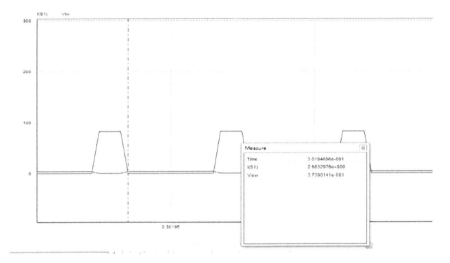

Fig. 16 Switching losses waveforms of DC–DC series resonant circuit

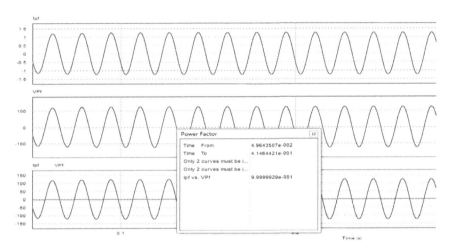

Fig. 17 Power factor waveforms of DC–DC series resonant circuit

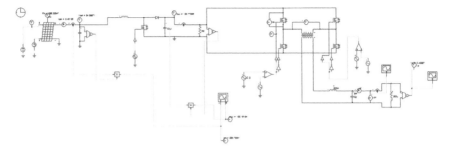

Fig. 18 DC–DC parallel resonant circuit

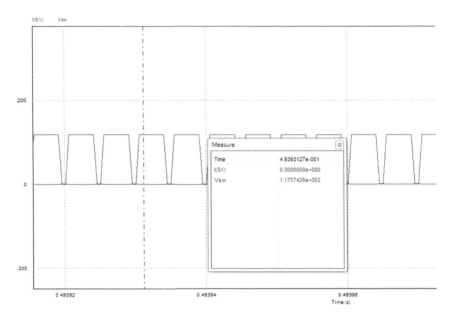

Fig. 19 Switching losses waveforms of DC–DC parallel resonant circuit

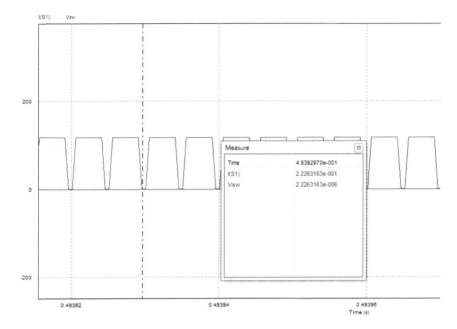

Fig. 20 Switching losses waveforms of DC–DC parallel resonant circuit

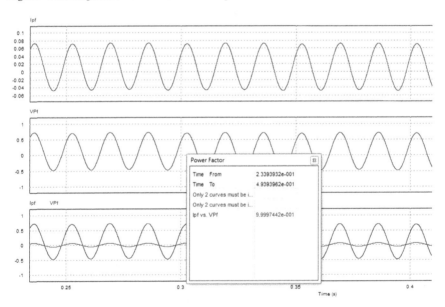

Fig. 21 Power factor waveforms of DC–DC parallel resonant circuit

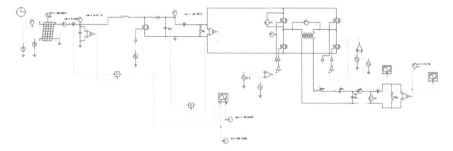

Fig. 22 DC–DC series–parallel resonant circuit

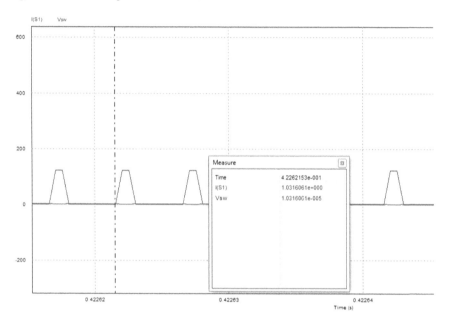

Fig. 23 Switching losses waveforms of DC–DC series–parallel resonant circuit

7   Conclusion

The power factor at the inverted output of solar PV panel has significantly improved from 0.76 to 0.99 with the introduction of resonant converter in all topologies. Switching losses are also minimized significantly as shown in the output waveforms. Hence resonant converter would be an efficient solution for improving the performance of solar PV system.

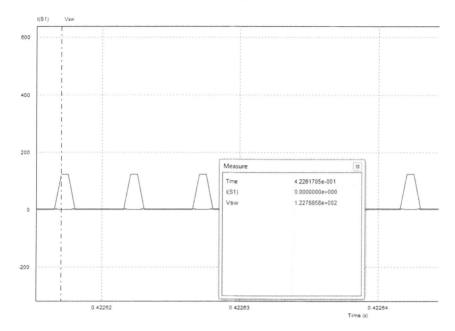

Fig. 24 Switching losses waveforms of DC–DC series–parallel resonant circuit

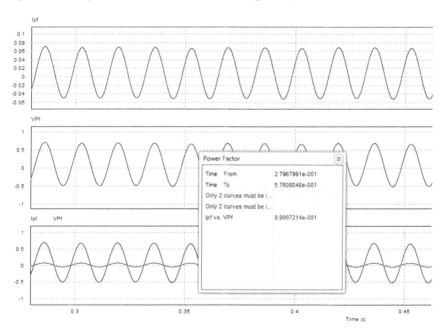

Fig. 25 Power factor waveforms of DC–DC series–parallel resonant circuit

8 Future Scope

We can future improve the efficiency by introducing MPPT technique, and also for better comparison of resonant converter topologies for performance analysis.

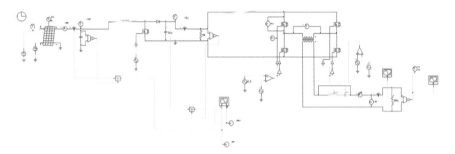

Fig. 26 DC–DC without resonant circuit

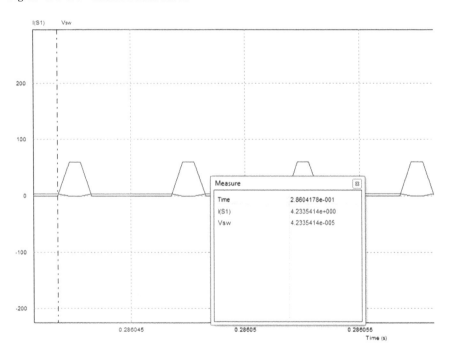

Fig. 27 Switching losses waveforms of DC–DC without resonant circuit

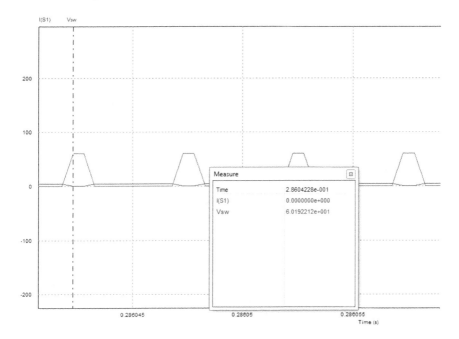

Fig. 28 Switching losses waveforms of DC–DC without resonant circuit

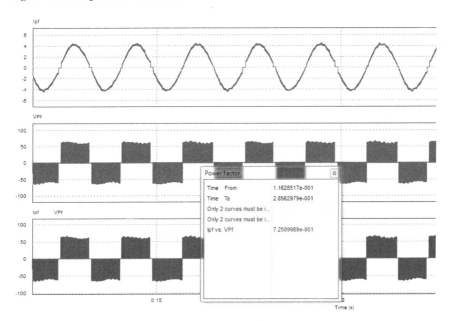

Fig. 29 Power factor waveforms of DC–DC without resonant circuit

References

1. Cross AM, Forsyth AJ. A high-power-factor, three-phase isolated AC-DC converter using high-frequency current injection
2. Seroji MN, Forsyth AJ. Small-signal model of a high-power-factor, three-phase AC-DC converter with high-frequency resonant current injection
3. Omar MF, Seroji MN, Hamzah MK. Analysis and simulation of phase-shift control for three-phase AC/DC full-bridge current injection series resonant converter
4. Omar MF, Seroji MN, Hamzah MK. Analysis and simulation of three-phase AC/DC full-bridge current injection series resonant converter (FBCISRC)
5. Gong G (2005) Comparative evaluation of three-phase high-power-factor AC–DC converter concepts for application in future more electric aircraft. IEEE Trans Industr Electron 52:727–737
6. Maldonado MA, Korba GJ (1999) Power management and distribution system for a more-electric aircraft (MADMEL). IEEE Aerosp Electron Syst Mag 14(12):3–8
7. IEEE recommended practices and requirements for harmonics control in electric power systems. IEEE Std.519 (1992)
8. Omar MF, Seroji MN, Hamzah MK (2010) Analysis and simulation of three-phase AC/DC full-bridge current injection series resonant converter (FBCISRC). IEEE symposium on industrial electronics and applications, ISIEA 2010, 3–5 October 2010, pp 159–164

Performance Analysis of SHEPWM Based on GA and PSO for CMLI

B. R. Vishwanath and P. S. Puttaswamy

Abstract Multilevel inverters are gaining much greater attention lately as a result of increasing demand for high power inverter units in the industrial applications. Reduction of harmonics and minimizing the THD from the MLI output is considered as a very important task in order to achieve the better performance and to prevent the device from getting damaged. This paper presents the performance study of different soft computing method for CMLI using SHEPWM technique. Genetic algorithmic (GA), Particle Swarm optimization (PSO) techniques are applied MLI to calculating the switching angles. The switching angles are determined such that the constraints of SHEPWM are met, which controls the switching of the CMLI thereby eliminating the lower order harmonics and minimizing the Total Harmonic Distortion (THD) while maintaining the required fundamental voltage. The switching angles are calculated offline and are then used in MATLAB to generate the pulses required for CMLI. A detailed simulation study work is carried out using MATLAB/SIMULINK.

Keywords Cascaded multilevel inverter (CMLI) · Total harmonic distortion (THD) · Selective harmonic elimination pulse width modulation (SHEPWM) · Genetic algorithm (GA) · Particle swarm optimization (PSO)

1 Introduction

As a result of increasing demand for high power inverter unit's multilevel inverters are gaining more attention in industrial applications. Multilevel inverter is a power conversion strategy in which output is obtained by adding the output of several inverter units, MLIs are used in many applications such as flexible AC transmission

B. R. Vishwanath (✉)
P.E.T. Research Center, PES College of Engineering, Mandya 571401, Karnataka, India
e-mail: br.vishwa@gmail.com

P. S. Puttaswamy
Department of Electrical and Electronics, PES College of Engineering, Mandya 571401, Karnataka, India
e-mail: psputtaswamy_ee@yahoo.com

© Springer Nature Singapore Pte Ltd. 2019
V. Sridhar et al. (eds.), *Emerging Research in Electronics, Computer Science and Technology*, Lecture Notes in Electrical Engineering 545,
https://doi.org/10.1007/978-981-13-5802-9_111

systems, laminators, compressors, UPS systems, STATCOM applications and so on [1].

The most widely used MLI topologies are (1) Diode clamped (2) Capacitor clamped (3) Cascaded H-bridge MLI (CHBMLI) [1]. Compared to the conventional inverter with transformer, there are several advantages using traditional MLI topologies i.e. smaller output voltage steps, lower harmonic components, increased electromagnetic compatibility and reduced switching losses. Among the three inverter topologies CHBMLI has several advantages such as same voltage levels can be achieved with lesser number of components compare with diode and capacitor clamped circuits and also achieved higher output voltage levels with less power circuit complexity [2].

The harmonics can be eliminated by controlling the switching action of the MLI which in turn could be done by the pulses applied to the MLI. There are several techniques are followed for eliminating the harmonics in the MLI. The most widely used controlling strategies for harmonic elimination are Sinusoidal PWM (SPWM), Space vector PWM (SVPWM), Selective Harmonic Elimination PWM (SHEPWM) and so on [3]. MLIs are usually operated with low switching frequency, thus SHEPWM which is a low switching frequency method is preferred over other techniques and also it offers several advantages such as low switching frequency with a wider converter bandwidth, and better DC source utilization [4].

In this paper Genetic algorithm (GA) [5, 6] and particle swarm optimization technique (PSO) which is a computational empirical search algorithm. This algorithm is used to find the switching angles from the non-linear equation of SHEPWM. By using GA and PSO provides optimization by finding the solution for the whole range of modulation index (M.I) compare to the conventional Newton-Rapson method and reduces the harmonics instead of eliminating them.

The main aim of this paper is to eliminate 5th, 7th, 9th and 11th order harmonics in the MLI. For experimental view developing the 9-level CMLI using SHEPWM based on GA and PSO by using MATLAB SIMULINK. The obtained simulation results shows that the SHEPWM efficiently remove the 5th, 7th, 9th, and 11th order harmonics and minimizes the Total Harmonic Distortion (THD).

1.1 Cascaded Multilevel Inverter

In this paper considering a three phase 9-level CHBMLI. A CHBMLI consists of an N number of H-bridge inverter units which are connected in series. Each basic H-bridge inverter unit can produce three different voltage levels i.e. +Vdc, 0, − Vdc through the cascaded of two basic cell with different combinations of the four switches. Each H-bridge unit generates a Sinusoidal staircase waveform by phase shifting its positive and negative phase leg's switching timings as shown in the Fig. 1. In this topology, the n-level output phase voltage levels is defined by $K = 2Si + 1$ where Si is the number of DC sources [2]. The Fig. 2 shows the n-level topology structure of CHBMLI.

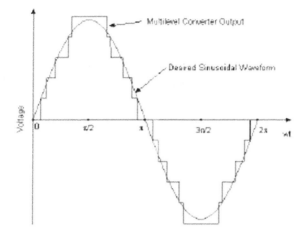

Fig. 1 Sinusoidal staircase waveform generated by CHBMLI

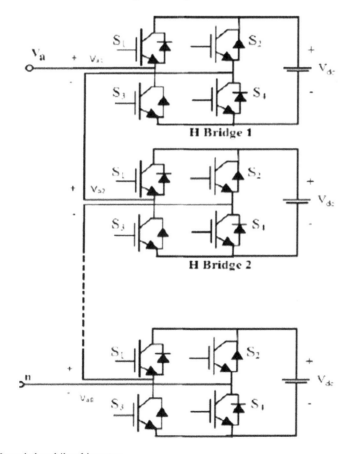

Fig. 2 Cascaded multilevel inverter

1.2 Selective Harmonic Elimination (SHE)

SHE is a fundamental switching frequency method which eliminates the selected lower order harmonics while retaining the required fundamental frequency. In this paper lower order harmonics 5th, 7th, 9th and 11th are eliminated.

SHE can be mathematically formulated as,

$$
\begin{aligned}
&\cos(\alpha 1) + \cos(\alpha 2) + \ldots + \cos(\alpha m) = mM \\
&\cos(5\alpha 1) + \cos(5\alpha 2) + \ldots + \cos(5\alpha m) = 0 \\
&\cos(7\alpha 1) + \cos(7\alpha 2) + \ldots + \cos(7\alpha m) = 0 \\
&\cos(11\alpha 1) + \cos(11\alpha 2) + \ldots + \cos(11\alpha m) = 0 \\
&\cos(13\alpha 1) + \cos(13\alpha 2) + \ldots + \cos(13\alpha m) = 0 \\
&\quad - \\
&\quad - \\
&\cos(n\alpha 1) \quad \cos(\alpha 2) + \ldots + \cos(n\alpha m) = 0
\end{aligned}
\tag{1}
$$

The Eq. (1) are nonlinear transcendental in nature. From the equation unknown switching angles $\alpha 1, \alpha 2, \alpha 3, \alpha 4, \alpha 5, \alpha 6, \alpha 7, \ldots, \alpha m$ are calculated by the soft switching techniques (GA and PSO) which are required to trigger the switching operation [3, 4].

1.3 Genetic Algorithm

Genetic algorithm is a computational heuristic search algorithm. The algorithm starts its search operation from a randomly generated population that is obtained over successive iterations.

To achieve optimization the algorithm uses three different operators. The first operator is the "Selection" operator which follows the Darwin's theory of "survival of the fittest" The second operator is the "crossover" operator, this operator passes on the best of the present population to the future population, thus achieving the required fitness value constraint given in the Eq. (2) The last operator is "mutation", this operator takes a particular individual alters its features so as to meet the required fitness value (FV) constraint. Figure 3 shows the flow chart of GA [7, 8].

$$
FV = \frac{\sqrt{\sum_{n=5,7,11,13} \left(\frac{1}{n} \sum_{k=1}^{5} \cos(n\alpha_k)\right)^2}}{\sum_{k}^{5} \cos \alpha_k}
\tag{2}
$$

The above equations are more important role to give the best solutions inside a large search space.

Fig. 3 Flow chart of GA [8]

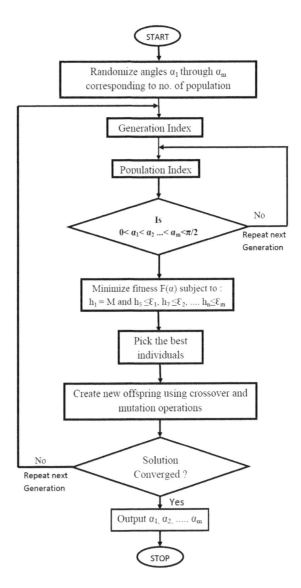

GA algorithm execute in different steps as follows,

1. Initialization of population size, i.e. by selecting initial individual switching angle randomly from the given population.
2. The reproduction operator decides how the origins are chosen to form the inheritor. This operation is a process in which parameters are traced consistently with corresponding utility values.

3. Crossover: after the reproduction part, method of intersection has been set up to generated new individuals.
4. Mutation works after crossover operation now have a new population full of individuals. Some of the individuals are directly copied, and others are selected from cross over. Mutation suggests that the selected part of individual population is modified because all the individuals are not equal, you allow for a slight chance of mutation. This method is repeated, up to optimum solution is obtained.
5. The FV perform plays a necessary role in guiding GA to induce the only solutions at intervals. To look out the specified resolution GA should run style of iterations. Once the first iteration, the obtained fitness values square measure won't to supply new successor.

1.4 Structures of PSO

Particle swarm optimization (PSO) was first introduced by Kennedy and Eberhart [9] based on bird flocking. PSO is motivated by social behavior of birds gathering or fish schooling. From the population of particles, PSO conducts the searching process. Each particle may become probable solution to the problem under investigation. The particle in a given population alters its position by moving in a multi-dimensional search space until rightest particle is encountered.

The N particles are involves from the population. For each iteration, the function 'f' measures the capability of individual particle 'i' in the given population then updated the each particle position, which is influenced by particles velocity, the difference of particle best and current position, and the difference of swarms best and current position. The last two conditions are multiplied with uniform random number from [0, 1] to get random influence of each other.

$$V_i \partial(t + 1) = [I_W \times V_i \partial(t)] + [A_1 \times rn_1 \times P_i \partial(t) - X_i \partial(t))]$$
$$+ [A_2 \times rn_2 \times (P_g \partial(t) - X_i \partial(t))] \tag{3}$$

$$X_i \partial(t + 1) = X_i \partial(t) + V_i \partial(t + 1) \tag{4}$$

where

Xi $(Xi1, Xi2, ..., Xin)T;$ ith particle position vector,
Vi $(Vi1, Vi2, ..., Vin)T;$ ith particle velocity vector,
Pi $(Pi1, Pi2, ..., Pin)T;$ pbest,
· Pg gbest, I_W = inertia weight, A_1 and A_2 = acceleration constant, $rn1$ and $rn2$ = random number in a range of 0–1

Pi is the best capability that particles have obtained. The first part in Eq. (3) is the inertia weight (I_W). The middle part is the cognitive part, which signifies the independent nature of the particle itself. Meanwhile the last part of the equation is

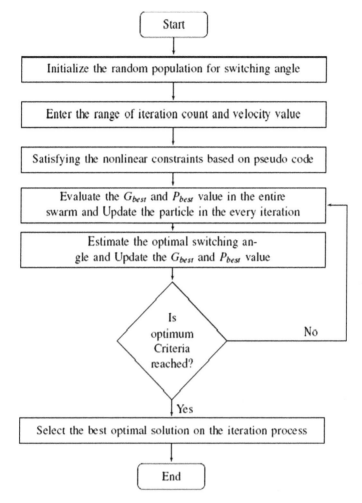

Fig. 4 shows the flow chart of PSO [13]

the social part. A_1 and A_2 denote the weighted value of the middle and last part of the Eq. 3; it helps to pull each particle towards gbest and pbest positions [10, 11, 13] (Fig. 4).

PSO algorithm execute in three steps they are [5],

Step 1: Initialization
For each particle $i = 1, ..., NP$, do
(a) Initialize the position of particle with a uniform distribution as $(0) \sim u(Lb, Ub)$, where Lb and Ub denote the lower and upper bounds of the search space.
(b) Set value to: $(, 0) = (0)$.
(c) Set value to: $(0) = \text{argmin } f[(0)]$.

(d) Set velocity to: $\sim (-Ub - Lb|, |Ub - Lb|)$.
Step 2: Repeat until a termination criteria is met
         For each particle = 1, …, , do
(a) Select random values: n1, n2 $\sim$ (0,1).
(b) Particle's velocity is updated by Eq. (3).
(c) Particle's position is updated by Eq. (4).
(d) (i) If [(,)] > [P()] Update the best known position of particle :(,) = ().
     (ii) If [gt (,)]> [P()], update the swarm's best known position: () = (). (+
     1)→t;
Step 3: Output () that holds the best found solution.

2 Implementation

2.1 Cascaded H-Bridge Multilevel Inverter

The cascaded H-bridge MLI (CHBMLI) is designed and implemented in MATLAB
SIMULINK as shown in the below diagram. Each inverter will generate 3 different
output voltag-es: +Vdc, 0, and −Vdc. The number of voltage levels at the output of
the CHBMLI is 2(Si) + 1, where Si is the number of DC sources. In this case number
of DC sources used is 4, so the output leg voltage levels of the CHBMLI is equal to
2(4) + 1 i.e. 9 levels. All three output voltage levels from different H-bridge units
will be added together to obtain the required staircase waveform (Figs. 5 and 6).

2.2 Selective Harmonic Elimination PWM

The Figs. 6 and 7 shows the execution of SHEPWM technique. A reference angle Θ
is generated from 0 to 2π using a clock signal with a frequency of 50 Hz and period
of 0.02 s. Θ is converted in to angle using the gain block. The reference angle and
the switching angles obtained using the GA will be compared using the relational
operators. When the reference angle is greater than or equal to a1 a pulse will be
generated until the reference angle is less than the switching angle a2. To limit the
pulse generation from a1 to a2 the AND logical operator is used. Similar process is
applied for switching angles a3 and a4. This is for the raising side. Similarly for the
falling side the reference angle will be compared with 180 − a4, if it is greater than
or equal to 180 − a4 a pulse will be generated until it is less than or equal to 180 −
a3. similar procedure is followed for the remaining switching angles.

For the negative cycle the reference angle is compared with 180 + a1, if the
reference angle is greater than 180 + a1 a pulse will be generated until it is less than
180 + a2. This is for the falling side and for the raising side the reference angle will
be compared with 180 − a4 + 180, if it is greater than 180 − a4 + 180 a pulse will be

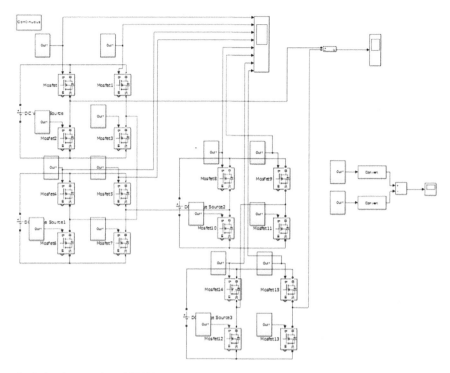

Fig. 5 Implementation of CMLI

generated until it is less than $180 - a3 + 180$. All the pulses will be added together and are viewed using scope window.

The pulse thus obtained using SHEPWM technique is applied to the normal pulse to achieve the required phase shift as shown in the Fig. 8.

2.3 Genetic Algorithm (GA)

The implementation code for the GA is written in MATLAB and the different steps are followed in GA is as follows:

Step1   Initialization of tournament number and population number.
Step2   Random generation of bits.
Step 3   Compute the value of strings.
Step 4   Define the upper and lower bounds.
Step 5   Fitness value calculation.
Step 6   Tournament selection.
Step 7   Parent and children selection for crossover and mutation.
Step 8   Fitness function evaluation.

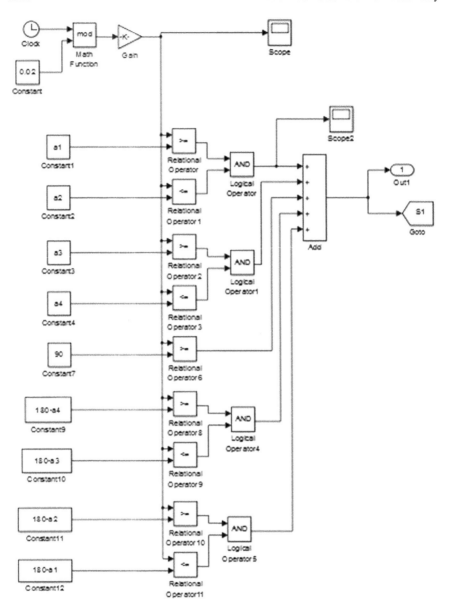

Fig. 6 Pulse generation for positive cycle using SHEPWM

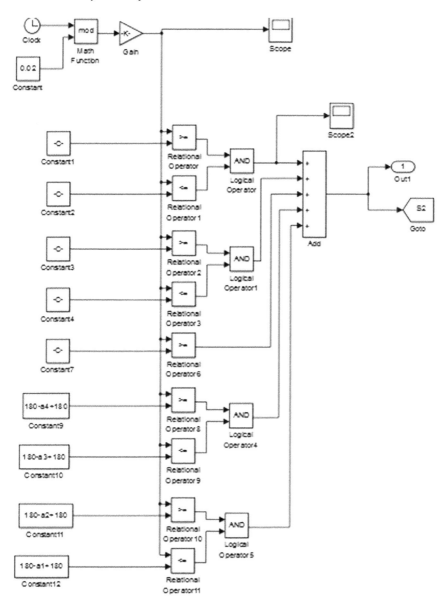

Fig. 7 Pulse generation for negative cycle using SHEPWM

Fig. 8 Application of
delayed pulse to the normal
pulse

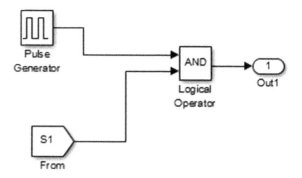

Step 9   Converged output (Switching angles).

2.4 Particle Swarm Optimization

Implementation of PSO Algorithm in Matlab.

The PSO algorithm consists of different steps which keep on repeating until it satisfies the required conditions:

- Find out the fitness value.
- Keep on finding each individual and find best value of fitness and position.
- Keep on evaluating the fitness and position of all variables.

2.5 Calculation of Switching

Before angles were calculated for single H-Bridge but now it is also applied for multilevel cascaded inverter with some conditions. The calculation depends on performance of components. In order to get high response and performance band control current method and PWM method technique for a MLI are observed.

Harmonic distortion of waveform is mainly observed switching angles for each voltage is calculated. Therefore switching angles of MLI are calculated by using both PSO and algorithms. When the angels are good, the corresponding THD will also be good.

For calculating the switching angle, the output waveform should be considered. The output is represented by the term r(t).

The equation for r(t) is given as

$$r(t) = \sum_{n=1}^{\infty}(p_n sin_n \alpha_n)(q_n cos_n \alpha_n) \tag{5}$$

Here even harmonics are zero, because it is not present therefore $q_n = 0$.
The switching angles are represented as $\alpha_1, \alpha_2, ..., \alpha_n$, therefore.

$$p_n = \left(\frac{4\pi vdc}{n\pi}\right) \sum_{n=1}^{m} cos_n \alpha_k \tag{6}$$

Here, $0 < \alpha_1 < \alpha_2 ... \alpha_k < \pi/2$.
For odd harmonics, the value of α ranges from α_1 to α_n
Therefore,

$$\alpha_1 = \left(\frac{4vdc}{\pi}\right) \sum_{k=1}^{m} cosn \alpha_k = M \tag{7}$$

$$\alpha_9 = \left(\frac{4vdc}{\pi}\right) \sum_{k=1}^{m} cos9 \alpha_k = 0 \tag{8}$$

2.6   Total Harmonic Distortion (THD)

The THD is given by the equation,

$$\%THD = \left(1/\alpha_1^2\right) \sum_{n=5}^{\infty} (b_n)^{1/2}] \times 100 \tag{9}$$

where,
n = 9i $\pm$ 1(i = 1, 2, 3,...)
Therefore $f(\alpha) = f(\alpha_1 + \alpha_2 ... \alpha_M)$
Here, $0 < \alpha_1 < \alpha_2 ... \alpha_k < 90$

3   Simulation Results

3.1   Cascaded Multilevel Inverter

The staircase waveforms obtained from the 5-level, 7-level and 9-level CMLI respectively. The number of DC sources used here is 2, 3 and 4 for 5, 7 and 9 levels respectively.

The leg voltage of the Multilevel inverter will be 2(2) + 1 i.e. 5 levels, 2(3) + 1 i.e. 7 levels and 2(4) + 1 i.e. 9 levels respectively.

Comparison between 5, 7 And 9 Level CMLI

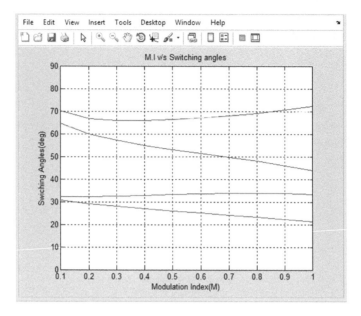

Fig. 9 M.I versus switching angles

From the simulation results obtained which is listed in the Table 1. It can be seen that as the number of levels of the cascaded multilevel inverter increases the Total Harmonic Distortion reduces and also the DC component will be reduced.

Simulation results for a nine-level CHBMLI operating with equal DC sources (50 V per H-Bridge) are shown in Fig. 9.

The above Figs. 10 and 11 shows the output wave form and FFT analysis of 9-level inverter, in that result it can be observed that the target harmonics are minimized with a THD of 13.67%.

Table 1 Comparison between 5, 7 and 9 level CMLI

CMLI	5th order harmonics (%)	7th order harmonics (%)	9th order harmonics (%)	THD IN (%)
Five level CMLI	12.1	14.9	9.8	33.32
Seven level CMLI	1.4	1.8	2.0	28.09
Nine level CMLI	0.7	0.01	0.07	13.67

Fig. 10 Output waveform of 9-level CMLI

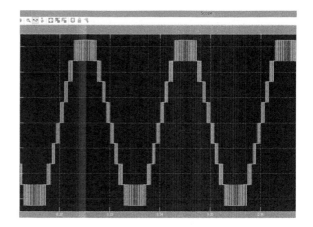

```
Sampling time      = 9.58128e-07 s
Samples per cycle  = 20874
DC component       = 0.001557
Fundamental        = 326 peak (230.5 rms)
THD                = 13.67%

      0 Hz  (DC):         0.00%      270.0°
     10 Hz                0.00%      246.3°
     20 Hz                0.00%      184.0°
     30 Hz                0.00%      179.8°
     40 Hz                0.00%      249.4°
     50 Hz  (Fnd):      100.00%       -0.0°
     60 Hz                0.00%        7.3°
     70 Hz                0.00%       26.2°
     80 Hz                0.00%       22.5°
     90 Hz                0.00%       28.7°
    100 Hz  (h2):         0.00%       12.3°
    110 Hz                0.00%       68.7°
    120 Hz                0.00%       63.7°
    130 Hz                0.00%       43.0°
    140 Hz                0.01%       30.5°
    150 Hz  (h3):         0.01%       13.3°
    160 Hz                0.00%      159.6°
    170 Hz                0.00%      201.1°
```

Fig. 11 FFT analysis of 9-level inverter

Table 2 9 level inverter Switching angles with different modulations Index (M.I)

M.I	a1	a2	a3
0.1	5	40	70
0.2	10	35	78
0.3	30	30	82
0.4	20	35	75
0.5	10	40	70
0.6	15	50	75
0.7	20	45	85
0.8	25	40	60
0.9	30	30	65
1	25	45	60

Table 3 Switching angles for different modulation index obtained from PSO

M.I	a1	a2	a3
0.1	10	50	80
0.2	10	35	78
0.3	30	30	82
0.4	20	35	75
0.5	25	0	70
0.6	15	0	75
0.7	10	50	85
0.8	25	45	60
0.9	30	40	65
1	25	30	55

3.2 Switching Angles Obtained Using GA Rule

The Table 2 represents the switching angle calculated by using the above mentioned equations. These are the angles obtained for genetic algorithm. Here the modulation index ranges from 0.1 to 1, these are normalized value, by using this THD reduction can be calculated and performance is analyzed.

3.3 Switching Angles Obtained Using PSO Rule

The Table 3 represents the switching angle calculated by using the above mentioned equations. These are the angles obtained for PSO algorithm. Here the modulation index ranges from 0.1 to 1, these are normalized value, by using this THD reduction can be calculated and performance is analyzed.

3.4   Simulation Result of Genetic Algorithm

The Fig. 12 shows the plotting of modulation index versus THD. The normalized value of modulation index is from 0 to 1. The graph shows the reduction of THD with modulation index. Here genetic algorithm is implemented and THD is reduced to 2.9. Switching angles are calculated and then THD is calculated by putting those angles in the equation.

The Fig. 13 shows the plotting of switching angles versus Modulation index and from the graph it can be seen that for modulation index 0.8 the best solutions are obtained. The main advantage of using GA is that the solutions for the whole range of Modulation index (MI) can be obtained and the best solutions can be used to achieve optimization.

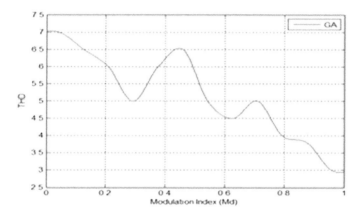

Fig. 12   Modulation Index versus THD of GA

Fig. 13   Modulation Index versus Switching Angles of GA

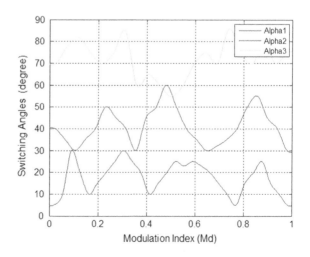

3.5 Simulation Result of PSO Algorithm

The Fig. 14 shows graph between the switching angles and the modulation index. In calculation of switching angle the firing angles as assumed as normalized values. Switching angles are then calculated by using the equation. Modulation index ranges from 0 to 1. PSO angle range is from 0 to 90. obtained angles are known as alpha 1, alpha 2, alpha 3 etc. When the obtained switching angles are good, there will be more THD reduction.

Comparison Result of GA and PSO Algorithm

The Fig. 15 shows the THD comparison found by applying genetic algorithm and particle swarm algorithm. In the paper PSO Method is the proposed method. THD reduction is more in PSO method than genetic algorithm. In GA, THD is almost reduced to 2.9%. In PSO, THD is reduced to 2.1%.

Fig. 14 Modulation versus switching angles of PSO

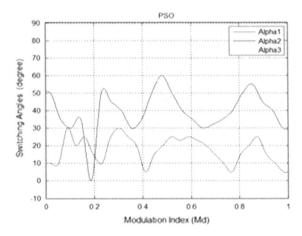

Fig. 15 Comparison of THD reduction of GA and PSO

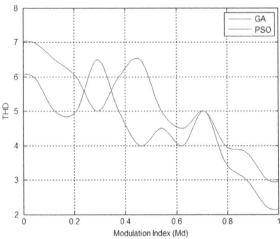

4 Conclusion

The paper demonstrates cascaded structure inverters area unit designed and enforced in MATLAB/SIMULINK. The pulses needed to drive the CMLI area unit generated by Selective Harmonic Elimination Pulse dimension Modulation technique. The shift angles for SHEPWM area unit calculated by Genetic rule and PSO rule. That the lower harmonics are eliminated efficiently using SHEPWM based on PSO and also the THD is minimized. The range of levels will increase the entire Harmonic Distortion reduces as discussed in the Table 1. It may be seen that THD reduction is more in PSO method than genetic algorithm. In GA, THD is almost reduced to 2.9%. In PSO, THD is reduced to 2.1% as discussed in the simulation results. By comparing both GA and PSO soft techniques it can be seen that PSO gives more THD reduction comparing with GA and PSO provides good performance than GA.

Some drawbacks are observe in the PSO algorithm like premature, computational complexity is more, convergence speed is less, sensitivity to parameters therefore improvement the PSO by Hybridization method, called hybridized PSO. This technique is helpful to in order to take the advantages of both methods and compensate the weaknesses of each other. [6, 12].

References

1. Rodriguez J, Lai JS, Peng FZ (2002) Multilevel inverters: a survey of topologies, controls, and applications. IEEE Trans Ind Electron 49(4):724–738
2. Lezana P, Rodríguez J, Oyarzún DA (2008) Cascaded multilevel inverter with regeneration capability and reduced number of switches. IEEE Trans Ind Electron
3. George and Anup Singh (2008) PWM techniques: a pure sine wave inverter. IEEE Trans
4. Anik et all, Selective harmonics elimination of PWM cascaded multi-level inverter. IJEST
5. Zhang Y, A comprehensive survey on particle swarm optimization algorithm and its applications. Hindawi Publishing vol 2015, Article ID 931256, pp 38
6. Hassan R, Cohanim B (2006) A comparision of PSO and GA. IEEE Trans
7. Whittley D (2009) A genetic algorithm tutorial. IEEE Trans Comput Appl
8. Riyadh M (2008) Gentic algorithm for harmonics elimination. J Kerbala Univ Sci 6(3)
9. Kennedy J, Eberhart R (1995) Particle swarm optimization. In: IEEE international conference on neural networks, vol 4, pp 1942–1948
10. Schutte JF (2008) The particle swarm optimization algorithm. IEEE Trans Struct Appl
11. Azli NA (2013) Particle swarm optimisation and its applications in power converter systems. Int J Artif Intell Soft Comput 3(4)
12. Singh A, Kumar V (2015) Introduction to GA and PSO. IEEE Trans
13. Ali SSA, et.al (2017) Exploration of modulation index in multi-level inverter using particle swarm optimization algorithm. Proc Comput Sci 105:144–152.

Induction Motor Internal and External Fault Detection

Kamalpreet Singh, Ruhul Amin Choudhury and Tanya

Abstract Induction motors are extensively used motor type for various industrial applications for the reason that they are robust, simple in structure, and efficient. On the other hand, induction motors are prone to different faults during their lifetime due to hostile environments. If the fault is not detected in its rudimentary phase, it may cause unexpected shut down of the entire system and colossal loss in industry. It is conspicuous that scope of this field is huge. This work presents detection of internal and external faults of induction motor. S-Transformation, which is superior as compared to CWT and STFT as it does not contain any cross terms, is used for bearing fault detection, and random forest, an algorithm which is easy to implement and requires minimum memory, is used for detection of external faults. The fault can be detected with more accuracy in premature state leads to improve the reliability of the system.

Keywords Fault detection · Induction motor · MLPNN · Random forest · S-Transform · Vibration analysis

1 Introduction

Induction motors (IMs) are usually mentioned as the drudges of industries. IMs account for almost 70–80% of the energy conversion [1, 2]. Because of this fact, fault detection of IMs is crucial. There are numbers of fault detection techniques proposed in recent decade. It has been found that some of the methods are not cost effective. Advancements in the technology and algorithms will lead to the effectives and efficient fault detection of IMs.

Fault detection of IMs is done by either invasive or non-invasive techniques. Non-invasive techniques are more preferred by the industry as it is an on-line study of the faults present in the system, while invasive techniques require the system to be offline

K. Singh (✉) · R. A. Choudhury · Tanya
Lovely Professional University, Phagwara, Punjab, India
e-mail: singhkamalpreet1996@gmail.com

© Springer Nature Singapore Pte Ltd. 2019
V. Sridhar et al. (eds.), *Emerging Research in Electronics, Computer Science and Technology*, Lecture Notes in Electrical Engineering 545,
https://doi.org/10.1007/978-981-13-5802-9_112

[3]. The production of the organization is not hampered by these methods, which leads to save both time and money [4]. The fault which occurs in the motor because of its internal structure is known as internal faults. It consists of faults related to rotor, stator, and bearing. Because of continuous operation, the inner parts of the motor face wear and tear which leads to the internal faults. The faults present in the supply are generally referred as external faults [5]. These are present due to power quality issues [6]. Faults in induction motors can be categorized as electrical, mechanical, and environmental faults [6, 7] (Fig. 1).

The common faults in any machine are electrical faults like stator and rotor winding faults and mechanical faults like air gap eccentricity and bearing faults. In a survey done by IEEE [8] & EPRI [9], it has been found that the failure percentage of IMs is shown in Fig. 2 (Table 1).

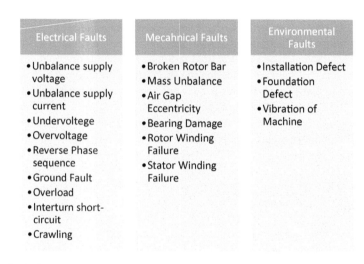

Electrical Faults	Mecahnical Faults	Environmental Faults
• Unbalance supply voltage	• Broken Rotor Bar	• Installation Defect
• Unbalance supply current	• Mass Unbalance	• Foundation Defect
• Undervoltege	• Air Gap Eccentricity	• Vibration of Machine
• Overvoltage	• Bearing Damage	
• Reverse Phase sequence	• Rotor Winding Failure	
• Ground Fault	• Stator Winding Failure	
• Overload		
• Interturn short-circuit		
• Crawling		

Fig. 1 Faults in induction motors

Fig. 2 Frequency of faults in induction motor

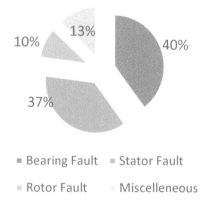

Table 1 Causes and effects of various faults in induction motor [5, 10–14]

Type of fault		Cause	Effect
Internal fault	Bearing fault	Fatigue failure due to long run of motor, corrosion, contamination of foreign particles, lubricant failure because of high temperature, misalignment of bearing due to wear of balls and races	Fracture of motor increase in noise and vibration, high wear of balls, overheating, increase in temperature and vibration
	Stator fault	Mechanical stress due to striking of rotor and stator coil due to shaft misalignment, electrical stress due to supply voltage transient due to lightning, LG, LL, LLL faults, and VFDs. Thermal stress caused by overload, higher ambient temperature, unbalanced voltage supply	Open circuit fault, turn to ground and turn to turn faults, insulation life is reduced
	Rotor faults	Broken rotor bar by reason of manufacturing defects, large centrifugal forces due to heavy end rings, thermal stresses, frequent start and stops, rotor mass unbalance as a result of shaft bending, internal misalignment, manufacturing defects	Overheating, ripple effect and increase in total harmonic distortion, dynamic eccentricity, increase in harmonic levels
External fault	Under voltage	Short circuit of transmission line, damage to the underground cables, connecting heavy loads, disconnecting capacitor banks	Shut down or burning of ASD, PLC, and controllers, reduction in efficiency of appliances, wear and tear of motor windings
	Over voltage	LG fault, switching on the capacitor banks, disconnecting heavy loads, loss of secondary neutral, poor voltage regulation, ferro resonance, high voltage circuit contact, lightning	Heating or burning of electronic equipment, insulation breakdown, flash over between phase and earth, failure of transformer and machines
	Single phasing	Broken or loose or oxidized terminal contact, melting of fuse	Melting of insulation, overloading of generators, increase in, vibrations and noise of motors, damage to motor winding, fluctuations in torque
	Voltage unbalance	Difference in reactance of the phases, connecting heavy loads to one of the phase	Reduction in efficiency of the motor, heating, melting of grease of bearings, excessive vibrations, increase in copper losses

2   External Fault Detection

External faults contains power quality-related faults, and classification techniques are used in this work for the detection of these faults.

2.1   Multi-layer Perceptron Neural Network

Inspired by the human brain, a neural network consists of highly connected networks of neurons that relate the inputs to the desired output [15]. The network is trained by iteratively modifying the strengths of the connections so that given inputs map to the correct response.

Best Used...

- For modeling highly nonlinear systems
- When data is available incrementally and you wish to constantly update the model
- When there could be unexpected changes in your input data.

One directional signal flow is allowed for feed forward neural networks (FFNN). FFNN are easy to implement, fast, and require small dataset for training. Because of these advantages of the FFNN, these are implemented in most of the scenarios [16] (Table 2).

Table 2 Existing techniques for induction motor fault detection

Type of fault	Method applied and year	Conclusion
Bearing fault	Fractal dimension theory using vibrations (2016)	OBD faults can be found with high efficacy by using KFD algorithm. But some industries do not use extra sensors [17]
	Stationary wavelet packet transformation and directed acyclic graph (2016)	Combining SWPT and DAG has reduced the number of descriptors [18]
	Neural network (2016)	Computer based technique thus requires less computations. Voltage and current both are considered to deal with voltage unbalance and various load conditions [19]
	Short-time Fourier transformation (2016)	Excessive lubrication can cause mechanical damage. Motor with excessive lubrication will cause new frequencies in the spectrum [20]
	MCSA (continuous wavelet transformation) (2016)	The amplitude of fault frequencies is very less in case of spectrum based techniques and can be mistaken as noise [21]

(continued)

Table 2 (continued)

Type of fault	Method applied and year	Conclusion
Stator fault	Radial flux sensing using observer coil (2016)	Faulty stator coil can easily be detected, but it needs to place the observer coil inside the machine [22]
	Sweep frequency response analysis (2016)	Able to detect even 1% of the fault, but it requires expert opinion to get repeatability [23]
	Fuzzy logic-based diagnosis (2016)	Park's vector transformation and PCA are used to make rule base and membership function. For inverter fed motors, having harmonics makes the diagnosis difficult [24]
	Extended Kaman filter (2016)	Resistance of the stator and rotor increases if fault occurs and by analyzing that fault can be detected [25]
	MCSA and MSCSA (2016)	MSCSA detects the faults with more accuracy, but on contrary, MCSA is simpler to apply [3]
Rotor fault	Stator dynamic deformation with optical fiber strain sensors (2017)	Even the voltage contains harmonics, the broken bar can be detected in two frequency spectrum regions [26]
	MCSA, MSCSA, and PCA (2016)	MSCSA is able to detect faults with more accuracy [27]
	Gabor transformation, Harmonic order tracking Analysis 2016	The position of the fault frequencies remain same and do not depend on supply frequency, load and rotor by using proposed technique [28]
	FFT, Hilbert transformation, envelope detection, DWT 2017	FFT using MCSA is unable to detect the fault for variable load and variable speed drives. DWT can easily identify the impacts of vibration and current signals of bowed rotor and unbalanced induction motor. ED, HT using vibration signals are used to provide diverse information of fault location [29]
	Sliding discrete Fourier transform 2016	At no load, MUSIC, ZMUSIC, FFT, and ZFFT are unable to detect fault whereas proposed method is able to detect the fault at no load and at load with more sensitivity in less time [30]
Compound fault	Modulation signal bi-spectrum analysis (2016)	An additional increase in the sideband amplitude occurs due to faults present together. MSBA is able to reduce the noise levels and also provides more accurate results as compared to traditional spectrum analysis [31]
External fault	Neural network and fuzzy logic (2016)	Unbalance of voltage, over voltage, under voltage, single phasing are detected using multi-layer perceptron and fuzzy logic [14]

Fig. 3 Structure of MLPNN

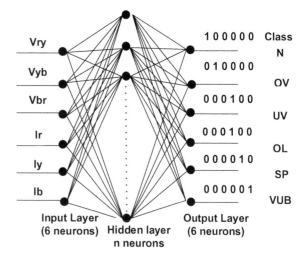

Fig. 4 Representation of random forest

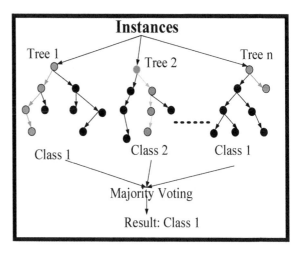

As the universal approximation theorem [32] states only single hidden layer is enough for a neural network to approximate any continuous mapping of the patterns to the output pattern for desired accuracy.

MLPNN can be used in cases the classes are nonlinear and complex. Minimum number of neurons and number of instances are required to program a given task. The number of neurons required in the hidden layer to achieve best accuracy can only be found by using hit and trial method because no analytical method exists for the same purpose.

There is no clear and exact rule due to complexity of the network [14]. Neurons depend on the function to be approximated, and its degree of nonlinearity affects the size of network. Large number of neurons and layers may cause over fitting and may cause decrease the generalization ability (Fig. 3).

2.2 Random Forest

A decision tree lets you predict responses to data by following the decisions in the tree starting from the root (beginning) down to a leaf node [33]. A tree consists of branching conditions where the value of a predictor is compared to a trained weight.

The number of branches and the values of weights are determined in the training process. Additional modification, or pruning, may be used to simplify the model.

Best Used...

- When you need an algorithm that is easy to interpret and fast to fit
- To minimize memory usage.

Random forests are extremely trendy tool for classification. Random forest is based on the decision trees (Fig. 4), and the classifiers are made greedily using the conditional entropy. In practice, random forest is quite attractive because of its advantages as decision trees are non-parametric and the model can be built between the input and the output by arbitrary complex relations [34]. It can handle heterogeneous data. Random forest is robust for noisy and irrelevant variables also to the outliers. This algorithm can be easily implemented even by a non-statistical person.

3 Internal Fault Detection

Surveys have revealed that bearing fault account for 75% of small and medium motor defects while 41% of large motor defects [35].

3.1 Fast Fourier Transformation

Fast Fourier transformation (FFT) is an algorithm which is used to calculate the discrete Fourier transform (DFT). It is an efficient algorithm and is used in many fields. DFT decomposes the sequence into the components based on the frequency. DFT is very useful as it reveals the presence of the periodic components in the input sequence. Generally, DFT of a real sequence results in a complex sequence of numbers of same length. The DFT of a sequence vector x can be calculated by [36].

$$y_{p+1} = \sum_{j=0}^{n-1} \omega^{jp} x_j + 1 \tag{1}$$

Here,

'n'   represents the length of the input sequence,
'ω'   is a complex unity, and

$$\omega = e^{-\frac{2\pi i}{n}} \tag{2}$$

'p' and 'j' are indices from 0 to n − 1.

The absolute value of y at index p + 1 represents the frequency present at f = p (f s/n) in the input data. The result sequence 'y' carries all the information about the frequency for the interested subspace. In classification, FFT forms a power matrix of special features.

Bearing data [37] is as followed:

Inside diameter = 0.9843 in.
Outside diameter = 2.0472 in.
Thickness = 0.5906 in.
Ball diameter = 0.3126 in.
Pitch diameter = 1.537 in.
Contact angle = 0°
Sampling rate = 12,000 samples/s

3.2 S-Transform

Stockwell Transformation is also termed as S-Transform is a time-frequency decomposition tool. It is developed to beat the drawbacks of the STFT. S-Transform is developed to overcome some of the disadvantages of the continuous wavelet transform. In S-Transform, the modulation sinusoidal is fixed with respect to the time axis. This transformation is based on the localization of the Gaussian window. S-Transform does not contain any cross term problem and results in a better signal clarity as compared to Gabor transform. Mathematically, S-Transform can be written as [38]:

$$S(\tau, f) = \int_{-\infty}^{\infty} x(t) \frac{|f|}{\sqrt{2\pi}} e^{-\frac{(\tau-t)^2 f^2}{2}} e^{-j2\pi ft} \tag{3}$$

S-Transform can also define multiple frequencies as one-dimensional function of frequency (f) and time scale (τ):

$$S(\tau, f_i) = A(\tau, f_i) e^{j\varphi(\tau, f_i)} \tag{4}$$

Local frequency and amplitude are computed, and these can be used to compute H (w, t). S-Transform has its own disadvantages as the clarity is worst for higher frequencies. In this work, the detection of fault is using the lower frequencies, so this limitation does not cause any problem in fault detection. If any how the use of S-Transform is required at higher frequencies, various adaptive forms have been developed.

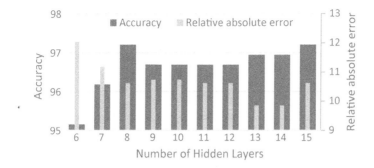

Fig. 5 Effect of hidden layers on the performance of MLPNN

In this work, DOST and DCST [39] are implemented. The DOST transform provides an efficient representation of the S-Transform by introducing orthogonal basis vectors. A set of $N\psi$ orthogonal unit-length basis vectors are constructed, each of which targets a particular region in the time-frequency domain. The regions are described by a set of parameters: $\psi\psi$ specifies the center of each frequency band, $\psi\psi$ is the width of that band, and $\psi\psi$ specifies the location in time. Using these parameters, the kth basis vector is defined as [40].

$$D[k]_{[v,\beta,\tau]} = \frac{1}{\sqrt{\beta}} \sum_{f=v-\beta/2}^{v-\frac{\beta}{2}-1} \exp\left(-i2\pi\frac{k}{N}f\right) \exp\left(i2\pi\frac{\tau}{\beta}f\right) \exp(-i\pi\tau) \quad (5)$$

Fourier transform DCST transform is a variation of the DOST. It may be defined by simply replacing the DFT with a DCT [41].

4 Results

In this work, MLPNN and random forest are used for external fault detection. Numbers of neurons in the input layer are equal to the number of variables. Variables to be fed to the input layer are voltages of three phases and current of three phases. The numbers of neurons in the output layer are equal to the number of classes. The classes are healthy, UV, OV, SP, OL, and VUB. Matlab is used for the implementation of MLPNN using nftool (Figs. 5 and 7). The comparison Table 3 is made to compare the performance of MLPNN for different hidden layers. Total numbers of instances are 393 in dataset [14]. For random forest, same dataset is used as the performance is analyzed in Figs. 6, 8 and Table 4.

Table 3 Performance of MLPNN

	Number of correctly classified instances	Accuracy	Percentage of incorrectly classified instances	Relative absolute error
6	374	95.16	4.83	12.08
7	378	96.18	3.81	11.18
8	**382**	**97.2**	**2.79**	**10.62**
9	380	96.69	3.3	10.73
10	380	96.69	3.3	10.73
11	380	96.69	3.3	10.62
12	380	96.69	3.3	10.62
13	381	96.94	3.05	9.85
14	381	96.94	3.05	9.85
15	**382**	**97.2**	**2.79**	**10.62**

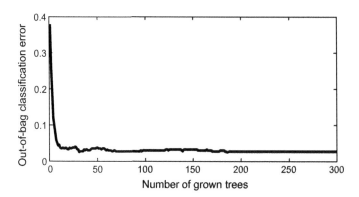

Fig. 6 Random forest classification error versus number of trees

For the detection of internal faults, i.e., bearing faults S-Transform is used. It can be seen that FFT Fig. 9 is able to detect inner race fault but not able to detect outer race fault, and it can easily be mistaken as noise. S-Transform by applying DOST and DCST is able to detect both type of faults. From the results, Fig. 10, it can easily be depicted that S-Transform is able to detect the faults as the fault causes new frequencies and the effect of these frequencies can easily be seen.

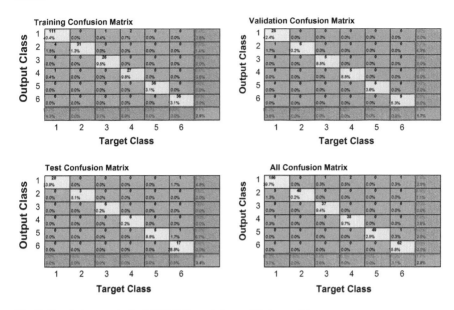

Fig. 7 Confusion matrix for MLPNN for training, validation and test cases

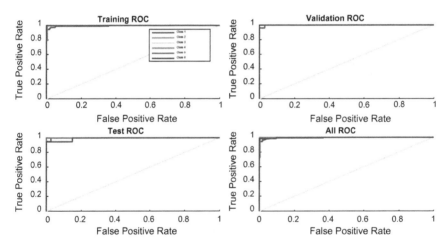

Fig. 8 ROC for MLPNN

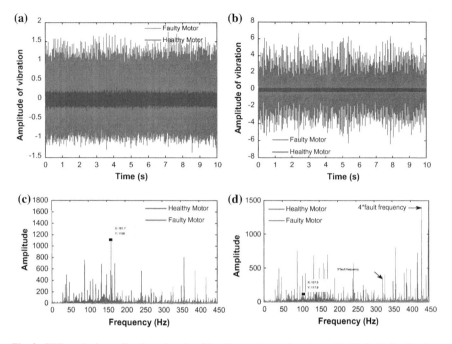

Fig. 9 FFT analysis **a** vibration signals of healthy motor and motor with IR fault, **b** vibration signals of healthy motor and motor with OR fault, **c** FFT analysis of IR fault, **d** FFT analysis of OR fault

5 Conclusion

In this work, the fault detection techniques for the internal and external faults of the induction motor are presented. From the results, it can be concluded that random forest provides best detection of the internal faults as compared to neural network. It has also been seen that S-Transform is able to detect the faults in premature state as the fault causes new frequencies, and the effect of these frequencies can easily be seen in the spectrum of S-Transform, whereas traditional FFT is not able to detect the faults efficiently. This technique is easy to implement as compared to flux sensing and other invasive techniques. The limitations of S-transform are that it provides less accuracy as the frequency increases. But in fault detection of induction motor, low frequencies are considered. The detection of the fault in premature state leads to increase the efficiency and reliability of the motors. However, broken bar, stator, and eccentricity faults are not discussed, and this is the future scope of the work.

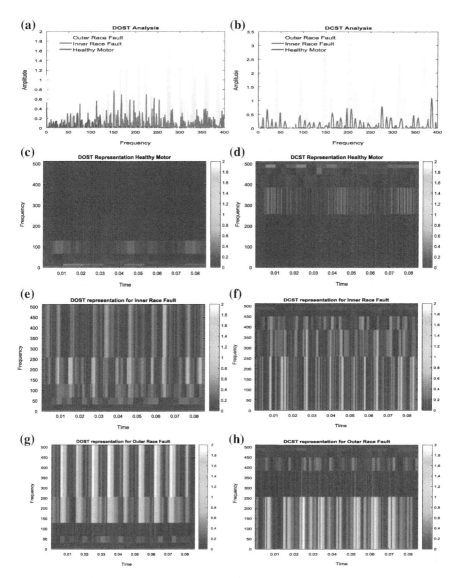

Fig. 10 S-Transform analysis **a** DOST analysis, **b** DCST analysis, **c** DOST of healthy motor, **d** DCST of healthy motor, **e** DOST of IR fault, **f** DCST of IR fault, **g** DOST of OR fault, **h** DCST of OR fault

Table 4 Performance of random forest

Number of features to be chosen randomly	Correctly classified instances	Accuracy	Percentage of incorrectly classified	Relative absolute error
1	384	97.7	2.29	7.98
2	384	97.7	2.29	7.25
3	**385**	**97.96**	**2.03**	**7.06**
4	379	96.43	3.56	7.22
5	380	96.69	3.3	7.32
6	380	96.69	3.3	7.44

References

1. Kumar KV, Kumar SS, Saravanakumar R, Selvakumar AI, ReddyK, Varghese JM (2011) Condition monitoring of DSP based online induction motor external fault detection using TMS320LF2407 DSP. In: International conference on process automation, control and computing, Coimbatore
2. García-Escudero LA, Duque-Perez O, Fernandez-Temprano M Morinigo-Sotelo D (2017) Robust detection of incipient faults in VSI-fed induction motors using quality control charts. IEEE Trans Ind Appl
3. Fontes AS, Cardoso CAV, Oliveira LPB (2016) Comparison of techniques based on current signature analysis to fault detection and diagnosis in induction electrical motors. In: 2016 Electrical engineering conference (EECon), Colombo
4. Bindu S, Thomas VV (2014) Diagnoses of internal faults of three phase squirrel cage induction motor—a review. In: 2014 International conference on advances in energy conversion technologies (ICAECT), Manipal
5. Masoum MA, Fuchs EF (2015) Power quality in power system and electrical machines, 2nd edn. Academic Press, Elsevier
6. Dash RN, Sahu S, Panigrahi CK, Subudhi B (2016) Condition monitoring of induction motor—a review. In: International conference on signal processing, communication, power and embedded systems (SCOPES)
7. Basak D, Tiwari A, Das SP (2006) Fault diagnosis and condition monitoring of electrical machines—a review. In: 2006 IEEE international conference on industrial technology, Mumbai
8. Singh G, Al Kazzaz S (2003) Induction machine drive condition monitoring and diagnostic research—a survey. Electr Power Syst Res 64(2)
9. Allbrecht P, Appiarius J, McCoy RM, Owen E (1986) Assessment of the reliability of motors in utility applications-updated. IEEE Trans Energy Convers EC 1(1)
10. Karmakar S, Chattopadhyay S, Mitra M Sengupta S (2016) Induction motor fault diagnosis. Springer Nature
11. Bhosale G, Vakhare A, Kaystha A, Aher A, Pansare V (2018) Overvoltage, undervoltage protection of electrical equipment. Int Res J Eng Technol (IRJET)
12. William K (2005) Causes and effects of single-phasing induction motors, vol 41, pp 1499–1505
13. Aderibigbe A, Ogunjuyigbe A, Ayodele R, Samuel I (2017) The performance of a 3-phase induction machine under unbalance voltage regime. J Eng Sci Technol Rev
14. Chudasama KJ (2016) To study induction motor external faults detection and classification using ANN and Fuzzy soft computing techniques. Gujarat Technological University, Ahmedabad
15. Ou G, Murphey YL, Feldkamp A (2004) Multiclass pattern classification using neural networks. In: Proceedings of the 17th international conference on pattern recognition, 2004. ICPR 2004

16. Haykin S (2009) Neural networks and learning machines, 3rd edn. Pearson Education
17. Perez-Ramirez CA, Amezquita-Sanchez JP, Valiterra-Rodriguez M, Dominguez-Gonzalez A, Camarena-Martinez D, Romero-Troncoso RJ (2016) Fractal dimension theory based approach for bearing fault detection in induction motors. In: 2016 IEEE international autumn meeting on power, electronics and computing (ROPEC 2016), Mexico
18. Abid FB, Zgarni S, Braham A (2016) Bearing fault detection of induction motor using SWPT and DAG support vector machines. In: IECON 2016—42nd annual conference of the IEEE Industrial Electronics Society, Florence
19. Gongora WS, Silva HVD, Goedtel A, Godoy WF, Silva SAOD (2013) Neural approach for bearing fault detection in three phase induction motors. In: 2013 9th IEEE international symposium on diagnostics for electric machines, power electronics and drives (SDEMPED), Valencia
20. Lopez-Ramirez M (2016) Detection and diagnosis of lubrication and faults in bearing on induction motors through STFT. In: 2016 International conference on electronics, communications and computers (CONIELECOMP), Choula
21. Singh S, Kumar N (2017) Detection of bearing faults in mechanical systems using stator current monitoring. IEEE Trans Ind Inform
22. Surya GN, Khan ZJ, Ballal M, Suryawanshi H (2016) A simplified frequency domain detection of stator turn fault in squirrel cage induction motors using observer coil technique. IEEE Trans Ind Electron
23. Vilhekar TG, Ballal MS, Umre BS (2016) Application of sweep frequency response analysis for the detection of winding faults in induction motor. In: IECON 2016—42nd annual conference of the IEEE Industrial Electronics Society, Florence
24. Aydin I, Karakose M, Akin E (2016) A new real-time fuzzy logic based diagnosis of stator faults for inverter-fed induction motor under low speeds. In: 2016 IEEE 14th international conference on industrial informatics (INDIN), Poitiers
25. Rayyam M, Zazi M, Hajji Y, Chtouki I (2016) Stator and rotor faults detection in Induction Motor (IM) using the Extended Kaman Filter (EKF). In: 2016 International conference on electrical and information technologies (ICEIT), Tangiers
26. Sousa KM, Costa IBVD, Maciel ES, Rocha JE, Martelli C, Silva JCCD (2017) Broken bar fault detection in induction motor by using optical fiber strain sensors. IEEE Sens J
27. Pires VF, Martins JF, Pires AJ, Rodrigues L (2016) Induction motor broken bar fault detection based on MCSA, MSCSA and PCA: a comparative study. In: 2016 10th International conference on compatibility, power electronics and power engineering (CPE-POWERENG), Bydgoszcz
28. Dybkowski M, Klimkowski K (2016) Stator current sensor fault detection and isolation for vector controlled induction motor drive. In: 2016 IEEE international power electronics and motion control conference (PEMC), Varna
29. Rahman MM, Uddin MN (2017) Online unbalanced rotor fault detection of an IM drive based on both time and frequency domain analyses. IEEE Trans Ind Appl
30. Moussa MA, Boucherma M, Khezzar A (2017) A detection method for induction motor bar fault using sidelobes leakage phenomenon of the sliding discrete fourier transform. IEEE Trans Power Electron
31. Shaeboub A, Lane UHM, Gu F, Ball AD (2016) Detection and diagnosis of compound faults in induction motors using electric signals from variable speed drives. In: 2016 22nd international conference on automation and computing (ICAC), Colchester
32. Quadri S, Sidek O (2014) Development of heterogeneous multisensor data fusion system to improve evaluation of concrete structures. Int J Image Data Fusion
33. Louppe G (2014) Understanding random forests. University of Liège
34. James G, Witten D, Hastie T, Tibshirani R (2015) An introduction to statistical learning. Springer, New York, Heidelberg, Dordrecht, London
35. Li DZ, Wang W, Ismail F (2015) A spectrum synch technique for induction motor health condition monitoring. IEEE Trans Energy Convers
36. Zhou J, Qin Y, Kou L, Yuwono M, Su S (2015) Fault detection of rolling bearing based on FFT and classification. J Adv Mech Des Syst Manuf

37. Case Western Reserve University Bearing Data Center Website. Case Western Reserve University. http://csegroups.case.edu/bearingdatacenter/home. Accessed 2018 Jan 21
38. Singh M, Shaik AG (2016) Bearing fault diagnosis of a three phase induction motor using Stockwell transform. In: 2016 IEEE annual India conference (INDICON), Bangalore
39. Battisti L, Riba L (2015) Window-dependent bases for efficient representations of the Stockwell transform. Appl Comput Harmon Anal
40. Wang Y, Orchard J (2009) Fast-discrete orthonormal. SISC 31:4000–4012
41. Battisti U, Riba L (2015) Window-dependent bases for efficient representations of the Stockwell transform. Appl Comput Harmon Anal

Comparison of Maximum Power Point Tracking—Perturb and Observe and Fuzzy Logic Controllers for Single Phase Photovoltaic Systems

P. S. Gotekar, S. P. Muley and D. P. Kothari

Abstract For effective utilization of irradiation's falling on the solar photovoltaic panel, several maximum power point (MPPT) techniques are used. The comparative analysis of perturb and observe (P&O) and fuzzy logic methods for MPPT is presented in this paper. The modeling technique employing fuzzy logic is simplified to enable it to track power efficiently.

Keywords MPPT · PV cell · P and O · Fuzzy logic

1 Introduction

Increasingly more and more countries are setting up high targets of renewable energy sources in their energy system as conventional sources are limited and have been causing environmental hazards with their usage. To achieve this aim, most of the countries are increasing renewable energy in their energy production mix as they are abundantly available, relatively cheaper, and cause less pollution. The applications of solar energy are increasing rapidly worldwide. Owing to the changing policies, India is all set to install 1.5 GW solar power capacity by 2019. Solar power, especially from photovoltaics, has increased after the launch of the Jawaharlal National Solar Mission in 2010. The unpredictable nature of solar power and its dependence on weather and climatic conditions are the limitations of solar energy.

Since irradiance of solar energy is continuously changing so, it is difficult to get the constant output voltage of a single phase photovoltaic system. The effort

P. S. Gotekar (✉) · S. P. Muley
Priyadarshini College of Engineering, RTMN University, Nagpur, India
e-mail: p_somkuwar@yahoo.com

D. P. Kothari
IIT Delhi, New Delhi, India

VIT Vellore, Vellore, India

VRCE, Nagpur, India

© Springer Nature Singapore Pte Ltd. 2019
V. Sridhar et al. (eds.), *Emerging Research in Electronics, Computer Science and Technology*, Lecture Notes in Electrical Engineering 545,
https://doi.org/10.1007/978-981-13-5802-9_113

1347

is made to maintain constant output power by using different techniques of MPPT. The conventional perturb and observe and advanced fuzzy logic-based MPPT are compared, and their analysis is presented in this paper. The rules designed for fuzzy logic controller can track the maximum power at high speeds.

A boost converter is connected to increase the output voltage when implementing a PV MPPT system for a single phase system, while taking into account residential applications.

Overall, this paper consists of modeling of PV cell, MPPT using conventional P and O technique and a fast implementing rule base for fuzzy logic controller. The system is analyzed using boost converter.

2   PV Cell Design

The photovoltaic cell uses the energy of the Sun and converts solar energy into electrical energy. This energy conversion has salient features since it is nontoxic, harmless, inexhaustible, and carbon dioxide-emission free. The output voltage of the PV panel is maintained constant for all changes in irradiance when using MPPT. This voltage is amplified using boost converter and is applied to the load. The structure of the system used for this analysis is as shown in Fig. 1.

The PV cell absorbs solar energy and converts it into electrical energy. PV module is the combination of solar cells. There are different configurations of PV cell-like single diode model, two diode model, and Rs-Rp model. The model selected in this research is single diode model.

The V-I curve of PV cell is a nonlinear equation which has many parameters classified as follows: constructors, constants, and the ones which must be calculated. Researchers develop simplified methods where some unknown parameters cannot be calculated. They are assumed to be constant. In some literature, these two have been identified more accurately. While designing the PV module—which is a combination of series and parallel resistance, ideality factor, photocurrent, diode current has also been considered. This designing is carried out so that at any time, the maximum power is achieved more precisely.

Fig. 1 Structure of the system

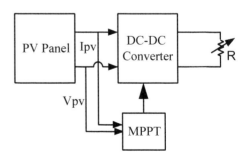

Fig. 2 Single diode model of PV cell

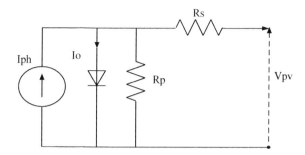

To predict the behavior of the solar cell under varying atmospheric conditions, mathematical modeling is required. The key factor that affects the accuracy of the simulation is the accurate representation of nonlinear characteristics of the PV system modeling as shown in Fig. 2.

3 Maximum Power Point Tracking

As the direction of the Sun changes, there is change in the insolation level, and hence, the output power of PV module also changes. The product of peak values of voltage and current represents the maximum power point 'P_{max}' of the solar module. The PV module should always be operated in MPPT region so that the maximum power is extracted for a given input conditions. For this purpose, various maximum power point algorithms are used. It is desirable that PV module operates near maximum power point.

The focus of the paper is on the tracking of maximum power point of PV module which in itself is a complex electro-energetic system. According to maximum power transfer theorem, the power output of a circuit is at its maximum when the Thevenin's impedance of the circuit (source impedance) matches with the load.

There are different techniques used to track the maximum power point. The conventional techniques are:

(1) Perturb and observe (hill climbing method).
(2) Incremental conductance method.

Some other techniques are:

(1) Fractional short-circuit current.
(2) Fractional open-circuit voltage.
(3) Neural networks.
(4) Fuzzy logic.

Perturb and observe and incremental conductance methods are conventional methods. The perturb and observe and fuzzy controllers are implemented in this research.

3.1 Perturb and Observe

Perturb and observe (P&O) is the simplest method with only one sensor used which is the voltage sensor to sense the PV array voltage. Hence, the cost of implementation is less and thus is easy to implement. The time complexity of this algorithm is very less, but on reaching very close to the maximum power point, it doesn't stop at the maximum power point and instead keeps on perturbing in both the directions. When this happens, the algorithm almost reaches to the maximum power point and this allows us to set an appropriate error limit.

In this method, the sign of the last perturbation and the sign of the last increment in the power are used to decide what the next perturbation should be on the left of the maximum power point; incrementing the voltage increases the power whereas on the right decrementing the voltage increases the power.

Figure 3 shows the flowchart of P&O algorithm. In this method, P&O shows how fast the maximum power point is reached depending on the size of the increment of the reference voltage.

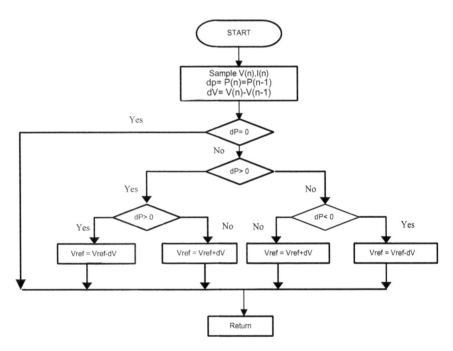

Fig. 3 Flow chart of perturb and observe algorithm

3.2 Fuzzy Logic Controller

Fuzzy logic was invented by Lofti A. Zadeh in 1965. Fuzzy logic uses the experience of human experiences by implementing it through membership functions and fuzzy rules.

3.2.1 Fuzzy Sets and Membership Functions

The extension of a crisp variable set where an element can only belong to a particular set (full membership) or does not belong at all (no membership). Fuzzy sets allow partial membership which means that an element may partially belong to more than one set.

3.2.2 Fuzzy Rules and Inferencing

The use of fuzzy sets allows the characterization of the system behavior through fuzzy rules between linguistic variables. A fuzzy rule is a conditional statement based on expert knowledge expressed in this form:

Rule: IF x is small THEN y is large

Where x and y are fuzzy variables, and small and large are labels of the fuzzy sets.

The flowchart in Fig. 4 represents the sequence of calculation of duty cycle. The general structure of a fuzzy logic controller is presented in Fig. 4 comprises four principal components.

3.2.3 Fuzzification Interface

The pieces of input data are converted into suitable linguistic values using a membership function. The equations associated with the calculation of error and change of error are given:

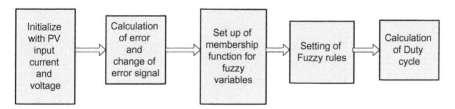

Fig. 4 Flow chart of the fuzzy logic controller

$$E(K) = \frac{\Delta I}{\Delta V} + \frac{I}{V} = \frac{\Delta P}{\Delta V} = \frac{\Delta P}{\Delta I} \tag{1}$$

$$CE(K) = E(K) - E(K-1) \tag{2}$$

$$\Delta I = I(K) - I(K-1) \tag{3}$$

$$\Delta V = V(K) - V(K-1) \tag{4}$$

$$\Delta P = P(K) - P(K-1) \tag{5}$$

3.2.4 Membership Function

The membership function selected is triangular membership functions. The graphical view of the membership function are NB, NM, NS, ZE, PS, PM, and PB, i.e., negative big, negative medium, negative small, zero, positive small, positive medium, and positive big.

For the setting of rules of fuzzy logic MPPT, different number of subsets has been used. But for this work, seven subsets based on forty-nine rules have been used. The tuning of forty-nine rules has been used. The fuzzy rules are indicated in Table 1 consists of a database with the necessary linguistic definitions and the control rule set.

3.2.5 Inference Engine

The simulation of a human decision-making process so as to infer the fuzzy control action from the knowledge of the control rules is done using inference engine.

Table 1 Set of 49 fuzzy rules of the fuzzy system

E	CE						
	NB	NM	NS	ZE	S	M	B
NB	ZE	ZE	ZE	NB	NB	NB	NB
NM	ZE	ZE	ZE	NM	NM	NM	NM
NS	NS	ZE	ZE	NS	NS	NS	NS
ZE	NM	NS	ZE	ZE	ZE	S	M
S	M	S	S	S	ZE	ZE	ZE
M	M	M	M	ZE	ZE	ZE	ZE
B	B	B	B	ZE	ZE	ZE	ZE

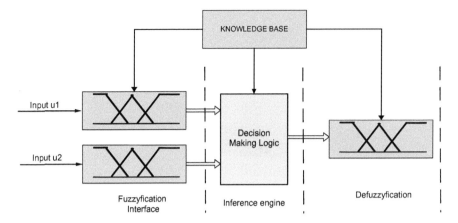

Fig. 5 Basic configuration of fuzzy logic controller

3.2.6 Defuzzification Interface

It converts the output obtained from fuzzy controller into a non-fuzzy output (Fig. 5).

4 Results

In simulation, the P&O controller and fuzzy logic controller were subjected to slow change in irradiance (15 W/m²s) and fast changing irradiance (50 W/m²s). Figures 6and 8 indicate the power output of P&O for slow and fast changing irradiance. Figures 7 and 9 indicate the power output for fuzzy logic controller for variation in irradiance. It is observed that fuzzy logic controller tracks the output faster and has better dynamic response (Table 2).

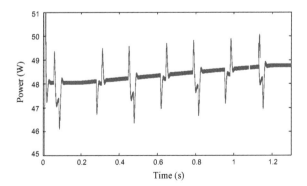

Fig. 6 Power with P&O with slow changing irradiance

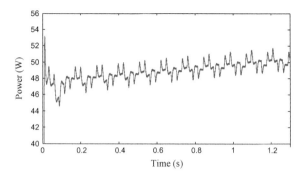

Fig. 7 Power with fuzzy logic controller for slow changing irradiance

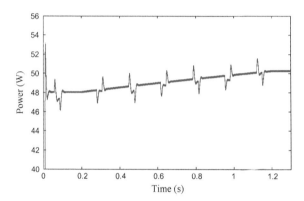

Fig. 8 Power due to perturb and observe controller for fast changing irradiance

Fig. 9 Power due to fuzzy logic controller for fast changing irradiance

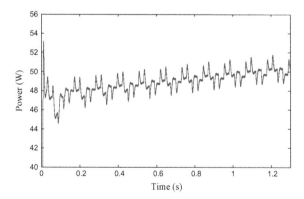

Table 2 Comparison between P and O and fuzzy logic controller

MPPT controller	Fast changing irradiance (W)	Slow changing irradiance (W)	No changing irradiance (W)
P and O	48.60	47.75	47.2
Fuzzy logic	48.81	48.12	48.0

5 Conclusion

The maximum power is dependent on temperature and solar irradiation. In order to improve efficiency, maximum power point tracker (MPPT) is used by PV systems to continuously extract the highest possible power and delivers it to the load.

This paper presents a comparison of perturb and observe technique and fuzzy logic controller to optimize the energy extraction in a photovoltaic power system. The efficient modeling of PV module with a fuzzy logic-based MPPT system has been implemented using MATLAB. The complexity of PV modeling was reduced, and implementation of the fuzzy technique is carried out to control the output of boost converter. It is observed that the system completes maximum power point tracking successfully.

References

1. Sera D, Kerekas T, Teodorescu R, Blaabjerg F (2006) Improved MPPT algorithms for rapidly changing environmental conditions. In: 12th International power electronics and motion control conference, pp 1614–1619
2. Al Nabusi A, Dhaouadi R (2012) Fuzzy logic controller based perturb and observe maximum power point tracking. In: European Association for development of renewable energies, environment and power quality
3. Ahmad A, Loganathan R (2013) Real time implementation of solar inverter with novel MPPT control algorithm for residential applications. Energy Power Eng
4. Mahamudul H, Saad M, Ibrahim Henk M (2013) Photovoltaic system modeling with fuzzy logic based maximum power point tracking. Int J Photoenergy 13
5. Bellia H, Youcef R, Fatima M (2014) A detailed modelling of photovoltaic module. NRIAG J Astron Geophys 3:53–61
6. El Khateb A, Rahim NA, Selvaraj J (2011) Fuzzy logic controller for SEPIC converter and PV single phase inverter. In: IEEE symposium on industrial electronics and applications, pp 182–187
7. Das SK, Panda PC, Samal S (2017) Grid connected PV systems with fuzzy logic controller. In: International conference on communication and signal processing (ICCSP), pp 1177–1181
8. Gotekar PS, Muley SP, Kothari DP, Umre BS (2015) Comparison of full bridge bipolar, H5, H6 and HERIC inverter for single phase photovoltaic systems. In: IEEE INDICON 2015, Jamia Millia Islamia, New Delhi, pp 1–6
9. Kothari DP, Singhal KC Ranjan R (2008) Renewable energy sources and emerging technologies, 2nd edn. PHI Learning Pvt Ltd

10. Jamil M, Rizwan M, Kothari DP (2017) Grid integration of solar photovolatic systems. CRC Press, Taylor and Francis, New York
11. Kothari DP, Subba Rao PMV (2009) Power generation. In: Grote KH, Antonsson EK (eds) Springer handbook of mechanical engineering. Springer, Germany

Comparative Study of Different High-Gain Converter

S. N. Bhavya and Uppara Rajesh

Abstract A DC–DC converter with high voltage gain is advantageous in most of the industrial applications such as uninterruptable power supply, vehicular system and conversion of low output renewable energy resources. Many DC–DC converters with high voltage gain are already available, but there are some issues need to be addressed like complexity of circuit, high ripple at input current, large stress across power semiconductor devices. In this paper, comparisons of different high-gain converters are carried out. Among all the compared converters, modified converter with dual output port has more gain, very useful and more advantageous compare to other converters. The results are carried out in the PSIM environment.

Keywords Dual ports · Low current ripple at input · Low switch stress · High gain · PSIM software

1 Introduction

DC–DC converter with high voltage gain is suitable for many industrial applications. To step-up the voltage, conventional boost converter is used. But it offers more stress across the switch which is same as the voltage at the output terminals. Converters with high gain are available but these converters are not efficient because of large ripple at the input current, number of component required is more, stress across switch is high, the number of power semiconductor devices required is more and hence the efficiency is less. Some of the converter uses large turn's ratio counts to get more gain, but this increases the cost and circuit complexity. Most of the high-gain converters do not have a multiple output. Here some of the different converter comparison has made.

S. N. Bhavya (✉) · U. Rajesh
Siddaganga Institute of Technology, Tumakuru, Karnataka, India
e-mail: bhavyasn1995@gmail.com

U. Rajesh
e-mail: rajeshu@sit.ac.in

© Springer Nature Singapore Pte Ltd. 2019
V. Sridhar et al. (eds.), *Emerging Research in Electronics, Computer Science and Technology*, Lecture Notes in Electrical Engineering 545,
https://doi.org/10.1007/978-981-13-5802-9_114

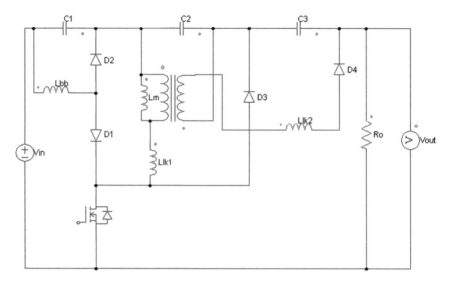

Fig. 1 Circuit diagram of buck-boost-flyback converter

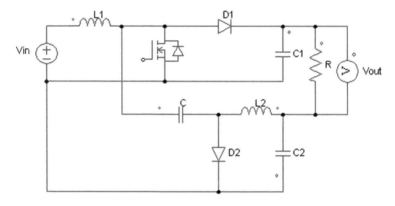

Fig. 2 Circuit diagram of Boost–Cuk DC–DC converter

A Buck-Boost-Flyback converter (Fig. 1) with one switch has more gain, but the stress across the switch is more. The overall gain of the system can be extendable by inserting buck-boost inductance, but complexity of circuit is more [1]. Boost–Cuk converter (Fig. 2) has high efficiency and low voltage gain [2]. Coupled inductor-based DC–DC converter has low ripple at input current, more voltage gain, more efficiency, less stress across power semiconductor devices [3].

Zeta-flyback (Fig. 3) converter has low gain, high stress across the switch with two transformers, this leads to more cost [4]. Highly efficient Sepic-Boost-Flyback (Fig. 4) has two transformers with turn ratio of 3 each, the gain is more but large ripple at the input current [5].

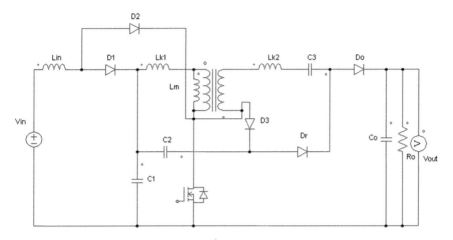

Fig. 3 Circuit diagram of converter with coupled inductor–diode–capacitor

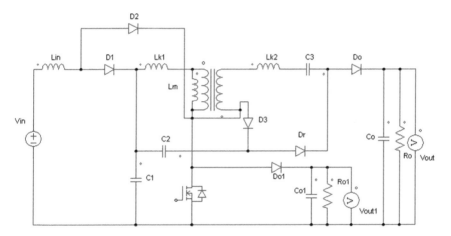

Fig. 4 Circuit diagram of modified dual port converter with coupled inductor–diode–capacitor

Modified converter with capacitor and diode has high voltage gain with less turns ratio that is 2:1, high efficient, less ripple at the input current, the stress across switch and other components is also less. Modified converter with dual output ports is useful for various applications like Thresher machines.

2 Analysis of Different Converter

Various converter comparisons have been carried out based on the converter parameters such as high gain, low input current ripple, efficiency, number of turn's ratio, number of output ports and voltage stress across the switch.

2.1 Buck-Boost-Flyback Converter

Tthe proposed converter (Fig. 1) has voltage gain of 10. By adding large number of buck-boost inductance, voltage gain can be still extendable. At the same time, it suffers from high stress across the switch, and current ripple at the input is high. To get a high voltage gain, number of turns used here are three, output voltage ripple is large and the efficiency is less. Also converter uses more number of inductors, hence the complexity of the circuit is increased.

Output voltage is given by

$$V_O = V_{in} + V_{C1} + V_{C2} + V_{C3}$$

Voltage across capacitor C1, C2, C3 can be given by

$$V_{C1} = \frac{D}{(1-D)} V_{in}$$

$$V_{C2} = \frac{D}{(1-D)^2} V_{in}$$

$$V_{C3} = \frac{nD}{(1-D)^2} V_{in}$$

Converter voltage gain can be given by

$$\frac{V_O}{V_{in}} = \frac{1+nD}{(1-D)^2}$$

where n = Number of turns ratio.

2.2 Boost–Cuk DC–DC Converter

The converter with Boost–Cuk DC–DC converter (Fig. 2), gain achieved is 3, converter consists of two inductors and a single switch. It's efficiency is 97% and the ripple at the input current is low and the stress offered across the switch is twice that of input voltage.

Voltage at the output of capacitor C1 and C2 is represented by

$$V_{O1} = \frac{V_S}{(1-D)}$$

$$V_{O2} = -V_S \frac{D}{(1-D)}$$

$$V_O = V_{O1} - V_{O2} = \frac{V_S}{(1-D)} - \frac{-V_S D}{(1-D)}$$

Voltage gain can be represented as

$$\frac{V_O}{V_{in}} = \frac{(1 + D)}{(1 - D)}$$

2.3   Converter with Coupled Inductor and Diode Capacitor

In the converter with coupled inductor–diode–capacitor (Fig. 3) has single switch, the input current ripple is low and the stress across switch is Vo/4, the turn's ratio is 2, bulkiness of the converter is less because of single inductor and has a high voltage gain around 15.

Voltage across capacitors C1, C2, C3 is given by

$$V_{C1} = \frac{V_{in}}{(1 - D)}$$

$$V_{C2} = \frac{DV_{in}}{(1 - D)^2}$$

$$V_{C3} = \frac{(N + 1 - DN)V_{in}}{(1 - D)^2}$$

By substituting capacitor voltages in output equation, gain can be obtained as

$$V_O = V_{C1} + (N + 1)V_{C2} + V_{C3}$$

$$\frac{V_O}{V_{in}} = \frac{(2 + N)}{(1 - D)^2}$$

2.4   Modified Converter with Coupled Inductor and Diode Capacitor

In the proposed modified dual port converter with coupled inductor–diode–capacitor has high gain. The gain value of the converter is 15, the ripple in the input current is 1.2, turn's ratio used in coupled inductor is 2, switching stress across the switch is less, i.e., is Vo/4, The number of inductors used is only limited to one hence, the complexity of the circuit is also reduced and it has a one more output port used for small power applications. So the proposed dual port converter with coupled inductor–diode–capacitor has more advantages in applications where we need both high-gain port and small power port.

Capacitors C1, C2, C3 voltage is given by

$$V_{C1} = \frac{V_{in}}{(1 - D)}$$

$$V_{C2} = \frac{DV_{in}}{(1-D)^2}$$

$$V_{C3} = \frac{(N+1-DN)V_{in}}{(1-D)^2}$$

By substituting capacitor voltages in output equation, gain can be obtained as

$$V_O = V_{C1} + (N+1)V_{C2} + V_{C3}$$

$$\frac{V_O}{V_{in}} = \frac{(2+N)}{(1-D)^2}$$

By inserting C1 and C2 capacitor voltages in second output equation, output voltage of the second port is given by

$$V_O = V_{C1} + V_{C2}$$

$$V_{O1} = \frac{V_{in}}{(1-D)^2}$$

3 Comparison of Different Converter

Table 1 shows the comparison of A) Buck-Boost-Flyback Converter, B) Boost–Cuk DC–DC Converter, C) Converter with Coupled Inductor and Diode Capacitor and D) Modified Converter with Coupled Inductor and Diode capacitor based on number of port, voltage gain, current ripple, efficiency, turns ratio.

Table 1 Comparative study of various converter parameter

Parameters	Converters			
	Converter A	Converter B	Converter C	Converter D
Voltage gain	$\frac{V_O}{V_{in}} = \frac{1+nD}{(1-D)^2}$	$\frac{V_O}{V_{in}} = \frac{(1+D)}{(1-D)}$	$\frac{V_O}{V_{in}} = \frac{(2+N)}{(1-D)^2}$	$\frac{V_O}{V_{in}} = \frac{(2+N)}{(1-D)^2}$
Current ripple at input	More	More	Less	Less
Number of turns	3	0	2	2
Efficiency (%)	<55	94	96	99.8
Multiple ports	Yes	No	No	Yes
Stress on switch	$\frac{V_O}{3}$	$\frac{V_{in}}{(1-D)}$	$\frac{V_O}{4}$	$\frac{V_O}{4}$

4   Simulations Results

All converters discussed above are simulated in PSIM environment. The converter simulated waveforms of output voltage, stress across the switch and ripple in the input current is shown in Figs. 5, 6, 7 and 8. Figure 5 indicates the stress across the switch is 164 V, the ripple in the input current is around 70 and output voltage of 390 and 4 V output ripple for 40 V supply. Figure 6 shows that for 30 V input, output is 90 V and stress offered is 60 V. Figure 7 indicates the 467 V output and 123 V stress on switch for 30 V supply. Figure 8 shows the 467 and 120 V are two outputs with ripple is 1.2 and switch stress is 120 V for 30 V input.

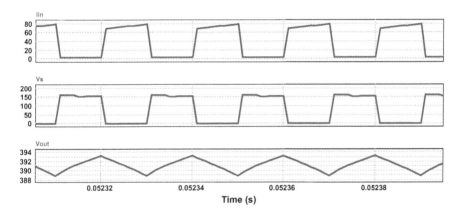

Fig. 5 Output representation of buck-boost-flyback converter

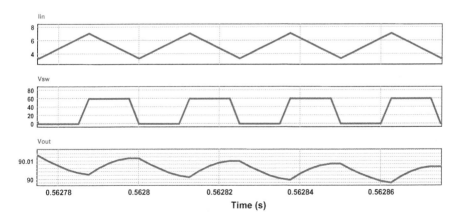

Fig. 6 Output waveform of Boost–Cuk converter

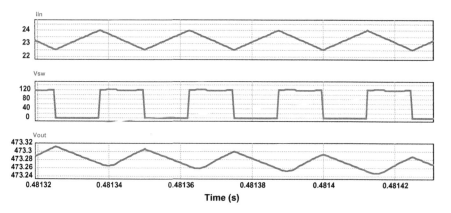

Fig. 7 Representation of waveform of converter with coupled inductor–diode–capacitor

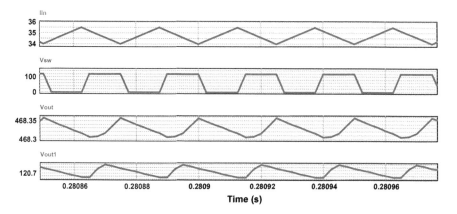

Fig. 8 Representation of waveform of modified dual port converter with coupled inductor–diode—capacitor

5 Conclusion

Based on the above comparison results, some converter has high gain but the stress across switch is more, the input current ripple is large, the efficiency is low. Some of the converters have good converter parameter but only single output port. The proposed modified coupled inductor–diode–capacitor converter explained above is more advantageous in all terms with two output ports. So modified dual port converter is best suitable for high-gain applications with low input current ripple, the stress across the switch is low, the efficiency of the converter is high, i.e., 99.8%. Among the two ports, the second port of converter is used for small-scale power applications and this converter replaces the diesel engine of crop machinery in future.

References

1. Shen CL (2015) Buck-boost-flyback converter with single switch to achieve high voltage gain for PV or fuel cell applications. IEEE Trans Ind Electron 55(2):749–757
2. Lodh T, Majumder T (2016) Highly efficient and compact single input multiple output DC-DC converters. IEEE Trans
3. Hu X, Gong C (2014) A high gain DC-DC converter integrating coupled inductor and diode capacitor techniques. IEEE Tran Power Electron 29(2)
4. Lodh T, Majumder T (2016) Highly efficient zeta-flyback DC-DC converter for high gain application with a compact structure. In: IEEE Application signal processing, communication, power and embedded system conference 2016, India, pp 71–78
5. Lodh T, Majumder T (2016) High efficient Sepic-Boost-Flyback converter with multiple output. IEEE Trans Power Embed Syst 57(2):505–514

Evolution in Solid-State Transformer and Power Electronic Transformer for Distribution and Traction System

Shivam Sharma, Ruhul Amin Chaudhary and Kamalpreet Singh

Abstract Power electronic transformer (P.E.T.) and solid-state transformer (SST) are one of the promising technologies in medium and high power conversion systems. In case of controlling power quality for the various load connected, P.E.T. and SST perform greatly in comparison with conventional line frequency transformer (CLFT) With advancements in high power switches and magnetic materials, P.E.T. can reach the efficiency almost equal to CLFT in distribution as well as traction system. P.E.T. eliminates all the limitation that CLFT faces in region of power quality maintenance and power transfer. Over the past two decades, researches and field trial studies are conducted to explore the challenges faced by conventional P.E.T. models and improved them to face all sort of applications in electrical systems. This paper aims to review the essential requirements of P.E.T. and SST modules both in traction and distribution systems. Basic design topologies of both SST and P.E.T. modules are also reviewed. There is also tabulation of all the models recently manufactured by companies for railways and distributions. Finally, this paper discusses the latest go-through in advanced topologies of P.E.T. and their architectural designs.

Keywords Power electronic transformer · Solid-state transformer · Conventional line frequency transformer · Alternating current · Direct current · Medium frequency · High frequency · Power electronic traction transformer · Modular frequency transformer

1 Introduction

Transformer is very essential component of modern power system. It not only provides transformation of voltage and current profiles but also provides isolation in between two systems. Basic principle behind the operation of line transformer is electromagnetic induction which was discovered independently by Michael Faraday

S. Sharma (✉) · R. A. Chaudhary · Kamalpreet Singh
Lovely Professional University, Phagwara, Punjab, India
e-mail: shivamsharmaeee@gmail.com

© Springer Nature Singapore Pte Ltd. 2019
V. Sridhar et al. (eds.), *Emerging Research in Electronics, Computer Science and Technology*, Lecture Notes in Electrical Engineering 545,
https://doi.org/10.1007/978-981-13-5802-9_115

in late 1831 known to be Faraday's law of electromagnetic induction, Joseph Henry in 1832 and other physicist [1–4]. In 1836, an Ireland physicist named Nicholas Callan designed first type of transformer with use of induction coil [4]. After going through experimental work, it was concluded that voltage at output side get increased and current get decreased by increasing number of turns at secondary side although transfer of power remains constant. Before 1880, all the transformer designs were carried forward with only arranging of coils; then in 1884, three engineers from Ganz factory come with a conclusion that open-circuit transformer is impractical and is not capable of regulating voltage [5]. In their joint paper, they provide a design of power transformer which includes inductive coils and core on which design of modern line transformer is based [6]. With good design and long history line, transformer still faces a large number of drawbacks termed:

1. Winding and core loss
2. Large size
3. Necessity of core cooling
4. Distortion in input and output current profile
5. No power factor correction.

All of these drawbacks of line frequency transformer lead to the introduction of solid-state transformer (SST) and power electronic transformer. The idea of solid-state transformer was initiated by Japanese engineer and named it as intelligent transformer [7]. Further in 1999, first patent was issued over the design of solid-state transformer which includes voltage conversion and power factor correction and provides overall efficiency of <75% [8]. Basic ideology behind solid-state transformer or power electronic transformer is to provide all functionality of line frequency transformer without the use of Faraday's law of electromagnetic induction. The P.E.T. provides functionality which includes power electronics and different design approach compared to conversional transformer. Features like instant voltage regulation, power factor correction, voltage, and current sag compensation come with basic P.E.T model. Rectification, inversion, and DC–DC conversion are the basic fundamental blocks of power electronic transformer. Many topologies have been presented for evaluating P.E.T. in recent years [9–14].

The basic configuration of S.S.T or P.E.T is shown in Fig. 1 [15]. It is basically a power electronic circuit that provides AC voltage profile step up/down via high-frequency isolation transformer. Therefore, weight and size of the overall system can be reduced potentially. As we know, $e_1 = N_1 \, d\Phi/dt$, where e_1 is induced emf, N1 is the number of turns in primary side, and Φ is the magnetic flux in core.

As we assume, Φ is sinusoidal in nature which can be represented as $\Phi = \Phi_m \sin(\omega t)$.

$e_1 = N_1 \, \omega \, \Phi_m \cos(\omega t)$; after arranging the above equation and making an assumption that induced emf is almost equal to applied voltage, then,

$$\Phi_m = V / \sqrt{2} \Pi f \, N_1;$$

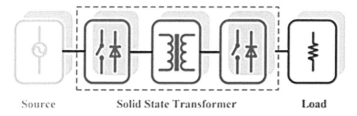

Source   **Solid State Transformer**   **Load**

Fig. 1 Configuration of solid-state transformer

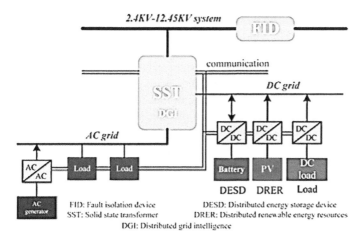

Fig. 2 SST as an energy router in FREEDM system

The above expression conclude that flux is directly proportional to voltage. Higher the value of applied voltage, more will be the working flux. With increase in flux, more core area will be acquired by transformer which leads to increase in weight and size of entire unit [10]. Above expression also describes that flux is inversely proportional to applied voltage frequency. With increase in frequency flux get reduced which leads to reduction in core size. Hence, in S.S.T. high frequency transformers are used which not only provide galvanic isolation but also reduce the weight and size of entire module [16]. With providing closed-loop control to the configuration of S.S.T. in Fig. 1, we can manage changeable power factor and reduction in load disturbances.

In the year 2008, an innovative distribution system architecture, called the future renewable electric energy delivery and management (FREEDM) system, was proposed as shown in Fig. 2 [17]. Instead of line frequency transformer, the S.S.T. is used to interface low-voltage AC domestic system with the distribution system. In addition, the distributed renewable energy source (DRES) and distributed energy storage device (DESD) are interfaced with DC link of S.S.T. through their individual DC–DC converters making a DC microgrid.

In [9], AC–AC buck converter has been presented to change the voltage profile directly without using any isolation transformer. In the second type, the input side AC waveform is modulated into medium–high-frequency square wave clubbed to the secondary of MF/HF transformer and again demodulated to sinusoidal AC form by secondary side converter coupled with low-pass filter [3]. Another type of P.E.T. design involves matrix converter which provides direct AC–AC power conversion using controlled valve switching [4].

In third type, it consists of three part parts involving input stage, isolation stage, and output stage [13, 14, 18, 19]. This type of design enhances not only functionality but flexibility of electronic transformer owning to availability of DC link. This type of approach can perform different power quality functions and galvanic isolation in between input and output system. With increase in stages, the number of switches will increase which leads to complex system and control topology.

All these years of research in power electronic transformer or S.S.T. lead to increasing overall efficiency of system and reduced switches number in converter units. This paper will provide you idea of basic merits and demerits of all P.E.T. designs. Many P.E.T. models are used in commercial applications such as traction system, distribution system, and wind energy systems. Currently, ABB is one of the manufacturers who are designing high-rated power electronic traction transformer (PETT). Many researchers demonstrate their P.E.T. prototypes both in software and hardware environment providing comparison and scale of change in between their models.

One of the biggest applications of power electronic transformer is in traction system. Railways are widely used in all kind of public and commercial transport and produce less CO^2 per passenger-Km in comparison to other transport systems. With increase in number of electric multiple units (EMUs) in railway system, demand of high efficiency and high power density traction system also is raised [20]. With reducing weight of the existing unit, efficiency will increase in comparison to former value. Size and weight of line frequency transformer somehow reduce the overall efficiency of traction system which is one of the biggest constraints in EMUs.

In railway vehicles, line frequency transformers (LFTs) are usually optimized for minimum power density (0.250–0.350 KVA/Kg) and provides efficiency of 94% for 25 kV/50 Hz traction system, respectively [21]. The increase in demand of railway vehicles strictly focused over size weight and efficiency of traction equipment. The effective use of upgraded insulation material, synthetic ester oil as dielectric, design of transformer winding may not fully help to address the issue [22]. A favorable alternative solution to increase power density and efficiency of traction system is the use of P.E.T. and S.S.T technologies [23, 24]. Another acronym synonymous with P.E.T. and S.S.T. technologies is medium-frequency transformer (M.F.T.). However, P.E.T-based traction system offers additional features such as multiple voltage interfacing, compactness, and capability of fault isolation. However, one of the biggest concerns in P.E.T. technology is interfacing converter with high-voltage (HV) side; on the other hand, M.F.T. (>500 Hz) requires complex controlling unit and master traction converter. Due to high power demand and architectural modification of pilot converter unit, the design of auxiliary power system has also become more challenging especially at the time of load fluctuations and sag in voltage and current profile [25]. In 2012, ABB successfully installed P.E.T.-based module in Swiss Federal Railways Ee 933 shunting locomotive [26]. Although some issues and challenges still need to be addressed, it is very important to carry forward an extensive review of requirements challenges and future scope for further improvement of P.E.T.-based system. This paper aims to review all the components related to P.E.T.-based system and its area of applications.

2 LFT and P.E.T. Technologies in Distribution System

2.1 LFT Distribution System

In India, primary distribution system comprises of 3-phase 3-line system with voltage rating of 11 kV which is further carry forward to secondary distribution system comprises of 3-phase 4-line system with voltage rating of 0.44 kV. In between the primary and secondary distribution system, LFT is installed with step-down voltage configuration. With advanced architectural modeling of LFT, still it lags with many issues like compensation of voltage sag, power factor correction, and size which are one of the biggest concerns. On the contrary, LFT comes with many advantages like easy installation, low operating cost, and less maintenance.

2.2 P.E.T. Distribution System

The limitation in LFT-based distribution system can be overcome by exploiting an alternative technology called P.E.T. distribution system as it provides better efficiency and higher power density in comparison to LFT distribution system [27]. The design of P.E.T.-based system is shown in Fig. 3 which describes the internal architecture of P.E.T. and its connection with the existing distribution system. MV defines medium-voltage system which is taken from secondary grid, and LV defines low-voltage system which will be provided to domestic users. Basic topology behind power electronic transformer comprises of three units: AC–DC conversion unit, DC–DC conversion unit, and DC–AC conversion unit.

Inside P.E.T., there are two compartments interconnected with each other through either DC link or high-frequency AC link which depend upon their basic working topology. The one with high-frequency AC link comes with two AC–AC converters, one connected to input terminal and other connected to output terminal shown in Fig. 4, and other with DC link modeling comes with four converter units shown in Fig. 5.

3 CLFT and P.E.T. Technologies in Traction System

3.1 CLFT Traction Technology

Electric power for railway vehicle is collected from high-voltage catenary, either single-phase AC (15 kV/16.5 Hz) or two-phase AC (25 kV/50/60 Hz) or DC (750/1500 V). Geographical location is one of the factors on which utilization of HV catenary depends and the type of rolling stocks [9]. The advanced-level connection and interface architecture of AC-powered CLFT-based traction power conversion chain are shown in Fig. 6. Basically, CLFT is heavy and big in size and consumes weight of rolling stocks about 10–18%. For making traction vehicles compact in size and more efficient, reduction of weight and size is mandatory for future consumptions. The future requirement imposed by transportation sector cannot be perfectly met by the use of CLFT traction systems.

3.2 P.E.T. Traction Technology

The architectural design of P.E.T-based traction system is shown in Fig. 7. In this new approach, the use of main transformer is avoided which in short reduces the size and weight of system and decreases load on rolling stocks. The HV catenary side is connected to a unit composed of several cells connected in cascade, and on the output side, unit cells are connected in parallel to get maximum power for traction equipment [13]. In comparison to CLFT-based traction systems, the configuration

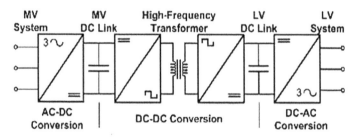

Fig. 3 Internal architecture of P.E.T-based distribution system

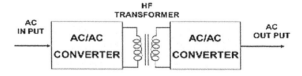

Fig. 4 Block diagram of electronic transformer using high-frequency AC link

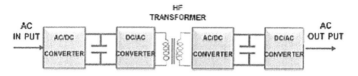

Fig. 5 Block diagram of power electronic transformer with DC link

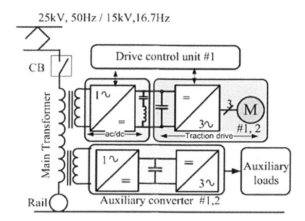

Fig. 6 Typical architecture of power conversion for CLFT-based railway traction

(shown in Fig. 6) requires an additional conversion stage (AC to HFAC) and direct interface of AFE to HV catenary. This will let AFE converters (which are connected in cascade) to employ maximum power to HV power switching devices. Due to the requirement of a large number of switching devices, overall cost of P.E.T. raised in comparison to CLFT. A list of key characteristics for comparison between CLFT- and P.E.T-based traction systems is shown in Fig. 8.

3.3 Essential Requirements for P.E.T.T. Technology

The further essential improvement required in P.E.T.T. is documented in [9, 10, 18, 28, 29] and summarized as: (a) reduction in size around 30–50% in comparison to CLFT; (b) at least 2–3% improvement in overall efficiency; (c) minimal injection of harmonic content at the input side or HV catenary side; (d) able to feed load under the circumstances of sag and fluctuation both in voltage and current profile; (e) stabilize DC voltage in case of interruption at catenary side and able to provide auxiliary power from battery source; (f) integrated converter topologies as well as integrated cooling mechanism for converter units as well as modular frequency transformers; (g) preferable triggering topologies for converter units in case of any failure event in one of the subassemblies; and (h) availability for onboard energy storage capability

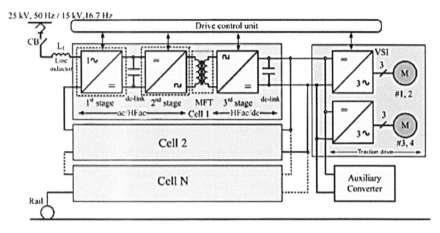

Fig. 7 Architecture of power conversion for P.E.T-based railway traction

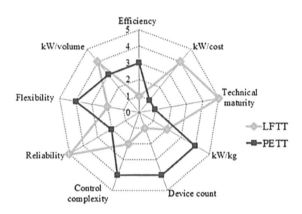

Fig. 8 Comparison between CLFTT and P.E.T.T. technologies

with the existing and upgraded topologies. Finally, the cost is the key consideration for ensuring the above requirements.

4 Converter Architecture and P.E.T. Technology

P.E.T. technology essentially covers the functionality of CLFT and AC/DC–DC/AC conversion system stage, providing greater power density and smooth output sinusoidal wave without having any harmonic content to distort it. However, it provides better power quality and additional functionality such as fault detection and isolation [12, 28, 29]. The minimum of three conversion stages are required for single-phase AC–AC, and maximum total of three stages are required for conversion of AC–DC (Fig. 7). The selection of pertinent technology for P.E.T. is the most important aspect.

Fig. 9 P.E.T. configuration: **a** single stage; **b** double stage with LVDC; **c** double stage with HVDC; and **d** multistage

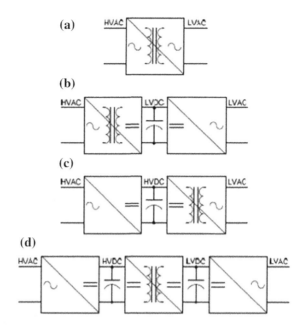

In [27], author addressed the issue of selecting the topology for desired system in support of bidirectional power flow as minimum requirement. In order to select perfect model of P.E.T. for suitable application, here are some proposed topologies shown in Fig. 9.

4.1 Two-Stage (AC/HVAC) Power Conversion Topologies

Two-stage conversion scheme basically consists of (a) single-phase AC–DC conversion as one stage and (b) DC-HFAC conversion as second stage with harmonic resonant filter. The input series and output parallel configuration-based P.E.T. model were first developed using H-bridge technique in cascaded manner. The switches used in configuration were high-voltage IGBTs in railways applications [30]. A 1200 KVA-rated P.E.T-based traction drive was developed and tested by ABB on shunting locomotive operated by Swiss Federal Railways. This P.E.T. architecture consists of nine cells cascaded with each other to cover up the entire input voltage of 15 kV and delivered 16.5 kV/ 400A of voltage and current to traction load with one cell redundancy [14, 28, 31]. The prototype provides the traction efficiency of about 92% and maintained unity power factor at KV side [32]. The output waveform of multilevel AFE converter as well as pulse width modulation technique provided by control unit maintains the harmonic injection by P.E.T. system under railways standards related to current and harmonics (IEEE 519) [28].

Fig. 10 Matrix converter
AC-HFAC

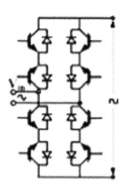

4.2 Single-Stage (AC-HFAC) Power Conversion Topologies

The single-stage topology is viable option to achieve higher efficiency and lower constant due to reduced number of stages as well as power switches and their control units.

(1) Cyclo-converter-based P.E.T. module: The early modules of P.E.T. only consist of frequency converters with only one working stage of AC–AC. The only reason behind this topology was to control the speed of traction motor and to make system look less complex and costly [16, 33]. These modules work on zero voltage switching technique to operate at high switching frequency with suitable RC snubber circuit to dissipate stored energy in leakage inductance of traction motors [34]. ABB also designed the P.E.T. prototype using single-stage frequency converter unit for 15 kV/16.7 Hz EMU application involving DC link. This architecture consists of 16 cells; each consists of series connected cyclo-converters having IGBTs as main power switches [34, 35]. ABB claimed to have improved efficiency of 3% with 50% and 20% reduction in weight and volume in comparison to the previous model of P.E.T. designed by ABB. A matrix-based P.E.T. model having rating of 4 KVA was developed by University of West Bohemia, in Czech Republic, shown in Fig. 9 [36].

(2) Current source converter (CSC): This module of P.E.T consists of flyback inductor for medium frequency as MFT and was designed by North Carolina State University, USA [37, 38]. Each converter consists of full-bridge current source converters and a medium-frequency flyback inductor shown in Fig. 10. The main use of this medium-frequency inductor is to provide galvanic isolation and voltage adaptation.

(3) Modular multilevel converter topology: These converters consist of ample number of submodules connected in series, which are termed as arms of converter. All these arms are further connected to multiwinding modular frequency transformer which provides four quadrant operations, harmonics elimination, and good power factor control at input side. With the use of high numbers of capacitors, these converters provide bidirectional power flow capability.

Fig. 11 Current source
converter AC-HFAC

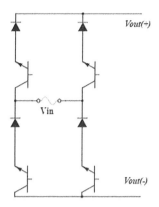

During motoring application, converter arm with highest value of capacitor will be consumed in order to get aspired voltage value and controlling action in braking mode. To get reliable operation from MMC, all the capacitors connected to converter arms must have same charging and discharging time period, and during operation, capacitors must work under high tolerance value. The algorithm used for balancing voltages of capacitors is clearly investigated in [17, 39]. The frequency of system can be increased in such a way to make modulation index an even number, so as to eliminate all even harmonics and make it easy to build redundant second-order harmonic filter. Siemens investigate a P.E.T.T. model having basic functionality of MMC with the rating of 5 MW [40]. This module comprises of 17-level MMCs with achieving efficiency of nearly 98% at nominal power and switching frequency of 10 kHz [41].

(4) Newly advanced power converter topologies: A single-stage AC–DC cascaded multilevel converter, with bidirectional power flow characteristics, is considered to be new module in the existing P.E.T. topologies and was developed and proposed by Federal University of Ceara, Brazil [42], shown in Fig. 11. In [19] three state switching cell C-type (TSSC-C) PWM DC–DC converter with nonsegregated state is presented and analysed. In this module multi-state switching cells are controlled with non-discrete (continuous) current mode operation. TSSC-C consists of pair of semiconductor switches, clubbed by diode connected to each phase of multi-interphase transformer (MIPT) which is considered to be a new type of three-phase switching. Sharing of current through two windings in MIPT is done due to demagnetization property of enhanced circuit configuration. To enhance current sharing and to reduce the factors of overloading, buck–boost converter is clubbed with TSSC-C topology.

In [41], P.E.T. having multifed topology is proposed with three-port active bridge converter (TAB). It provides flexibility with connection to grid, power generating units and loads by used of triple port. This module is also used as power efficiency enhancer and energy router to interface model with outside world having loads and sources for DFACTS. The prototype comparison of various P.E.T-based traction

Table 1 Comparison of present topologies of P.E.T. modules by worldwide manufacturers

Manufacturer	First stage	Second stage	MFT type	Third stage	Switching device rating
ABB 1, (1.2 MVA)	16-cell cyclo-converter (AC/HFAC)	–	400 Hz, 1:1 multicell	Full-bridge inverter	3.3 kV/400 A
ABB 2, (1.2 MVA)	8-cell cascaded H-bridge	Half bridge	1.7 kHz, 1:1 multicell	Half-bridge inverter	6.5 and 3.3 kV
ABB 3, (4.2 MVA)	12-cell cascaded CHB	Half bridge	10 kHz, 1:1 multicell	Full-bridge inverter	1.7 kV
Siemens 1 (5 MW)	MMC (AC/HFAC)	–	Single multiwinding	Full-bridge inverter	1.2 kV/400 A
Siemens 2 (2 MW)	17-level MMC (AC/HFAC)	–	10 kHz, single multiwinding	Full-bridge inverter	1.2 kV
Bombardier (5 MW)	8-cell cascaded H-bridges	Full bridge	8 kHz, 1:1 multicell	Full-bridge inverter	6.5 kV
Alstom 1 (2MVA)	12-cell full bridge	Half bridge	2 kHz, single multiwinding	Half-bridge inverter	6.5 and 3.3 kV
Alstom 2 (2MVA)	Current source converter	Half bridge	5 kHz, single multiwinding	Half-bridge inverter	6.5 kV

systems manufactured and designed by various companies is shown in Table 1. Most of the manufacturers designed their module only with stage conversions including H-bridge multilevel converters [43].

4.3 P.E.T-Formed Auxiliary Power Converters

It is very essential to feed all the auxiliary loads and charge batteries of vehicles or domestic loads for basic and reliable operations. It is important to generate onboard supply for three-phase system with 415 V/50 Hz to light up the domestic loads with providing unity power factor no matter what kind of load and output profiles with pure sinusoidal wave nature is. The basic architecture of auxiliary power converter for CLFT-based and P.E.T-based railways systems is shown in Fig. 8 and Fig. 12, respectively [25].

Fig. 12 AC–DC three-state switching cell

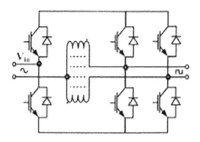

In [26], an electronic power transformer is presented along with super capacitor bank and bidirectional DC–DC converter. The only reason to provide capacitor bank is to withstand voltage momentary interruptions and to dissipate the outcome of voltage sag and swell. This module of P.E.T. is designed to work in domestic load environment. With the connection of electronic power transformer in cascaded with super-charged capacitors eliminates all types of urges in input supply and provide clean uninterrupted power supply to load.

5 Advancement in P.E.T. Modules and Medium-Frequency Design Consideration

In recent years, advancement in P.E.T. modules achieves new stages of designs. With increased number of P.E.T. applications, modification of control unit and basic design is increasing too. For uninterrupted power supply, P.E.T. is installed in domes-

Table 2 Comparison of present topologies of P.E.T. modules by universities and institutes

Universities	First stage	Second stage	Third stage	Conclusion
Royal Institute of Technology, Sweden	Matrix converter	–	Dual converter	Thyristors are used as switching device to overcome power rating. Natural and forced commutation is carried forward
Ecole Polytechnique Federale De Lausanne (EPFL), Switzerland (Prototype-I)	Full bridge	Full bridge	Full bridge	Bidirectional DC–DC converter is used for voltage control and power flow control

(continued)

Table 2 (continued)

Universities	First stage	Second stage	Third stage	Conclusion
Ecole Polytechnique Federale De Lausanne (EPFL), Switzerland (Prototype-II)	Full bridge	CSI full bridge	Full bridge	This P.E.T. module is used for the application of multisystem power supplies (15 kV/16.7 Hz and 3 kV DC)
University of West Bohemia, Czech Republic (Prototype-I)	Full bridge	Full bridge	Full bridge	Multicell primary and secondary winding MFT is used with operating frequency of 400 Hz
University of West Bohemia, Czech Republic (Prototype-II) (4 kVA)	Matrix converter	Full bridge	Half bridge	Good dynamic tolerance under any fault condition and certainly in voltage imbalance fault
Tsinghua University, China (6 KVA)	Full bridge	–	Full bridge	Soft-switching phase shift PWM technique is used for 23-cell converter with 1 kHz operating multiwinding MFT
Federal University of Ceara, Brazil	TSSC-C	–	Full bridge	Uses multi-interphase transformer with new type of three-phase switching; this enhances current handling capability of entire module
FREEDM System Center, North Carolina State University, USA	CSI Full bridge		CSI Full bridge	Flyback inductor is used as MFT to get all functionality of CLFT with reduced size and weight

tic applications. Table 2 will describe the topologies presented by universities and institutes with their rating and drawbacks [43].

6 Conclusion

This paper presents the analytical discussion regarding different topologies of power electronic transformer both in distribution and traction systems with recent researches. P.E.T-based system provides greater reliability and a huge control area. It will not only provide changeable current and voltage values but also occupied less area and volume in comparison to conventional line frequency transformer. It is also concluded in this paper how weight of P.E.T. is less in comparison to CLFT. However, P.E.T. system is more expensive and complex which leads to only drawback of P.E.T. It can be concluded that with use of P.E.T. in any application, overall efficiency of system will be increased and desired voltage or frequency can be carried forward for any sort of application.

References

1. A Brief History of Electromagnetism (PDF)
2. Electromagnetism. Smithsonian Institution Archives
3. MacPherson RC. Joseph Henry: The Rise of an American Scientist
4. Guarnieri M (2013, December) Who invented the transformer? [Historical]. In: IEEE industrial electronics magazine, vol 7, no 4, pp 56–59
5. Hughes TP (1983) Networks of power: electrification in Western society, 1880–1930. Johns Hopkins University Press, Baltimore
6. Uppenborn F (1889) History of the transformer, original translated from German. E & F.N. Spon, New York
7. Harada K, Anan F, Yamasaki K, Jinno M, Kawata Y, Nakashima T (1996) Intelligent transformer. In: PESC Record. 27th annual IEEE power electronics specialists conference, vol 2, Baveno, pp 1337–1341
8. De Keulenaer H, Chapman D, Fassbinder S, McDermott M (2001) The scope for energy saving in the EU through the use of energy-efficient electricity distribution transformers. In: 16th International Conference and Exhibition on Electricity Distribution, 2001. Part 1: Contributions. CIRED. (IEE Conf. Publ No. 482), Amsterdam, Netherlands, vol 4, p 5
9. Mermet-Guyennet M (2010) New power technologies for traction drives. In: Proceedings of the IEEE international symposium on power electronics electrical drives, automation and motion, Pisa, pp 719–723
10. Drofenik U, Canales F (2014) European trends and technologies in traction. In: Proceedings of the IEEE international power electronics conference (ECCE-ASIA), Hiroshima, pp 1043–1049
11. Andre-philippe C, Didier F (2015) Evolution and future of traction transformer on rolling stocks. In Proceedings of the IEEE international conference on electrical system for aircraft, railway, ship propulsion and road vehicles, Aachen, pp 1–6
12. Steiner M, Reinold H (2007) Medium frequency topology in railway applications. In: Proceedings of the European conference power electronics and applications, pp 1–10
13. Besselmann T, Mester A, Dujic D (2014) Power electronic traction transformer: efficiency improvements under light-load conditions. IEEE Trans Power Electron 29(8):3971–3981
14. Claessens M et al (2012) Traction transformation: a power-electronic traction transformer (PETT). https://library.e.abb.com
15. Oliveira DS, Honorio DDA, Barreto LHSC, Praca PP (2015) A single-stage AC-DC modular cascaded multilevel converter feasible to SST applications. In: Proceedings of the IEEE international exhibition and conference for power electronics, intelligent motion, renewable energy and energy Management, Nuremberg, Germany, pp 1–8

16. Wang H, Blaabjerg F, Reliability of capacitors for DC-link applications in power electronic converters an overview. IEEE Trans Ind Appl 50(5):3569–3578
17. Martin J, Ladoux P, Chauchat B, Casarin J, Nicolau S (2008) Medium frequency transformer for railway traction: soft switching converter with high voltage semi-conductors. In: Proceedings of the IEEE international symposium on power electronics, electrical drives, automation and motion, Ischia, pp 1180–1185
18. Yano M, Kurihara M, Kuramochi S (2009) A new on-board energy storage system for the railway rolling stock utilizing the overvoltage durability of traction motors. In: Proceedings of the European conference on power electronics and applications, pp 1–10
19. Farnesi S, Marchesoni M, Vaccaro L (2016) Advances in locomotive power electronic systems directly fed through AC lines. In: Proceedings of the international symposium on power electronics, electrical drives, automation and motion, Anacapri, pp 657–664
20. Samadaei E, Gholamian SA, Sheikholeslami A, Adabi J (2016) An envelope type (E-Type) module: asymmetric multilevel inverters with reduced components. IEEE Trans Ind Electron 63(11):7148–7156
21. Hu Y, Xie Y, Fu D, Cheng L (2016) A New Single-Phase π-type 5-level inverter using 3-terminal switch-network. IEEE Trans Ind Electron 63(11):7165–7174
22. Burguete E, López J, Zabaleta M (2016) A new five-level active neutral-point-clamped converter with reduced overvoltages. IEEE Trans Ind Electron 63(11):7175–7183
23. Alishah RS, Hosseini SH, Babaei E, Sabahi M (2016) A new general multilevel converter topology based on cascaded connection of sub-multilevel units with reduced switching components, DC sources, and blocked voltage by switches. IEEE Trans Ind Electron 63(11):7157–7164
24. Sun X, Wang B, Zhou Y, Wang W, Du H, Lu Z (2016) A single DC source cascaded seven-level inverter integrating switched-capacitor techniques. IEEE Trans Ind Electron 63(11):7184–7194
25. Le QA, Lee DC (2016) A novel six-level inverter topology for medium-voltage applications. IEEE Trans Ind Electron 63(11):7195–7203. https://doi.org/10.1109/TIE.2016.2547909
26. Li B et al (2016) An improved circulating current injection method for modular multilevel converters in variable-speed drives. IEEE Trans Ind Electron 63(11):7215–7225
27. Proof of the principle of solid-state transformer and the AC/AC switch-mode regulator. EPRI TR-105 607. San Jose State University, San Jose
28. Dujic D, Chuanhong Z, Mester A, Steinke JK, Weiss M, Lewdeni-Schmid S, Chaudhuri T, Stefanutti P (2013) Power electronic traction transformer-low voltage prototype. IEEE Trans Power Electron 28(12):5522–5534
29. Feng J, Chu WQ, Zhang Z, Zhu ZQ (2017) Power electronic trans-former based railway traction systems: challenges and opportunities. IEEE J Emerg Sel Top Power Electron 5(3):1237–253
30. Zhao C, Lewdeni-Schmid S, Steinke JK, Weiss M (2011) Design, implementation and performance of a modular power electronic transformer (PET) for railway application. In: Proceedings of the European conference on power electronics and applications (EPE), Birmingham, pp 1–10
31. Zhao C, Dujic D, Mester A, Steinke JK, Weiss M, Lewdeni-Schmid S, Chaudhuri T, Stefanutti P (2014) Power electronic traction transformer-medium voltage prototype. IEEE Trans Ind Electron 61(7):3257–3268
32. Schmid T, Chaudhuri, Stefanutti P (2014) Power electronic traction transformer- medium voltage prototype. IEEE Trans Ind Electron 61(7):3257–3268
33. Yang S, Bryant A, Mawby P, Xiang D, Ran L, Tavner P (2011) An industry-based survey of reliability in power electronic converters. IEEE Trans Ind Appl 47(3):1441–1451
34. Kjaer PC, Norrga S, Ostlund S (2001) A primary-switched line-side converter using zero-voltage switching. IEEE Trans Ind Appl 37(6):1824–1831
35. Norrga S (2002) A soft-switched bi-directional isolated AC/DC converter for AC-fed railway propulsion applications. In: Proceedings of the international conference on power electronics, machines and drives, pp 433–438
36. Hugo N, Stefanutti P, Pellerin M Akdag A (2007) Power electronics traction transformer. In: Proceedings of the European conference power electronics and applications (EPE), Aalborg, pp 1–10

37. Pittermann M, Drabek P, Bednar B (2015) High voltage converter for purpose to minimizing of weight of traction transformer. In: Proceedings of the IEEE international symposium on applications electronics, Pilsen, pp 197–200
38. Pittermann M, Drabek P, Bednar B (2015) Single phase high-voltage matrix converter for traction drive with medium frequency transformer. In: Proceedings of the international 41st IEEE annual conference of the industrial electronics, Yokohama, pp 005101–005106
39. Zadeh MB, Fazel SS (2013) A new simple control approach of M2LC for AC railway applications. In: Proceedings of the IEEE international conference on power electronics, drive systems and Technologies, Tehran, pp 407–415
40. Liu W, Zhang K, Chen X, Xiong J (2016) Simplified model and sub-module capacitor voltage balancing of single-phase AC/AC modular multilevel converter for railway traction purpose. IET Power Electron 9(5):951–959
41. Jakka VNSR, Shukla A (2016) A triple port active bridge converter based multi-fed power electronic transformer. In: 2016 IEEE energy conversion congress and exposition (ECCE), Milwaukee, WI, pp 1–8
42. Honrio D, Oliveira D, Barreto LH (2015) An AC-DC multilevel converter feasible to traction application. In: Proceedings of the IEEE international conference on power electronics and applications (EPE'15), Geneva, pp 1–9
43. Ronanki D, Williamson SS, Evolution of power converter topologies and technical considerations of power electronic transformer based rolling stock architectures. IEEE Trans Transp Electrif (99):1–1

Optimized Control of VAR/Voltage in the Off-grid Hybrid Power System

Harsha Anantwar, Shanmukha Sundar and B. R. Lakshmikantha

Abstract Voltage is a fundamental element in the quality of power supply, may rise/drop depending on the reactive power balance; hence, it has become extremely important to manage the reactive power balance for voltage control in the off-grid hybrid power system (OGHPS). This paper investigates the application of bacteria forging algorithm and genetic algorithm optimization algorithm to design an optimal control for voltage stability of off-grid hybrid power system. The off-grid hybrid power system considered in this work consists of an induction generator for wind power system, photovoltaic (PV) system with inverter, synchronous generator for diesel power generation, and composite load. The over-rated PV inverter has ample amount of VAR capacity while sourcing PV real power. Two control structures are incorporated in this work, to regulate load bus voltage. The first control structure is for controlling the total reactive power requirement of the system that by controlling inverter voltage magnitude for sourcing required reactive power to the system, and the second control structure is for controlling the SG excitation and hence the load bus terminal voltage. Both control structures have proportional-integral (PI) controller with a single input. In order to coordinate VAR/voltage control, the controller parameters tuned optimally and simultaneously using bacterial forging and genetic algorithm-based optimization method. Small signal model of all components of OGHPS is simulated in Simulink, tested for reactive load disturbance, and/or wind power input disturbance of different magnitudes for voltage stability. All system state variables are examined to evaluate the effectiveness of proposed optimal coordinated controls.

Keywords Reactive power control · Voltage regulation · Off-grid hybrid power system

H. Anantwar (✉) · S. Sundar
Dayananda Sagar College of Engineering, Bangalore, India
e-mail: hanantwar@yahoo.com

B. R. Lakshmikantha
Dayananda Sagar Academy of Technology and Management, Bangalore, India

© Springer Nature Singapore Pte Ltd. 2019
V. Sridhar et al. (eds.), *Emerging Research in Electronics, Computer Science and Technology*, Lecture Notes in Electrical Engineering 545,
https://doi.org/10.1007/978-981-13-5802-9_116

Nomenclature

VAR	Volt-ampere reactive
BFA, *GA*	Bacteria foraging algorithm and genetic algorithm
SG, *IG*	Synchronous generator, induction generator
DE, *PV*	Diesel generator and photovoltaic
P_{IN}, Q_{IN}	Inverter active and reactive power
V	Load voltage
V_{IN}, δ	Inverter output voltage and phase angle
$\delta 1$	Power angle between terminal voltage and internal EMF of armature of SG
Q_{CP}, Q_{SG}, Q_{IG}	Reactive power of capacitor bank, synchronous generator, and induction generator
Δ	Small change in variable
Q_L	Reactive power load demand
P_{WD}	Wind power input to IG
X_m	Magnetizing reactance of IG referred to stator

1 Introduction

To meet the demand of electrical energy in far-off communities and small islands where there is difficult to have a connection from the central public utility, it is essential to have energy solution which is cost-effective and environment friendly. Mix of different renewable energy sources called as hybrid power system is very hopeful solutions. Presence of large quantity of wind and solar energy observed in remote territories presents prospect to utilize them to fulfill their energy requirement [1, 2]. The concern with renewable sources is that they are undependable, to realize dependable and quality power supply, requires suitable and efficient control techniques. The test system considered in this work is off-grid hybrid power system (OGHPS), having power generation from diesel, wind, and PV system. The isolated power systems similar to test system have been already in existence in several small islands/isolated communities [3]. The IEEE type 1 excitation system is employed for SG coupled to diesel engine, and the IG is used for wind power generation. An IG has poor voltage characteristic as they absorb magnetizing current from the system, the reactive power required by the IG varies with slip (wind speed). The reactive power required by OGHPS varies with varying reactive power load demand and/or input wind power to IG. For VAR management and voltage control, system reactive power is needed to be balanced by its sources and sinks under all operating conditions. Deficient reactive power in the system can cause severe drop in voltage and results in poor voltage profile stability. If voltage variation may go outside the tolerable limits, condition of power supply will not be acceptable for consumers. Hence, it is obligatory to have a sufficient reactive power source to be present in the system.

The earlier works reported in [4–8] for voltage and reactive power control of the wind diesel hybrid power system are based on static VAR compensator (SVC) and static synchronous compensator (STATCOM)] with load either static (exponential) or static plus dynamic is investigated, some very good works have been reported, but, the parameters of the SVC/STATCOM controllers were optimized while the controller parameters of AVR were fixed, hence cannot assure the proper cooperative control.

The work in [9] proposed voltage control of wind diesel hybrid power system based on H∞ loop-shaping control of SVC and AVR with static load only. In their work, SVC and AVR controller parameters were optimally tuned at the same time and the proposed voltage control strategy performed agreeably. However, the parameters of the SVC and AVR controllers were optimized under the arbitrary load change with a fixed reactive power request by the IG, which is not reasonable. The work in [10] investigated the application of the model predictive for control of SVC and AVR for voltage stability of an isolated hybrid wind–diesel power system based on reactive power control with the static type of load.

A PV inverter can control the active and non-active power within the bounds obliged by its apparent power, fast reacting and has superior transient performance, put off the need of a reactive power compensator, extra investment, hence is a convincing answer to address voltage regulation problem in OGHPS. PV inverter with surplus VAR capacity as a reactive power compensator for voltage control in OGHPS is proposed by the author in the previous work [11].

This work presents coordinate control of PV inverter and AVR to control the load voltage in OGHPS considering composite load model. Two control structures are incorporated in this work, to regulate load bus voltage. The first control structure is for controlling the total reactive power requirement of the system by controlling inverter voltage magnitude for sourcing required reactive power to the system, and the second control structure is for controlling the SG excitation and hence the load bus terminal voltage. Both control structures have PI controllers with a single input. To incorporate realistic features in this study, the parameters of the PI controller in both control structures have been optimized at the same time.

With the requirement of optimization of several parameters simultaneously under change reactive load demand as well as wind input power (wind speed), tuning strategies for PI controller of the system become very important. If PI parameters are not tuned properly, it may lead to oscillatory, sluggish recovery and in the worst case situation would result in the collapse of system operation. For PI tune, many conventional methods are based on minimizing performance index criteria available in the literature, which does not give satisfactory result when the requirement is to optimize several gains of the controllers under changing operating condition [13–16].

In the recent years, optimal tuning of controller parameters using intelligent computing technology has gained much attention [15–18]; therefore, control optimization algorithms such as genetic algorithm (GA) and bacterial foraging algorithm (BFA) are suggested in this work for tuning two controllers simultaneously. Optimal PI controller designing is mainly the outcome of minimizing a mathematical function (fitness function), which decides necessary control action.

In the view of the above discussion, this work focuses on VAR/voltage control of OFHPS considering the composite load model, with control parameters of the inverter and AVR tuned in coordination using BFA and GA when the system is subjected to varying disturbances.

The main contributions of this paper are as follows: (i) development of optimal controller for inverter and AVR using BFA and GA, (ii) comparison of performance of optimal controllers for voltage control in the incident of perturbation in composite reactive load or/and reactive power absorbed by IG due to fluctuation in mechanical input wind power, and (iv) time domain performance analysis of the system when subjected to step change and random varying step change of the load and wind power disturbances.

2 Off-grid Hybrid Power System Configurations and Voltage–Reactive Power Equation with Composite Load

The OGHPS considered for the study is shown in Fig. 1 and consists of SG (diesel engine) with PI-based excitation control and IG (variable wind speed turbine). Single stage PV system interfaced with an inverter and a fixed capacitor bank are connected to a common load bus. Mathematical model of system components based on the power balance equation is implemented in Simulink to analyze voltage profile stability and VAR control under different disturbances. In this configuration, power sources and load are assumed to be close to each other.

2.1 Voltage–Reactive Power Equation of the OGHPS, Considering Composite Load

When the system is in a steady-state condition, the system power balance equation will be governed by [4]

$$Q_{SG} + Q_{IN} + Q_{CP} = Q_L + Q_{IG} \tag{1}$$

Under the varying operating condition such as change in reactive power load demand Q_L and/or change in wind power input (P_{WD}), the system reactive power generation increases by an amount of $\Delta Q_{IN} + \Delta Q_{SG}$, due to the inverter and AVR controllers. The required reactive power will also change because of the change in the voltage by ΔV. Then, the excess reactive power in the system can be expressed as

$$\Delta Q_N = \Delta Q_{SG} + \Delta Q_{IN} + \Delta Q_{CP} - \Delta Q_L - \Delta Q_{IG} \tag{2}$$

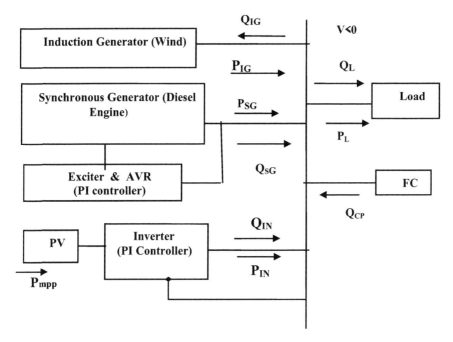

Fig. 1 Schematic of OGHPS (test system)

The net surplus reactive power Q_N increases the voltage and hence increases the electromagnetic energy absorption (Em) of the induction generator at a rate $\frac{dEm}{dt}$ as well as reactive load consumption of the system, which can be expanded as [4, 8, 9]

$$\Delta Q_N = \frac{dEm}{dt} + D_{lvq}\Delta V(s) \tag{3}$$

$$Em = \frac{V^2}{\omega Xm} \tag{4}$$

With the increase in voltage, the reactive power loads connected to the system experience an increase in its reactive power requirement by D_{lvq} (reactive power change with voltage change (p.u. VAR/p.u. Volt) is given by

$$D_{lvq} = \frac{\partial Q_L}{\partial V} \tag{5}$$

Using Eqs. (3) and (4), Eq. (3) can be written as

$$\Delta V(s) = \left(\frac{1}{S\left(\frac{V}{\omega Xm}\right) + D_{lvq}}\right)\Delta Q_N \tag{6}$$

Fig. 2 Composite load structure

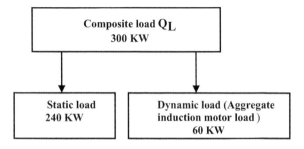

The above Eq. (6) is derived for static load, which is suitable for steady-state condition and does not involve the dynamics of load. Static load Q_{Lst} represented by exponential function is given by [19]

$$Q_L = Q_{Lst} = CV^q \tag{7}$$

where C is constant of the load and q is exponent which describes the voltage sensitivity of load.

In power system, voltage stability is affected by choice of the load model and its parameter. Dynamic load models are essential for examining the effect of nonlinear loads in dynamic studies due to load and input disturbances [20]. The composite load provides a much more accurate representation of load response to voltage [21]. Composite load represents the combined effect of aggregate of static and dynamic load (induction motor) as shown in Fig. 2 and is considered for investigation of voltage profile stability through reactive power management in OGHPS. The participation ratio of static to dynamic load in composite load presentation for remotely located OGHPS is suggested as 4:1 in literature [22–24]. The test system has a generation capacity of 400 KW with a load of 300 KW. Total 300 KW load consists of static load of 240 KW and dynamic load of 60 KW. An aggregate dynamic load model is developed considering group of seven induction motors of ratings ranging from 4 to 20 KW.

In order to incorporate the effect of composite load in the system voltage-reactive power, given Eq. (2), load voltage characteristic D_{lvq} has two parts, one for static load and one for dynamic load, and is governed by

$$D_{lvq} = D_{lvq-st} + D_{lvq-dy} \tag{8}$$

$$D_{lvq-st} = \frac{\partial Q_{Lst}}{\partial V} = q(Q_{Lst}/V) \tag{9}$$

Reactive power-voltage characteristic of dynamic loads on the system D_{lvq-dy} is developed based on the detailed fifth-order model of induction motor load [25] for 60 KW and is obtained as in Eq. (9).

$$D_{lvq-dy} = \frac{\partial Q_{Ldy}}{\partial V}$$

$$= \frac{0.0129s^5 + 169s^4 + 6.86e4s^3 + 2.9e8 + 2.17e10s + 1.7e11}{s^5 + 1.326e4s^4 + 3.81e6s^3 + 1.568e9s^2 + 1.8e11s + 3.88e12} \quad (10)$$

Using Eqs. (2), (8), (9), (10) and (6), reactive power-voltage equation of test system with a composite load model can be expanded as

$$\Delta Q_{sG} + \Delta Q_{IN} + \Delta Q_{CP} - \Delta Q_L - \Delta Q_{IG}$$
$$= \Delta V(s) \left\{ s \left(\frac{V}{\omega Xm} \right) + \left(D_{lvq-st} + D_{lvq-dy} \right) \right\} \quad (11)$$

The small signal model of other system components such as SG, IG, and FC for incremental change in reactive power and small signal linear equation of exciter output voltage ΔEf are available in articles [4, 5, 8–10, 26] and mathematics of PV system inverter for its incremental change in reactive power ΔQ_{IN} to support the system for reactive power balance is explained in authors' previous work [11] and is employed in this work for developing a simulation model of the test system.

3 PI Controller Parameter Optimization by BFA and GA

PI controller gain parameters of PV inverter and AVR are optimized simultaneously. The two gain parameters (K_P and K_i) of each controller make the optimization problem four dimensional. To obtain the optimal values of controller parameters (K_P and K_i), optimization task is used to minimize the objective function. The objective function considered here is an integral of time multiplied squared error (ITSE) as mentioned below.

$$Min(OB) = Min(ITSE) = Min \left[\int_0^\infty \left[t \times \Delta V(t)^2 \right] \right] \quad (12)$$

$$\text{Subjected to :} \quad Kpx_{min} \leq Kpx \leq Kpx_{max}$$
$$Kix_{min} \leq Kix \leq Kix_{max} \quad (13)$$

where $x = 1$ for inverter controller and $x = 2$ for AVR controller and ΔV is voltage deviation from steady state during disturbances in the system.

Conventional parameter tuning methods are based on performance index criteria such as IAE, ITAE, ISE, and ITSE. The ITSE has more mathematical tractableness especially for higher order systems. In this work, conventional method of PI tuning based on ITSE is employed due to its advantage that it penalizes less to initial errors to support rapid settling of the controlled output [27]. BFA and GA techniques are applied in this work to solve optimization problem presented in Eqs. (12) and (13);

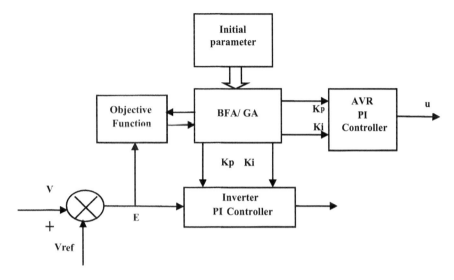

Fig. 3 BFA-/GA-based optimal tuning of PI controller

and the constraints in Eq. (10) are chosen according to the earlier published work [11]. The optimal controller structure based on BFA/GA is shown in Fig. 3.

The control output from PI shown in Fig. 3 is given by

$$U = K_P \, \Delta V + K_I \int \Delta V \, dt \tag{14}$$

K_p and K_i are optimized gains obtained by applying GA and BFA to achieve desired control output (U) to balance out the reactive power demand to control load voltage. BFA and GA methods applied for tuning of PI controllers are explained in the following subsection.

3.1 Bactria Foraging Algorithm (BFA)

BFA is a social system-based algorithm. A BFA is an intelligent method of optimization inspired from the communal. BFA is based on foraging technique of *E. Coli* bacteria [28]. Foraging property of bacteria is modeled as optimization process. The forging activity of E. coli bacteria is explained by chemotaxis, reproduction, and elimination dispersal [29]. BFA mimics forging principle to find optimal values of controller parameters. Optimization steps models how *E. Coli* bacteria locate food is divided into chemotactic, reproduction, and elimination-dispersal are as explained below.

Steps for the implementation of BFA to obtain optimal parameters of the controller

Step 1 Initialize the BFA parameters
(Number of bacteria (S), Number of chemotactic steps (N_C), Limit of a swim
(N_s) Number of reproduction steps (N_r), Number of elimination-dispersal
events (N_{ed}), The probability that each bacteria will be eliminated/dispersed
(P_{ed}), step-size C(I)) and define objective function to be optimized.
Step 2 Elimination-dispersal loop counter for $L = 1$ to N_{ed}, do $L = L + 1$
Step 3 Reproduction loop counter for $K = 1$ to N_r, do $K = K + 1$
Step 4 Chemotactic loop counter for $J = 1$ to N_C, do $J = J + 1$
For $I = 1$ to S, obtain the chemotactic step for bacterium 'me,'

a. Compute the objective function OB(I, J, K, L), Save as OBlast = OB(I,
J, K, L), to compare this values with other values of objective function
which may found during a run
b. Tumble-Generate a random vector $\Delta(\mathbf{I}) \in \mathcal{R}^S$, for each bacterium $\Delta_{\mathbf{MS}}(\mathbf{I})$, MS = 1, 2, ..., S, and move form position P(I,
J, K, L) in with step of size C(I), compute $P(I, J + 1, K, L) =$
$P(I, J, K, L) + C(I) \left(\dfrac{\Delta(I)}{\sqrt{\Delta^T(I) \times \Delta(I)}} \right)$ and compute $OB(I, J, K, L) =$
$OB(I, J + 1, K, L)$,
c. Initialize swim loop counter m = 1 to N_S,
    • While m < N_S, do m = m + 1; and if OB (I, J, K, L) < OBlast (if
    doing better) then OBlast = OB(I, J + 1, K, L), compute new position
    of a bacteria

$$P(I, J + 1, K, L) = P(I, J + 1, K, L) + C(I) \times \left(\frac{\Delta(I)}{\sqrt{\Delta^T(I) \times \Delta(I)}} \right)$$

    Compute the new OB(I, J + 1, K, L) for the new position of a bacteria
    P(I, J + 1, K, L)
    • Else m = N_S (end of while loop)
d. Go to next bacterium (I + 1), If I ≠ S, go to step 4b to process next
bacterium

Step 5 If J < N_C, go to step 4.
Step 6 Reproduction loop start from here

• For the given K and L and for each bacterium (1 to S), compute the health of
the bacterium $OB^I_{health} = \sum_{J=1}^{NC+1} OB(I, J, K, L)$ (OB^I_{health} indicates how
ineffectively bacteria searches food) and sort the bacteria in ascending
order of OB_{health} values. (The higher objective function value indicates
the weaker health of bacteria.)
• The bacteria with the higher OB_{health} value will die, and other healthy
bacteria undergo processes of splitting up to the maintain population.

Fig. 4 BFA search plot for
obtaining an optimal solution
(objective function
value–steps)

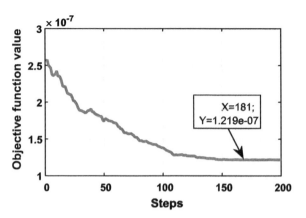

Step 7   If $K < N_r$, then go to step (2),

Step 8   Elimination-dispersal, for $I = 1$ to S, eliminate and disperse each bacterium
which has probability value less than P_{ed}. This process maintains the population of bacteria.

Step 9   If $L < N_{ed}$, go to step 2, else end.

The BFA algorithm based on above steps is implemented in MATLAB. The parameters defined in the MATLAB program are as follows: $S = 6$; $N_C = 4$; $N_S = 4$;
$N_r = 4$; $N_{ed} = 2$; $Sr = 3$; $P_{ed} = 0.25$. The convergence plot of objective function
values (nutrient value) against the number of steps taken by bacteria to reach nutrient value is as illustrated in Fig. 4. The small population of bacteria is considered
to reduce the computational execution complexity for the BFA, which is highly an
iteration-based algorithm.

3.2   Genetic Algorithm (GA)

Genetic algorithm is well known for finding optimal solutions to optimization problems. GA is popular due to its diversity of application. GA operator is selected;
crossover and mutation decide the performance of the GA. In the application of GA
for solving an optimization problem, the fitness of chromosomes is calculated using
an objective function in every iteration. Fittest chromosomes are chosen according
to their fitness value to make sure that the child carries the best mix of the genes
of their parents, and some of the chromosomes are adapted through crossover and
mutation results into new population for the next generation [30].

The stepwise applications of GA algorithm for optimizing PI parameters of the inverter and AVR simultaneously are explained below,

Step 1 Initialize the GA search parameters such as population size of chromosomes, crossover—fraction, mutation, maximum generation, and elite count.

Step 2 Generate a random population of 'I' chromosomes, each chromosome comprises of the four parameters (Kp1, Ki1, Kp2, and Ki2) of both PI controllers.

Step 3 Evaluate the fitness (objective) function of individual chromosome in the population.

Step 4 Assess the evaluated objective function for each chromosome (PI parameters). If the stopping condition is met, then the GA program ends and gives the best chromosomes (PI parameters) else it continues to the next step.

Step 5 Selection: choose parent chromosomes from a population in consistent with their fitness rank (the more the value of fitness, the higher its possibility for the selection of chromosomes)

Step 6 Crossover: with a crossover probability cross over the parents to produce new Children.

Step 7 Mutation: mutation probability alters new offspring to make new population.

Step 8 Replace old population with new generated population and go to step 2

Based on the above steps, GA parameters are defined in the program as follows: selection function: stochastic uniform, population type: 'double vector', crossover function: crossover scattered, mutation function: adaptive feasible, crossover fraction: 0.6, generations: 50, population size: 6, tolerance functions: $1.0\,e-06$, migration direction: 'forward'. The size of population in GA and the number of bacteria in BFA are considered same to evaluate the performance of both algorithms.

Table 1—Optimal values of PI controller parameters obtained by GA and BFA.

The fitness value plot is illustrated in Fig. 5, is steadily getting lesser, and is an indication that optimization reached. The mean fitness of the population is also decreased and indicates that the entire population is improved to have better solutions. The optimal values of controller parameters obtained by BFA and GA are given in the following Table 1.

Table 1 Optimal controller parameters obtained by GA and BFA

Method	Optimum value of fitness function	Inverter		AVR	
		kp	ki	kp	KI
GA	1.37E−07	16.5	2776.2	31.3	46.3
BFA	1.219E−07	21.1	2842.99	44.224	50.4913

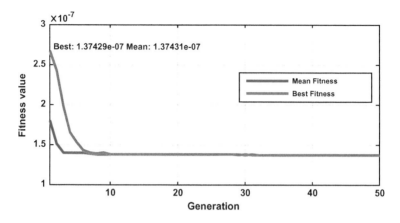

Fig. 5 GA search plot for obtaining an optimal solution (fitness value–generation)

4 Simulation Results and Discussion

The mathematical model of OFHPS based on the reactive power balance equation is simulated in Simulink considering various operating conditions and time domain responses of the system variables when PI controller parameters are optimally tuned by conventional method (based on performance index); GA and BFA under four different disturbance case studies are illustrated as follows:

Case 1—Step disturbance of 5% of reactive load demand Q_L

The time domain responses of deviation in system state variables such as voltage, inverter reactive power, and SG reactive power for step increase of 0.05 p.u., in reactive loading at t = 0.025 s, at the constant wind power input to IG are illustrated in Fig. 6a–c. The system is in steady state till = 0.025 s, prior to change in reactive load demand. From the Fig. 6a–c, it is observed that inverter provides dynamic support of reactive power to mitigate the load disturbance, while the AVR of synchronous generator initially supports by taking action to maintain voltage levels following the disturbance (according to its size). From the time responses shown in Fig. 6a–c, it is clear that control characteristics such as peak value, oscillation, and settling of state variables are improved considerably in the case of BFA and GA-based optimal PI controllers compared to conventional tuned PI.

Case 2—Step disturbances of 10% of both wind power input to IG and reactive power load

The time domain response of deviation in system state variable such as voltage and reactive power of the inverter, SG for the step increase of 0.1 p.u. (10%) in both reactive loading and wind power input to IG, at t = 0.025 s is illustrated in Fig. 7a–c.

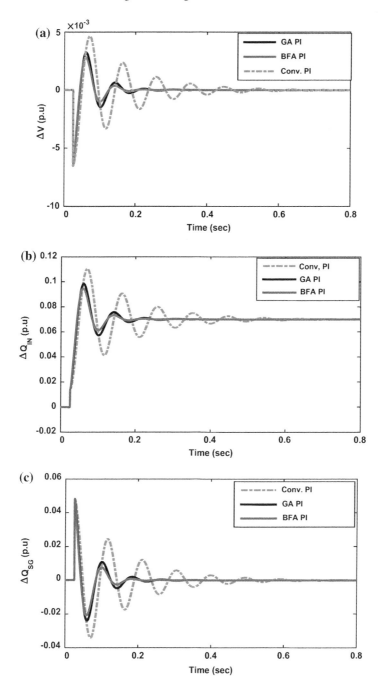

Fig. 6 **a** Time response of voltage deviation (ΔV) for 5% step change in reactive load demand, **b** Time response of ΔQ_{IN} for 5% step change in reactive load demand. **c** Time response of ΔQ_{SG} for 5% step change in reactive load demand

When mechanical wind power input to IG increases, the slip of IG increases; hence, its reactive power demand increases, SG supports initially the following disturbance, SG equipped with AVR is incapable to suppress the voltage deviation and to maintain voltage; hence, inverter contributes additional reactive power following disturbance. From Fig. 7a–c, it is clear that the system parameters regain steady-state condition rapidly with a BFA and GA control compared to conventional. The state variables ΔV and ΔQ_{SG} become zero as shown in Fig. 7b, c. The peak value and oscillation of state variables are reduced considerably in the case of BFA and GA-based optimal PI controllers compared to conventional.

Case 3—Random step disturbance in reactive load demand

The test system is investigated for time domain responses of deviation in system state variables (voltage, reactive power of the inverter, and reactive power SG) for random step disturbance in reactive loading which are illustrated in Fig. 8b–d. Reactive load is randomly changed in steps to 0.1 p.u. (10%), mechanical input wind power to IG remained the same, hence no change in reactive power demand of IG.

It is observed from random loading condition, the first peak values of state variables which depend upon the magnitude of disturbance have been reduced for BFA and GA-based optimal PI controllers than conventional tuned PI.

Case 4—Random step change in both input wind power to IG and reactive load demand.

The state variables (ΔQ_{IN}, ΔQ_{SG}, and ΔV) which are used in time domain analysis for randomly changing step disturbances in both reactive loading and wind power supply to IG are illustrated in Fig. 9b–d. Reactive load is randomly changed in steps 0.1 p.u. (10%), and mechanical input wind power to the IG is randomly changed in steps from 0.014 p.u. (1.4%) to 0.08 p.u. (8.0%) as shown in Fig. 9a. SG with AVR control supports to maintain SG terminal voltage, while inverter provided required reactive power under a random change in load to balance VAR in the system to maintain a flat voltage profile. It is clear from Fig. 9b–d that coordinately optimized PI controllers by GA and BFA exhibited better dynamic reactive power control outcome and hence improved stability of voltage, compared to conventional tuning of the PI controller under random disturbance condition.

In order to assess the effectiveness of optimization method GA and BFA for optimal control, the step response characteristic for voltage for 10% reactive loading disturbance and 10% wind power change (Case study 2) is presented in Table 2.

The control characteristics data on time response of state variables obtained from a simulation using MATLAB command 'stepinfo' presented in Tables 2 and 3 pointed out that control output for BFA-tuned PI is better than GA-tuned PI.

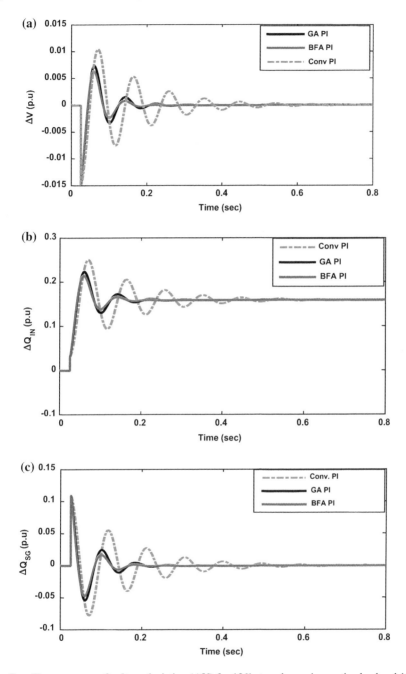

Fig. 7 **a** Time response of voltage deviation (ΔV) for 10% step change in reactive load and 10% step change in wind power input to IG. **b** Time response of ΔQIN for 10% step change in reactive load and 10% step change in wind power input to IG. **c** Time Response of ΔQSG for 10% step change in reactive load and 10% step change in wind power input to IG

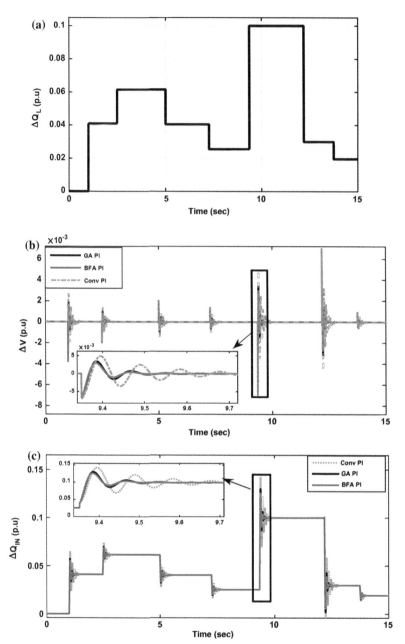

Fig. 8 **a** Random step disturbance in reactive load demand with constant wind power input to IG. **b** Time response of voltage deviation for random step change in reactive loading with constant wind power input to IG. **c** Time response of ΔQ_{IN} under random step disturbance in reactive loading Q_L with constant wind power input to IG. **d** Time response of ΔQ_{SG} under random step disturbance in reactive loading Q_L with constant wind power input to IG

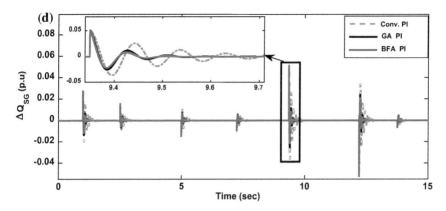

Fig. 8 (continued)

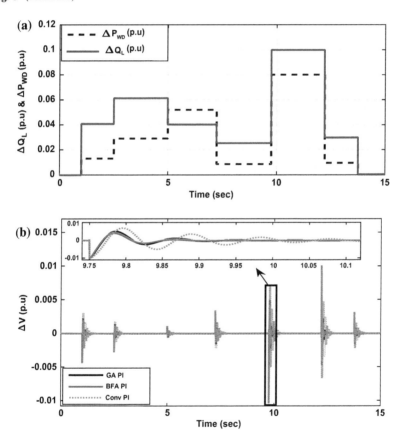

Fig. 9 **a** Random step disturbances of reactive load and wind power PWD. **b** Time response of voltage deviation for random step disturbances. **c** Time response of ΔQ_{IN} for random step disturbances. **d** Time response of ΔQ_{SG} for random step disturbances

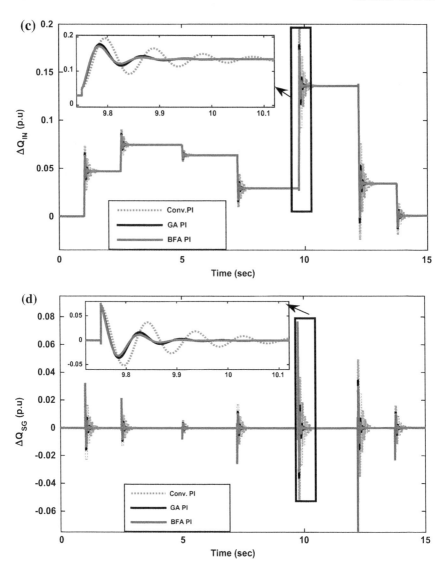

Fig. 9 (continued)

Table 2 Step response characteristic for voltage deviation (ΔV) for 10% ΔQ_L and 10% ΔP_{WD} disturbances (Case study 2)

Optimization algorithm	Rise time (s)	Settling time (s)	Peak (V/unit)	Peak time (s)
BFA	22.0691e−06	0.1507	0.0278	2.9714e−04
GA	8.3016e−06	0.1773	0.0373	3.2191e−04

Table 3 Maximum deviation in p.u. for state variables ΔQ_{IN}, ΔQ_{SG}, and ΔQ_{IG}

Disturbances in %		BFA-PI			GA-PI		
ΔQ_L	ΔP_{WD}	ΔQ_{IN}	ΔQ_{SG}	ΔQ_{IG}	ΔQ_{IN}	ΔQ_{SG}	ΔQ_{IG}
5%	0	0.1172	0.06868	0.0012	0.1208	0.0687	0.0012
10%	5%	0.1696	0.0992	0.0450	0.1748	0.0993	0.0451

5 Conclusion

Voltage/VAR control of OFHPS considering a composite load model with optimally designed controllers for inverter and AVR is studied in this work. The system model based on reactive power–voltage characteristics is simulated in Simulink and tested considering uncertainties such as varying reactive loading and wind power supply to IG. These uncertainties significantly affect the system voltage.

The dynamic model of OGHPS considering more realistic composite load model with optimal controllers is built in Simulink and is tested for designed optimal controllers under changing operating conditions to investigate the voltage profile stability. Simulation results are compared with the following step and random step disturbances with reactive load demand and wind power. The performance of BFA and GA tuned controller is compared for fixed step disturbance as well as randomly varying step disturbances.

The simulation results revealed that the BFA tuned optimum of controller parameters is worked robust even for uncertainties like considerable changes in the reactive loading and variable reactive power demanded by IG.

From this work, it can be concluded that BFA and GA optimal tuned PI controller of inverter and AVR controllers have a better control effect, but the overall performance BFA tuned PI controllers outperformed the GA tuned PI controllers BFA provided better optimal solution. BFA needs more computational effort to search for an optimal solution. The number of steps/iteration required for BFA to solve the optimization problem is more compared to GA.

Appendix

Test system data

Base quantities − KVA = 400, Voltage = 400 V,
Frequency = 50 Hz,
Generation capacity (kW)
Wind generation = 150;
Diesel generator = 150;
PV system = 100,
Load = 300 KW, Load power factor = 0.9,

Load parameters − nq = 3, Dlvq-static = 0.86,
% Oversizing factor for inverter sizing = 40% of PV panel-rated capacity.

References

1. Kaldellis J et al (2010) Stand-alone and hybrid wind energy systems technology, energy storage and applications. Woodhead Publishing Limited and CRC Press LLC
2. Patel MR (2005) Wind and solar power system: design, analysis, and operation, 2nd edn. CRC Press, Boca Raton, FL, USA
3. Mickal HI (1983) 100 kW Photovoltaic power plant for Kythnos Island. In: Proceeding of fifth EC photovoltaic conference, pp 490–494, Oct 1983
4. Bansal RC (2006) Automatic reactive-power control of isolated wind–diesel hybrid power systems. IEEE Trans Ind Electron 53(4)
5. Sharma P, Saxena NK, Bhatti TS (2009) Study of autonomous hybrid power system using SVC and STATCOM. In: Proceedings of ICPS 2009, Kharagpur, India, 27–29 Dec 2009
6. Liu J, Zhang L, Cao M (2014) Power management and synchronization control of renewable energy microgrid based on STATCOM. In: IEEE conference and expo on transportation electrification Asia-Pacific (ITEC Asia-Pacific)
7. Menniti D, Pinnarelli A, Sorrentino N (2010) An hybrid PV-wind supply system with D-Statcom interface for a water-lift station. In: International symposium on power electronics electrical drives automation and motion (SPEEDAM), June 2010
8. Saxena NK, Ashwani K (2014) Analytical comparison of static and dynamic reactive power compensation in isolated wind diesel system using dynamic load interaction model. Electric Power Compon Syst 53(5):508–519
9. Vachirasricirikul S, Ngamroo I, Kaitwanidvilai S (2010) Coordinated SVC and AVR for robust voltage control in a hybrid wind-diesel system. Energy Convers Manage 51(12):2383–2393
10. Kassem AM, Abdelaziz AY (2014) Functional predictive control for voltage stability improvements of autonomous hybrid wind–diesel power system. Electric Power Compon Syst 42(8):831–844. https://doi.org/10.1080/15325008.2014.896431
11. Anantwar H, Lakshmikantha BR, Sundar S (2017) Fuzzy self tuning PI controller based inverter control for voltage regulation in off-grid hybrid power system. Energy Procedia 117:409–416
12. Liao Y, Fan W, Cramer A, Dolloff P, Fei Z, Qui M, Bhattacharyya S, Holloway L, Gregory B (2012) Voltage and var control to enable high penetration of distributed photovoltaic systems. In: North American power symposium (NAPS), 9–11 Sept 2012
13. Wang Y, Shao H (2000) Optimal tuning for PI controller. Automatica 36:147–152
14. Zhuang M, Atherton DP (1991) Tuning of PID controllers with integral performance criteria. In: Proceedings of IEE Control '91, no 332, vol 1, pp 481–486
15. Chopra V, Singla SK, Dewan L (2014) Comparative analysis of tuning a PID controller using intelligent methods. Acta Polytechnica Hungarica 11(8):235–249
16. Kim DH, Dong C, Tran CT, Duy VH (2016) Optimal tuning of PI controller for vector control system using hybrid system composed of GA. In: AETA 2015: recent advances in electrical engineering and related sciences. Lecture notes in electrical engineering, vol 371. Springer, Cham
17. Ma J, Bi Z, Ting TO, Hao S, Hao W (2016) Comparative performance on photovoltaic model parameter identification via bio-inspired algorithms. Solar Energy 132:606–616
18. Chen Y-P, Li Y, Wang G, Zheng Y-F, Xu Q, Fan J-H, Cui X-T (2017) A novel bacterial foraging optimization algorithm for feature selection. Expert Syst Appl 83:1
19. IEEE Task Force on load representation for dynamic performance (1993) Load representation for dynamic performance analysis. IEEE Trans Power Syst 8:472–482
20. Stojanovi DP, Korunovi LM, Milanovi JV (2008) Dynamic load modeling based on measurements in medium voltage distribution network. Electric Power Syst Res 78:228–238

21. Kosterev D, Meklin A (2006) Load modeling in WECC. In: Power systems conference and exposition, pp 576–581
22. Parveen T (2009) Composite load model decomposition: induction motor contribution. PhD dissertation, Faculty of Built Environment and Engineering, School of Engineering Systems, Queensland University of Technology
23. Fahmy OM, Attia AS, Badr MAL (2007) A novel analytical model for electrical loads comprising static and dynamic components. Electr Power Syst Res 77:1249–1256
24. Kim BH, Kim H, Lee B (2012) Parameter estimation for the composite load model. J Int Council Electr Eng 2(2):215–218. https://doi.org/10.5370/jicee.2012.2.2.215
25. Krause PC, Wasynczuk O, Sudhoff SD (2002) Analysis of electric machinery and drive systems, 2nd edn. Wiley-IEEE Press, New York
26. Kothari DP, Nagrath IJ (2006) Electric machines. Tata-McGraw-Hill, India
27. Carrasco DS, Salgado ME (2010) Optimal multivariable controller design using an ITSE performance index. Int J Control 83(11):2340–2353. ISSN 0020-7179 Print. https://doi.org/10.1080/00207179.2010.520033
28. Chen Y-P, Li Y, Wang G, Zheng Y-F, Xu Q, Fan J-H, Cui X-T (2017) A novel bacterial foraging optimization algorithm for feature selection. Expert Syst Appl 83:1–17
29. Zhu G-Y, Zhang W-B (2017) Optimal foraging algorithm for global optimization. Appl Soft Comput 51:294–313
30. Houck C, Joines J, Kay M (1995) A genetic algorithm for function optimization: A MATLAB implementation. North Carolina State University, Raleigh, NC, Technical report NCSU-IE-TR-95-09

Methods to Optimize the Performance of an Existing Large-Scale On-grid Solar PV Plant

Suma Umesh, J. Chaithra, G. Deborah, J. Gayathri and N. Pruthvi

Abstract There are a plethora of challenges faced due to the usage of conventional energy sources. Our objective is to optimize the performance and working of an existing on-grid solar power plant by focusing on common problems found in such large-scale installations. The suggested proposals for improvements were based on three identified areas: power generation and performance ratio (PR), running costs, and maintenance costs. We have used PVsyst, a software package, for simulating and analysing the working of the power plant. SCADA data was obtained from the plant along with generated sets of data from PVsyst and was further used to develop our proposals for improvement. Four improvements were suggested, which are "method to improve PV panel cleaning efficiency for dry tropical regions", "Simulink-based estimation of partial shading loss reduction using herbicides for vegetation management", "procedure to suggest new optimum tilt for a seasonal tilt arrangement", and "automated switching and lighting circuit using two-way relay switch".

Keywords Energy management · Resource management · Renewable energy · Solar · Photovoltaic · Power plants · Large scale · Optimization · Performance ratio · Seasonal tilt

S. Umesh (✉) · J. Chaithra · G. Deborah · J. Gayathri · N. Pruthvi
BMS Institute of Technology and Management, Bangalore, India
e-mail: sumaumesh@bmsit.in

J. Chaithra
e-mail: jchaithra@gmail.com

G. Deborah
e-mail: debbie45.9@gmail.com

J. Gayathri
e-mail: gayathreejagadeesh@gmail.com

N. Pruthvi
e-mail: rjpruthvi@gmail.com

© Springer Nature Singapore Pte Ltd. 2019
V. Sridhar et al. (eds.), *Emerging Research in Electronics, Computer Science and Technology*, Lecture Notes in Electrical Engineering 545,
https://doi.org/10.1007/978-981-13-5802-9_117

1 Introduction

For the efficient functioning of a utility-scale solar photovoltaic plant, it is a necessity to optimize the operational and maintenance activities of the plant. PV plants that have been in operation for more than a few years may receive changed insolation, vary in soiling loss trends or other plant parameters which affect the working of the plant or its upkeep and running costs. The performance of the plant should thus be continually optimized and its maintenance requirements kept minimal. Areas for incorporation of new technology to improve power plant control are also identified as required

This paper identifies and presents solutions to common operational and maintenance-related problems found in PV plants through the performance evaluation of a 100 MW on-grid PV plant in South India. These improvements can be incorporated in an already existing plant to enhance its overall performance, improve its resource management, and improve plant control.

2 Method to Improve PV Panel Cleaning Efficiency for Dry Tropical Regions

The environmental conditions that the modules are installed in play an important role in determining the energy output. PV panels that have not been cleaned properly have an overall decreased yield as well as an increased possibility of module-level failures, due to hot spots, found in unclean modules [1]. Degradation in PV system performance takes place when PV panels are not properly cleaned. For a dry tropical Temperature range (20–49 °C) with an annual precipitation 15 cm and latitude range of 15°–25° N and S Regions which is prone to dusty desert environment and frequent dust storms (for any PV configuration), cleaning systems must respond to intensity of dust accumulation, and a minimum weekly cleaning is recommended [2].

Soiling losses may be due to dust, bird excreta, pollution, particulate matter and salt water, among others, and timely cleaning of the modules is required based on the specific environmental concern [3–5]. Manual cleaning of the modules PV array field, especially in large capacity plants, takes considerable time and effort, along with large quantities of materials used. Also, at many PV plant sites, especially in dry tropical regions, water is a scarce resource, and a general minimization of water usage is preferable as well as economical.

A PV module cleaning proposal to minimize the amount of water usage involved in cleaning of the solar panels in the grid-connected system is suggested. The proposal is an addition to manual cleaning system of PV panels that are currently used in many large-scale PV installations. The addition of a mist nozzle is explored based on a 3-D CAD model of the same, and flow simulation is then performed using SolidWorks software. An estimated amount of water saved using this system is calculated.

2.1 Mist Nozzle

Dispersal of water droplets into air is characterized as a spray or mist formation. A spray is formed by pressurizing water in a nozzle in order to atomize it. A mist nozzle facilitates dispersion of liquid into a spray. Mist jet uses air pressure to atomize water. These nozzles break up the fluid into droplets. A small orifice nozzle is modelled here. It operates at high-pressure and pushing the fluid through a very small opening to break it apart into fog.

The parameters that affect spray nozzle are pressure, spray pattern type, spray angle, nozzle type, specific gravity of the fluid, viscosity and surface tension, impact and reach of the spray.

For cleaning, impact of a spray is an important characteristic and the spray should have sufficient reach to ensure that it hits the target area and gets well distributed. Spray drift can result in the target being missed or reduced effectiveness if sprayed into a gas flow or in windy conditions [6]. Higher the flow rate, greater the impact of the spray, and by increased pressure, the impact reduces in certain nozzles. To be noted is that by increasing the pressure, water droplets are atomized to finer droplets which have less momentum. For maximum impact, fluid pressure is kept to an acceptable constant while allowing for a higher flow rate in this design.

Mist Nozzle Design. A 3-D CAD drawing of a mist nozzle of acceptable size was used for SolidWorks flow simulation. Type of fluid is chosen as water, and analysis type is set as internal. Boundary conditions and flow rate are chosen as required. The static pressure and pressure difference between the inlet of the swirl cylinder and the outlet of the orifice exposed to the surrounding environment are obtained (Table 1).

Table 1 Nozzle specification

Nozzle type	Mist nozzle
Length of swirl chamber (L_S) in mm	41.5
Diameter of swirl chamber (D_S) in mm	22
Length of orifice (L_0) in mm	14.5
Diameter of orifice (D_0) in mm	3
Number of inlet slots (n) in mm	2
Swirl chamber convergent angle (α) in °	30
Inlet slot diameter (D_P)	1

Design Flow Simulation

- **Wizard Set-up**: A project is created under the set-up where the fluid and analysis type are set. This creates a mesh around the structure consideration.

- **Boundary Conditions and Goal Setting**: Boundary conditions are set indicating the inlet pressure and outlet conditions. The flow rate is set to a desired value. Surface goals are set at the inlet and outlet of the nozzle to observe the static pressure. Equation goals are obtained to observe the pressure difference between the inlet of the swirl cylinder and the outlet of the orifice exposed to the surrounding environment.
- **Running the Simulation**: The simulation runs, and the simulation result is obtained. A flow trajectory is obtained to observe the water flow within the nozzle. A cut plot model is obtained to observe the differential pressure and velocity of the fluid inside the nozzle.

A model is designed on SolidWorks 3-D software (Figs. 1, 2, and 3). Flow rate trajectory and cut plot of the velocity variation in the model were obtained for analysis purposes (Figs. 4 and 5).

Design Results:
The water consumption of this nozzle is compared with water consumption of regular spray nozzles commonly used in manual cleaning of PV panel installations. The water consumption of a 50 MW PV plant in South India with 199,992 panels, with an average of 13,333 panels cleaned per day, requires around 10,000 L. The water savings compared with a mist nozzle based on design is seen in Tables 2 and 3.

A mist nozzle therefore saves 89.33% more energy than a regular spray nozzle. The additional use of a mist nozzle into manual PV panel cleaning procedures for light layers of dust can be used in combination with a spray nozzle.

Fig. 1 Mist nozzle model—front view

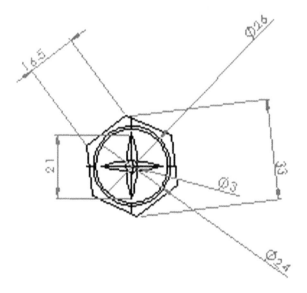

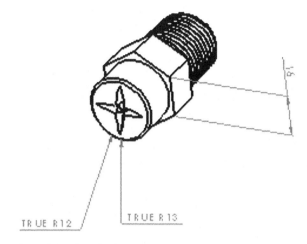

Fig. 2 Mist nozzle model—trimetric view

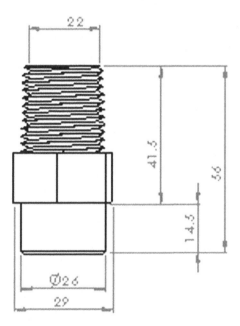

Fig. 3 Mist nozzle model—front view

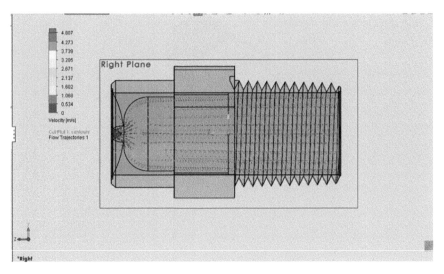

Fig. 4 Flow trajectory

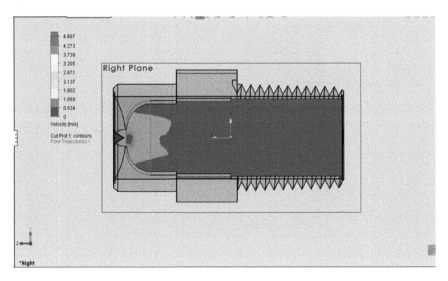

Fig. 5 Cut plot—velocity variation

2.2 Cleaning System Design

The collector pipe used is three inch in diameter and one metre in length. At one end of the collector, one-inch diameter hole along with a sieve to filter the collected water after cleaning the panel. This forms a re-circulating closed water loop. The nozzle pipe along with the collector module is detachable, and they do not affect

Table 2 Mist nozzle flow trajectory simulation results, for iterations: 40; analysis interval: 20

Goal name	Unit	Value	Averaged value	Minimum value
GG Av velocity 1	(m/s)	1.044831918	1.044572542	1.042092729
SG Av static pressure 1	(Pa)	7619675.872	7656380.568	7617008.555
SG Av static pressure 2	(Pa)	−185619.6709	−192080.0655	−216959.0958
Equation goal 1	(Pa)	7805295.543	7848460.634	7804947.656

Table 3 Water savings comparison of spray nozzle with mist nozzle

Nozzle type	Water used per panel (ml)	Water used per day (l)
Regular nozzle	750	10,000
Mist nozzle	80	1066.64

the mechanical stability of the mounted PV panels. The pressure of the mist can be adjusted, and the flow rate can be controlled. A microfibre cloth can be used to scrub off the dirt on the PV panels. The water collected is filtered to separate the dust particles, and the filtered water is reused to clean other PV modules.

2.3 Cleaning Procedure Working

A tank filled with water is initially connected to a spray nozzle where pressurized water is aimed at adhesive layers of dust, muddy spots, and other precipitations on panel which are hard to remove. A nozzle pipe where the water gushes into the nozzle and the atomized water in the form of mist is then used to clean the entire PV panel. The inlet pressure is maintained at 75–80 bar pressure to obtain a flow rate of 250 ml/min. A microfiber cloth can be used to scrub off the dirt on the panel after moistening the surface of the panel. A small quantity of water along with the particulate matter flows down the panel and is collected in a collector attachment, shown in Fig. 6, similar to a half-cut steel pipe clipped on at the bottom. The water collected can filter to remove dust particles and the filtrated water thus obtained can be used to clean other PV panels. This forms a re-circulating closed water loop. The water used can be recycled and used again.

2.4 Conclusion

A PV module cleaning system with greater efficiency can be obtained. A spray nozzle is used for pressured streams of water aimed at hard to clean spots on the PV panel, which is followed with a mist nozzle spray and microfiber cloth system. Overall

Fig. 6 SolidWorks model of clip-on collector through system at PV panel

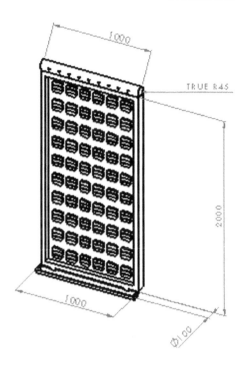

water consumption is drastically reduced by this method. This saves costs and is environmentally beneficial.

3 Simulink-Based Estimation of Partial Shading Loss Reduction Using Herbicides for Vegetation Management

A common operational and maintenance problem faced in PV plants is due to tall weeds or vegetative growth around the installation which can create shading and can also lead hot spot heating which can negatively impact system production and module damage. This problem is exacerbated in large PV plants as weed removal for a huge land area of PV arrays is complex. There are difficulties faced in effective weed removal in all areas of the plant due to time constraints, large surface area, costs in manual labour, difficulty in finding eco-friendly methods as well as continuous re-growth of weeds.

A method to reduce rate of weed re-growth is suggested through the usage of 10% acetic acid and salt to change the soil's salinity. The partial shading loss reduction through the usage of such a method is estimated using Simulink [7] and compared with the loss reduction due to grass cutting.

3.1 Partial Shading

The output current of a PV module is a function of solar irradiance [7]. If there is a reduction in solar irradiance as a result of partial or complete shading, the performance of the PV module will be affected. According to statistical studies, power losses due to partial shading can vary from 10 to 70% [8].

Types of shadings are near shadings and far shadings. Shadings from objects that act on the PV array field in a global way are known as "far" shadings, such as when the sun is visible or not visible for an instant on the PV panels, and typically occur when the shading object is more than 10 times the size of the PV field size.

Far shading is generally compensated for the most well-designed PV plants. The design of the site is usually such that shading done due to mountains or far away objects are prevented from casting shadows on the PV panel surface area.

Near shading caused due to shadows of the mounted panel structures falling on nearby panels is also generally minimized. However, vegetation growth consisting of wild grass and other weeds are difficult to prevent.

3.2 Site-Specific Details

From plant observation, an estimated 5–20% of all PV panels' surface area is covered by grass at any given time, attributed to varying rates and patterns of grass growth over the year. The maximum and minimum partial shading losses for the estimated percentage of grass coverage are calculated. This is done by considering various shading patterns that be cast on panel surface area and the ensuing partial shading losses [8].

1. PV panel temperature during grass cutting operation at site (usually done during afternoon hours) is an average of 35°.
2. Grass cutting is done for PV panel arrays connected to a single inverter room on a bimonthly basis. This process is repeated throughout the year.
3. The PV array field does not have levelled land, and therefore, completely automated grass cutting machines cannot be used.
4. Herbicide usage that can modify the surrounding habitat or can cause health problems cannot be used according to land usage rights set by the government.
5. The site must maintain environmental standards set by the government, and as part of its balance of systems is kept operational in a way such that operational and maintenance activities at the plant do not disturb the ecological balance of the surrounding area.
6. Methods to reduce grass growth over time such as the use of rubber sheets or landscape sheets cannot be used in such large plant areas
7. Usage of herbivorous animals like cows or sheep is not used due to potential chances of electrocution as well as non-reliability for larger plant areas.

3.3 Simulink-Based Estimation of Partial Shading Loss in a PV String

Components Selected

1. A TP250MZ PV panel is used.
2. The system consists of a string containing 2 sets of 24 panels connected in series which is then connected parallel to each other.
3. DC voltage and DC current measurement blocks are used to measure current and voltage parameters of PV string.
4. Ramp irradiation and temperature input blocks are given to PV array.
5. Relevant scope blocks are connected to measure output current and voltage from each block.

Simulink Model Design

1. Due to the dynamic nature of grass growth along with the overall shape of the near shading, shading losses will vary at any given time among different PV strings.
2. Thus, only the partial shading falling on one array string is simulated and the general range of partial losses is calculated.
3. The 48-panel arrangement is split into 6 blocks of 8 cells each. The 6 blocks are connected with 3 blocks in series connected in parallel to another 3 blocks in series, i.e., modelled as 6 modules with 8 cells each.
4. The lower blocks are susceptible to partial shading due to vegetation.
5. Partial shading can be simulated by showing the corresponding reduction in irradiance received on panel surface due to grass cover.
6. The pattern of partial shading can vary in shape and size throughout the year. The shaded area can cover the bypass diodes or not according to which output V-I and P-V curves vary.

Assumptions Made in Design

1. Upper line of string is not affected by grass growth and resultant near shading.
2. Irradiance at upper line of string is taken as 1000 W/m^2 at S.T.C.
3. A comparison is made of output at MPP at STP. conditions ($25°$) and for $35°$, where losses occur due to temperature coefficient of PV cell.
4. Partial shading patterns are taken assuming various grass growth locations and heights. Irradiance received at each block is always assumed to be a minimum of 200 W/m^2 during working conditions.

Simulink Results:

Peak performance

The MPP power when peak irradiance (taken as 1000 W/m^2) is received at the cell is 11,950 W at STP.

MPP power is 11,450 W when at 35 °C (Figs. 7 and 8).

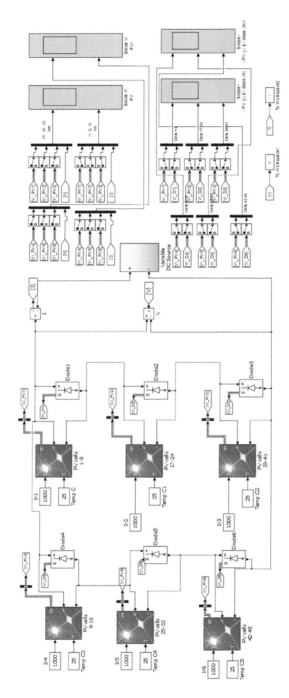

Fig. 7 Simulink model under STP conditions and peak irradiance to all cells

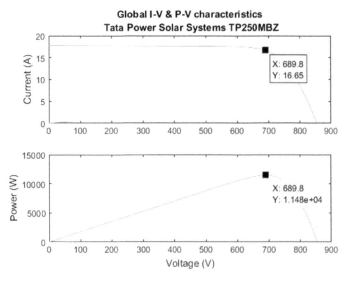

Fig. 8 V-I and P-V characteristics at 35 °C and irradiance of 1000 W/m^2

Partial shading loss due to minimum coverage of PV string area (5%)

Here, for an estimated minimum of 5% of string covered due to grass growth, the resultant partial shading losses are shown, both for STP conditions and for plant working temperatures of 35 °C. Table 4 shows the power, current, and voltage at MPP for the PV string. Multiple possible shadows caused due to grass growth coverage of 5% of the panel are considered, and maximum and minimum ranges of partial shading losses are obtained, shown in Figs. 9, 10, and 11.

Partial shading loss due to maximum coverage of PV string area (20%)

Here, for an estimated minimum of 20% of string covered due to grass growth, the resultant partial shading losses are shown, both for STP conditions and for plant working temperatures of 35 °C. Table 5 shows the power, current, and voltage at MPP for the PV string. Multiple possible shadows caused due to grass growth coverage of 20% of the panel are considered, and maximum and minimum ranges of partial shading losses are obtained, shown in Figs. 11, 12, and 13.

Table 4 Power, current, and voltage at MPP for multiple possible grass growth shapes that cover 5%

Type of shading	Lower line of string (24 cells)			At MPP (STP)			MPP at 35 °C			Partial shading losses (W)	
	W/m²			V(V)	I (A)	P(W)	V(V)	I(A)	P(W)	At STP (25°)	At 35°
	(9–16)	(25–32)	(41–48)								
Equal	900	900	900	721	15.78	11,380	691	15.82	10,940	570	510
Ramp	950	900	850	710.4	15.65	11,117	695.4	15.58	10,830	833	620
Two blocks (Equal)	1000	850	850	726	15.45	11,210	695.1	15.5	10,770	740	680
Two blocks	1000	900	800	727.9	15.79	11,120	683.3	15.43	10,540	830	910
One block	1000	1000	700	736	14.2	10,450	709.5	14.17	10,060	1500	1390

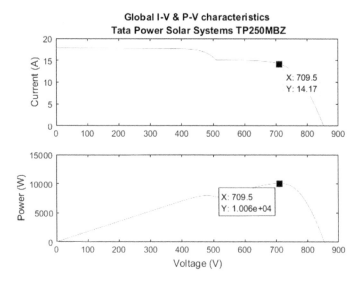

Fig. 9 Resultant I-V and P-V characteristic curve for shape with maximum partial shading losses at 5%

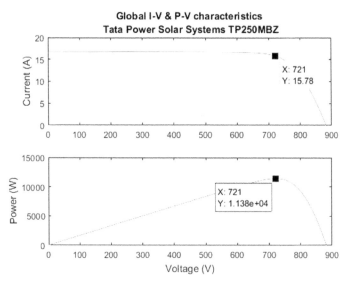

Fig. 10 Resultant I-V and P-V characteristic curve for shape with minimum partial shading losses at 5%

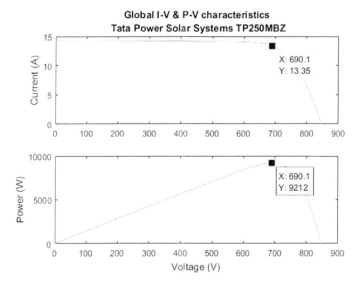

Fig. 11 Resultant I-V and P-V characteristic curve for shape with maximum partial shading losses when shaded (20%)

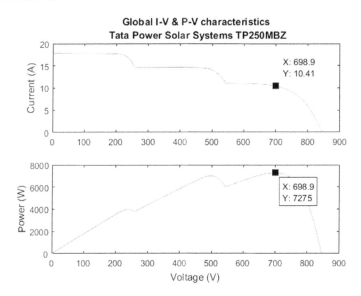

Fig. 12 Resultant I-V and P-V characteristic curve for maximum partial shading losses when shaded (20%)

Table 5 Power, current, and voltage at MPP for multiple possible grass growth shapes that cover 20% of the string panel area

Type of shading	Lower line of string (24 cells)			At MPP (STP)			MPP at 35 °C			Partial shading losses (W)	
	W/m²			V (V)	I (A)	P (W)	V (V)	I (A)	P (W)	At STP	At 35°
	(9–16)	(25–32)	(41–48)								
Equal	800	800	800	721.6	13.29	9588	690.1	13.35	9212	2362	2238
Ramp	900	750	350	730.7	11.23	8204	702.1	11.23	7893	3746	3557
Two blocks (Equal)	900	450	450	727.2	12.11	8803	698.9	12.1	8456	3147	2994
Two blocks	1000	650	250	728.6	10.38	7286	727.2	12.11	8803	4664	2647
Two blocks	1000	800	200	506.1	15.26	7754	698.9	10.41	7275	4196	4175

Result:

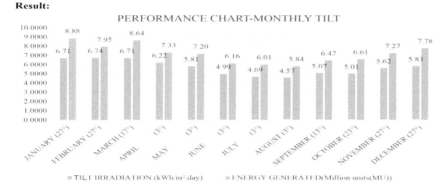

Fig. 13 Graph representing the performance of the plant with a monthly change in the tilt

3.4 Organic Contact Herbicide and Salt Spraying System to Reduce Vegetative Growth

Solution Constraints

1. Site conditions preclude the usage of systemic herbicides as they have a permanent effect on the environment. Any external herbicide used can only be used after multiple studies proving its long-term harmlessness on the environment.
2. Contact herbicides that are corrosive in nature or affect surrounding human or animal life on direct or indirect contact can also not be used.
3. The herbicides used must also be relatively inexpensive in nature with respect to auxiliary costs in running mowing equipment or paying for manual labour.
4. With respect to the constraints, acetic acid (Vinegar) and salt mixture can be used along with a fertilizer sprayer to cull vegetative life in and around PV panel arrays. 10% acetic acid is non-hazardous to plant and animal life and works by breaking down plant tissue on contact [9].
5. Salt application increases sodium levels in the soil due to which plant roots wither due to osmotic pressure increase. The reductions in growth and photosynthesis are greater under NaCl stress, and the effect is additive [10].

Procedure

1. Initial grass cutting around a single inverter room is followed by 10% vinegar solution application.
2. Since a contact herbicide deals with breakdown of plant tissue at surface level, roots of the grass will remain.
3. Salt is further sprinkled on the same area. This creates NaCl stress along with killing the remaining grass roots.
4. Further grass growth in the same area is also drastically reduced.
5. Grass will not thus re-grow to a height that will cause partial shading on module using this procedure.

6. This procedure reduces also overall grass growth over a year's period drastically. Repeated applications cause a cumulative effect over a period of years and cause further and further decrease in grass growth.
7. An additional precautionary method can be taken by slowly replacing cut grass area with low lying grass species that are drought resistant as well as inexpensive, which will reduce surface area for normal grass to grow.
8. Cost estimates suggest that over a five-year period this method is as cost-effective as single application herbicides, while posing fewer concerns over impacts on human and ecosystem health [8].

3.5 Results

After a year of application of grass removal methods:

Original System

Bimonthly improvement due to grass cutting will only eliminate partial shading losses due to PV strings that go to a single inverter room.

From site observation, grass takes 2–3 months to re-grow and causes partial shading again after being cut, due to which only 6–7 PV field arrays connected to inverter rooms remain completely unshaded at any given time. This means a minimum of 2000 out of 4187 strings have various portions of their PV panel shaded in a range of 5–20%.

The overall partial shading losses at peak irradiance lie between a range of 1140–8392 KW (at STP) and 2020–8350 KW (at 35°).

Improvement Proposal

Using the suggested improvement, if a minimum of 5–6 months is taken for grass to re-grow to original height after herbicide usage, only about 800–1000 strings will be shaded after one year, and the partial shading will further decrease in future years.

The overall partial shading losses at peak irradiance lie between a range of 456 KW and 3356 KW, excluding at STP and 408–3340 KW at 35°.

3.6 Conclusion

Array power improvement in the range of 600–5036 KW is estimated (for STP conditions) at any given time depending on real-time grass growth patterns at site.

During the afternoon (for an average panel temperature of 35°), when grass cutting takes place, array power improvement in the range of 1612–5010 KW is estimated.

4 Procedure to Suggest New Optimum Tilt for a Seasonal

Tilt Arrangement

A PV plant must be continuously evaluated to ensure optimum working and generation of the plant over the years due to changing environmental parameters [11]. The original optimal tilt angle in a seasonal tilt arrangement may be modified for increased power generation after few years of plant operation [11]. In order to maximize the absorption of solar radiation, it is necessary that the panels are tilted at an angle from the horizontal surface such that they are perpendicular to the sun's rays [12, 13].

From the analysis of the insolation data obtained from the plant site, it is evident that the plant is receiving very good insolation throughout the year. The current tilt arrangement is a two-tilt arrangement system where the panel tilts are changed twice a year, i.e., 3° during summer months and 27° during the winter month, and are shown in Table 6.

With the aim of suggesting optimum tilt angles other than the existing tilt arrangement (3° and 27°), an analysis is carried out on the simulated reports generated for various tilt angles ranging from 3° to 27° using PVsyst PC software package [14].

4.1 Suggestion of Additional Tilts Changing Tilt Angles Monthly

Calculations are done based on the experimental data obtained from PV syst PC software package. A table comparing the tilt irradiance received, energy generated, and the resultant performance ratio is shown along with the yearly percentage improvement for each parameter. Here, the tilt suggested is changed on a monthly basis: April–August (3°), March (17°), September (13°), October (23°), November–February (27°) (Tables 7 and 8).

To get the most from solar panels, they should be aligned in the direction that captures the most sun. In an attempt to tap more solar energy, a suggestion to increase the number of tilt angles is made. The effect of varying the tilt angle on collected monthly solar radiation can be seen in terms of the total output power generated.

Table 6 Performance of the plant with the current tilt arrangement available at the plant

Current tilt arrangement		Tilt irradiation KWh/m² day	Energy generated Million Units (MU)	Performance ratio (%) (PR)
Month	Tilt used (°)			
March–September	3	5.252618452	35.739749	81.68
October–March	27	5.98111747	42.349402	82.77
		5.616867961	78.089151	82.22

Table 7 Table indicating the performance of the plant with a monthly change in the tilt

Monthly tilt		Tilt irradiation	Energy generated	PR (%)
Month	Panel (°)	KWh/m^2/Day	(MU)	
January	27	6.712	8.88	85.60
February	27	6.7438	7.9512	84.43
March	17	6.7146	8.6419	83.28
April	3	6.2208	7.3291	79.05
May	3	5.8146	7.1988	80.42
June	3	4.9878	6.1559	82.74
July	3	4.6868	6.0142	83.13
August	3	4.5702	5.8418	82.99
September	13	5.0711	6.4738	85.39
October	23	5.0053	6.61	85.72
November	27	5.617	7.2666	86.55
December	27	5.8298	7.7846	86.49
		5.6645	86.1479	83.82
Percentage improvement		0.85%	10.32%	1.94

Table 8 Table indicating the performance of the plant with a seasonal change in the tilt 7° for the months of March–May

For a summer tilt of 7°

Suggestion 2: Changing tilt angles seasonally

Month	Tilt suggested (°)	Tilt irradiation	Energy generated	Performance ratio (%)
		KWh/m^2 day	Million Units (MU)	
March–May (Summer)	7	6.18436087	23.612855	83.26
June–September (Monsoon)	3	4.818755738	24.202588	82.84
October–February (Winter)	27	5.968774834	38.492886	85.79
		5.657297147	86.308329	83.96
Percentage improvement		0.72%	10.53%	2.12

Improvements:

1. There is an increase in the amount of solar irradiation received throughout the year by changing the tilt angles every month, hence resulting in an increase in the performance ratio.
2. Total number of million units generated throughout the year is greater when compared to the existing tilt arrangement.

Potential problems:

1. The installation and maintenance of this arrangement are more complex than a two-tilt arrangement.
2. For a huge solar PV plant the changing of tilts of the panels, the losses incurred due to damage of panels caused by stresses and miss handling by personnel during frequent change of tilts of the panels is significant.
3. Practically feasibility must be determined by doing a cost–benefit analysis, as monthly tilt variation is usually not practised in larger PV plants.

Changing tilt angles seasonally

Calculations are done and a table comparing the tilt irradiance received, energy generated and the resultant performance ratio is shown along with the yearly percentage improvement from each parameter. Here, the tilt suggested is changed seasonally during summer (7°/10°), monsoon (3°), and winter (27°) (Figs. 14, 15, 16, and 17). **Selecting 7° tilt for the summer months (March–May)**:

1. It is observed that for the proposed three-tilt arrangement with a 7° summer tilt, the average solar irradiation received throughout the year increases by 0.72%. When compared to the value obtained using two-tilt arrangement, the performance ratio increases by 2.12%.
2. Total number of million units generated also increases by a significant 10.53%.

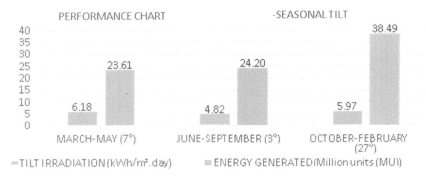

Fig. 14 Graph representing the performance of the plant with a seasonal change in the tilt (7° for the months of March–May)

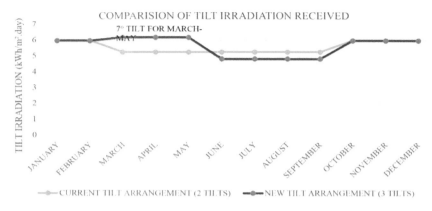

Fig. 15 Graph indicating a comparison between the current two-tilt arrangement and the proposed three-tilt arrangement (7° for the months of March–May) for the tilt irradiation received

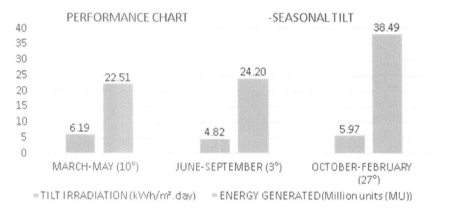

Fig. 16 Performance of the plant with a seasonal change in the tilt (10° for the months of March—May)

Selecting 10° tilt for the summer months (March–May):

1. It is observed that the average solar irradiation received throughout the year increases by 0.74% compared with the value obtained using two-tilt arrangement, and the performance ratio increases by 0.64%

2. The total number of million units generated increases by 9.12%.

Advantage of using this mechanism: A summer tilt of 7° is clearly preferable to a 10° tilt according to the overall energy generated as well as the PR of the plant over a year from a comparative analysis of Tables 3 and 4. However, a greater tilt irradiance is received on solar panels due to a 10° tilt during summer months compared to a 7° tilt (Tables 9 and 10).

It is realized that an increase in the solar irradiation does not have a linear relation with number of tilt angles as environmental factors also play a major role in impact-

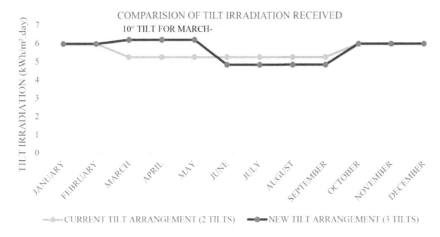

Fig. 17 Comparison between the current two-tilt arrangement and the proposed three-tilt arrangement (10° for the months of March–May) for the tilt irradiation received

Table 9 Plant performance with a seasonal change in the tilt 10° for the months of March–May

For a summer tilt of 10°				
Suggestion 2: Changing tilt angles seasonally				
Month	Tilt suggested	Tilt irradiation	Energy generated	Performance ratio (%)
		KWh/m^2 Day	Million Units (MU)	
March–May (Summer)	10°	6.186970652	22.513363	79.62
June–September (Monsoon)	3°	4.818755738	24.202588	82.84
October–February (Winter)	27°	5.968774834	38.492886	85.79
		5.658167075	85.208837	82.75
Percentage improvement		0.74%	9.12%	0.64

Table 10 NODE MCU specifications

Operating voltage	3.3 V
Input voltage (recommended)	5 V
Digital I/O pins	9
PWM digital I/O pins	8 (all pins except D0)
Analog input pins	1
DC current per I/O pin	12 mA
DC current for 3.3 V pin	50 mA
EEPROM	4 MB
Clock speed	80 MHz

ing the net million units generated. By changing the tilt arrangement from a two-tilt system to a three-tilt system, a significant improvement in average irradiation, performance ratio, and net million units generated is observed; the installation complexity and maintenance for the this tilt arrangement increase slightly but the performance improvement outweighs the challenges faced to adopt a three-tilt arrangement.

4.2 Conclusion

For the optimization of the system with an increment in the overall output of the plant, a three-tilt arrangement system can be opted for. Based on a cost–benefit analysis and the overall increase in power generation and irradiation received along with considerations of safety factor and environmental factors, this method can be used to suggest new optimum tilts through PVsyst.

5 Automated Switching and Lighting Circuit Using Two-Way Relay Switch

An additional area for plant optimization is the incorporation of new technology to improve plant control. Automated control of auxiliary circuits such as fan and light circuits can allow for remote access control of the plant and will improve the plant's operation, safety, and reliability [15].

The power plant is spread widely over 504 acres of land consisting about 26 pre-engineered buildings (PEBs) which have connected lighting and fan circuits along with other auxiliary supply needs. These buildings are placed at a significant distance from each other as well as the main control room. In order to address this issue, a control module was designed and a prototype was developed [16], based on the layout and existing wiring scheme of the inverter rooms (Figs. 18 and 19).

5.1 Prototype Design

Components Required

1. Node MCU
2. Buck converter (12–3.3 V)
3. 4 channel 12 V relay
4. Wires
5. PCB.

Code

```
#define BLYNK_PRINT Serial
#include <ESP8266WiFi.h>
#include <BlynkSimpleEsp8266.h>
Char auth[]="Authentication Token"; // Enter WiFi credentials
Char ssid[]= "Network Name"; // Enter the name of the network
Char pass[] "Password"; // Enter a password
void setup()
{
  Serial.begin(9600);
  Blynk.begin(auth,ssid,pass);
}
Void loop()
{
Blynk.run();
}
```

5.2 *Working*

The code is dumped on the NodeMCU, and connectivity is checked. The prototype has a client and the host. The client is being the NodeMCU and host is being the device on which blynk is installed.

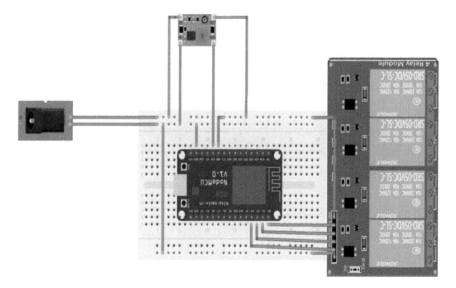

Fig. 18 Schematic diagram of prototype

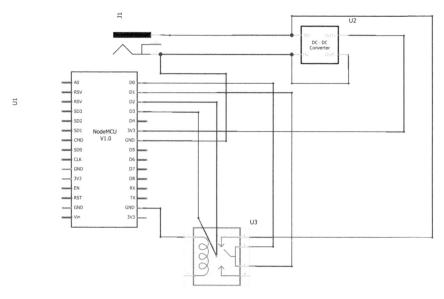

Fig. 19 Pin connections of the prototype

Table 11 Load point calculations

Sl. No.	Load type	Wattage (W)	Load points	Total load (W)
1.	Lighting fixtures	56	8	448
2.	Exhaust fans	200	4	800
	Total		12	1248

The client needs a dedicated Wi-fi network to work on. The best advantage that blynk offers is the client and the host needs not necessarily be on the same network thereby giving a remote access. The relays of the prototype are connected to the appliances via two-way switch mechanism to have a manual override in case the prototype is down.

The prototype has been tested out for both AC and DC loads. We can observe delay if the signal strength is less but the delay is minimal.

Wiring Diagram

A wiring diagram as well as 3-D layout of inverter rooms where the circuit will be used is drawn using AutoCAD (Table 11).

Calculations

Let the number of load points which can be controlled using the prototype in the inverter room be 12. (Refer Figs. 20 and 21). The calculations are as follows:

For a supply voltage of 240 V, with two sub-circuits are required.

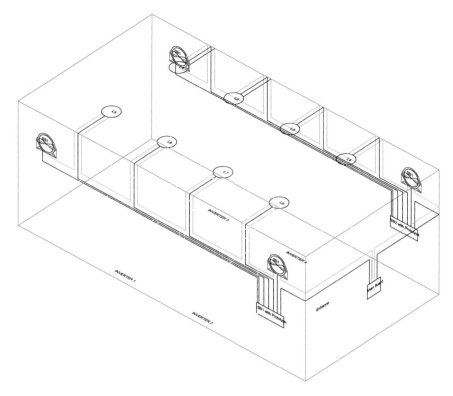

Fig. 20 AutoCAD 3-D layout of inverter room

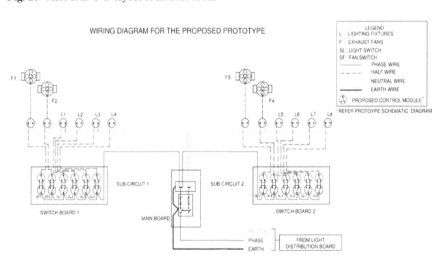

Fig. 21 Wiring diagram for the proposed prototype

Table 12 Total load in sub-circuit 1 and sub-circuit 2

Sub-circuit 1					Sub-circuit 2				
Sl. No	Load type	Wattage (W)	Load points	Total load (W)	Sl. No.	Load type	Wattage (W)	Load points	Total load (W)
1.	Lighting fix-tures	56	4	224	1.	Lighting fix-tures	56	4	224
2.	Exhaust fans	200	2	400	2.	Exhaust fans	200	2	400
	Total		6	624		Total		6	624

(As maximum load in a sub-circuit of 800 W and the total load present of 1248 W). [Refer Tables 11 and 12].

Rating of Main Switch Board and Distribution Board is calculated as:

Line Current = Connected Load/Supply Voltage

Line current = 1248/240 = 5.2 A

Therefore, full load current in each sub-circuit = 2.6 A (from Table 12).

Results. For a given inverter room, procedure to incorporate an automated relay switch is elaborated. This prototype can be expanded for higher rated appliances by changing relays of higher rating.

6 Conclusion

A set of viable, site-specific proposals are presented to optimize the long-term performance of an existing 100 MW solar photovoltaic plant.

The paper presents methods for

- Water resource management and improvement of efficiency of a manual PV panel cooling system
- Partial shading loss reduction and PV array power generation improvement through vegetation growth management
- Improvement in power generation using a seasonal tilt arrangement and a method to suggest and evaluate additional tilt angles
- Proposal to automate control of auxiliary equipment in power plant for remote access control, improvement in plant reliability and safety.

An overall enhancement of the performance of the power plant was attained along with a projected reduction in running costs.

7 Future Scope

The suggested improvements can also be adapted for use in similar already existing solar PV installations. Common operational and maintenance problems faced in such systems will have viable solutions, and an overall optimization of the PV plant performance along with operational loss reduction can be attained. Plant performance can be evaluated and modified to suit changing environmental conditions of the site over time.

Acknowledgements The authors would like to extend their gratitude towards Tata Power Solar Systems Limited (TPSSL) for permitting us to carry out our study at the plant site. The author would also like to thank Mr. Seshadri Devanadhan, at TPSSL, for his support.

References

1. Maghami MR, Hizam H, Gomes C, Radzi MA, Rezadad MI, Hajighorbani S (2016) Power loss due to soiling on solar panel: a review. Renew Sustain Energy Rev 59:1307–1316
2. Mani M, Pillai R (2010) Impact of dust on solar photovoltaic (PV) performance: research status, challenges and recommendations. Renew Sustain Energy Rev 14(9):3124–3131
3. Hassan AH, Rahoma UA, Elminir HK, Fathy AM (2005) Effect of airborne dust concentration on the performance of PV modules. J Astron Soc Egypt 13(1):24–38
4. Rao A, Pillai R, Mani M, Ramamurthy P (2014) Influence of dust deposition on photovoltaic panel performance. Energy Procedia 54:690–700. ISSN 1876-6102. https://doi.org/10.1016/j.egypro.2014.07.310
5. Maghami MR, Hizam H, Gomes C, Radzi MA, Rezadad MI, Hajighorbani S (2016) Power loss due to soiling on solar panel: a review. Renew Sustain Energy Rev 59:1307–1316. ISSN 1364-0321
6. Hemsath KH, Vereecke FJ (1977) Spray mist cooling arrangement. US Patent 4,065,252, 27 Dec 1977
7. Patel Hiren, Agarwal Vivek (2008) MATLAB-based modeling to study the effects of partial shading on PV array characteristics. IEEE Trans Energy Convers 23(1):302–310
8. Ishaque Kashif, Salam Zainal (2013) A review of maximum power point tracking techniques of PV system for uniform insolation and partial shading condition. Renew Sustain Energy Rev 19:475–488
9. Booth AL, Skelton NW (2009) The use of domestic goats and vinegar as municipal weed control alternatives. Environ Pract 11(1):3–16
10. Brosnan JT, DeFrank J, Woods MS, Breeden GK (2009) Sodium chloride salt applications provide effective control of sourgrass (Paspalum conjugatum) in seashore paspalum turf. Weed Technol 23(2):251–256
11. Nadim M, Rashed MRH, Muhury A, Mominuzzaman SM (2016) Estimation of optimum tilt angle for PV cell: a study in perspective of Bangladesh. In: 2016 9th international conference on electrical and computer engineering (ICECE). IEEE, pp 271–274
12. https://needsolarsystem.wordpress.com/2013/08/21/types-of-solar-panel-array-mountingsfixed-adjustable-tracking/
13. PV Education. http://www.pveducation.org/pvcdrom/properties-of-sunlight/elevation-angle
14. Yadav P, Kumar N, Chandel SS (2015) Simulation and performance analysis of a 1 kWp photovoltaic system using PVsyst. In: 2015 international conference on computation of power, energy information and communication (ICCPEIC). IEEE

15. Walia NK, Kalra P, Mehrotra D (2016) An IOT by information retrieval approach: smart lights controlled using WiFi. In: 2016 6th international conference cloud system and big data engineering (Confluence). IEEE, pp 708–712

16. Iwaki K (1990) Control room design and automation in the advanced BWR. In: Proceedings of the annual international symposium balancing automation human action in nuclear power plants

Application of Hilbert–Huang Transform and SVM Classifier to Monitor the Power Quality Disturbances

R. Shilpa and P. S. Puttaswamy

Abstract Electrical power quality portrays an imperative part of providing power effectively to the consumers. As power turns out to be more fundamental and significant asset for the whole world, the quality used at all its level will be critical for the steady and also for the efficient working of the equipment. As there is an increase in the consumption of power, the production of quality power is a challenge in power engineering. Therefore, it is important to address the issues that affect the quality of the power. Hence, to address these issues, distinctly voltage swell, sag, transients, and distortions due to harmonics, Hilbert–Huang transform is utilized for identification of distortions and support vector machine is employed for classification. The data is also collected from the substation and the analysis is accomplished by estimating the performance of empirical mode decomposition, ensemble empirical mode decomposition, and complete ensemble empirical mode decomposition.

Keywords Empirical mode decomposition · Ensemble empirical mode decomposition · Complete ensemble empirical mode decomposition · Support vector machine

1 Introduction

In the modern society, the quality of the power has increasingly become an important factor together with the information related to requirements and also the expectations that are associated with the power. The reason for this issue is due to increased

R. Shilpa (✉) · P. S. Puttaswamy
Department of Electrical and Electronics Engineering, PES College of Engineering, Mandya 571401, Karnataka, India
e-mail: shilpa.r@vvce.ac.in

P. S. Puttaswamy
e-mail: psputtaswamy_ee@yahoo.com

© Springer Nature Singapore Pte Ltd. 2019
V. Sridhar et al. (eds.), *Emerging Research in Electronics, Computer Science and Technology*, Lecture Notes in Electrical Engineering 545,
https://doi.org/10.1007/978-981-13-5802-9_118

requirements and prerequisites for the power quality by customers, regulators, and network utilities. Many industrial and commercial customers possess equipment that is very sensitive to the power disturbances. Hence, it is more essential to understand the importance of the power quality that is being supplied through the powers system, dynamic operations, faults, and also the nonlinear loads that often cause a various kinds of power quality disturbances (PQD) like voltage swell, voltage sag, impulses, flickers, switching transients, harmonics, and notches. One of the critical aspects in the power quality study is that its ability to achieve an automatic monitoring of power quality and also the data analysis. Generally, utilities install the power quality digital meters or the fault recorders in certain locations to record some of the power quality events and store these data for the further analysis. The process of collecting, investigating, and understanding unprocessed measured data into useful information is power quality monitoring. The collection of data is typically done by continuous estimation of both voltages as well as current over a period of time. The procedure for investigation and also an interpretation of the same is performed manually, yet the late advances in artificial intelligence and also in signal processing fields have made it feasible to design the intelligent systems and also implement the same to automatically investigate and analyze the raw data to beneficial information with least human interference. It is important to figure out the quality of power that is supplied to various industries and commercial consumers that have appliances which are sensitive to the power disturbances. Hence, feasible algorithms known as empirical mode decomposition (EMD) and particularly ensemble empirical mode decomposition (EEMD) which are the noise-assisted version of EMD are conferred, for assimilation of statistical characteristics like minimum, mean, maximum values of first instantaneous frequency (IF) and also the value of instantaneous amplitude (IA), singular value decomposition values of both IA, IF [1]. Consequently, the classification is employed by the multi-class support vector machine.

2 Literature Review

An approach of recognizing distorted events by separating the signals into its basic features called empirical mode decomposition (EMD) and gathering it appropriately was presented by Manjula and Sarma [2]. The essential attributes of these distortions like in each distorted signal, these intrinsic mode functions (IMFs) are trained using the probability neural network (PNN). This approach can distinguish the mutilated signals more precisely, yet the PNN requires large memory space to store the model. Dash et al. [3] have proposed a Fourier linear combiner which is used to construct a system that possesses features of power disturbances like magnitude and slope values. The fuzzy expert system is used to train these acquired values. The class of disturbances was tested using pre-defined commands. The approach is predominant in furnishing the most accurate results for prominent voltage distortions, but the disadvantages like higher total classification time and the computational time needed for classifications based on fuzzy logic. To ascertain the momentary time distortions like swell, sag, and transients, an approach on the basis of filtering and math formats was discussed by Radil Tomas et al. [4]. The signals distorted are sectioned followed by normalization process. In this method, every distorted event is recognized using root mean square threshold methodology. Based on the time length of the determined signal, the classification is performed. The merits of this system are uncomplicated but the demerit is that only sag and transients can be classified. The significance of support vector machine (SVM) and radial basis function (RBF) network as artificial neural systems (ANN) along with classical learning algorithms demonstrated through some critical detriments featured in Janik and Lobos [5] work. Primarily, the error function is limited to be a multi-modal with several local minima where the learning process can stall out. Secondly, the complexity of the neural network architecture has not been able to control by machine learning algorithm. Hence, the selected architecture influences the generalization abilities. Zhang et al. [6] presented an approach to identify the voltage distortions by decreasing the input feature size employing the entropy-based method. A comparative analysis of the performance of wavelet transforms and the entropy-based algorithm is done. An easy and beneficial learning method known as RBF is used as a classifier. The entropy-based algorithm is utilized for extricating the input features of the network. However, the approach requires much more computational effort, even though its accuracy level is high. The timing of the central processing unit (CPU) and its potential is superior to the ANN but suffers from the absence of sparseness of solutions. Thus, this work is proposed based on the emerging, potential algorithm called Hilbert–Huang transform (HHT) and SVM classifier. The nonlinear, non-static univariate data like PQ disturbances are analyzed using the empirical mode decomposition algorithm. HHT is a combined version of EEMD and Hilbert spectrum. The extracted features using HHT are classified using radial basis function (RBF) based multi-class SVM classifier.

3 Methodology

The fundamental phases of proposed method subsist of the below-mentioned stages, shown in Fig. 1.

- Power quality distortions generation
- PQD feature detection followed by extraction
- SVM for disturbance classification

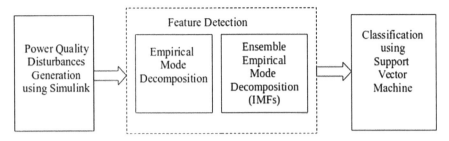

Fig. 1 Classification stages of the presented approach

3.1 Generation of PQDs

(1) *Voltage Sag*

The AC voltage reduced at a specified frequency for the period of 0.5 cycle to 1 cycle time is called as sag. The complete wave generated is for a 0.4 s duration and the sag is introduced in the period of 0.10–0.25 s as shown in Fig. 2. The AC power supply is set to 230 V, 50 Hz value with the transmission line parameter of 40 km, load resistance of 10 Ω and inductance of 0.005 H. The type of fault used in the network and the distance between the load and fault result in different ranges of changes in voltage. Initially, the fault generator is open before 0.10 s. The respective phase will be interrupted during its closure time (between 0.10 and 0.25 s) [13].

(2) *Voltage Swell*

The swell in the circuit is introduced by increasing the distance between the load point and the fault, as there will be a rise and drop in the voltage values, which is shown in Fig. 3. The AC power supply is set to 230 V, 50 Hz values, transmission line parameter line of 40 km, load voltage of 10 Ω and inductance value of 0.005 H.

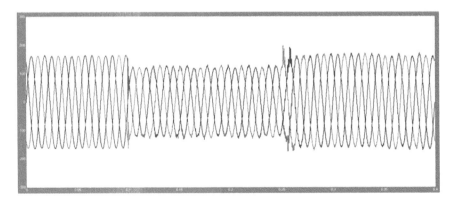

Fig. 2 Generated voltage sag

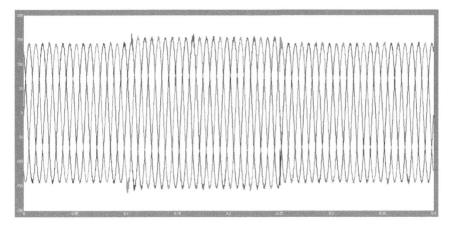

Fig. 3 Generated voltage swell

The complete waveform is simulated for a duration of 0.4 s and the swell wave is introduced in the duration of 0.1–0.25 s [13].

(3) *Voltage Harmonics*

The harmonic circuit model consists of three-phase source voltage, voltage–current measurement block (V–I), a bridge rectifier, transmission line, and combination of resistor–capacitor linear load. Removing the fault generator and replacing it by a bridge rectifier will introduce harmonic disturbance in the signal as shown in Fig. 4. The waveform is simulated for 0.4 s for which the power supply is set to 230 V, 50 Hz frequency, transmission line of 40 km long [13].

(4) *Voltage Transients*

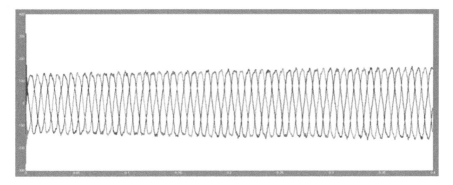

Fig. 4 Generated voltage harmonics

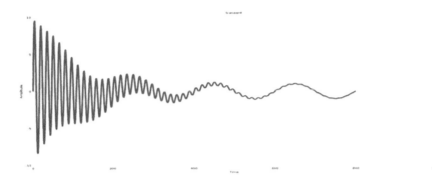

Fig. 5 Octave programmed voltage transient

The unexpected change in the enduring state of a typical voltage data to which it
decays to zero within a cycle is described as transients. The transient signal as shown
in Fig. 5 is generated using an Octave program based on the mathematical model
given in (1).

$$a(t) = amplitude * \left[\sin(\omega t) + C * e^{(-80*(t-T_{d1})} * \sin(\omega(t - T_{d1})(u(t))) \right] \quad (1)$$

where 'Amplitude' value is set to 1, constant $C = 0.4$, 'T_{d1}' is the time duration of
which transient occurs, i.e., 0.04 [14].

4   Feature Detection

The unstable PQ disparities are identified by the application of EMD and EEMD
algorithms which can also be utilized for univariate signals [7, 8].

4.1   Empirical Mode Decomposition

The significant part of utilizing EMD is to disintegrate the non-stationary random
input voltage distortions into its monocomponents and the generated monocom-
ponent functions employing this algorithm are termed as intrinsic mode function
(IMF). The monocomponents can be called as the functions for which the positive
instantaneous frequencies are ascertained. This adaptive algorithm disintegrates the
non-stationary PQ disturbances into intrinsic mode function and residue that illustrates the magnitude and frequency modulation depending on the sort of time signals

being investigated [7]. The algorithm involves various steps in breaking the non-linear, non-stationary input signals into its monocomponents given below with the various steps involved. The whole process is iterated until the residue obtained is a monotonic function. This iterated process is termed as sifting. A critical step in this algorithm is stopping the process of sifting. The process of sifting can be terminated by using several criteria and two such techniques are utilized in this research work and they are standard deviation and Rilling's criteria.

Step 1: Consider a univariate signal, $input(t)$
Step 2: Identify the nearby most extreme and nearby least minimum peaks from this signal.
Step 3: The upper and lower envelopes employing the cubic spline interpolation are extracted.
Step 4: Determine the mean, mean (t) of the envelopes by Eq. (2):

$$mean(t) = (Upper\,Envelope + Lower\,Envelope/2) \qquad (2)$$

Step 5: Obtain the difference between mean and the signal as given by Eq. (3):

$$Difference(t) = input(t) - mean(t) \qquad (3)$$

Step 6: The difference (t) is named as intrinsic mode function IMF1(t), which is the difference among the signal and mean.
Step 7: Calculate the residue as shown in Eq. (4):

$$residue(t) = residue(t) - IMF1(t) \qquad (4)$$

Step 8: If the residue, residue (t) is a monotonic function, then process is stopped, otherwise input variable input (t) will be replaced by residue(t) and go to step 2 to get the IMF, residue.

4.2 Ensemble Empirical Mode Decomposition

EEMD is an advanced technique for sifting the input signal. The signal input is a mix of univariate power quality disturbance signal and white noise. The signal is analyzed in both time and space domain by the algorithm. The integrated white noise signal function is treated as referral frame both in the time and frequency domain. The sifting process is carried out with input and white noise signal [15]. The EEMD algorithm steps include the following:

Step 1: Let white noise $N(t)$ is added to the univariate signal $input(t)$ as shown in Eq. (5) to have

$$input_j(t); \; input_1(t) = input(t) + N_1(t) \tag{5}$$

Step 2: Decompose the signal $input_1(t)$ by using proposed EMD algorithmic approach
Step 3: The new IMF set is acquired after iterating the steps 1 and 2 for a number of trials added with different series of noise.

The performance evaluation of two algorithms has been evaluated [8, 9]. The Pearson's product-moment correlation coefficient between the input signal and first IMF is higher for EEMD algorithm.

4.3 Complete Ensemble Empirical Mode Decomposition with Adaptive Noise

Since, EEMD produces noise where a little amount of noise is found in the residue, the reconstruction of signal differs. To overcome this, particular noise is added to each stage of decomposition and unique residue with less noise. The CEEMD algorithm can be described [11, 12] as follows:

1. White noise is added to the original signal $i(t)$
2. Obtain the first decomposed component applying EMD
3. Repeat the decomposition and add white noise of different realizations
4. Obtain an average over the ensemble to obtain the IMF_1
5. Compute the residue
6. Compute the second IMF component IMF_2
7. Repeat the above steps to obtain the $(m + 1)$th IMF Component

4.4 Classification of Voltage Disturbances by Cross-Correlation

The classification of disturbances by ascertaining the cross-correlation values is demonstrated and the method is explained below. The first IMF obtained from the Hilbert transformation provides the disturbance duration of the input signal and the distortion's origin is given by the obtained IA. The method is applied to disturbances such as voltage sag, transients, and multiple event interruption. The homogeneity connecting the two waveforms is given by Eq. (6);

$$[w_1(t) * w_2(t)] = \int w_1(\Gamma) w_2(t + \Gamma) d(\Gamma) \qquad (6)$$

The event whether it is single or multiple is decided by the cross-correlation operator '*'. The input considered is a sine wave with a frequency of 50 Hz and the Hilbert Spectrum for the same is obtained. Then cross-correlation is computed between the two waveforms which provides the cross-correlation coefficients (CCF). If CCF values lie between 0.5 and 0.95, then the input signal is classified as single event and if the CCF values lie between 0.1 and 0.95 then it is identified as multiple event, i.e., signal possessing multiple disturbances. The classified signal will be interrupted if the CCF value is less than or equal to 0.1 and if the value of CCF is greater than or equal to 0.95 then the signal is classified as an input sine signal without any disturbances and hence no event. Table 1 [9] gives the conditions summarized.

5 Results

Table 1 represents the cross-correlation results [9] by which the disturbance classification is accomplished. The performance analysis of EMD and EEMD is carried out depending on the first IMF and input signal coefficient (Table 2).

Figures 6 and 7 depict the obtained IMFs for harmonic signal from EMD and also EEMD algorithms. Analysis of real-time data signals from various substations shows the location of fault in the gathered data by visualizing the largest singular peak in the first instantaneous amplitude. Figure 8 illustrates the signal plotted from the

Table 1 Cross-correlation classification results

Sl. No	Power quality disturbances	Cross-correlation coefficient	Interval detected
1.	Transients	0.8006	0.01–0.08
2.	Interruption	0.05	0.02–0.06
3.	Multiple Events	0.1996	0.2–0.3

Table 2 Comparison of Pearson product-moment correlation coefficient between EMD and EEMD

Sl. No	Correlation coefficient values		
	Power quality disturbances	EEMD	EMD
1.	Voltage sag	0.0236	0.0021
2.	Transients	0.9493	0.9407
3.	Voltage swell	0.07048	0.0240
4.	Harmonics	0.0504	0.0184

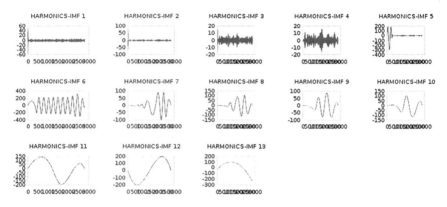

Fig. 6 Harmonics IMFs obtained by EMD

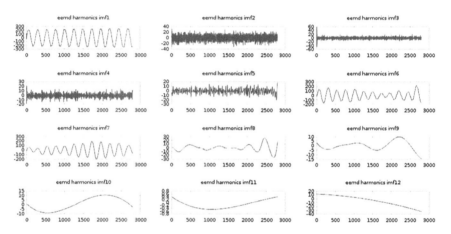

Fig. 7 IMFs of harmonics using ensemble empirical mode decomposition

data collected by Jaipura 66 kV substation. Figures 9 and 10 depict the decomposed components using EEMD and the first instantaneous amplitude indicating the fault origin, respectively. Table 3 encloses the tabulated values of the two most significant features that are extracted out of eleven using EEMD from four PQDs. The execution assessment of the proposed algorithms utilizing correlation coefficient values between the first IMF and the univariate input is evaluated. The results of comparison between two stoppage criteria shown in Table 4 which exhibits that the Rilling's criterion is found to be superior to standard deviation criterion.

This method of classification is applied on programmed generated data and is able to classify the distortions only for single or multiple events.

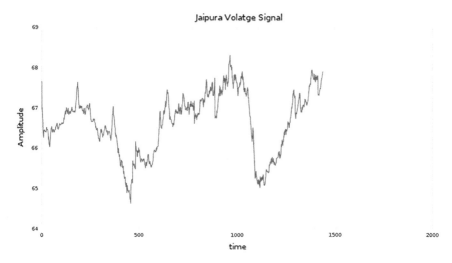

Fig. 8 Jaipura voltage signal collected 66 kV

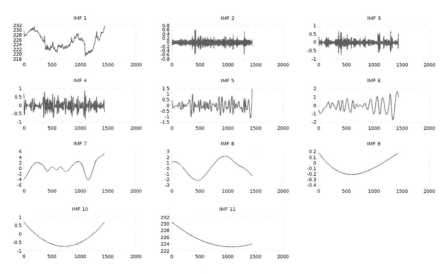

Fig. 9 Decomposed wave of Jaipura voltage signal

5.1 Classification by Support Vector Machine

HHT is a combined form of EEMD and Hilbert analysis. The Hilbert transformation is utilized to identify the instantaneous frequency values (IF) with instantaneous amplitude (IA) of first IMF. IA is obtained by Hilbert transformations of IMF [7]. Support vector machines (SVM) [10] are a group of learning machines. The goal of

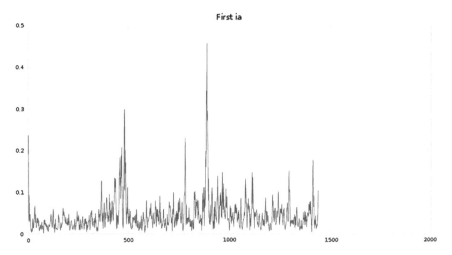

Fig. 10 First instantaneous amplitude indicating the fault origin near the sample 500

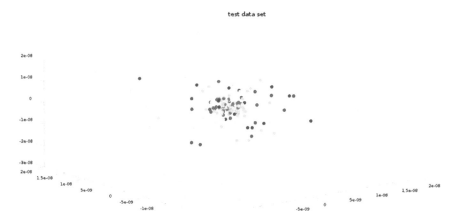

Fig. 11 Scattered plot of data set and classified data

the SVM is to find the optimal hyperplane that isolates the input. The features that are extracted using the EEMD algorithm are trained and tested using the SVM algorithm. Eleven features are extracted using EEMD-based Hilbert–Huang transform for voltage sag, transients, swell and harmonics, etc. and they are the first IMF values, maximum values of instantaneous frequency(IF) and instantaneous amplitude (IA), minimum values of IF and IA, singular value decomposition values, mean and standard deviation values of first IF and first IA. The two important features out of eleven that are extracted using EEMD are first IF and IA from four PQDs and are tabulated in Table 3. The Octave interface LIBSVM tool is used for classification purpose [10].

The features that are extracted using the EEMD algorithm are trained and tested using the SVM algorithm. Eleven features are extracted using EEMD-based Hilbert–Huang transform for voltage sag, transients, swell, and harmonics and they are the first IMF values, maximum values of instantaneous frequency and instantaneous amplitude, minimum values of IF and IA, singular value decomposition values, mean and standard deviation values of first IF and first IA. The scattered plot of the classified data is shown in Fig. 11. The classification of extracted features is done using SVM with RBF kernel, resulting in 76.74% overall accuracy of the result for 250 data set. The cost parameter is set to 100 and gamma to 0.2 values for which the resulting classification accuracy is higher than other values and requirement of support vectors is also less. One-versus-rest approach is used for the multi-class classification. Figure 11 displays the predicted, examined data with its label and the vacant rings as the training set. The unfilled rings represent the training data and filled rings depict the tested-predicted class of each and every disturbance with the green color means harmonics, red color indicating voltage sag, purple portraying voltage swell and transients are represented by blue color.

Classification is also done for the data collected from Jaipura substation 66 kV, Kadakola substation 230 V, Hootagalli substation 230 V, and Malavalli substation 66 kV. The classification results displayed showed that the signal contained is harmonics as shown in Fig. 12.

Figure 13 depicts the voltage signal which was collected from JP Nagar substation 66/11 kV.

Figure 14 shows the decomposed wave of JP Nagar substation after applying CEEMD algorithm. As it can be observed from the figure, the number of siftings is reduced when compared to EEMD.

Table 3 Features extracted using EEMD

Sl. No	Power quality disturbances	Maximum value of first IA	Maximum value of first IF
1.	Voltage sag	22.6360	0.4872
2.	Voltage swell	56.3960	0.4916
3.	Transients	22.0240	0.4910
4.	Harmonics	84.3660	0.4954

Table 4 Estimation of the standard deviation criteria and Rilling's criterion performance by correlation values

Sl. No	Power quality disturbances	Rilling's Criteria	Standard deviation criteria
1.	Voltage swell	0.6254	0.5863
2.	Transients	0.9390	0.9235
3.	Voltage sag	0.0176	0.0203
4.	Harmonics	0.0127	0.0181

```
nSV = 89, nBSV = 18
Total nSV = 89
Accuracy = 85.7143% (78/91) (classification)
Accuracy = 92.3077% (84/91) (classification)
Accuracy = 81.3187% (74/91) (classification)
Accuracy = 93.4066% (85/91) (classification)
acc = 0.81319
Test data is Harmonics
Test data is SAG
Test data is SWELL
Test data is SAG
Test data is SWELL
Test data is SWELL
Test data is SAG
Test data is Harmonics
Test data is SWELL
Test data is Harmonics
Test data is SAG
Test data is SAG
Test data is Harmonics
Test data is SAG
Test data is Harmonics
Test data is SAG
ans =
Test data is TRANSIENTS
ans = 1
```

Fig. 12 Classification result for the signal collected from Jaipura Substation

Figure 15 illustrates the first IA obtained from the IMF indicating the origin of the disturbance/fault.

6 Conclusion

The Simulink generated power quality distortions such as transients, swell, voltage sag, and harmonics and the substation data collected is analyzed. EMD and EEMD algorithms performance is compared which is employed to extract the statistical features. The real-time data analysis is accomplished utilizing EEMD and CEEMD. Support vector machine used for classification provides higher accuracy. EEMD and CEEMD algorithms work well for the non-stationary, nonlinear signals. The root cause for tripping of substation, total loss of power, and reduced electric efficiency can be identified by classification. The fundamental issue of the EMD is

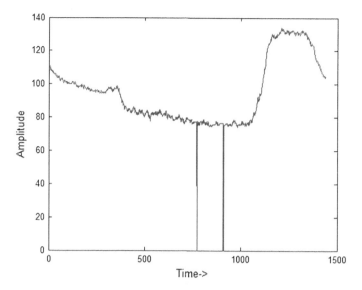

Fig. 13 Voltage signal collected from JP Nagar Substation, 66/11 kV

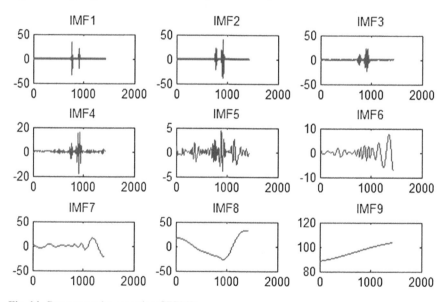

Fig. 14 Decomposed wave using CEEMD

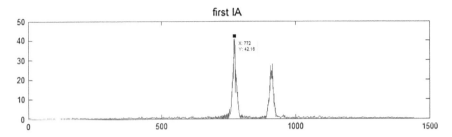

Fig. 15 First instantaneous amplitude indicating the fault origin near the sample 772

over-filtering, which can be overcome by utilizing Rilling's criteria. Analysis of constant information demonstrates the flaw area by utilizing first IA. Computation time of the calculation lessens contrasted with that of conventional EMD calculation. The software used to program the algorithms is freely available. CEEMD is used to obtain better spectral separation of modes and to reduce the number of siftings needed.

References

1. Yalcin T, Ozgonenel O, Kurt U (2011) Multi-class power quality disturbances classification by using ensemble empirical mode decomposition based SVM. In: ELECO international conference on electrical and electronics engineering. Turkey, Dec 2011
2. Manjula M, Sarma AVRS (2012) Assessment of power quality events by empirical mode decomposition based neural network. Proc World Congress Eng 2012:4–6
3. Dash PK, Jena RK, Salama MMA (1999) Power quality monitoring using an integrated Fourier linear combiner and fuzzy expert system. Int J Electr Power Energy Syst 21(7):497–506
4. Tomas R, Ramos PM, Janeiro FM, Cruz Serra A (2008) PQ monitoring system for real-time detection and classification of disturbances in a single-phase power system., IEEE Trans Instrum Meas 57(8):1725–1733
5. Janik P, Lobos T (2010) Automated classification of power quality disturbances using SVM and RBF networks
6. Zhang M, Li K, Hu Y (2010) Classification of power quality disturbances using wavelet packet energy entropy and LS-SVM. Energy Power Eng 158
7. Huang NE, Shen Z, Long SR, Wu ML, Shih HH, Zheng Q, Yen NC, Tung CC, Liu HH (1998) The empirical mode decomposition and Hilbert spectrum for nonlinear and non-stationary time series analysis. Proc R Soc Lond 903–995
8. Shilpa R, Prabhu SS, Puttaswamy PS (2015) Analysis of power quality disturbances using empirical mode decomposition and SVM classifier. Int J Adv Res Electron Commun Eng (IJARECE) 4(5)
9. Shilpa R, Puttaswamy PS, Detection and classification of short transients and interruption using Hilbert transform. Glob J Res Eng Electr Electron Eng 15(4), Version 1.0 (2015)
10. Chang C-C, Lin C-J (2011) LIBSVM: a library for support vector machines. ACM Trans Intell Syst Technol
11. Torres ME, Colominas MA, Schlotthauer G, Flandrin P (2011) A complete ensemble empirical mode decomposition with adaptive noise. In: IEEE International conference on acoustic, speech and signal processing, (ICASSP), pp 4144–4147
12. Sourav MdSG (2016) Implementation of complete ensemble empirical mode decomposition to analyze EOG signals for eye blink detection. Glob J Res Eng 16(3), Version 1.0

13. Zhu W, Ma W-Y, Gui Y, Zhang H-F (2012) Modelling and simulation of PQ disturbance based on Matlab. Int J Smart Grid Clean Energy
14. Dandwate A, Khanchandani KB. Generation of mathematical models for various PQ signals using MATLAB. Int J Eng Res Appl (IJERA). ISSN 2248-9622
15. Yalcin T, Ozgonenel O, Kurt U (2011) Multi-class power quality disturbances classification by using ensemble empirical mode decomposition based SVM. In: 7th International conference electrical and electronics engineering (ELECO), 2011. IEEE, pp 1–122

Voltage Stability Enhancement in Radial Distribution System by Shunt Capacitor and STATCOM

Mala and H. V. Saikumar

Abstract Voltage stability has a major concern in power system operation. It is the ability of the power system to maintain acceptable voltages at all buses in the system under normal conditions and after being subjected to a disturbance. Voltage instability may result in voltage collapse of the system. Hence, assessment of voltage stability is important. Implementation of new equipment including high-power electronics-based technologies such as flexible AC transmission systems (FACTS) has become essential for improvement of operation and control of power systems. The project work aims at the enhancement of voltage stability in the radial distribution system by using shunt capacitor and FACTS controller. A stability index named line stability indicator (LSI) is formulated for voltage stability analysis. This indicator is tested on a standard IEEE 33 bus radial distribution system. The indicator is used to find the weak lines in the system. Placement of shunt capacitor and FACTS controller at the receiving end side of the weak bus results in improvement of voltage profile of the system. Cuckoo search (CS) algorithm is applied for optimal sizing of shunt capacitor and FACTS controller. Program is coded in MATLAB for the enhancement of voltage stability in the radial distribution system.

Keywords Radial distribution system (RDS) · Voltage stability · Line stability indicator (LSI) · STATCOM · Cuckoo search (CS)

1 Introduction

An electric power system consists of electrical components which are deployed to supply, transfer, and distribute electric power. Distribution system is the main point of link between bulk power generators and consumers; it holds very significant

Mala (✉)
Power Systems, NIE Mysuru, Mysuru, India
e-mail: malamh02@gmail.com

H. V. Saikumar
Department of EEE, NIE Mysuru, Mysuru, India
e-mail: Saihv2003@yahoo.com

© Springer Nature Singapore Pte Ltd. 2019
V. Sridhar et al. (eds.), *Emerging Research in Electronics, Computer Science and Technology*, Lecture Notes in Electrical Engineering 545,
https://doi.org/10.1007/978-981-13-5802-9_119

position in the power system. It is the part of power system which distributes power to various consumers in ready to use form at the place of consumption [1]. Distribution system is classified into radial distribution system, ring main distribution system, and interconnected system. In the radial distribution system, separate feeders radiate from a single substation and feed the distributors at one end only. Electric power flows along a single path, if the power flow is interrupted it results in complete loss of power to the customers.

Voltage stability of the system is characterized by the capability of the system to remain in synchronism and to maintain voltage close to the rated values even in the presence of disturbances [2]. The voltage stability problem of distribution networks is associated with a rapid drop of voltage because of heavy system load. Voltage instability may result in voltage collapse of the system. To meet the reactive power demand and to increase the power transmittable capability of lines reactive power, compensation is provided. Either shunt or series reactive power compensation can be provided. As most of the loads are inductive, compensation is given by connecting shunt capacitors to the line [3].

With the invention of thyristor devices, power electronic converters are developed that led to the implementation of flexible AC transmission systems (FACTS). In FACTS, controllers various power electronic controllers are employed to regulate power flow, transmission voltage and to reduce system losses. STATCOM a shunt connected FACTS controller used to increase the reliability and efficiency of distribution systems due to its various advantages. STATCOM plays an important role in improving voltage regulation, voltage stability, and reduction of system loss of distribution systems under both steady and dynamic conditions [4].

An immense pact of literature work has been reported for placement of shunt facts controllers considering reactive power, improvement in voltage profile, and reduction of loss. Formulation of a stability index named line stability indicator for identifying weakest line in the system is given in [3]. A nature inspired evolutionary computing approach namely cuckoo search (CS) optimization method is applied for optimal capacitor placement in distribution systems [5].

In the work reported in this paper, voltage stability enhancement is done by the use of shunt capacitor and STATCOM. The test system is IEEE 33 bus radial distribution system. The location of the compensating devices has been found by line stability indicator and rating of capacitor and STATCOM independently determined by cuckoo search. The improvement in the voltage profile with these devices has been observed.

2   Line Stability Indicator (LSI)

In the work reported in this paper, LSI is used as an index for determining the weakest bus of the system. LSI is the indicator of line stability, in which the discriminant of the voltage quadratic equation is set to zero to achieve stability [3].

Fig. 1 Two bus equivalent network

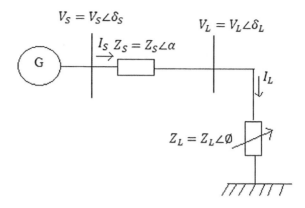

$$V_S = V_S \angle \delta_S$$

$$I_S \ Z_S = Z_S \angle \alpha$$

$$V_L = V_L \angle \delta_L$$

$$Z_L = Z_L \angle \emptyset$$

For the system in Fig. 1, the LSI is given by:
For real roots, the discriminant can be written as,

$$\frac{2\sqrt{Q_L\left(\frac{1}{X} - \frac{\cos\delta}{X}\right)}}{I \cos\delta} \leq 1$$

so, the line stability indicator (LSI) can be writter as

$$LSI = \frac{2\sqrt{Q_L\left(\frac{1}{X} - \frac{\cos\delta}{X}\right)}}{I \cos\delta} \tag{1}$$

where Q_L is the load side reactive power, X is the line reactance, I is the line current, and $\cos\delta$ is the cosine of the phase angle difference of sending end and receiving end voltages.

3 Shunt Capacitor and STATCOM

Shunt capacitors are commonly used at the load side of the distribution feeders for reactive power compensation, because the feeders with large reactive power demands are subjected to large voltage variation as the loading levels change significantly [6]. There are many advantages that can be obtained from placing capacitor like reduction in power loss and regulate the voltage profile at acceptable levels. The capacitor can be modeled as the admittance at the weakest bus. The reactive power injected by the capacitor is directly proportional to the square of the bus voltage for any load condition [7].

Static synchronous compensator (STATCOM) a shunt connected FACTS controller, which uses various power electronic switches to control the reactive power flow through a power network and thereby increasing the stability of power network. STATCOM can generate or absorb reactive power at a faster rate.

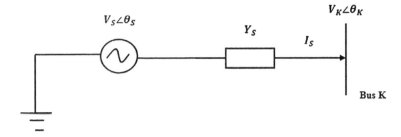

Fig. 2 Equivalent circuit of STATCOM

The STATCOM is represented as voltage source for the full range of operation. The STATCOM equivalent circuit is as shown in Fig. 2.

The power flow equations with STATCOM [7] at bus K can be used to model STATCOM.

4 Problem Formulation

The objective of the optimization problem is to find the optimal size of the capacitor and STATCOM to reduce the power loss and improve the voltage profile of the system under consideration subjected to certain constraints. The objective function of the problem formulation can be expressed as follows:

$$\min f(x_1, x_2) = \sum_{i=1}^{n} P_{loss,l}, Q_{loss,l}, \Delta V \tag{2}$$

Such that the following bus voltage and total reactive power constraints must ensure that all the parameters in the radial distribution system are within their acceptable limit.

Bus voltage constraint:

$$V^{min,i} \leq V_i \leq V^{max,i}$$

where $V^{min,i}$ and $V^{max,i}$ are the minimum and maximum voltage at bus i.

Total reactive power constraint: The total reactive power injection Q_C^{Total} must be less than or equal the total load reactive power Q_L^{Total} as,

$$Q_C^{Total} \leq Q_L^{Total}$$

where $x1$ and $x2$ are the sizes of shunt capacitors in the system, n is the number of branches, $P_{loss,l}$ is the active power loss at each line l and is given by:

$$P_{loss,l} = \sum_{l=1}^{nbr} R_l I_l^2 = \sum_{i=1}^{b} \sum_{\substack{j=1 \\ i \neq j}}^{b} G_{ij}\left[V_i^2 + V_j^2 - 2V_i V_j \cos(\delta_i - \delta_j)\right] \qquad (3)$$

$Q_{loss,l}$ is the reactive power loss at each line l and is given by

$$Q_{loss,l} = \sum_{l=1}^{nbr} X_l I_l^2 = \sum_{i=1}^{b} B_{ij}\left[V_i^2 + V_j^2 - 2V_i V_j \sin(\delta_i - \delta_j)\right] \qquad (4)$$

where n and b are the number of branches and buses, respectively, Il is the line current through the line l, Rl, and Xl are resistance and reactance of the line, G_{ij} is the conductance of the line l between buses i and j, B_{ij} is the susceptance of the line l between buses i and j, V_i and δ_i are the magnitude and angle of voltage at bus i, V_j and δ_j are the magnitude and angle of voltage at bus j. ΔV is the voltage deviation which is the difference between nominal voltage and actual voltage. The formula for voltage deviation is given by:

$$\Delta V = \sum_{i=1}^{n} |V_n - V_i|^2 \qquad (5)$$

where n is the number of buses, V_i is the actual voltage at the ith bus, and V_n is the nominal voltage. The weakest lines are identified by the LSI. The shunt capacitor and STATCOM [8] are optimally sized for improvement of voltage stability and placed at the weakest buses [9]. The objective function and constraints for optimal sizing STATCOM are the same as that of shunt capacitor.

5 Cuckoo Search with Levy Flight

Cuckoo search technique contains a population of eggs and nests. The following representations are used, where each egg in a nest is considered as a solution and a cuckoo egg as a new solution. The cuckoo egg is less likely to be discovered, if it is very similar to the host egg, then the fitness value is related to the difference in solutions. For simplicity in describing the algorithm, there are three idealized rules that are utilized [10]. There are two stages in the process of cuckoo search algorithm. Cuckoo eggs are created and laid into the host bird's nest in the first stage, the other stage includes the probability of abandonment of cuckoo eggs. Levy flight is used to create the cuckoo eggs. The levy flight provides a random walk while the random step length is drawn from the levy distribution. Mantegna equations are used to create the step length for levy flight [11].

In the applied CS algorithm, each cuckoo egg is the objective function, and nest represents size of the capacitor during optimal sizing of capacitor. Objective function (fitness function) is to reduce the total real and reactive power loss and improve voltage profile of the radial distribution system. Nests lie between the specified minimum and maximum range. In general, each cuckoo egg is placed in a random nest, one at a time. When the host bird discovers the alien egg, it is abandoned. In the same way for each size of the capacitor in the specified range, objective function is evaluated using data obtained from the Newton Raphson load flow solution. The obtained fitness function is saved and compared with the values of base case. If the fitness function (voltage and total loss of the system) is better than the base case values then current size of the capacitor, current fitness values are saved. Next step is to choose a next random size of the capacitor and calculating the fitness values using new capacitor size. The new fitness values and size of the capacitor are compared with a saved fitness and size of capacitor, the better results are saved. The procedure is carried out until the objective function, i.e., the total real and reactive power losses of the system are minimized and voltage profile of the system is improved. Best nest implies best size of capacitor and best fitness function is the best objective function where total system losses are minimized and voltage profile of the system is improved. Similarly in the optimal sizing of STATCOM, each nest represents size of the STATCOM and cuckoo egg is the objective function.

6 Proposed Methodology

Newton Raphson load flow analysis is carried out on the IEEE 33 bus system. Line flows, losses, magnitude, and angle of the voltage are obtained from the load flow. From the parameters obtained from load flow, the proposed index, i.e., Line Stability Indicator (LSI) for all lines is calculated. The weakest line is found by the value of LSI. The line with the largest index with respect to a bus is considered the most critical line of that bus and the reactive power control device is placed in the load side of the critical line, so that total real and reactive power losses will decrease and voltage level of the buses will increase. Cuckoo search optimization is applied for the optimal sizing of shunt capacitor and STATCOM. The optimal sizing of the capacitor and STATCOM is done such that it results in improvement of voltage profile of the system and reduction of loss. The solution methodology is tested on system under consideration.

7 Results and Discussion

The solution methodology is tested on standard IEEE 33 bus system. Newton Raphson load flow analysis is carried out and results are given in Table 1.

Table 1 Base case load flow result

Total active power generation	3.918 MW
Total reactive power generation	2.435 MVar
Total active load	3.715 MW
Total reactive load	2.3 MVar
Total active power loss	203 kW
Total reactive power loss	135 kVar

Fig. 3 Base case voltage profile

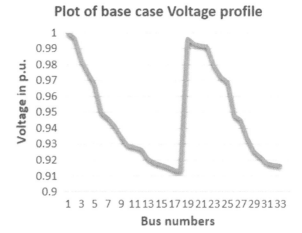

Plot of base case Voltage profile

Table 2 LSI values for critical lines

Line No.	Connected between buses	LSI
17	17–18	1.0928
32	32–33	1.0967

Figure 3 gives the voltage values at all the buses in the test system. The minimum voltage of proposed system is 0.9130 p.u. at node 18 (Fig. 4).

Load flow program is done in MATLAB to obtain various parameters of the system under consideration. From these parameters, the value of LSI for all lines is obtained. Table 2 gives the LSI values for critical lines. The index can have a value above 1 if the system is about to suffer a voltage collapse. The line that presents the largest index with respect to a bus is considered the most critical line of that bus. From Table 2, it is clear that weakest lines are line number 17 which is connected between buses 17 and 18 and line number 32 which is connected between buses 32 and 33. Reactive power control device is placed in the load side of the most critical line, so that total real and reactive power losses will reduce and voltage level of the buses will improve.

Table 3 shows the candidate locations and sizes of capacitors. The improvement in the voltage profile of the system before and after placing the shunt capacitors at the weakest buses is given in Tables 4 and 5.

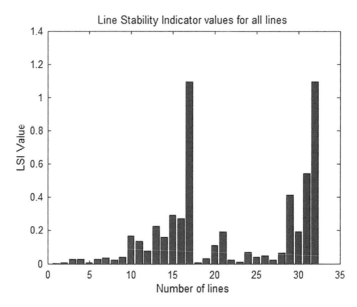

Fig. 4 Bar chart showing LSI values of all lines

Table 3 Optimal sizes of capacitors obtained from cuckoo search

Candidate buses	Capacitor size (kVar)
18	318
33	838

Table 4 Line losses with and without capacitor at buses 18, 33, and both

Parameter	Base case	At bus 18	At bus 33	At buses 18 and 33
Total reactive Power Loss (kVAR)	135	124	106	100
Total active Power Loss (kW)	203	185	155	146

Table 5 Voltage profile improvement before and after capacitor placement

Bus No	Voltages before capacitor placement	Voltages after placing capacitor	Voltages after placing capacitor	Voltages after capacitor placement
		At bus 18	At bus 33	At buses 18 and 33
1	1	1	1	1
2	0.99703	0.99714	0.99733	0.99743
3	0.98294	0.98362	0.9848	0.98545
4	0.97545	0.97657	0.97848	0.97953
5	0.96806	0.96961	0.97228	0.97376
6	0.94965	0.95279	0.95817	0.96118
7	0.94617	0.95063	0.95472	0.95905
8	0.94132	0.94632	0.94992	0.95477
9	0.93506	0.94167	0.94371	0.95017
10	0.92924	0.93749	0.93795	0.94602
11	0.92838	0.93677	0.93709	0.94532
12	0.92687	0.93555	0.9356	0.94411
13	0.92076	0.93198	0.92954	0.94057
14	0.91849	0.93128	0.9273	0.93987
15	0.91708	0.93102	0.9259	0.93962
16	0.91571	0.93084	0.92455	0.93944
17	0.91368	0.93257	0.92254	0.94115
18	**0.91308**	**0.93322**	**0.92194**	**0.9418**
19	0.9965	0.99661	0.9968	0.9969
20	0.99293	0.99304	0.99322	0.99332
21	0.99222	0.99233	0.99252	0.99262
22	0.99158	0.99169	0.99188	0.99198
23	0.97935	0.98004	0.98122	0.98187
24	0.97268	0.97337	0.97456	0.97522
25	0.96935	0.97004	0.97124	0.97189
26	0.94773	0.95086	0.95687	0.95988
27	0.94516	0.94831	0.95518	0.9582
28	0.93372	0.93691	0.94932	0.95236
29	0.9255	0.92872	0.9453	0.94835
30	0.92195	0.92517	0.94329	0.94636
31	0.91778	0.92103	0.94478	0.94783
32	0.91687	0.92011	0.94597	0.94903
33	**0.91659**	**0.91983**	**0.94876**	**0.95181**

Fig. 5 Plot of voltage profile before and after capacitor placement

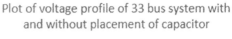
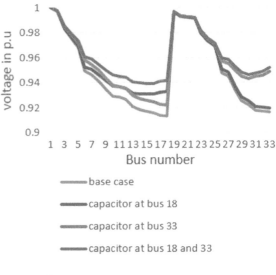

Fig. 6 Plot of voltage profile before and after STATCOM placement

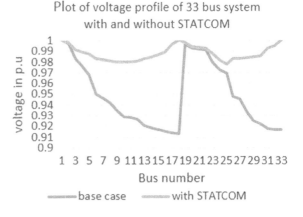

The voltage profile of the system under consideration when shunt capacitor is placed at bus 18, bus 33, and both weakest buses is given in Figs. 5 and 6.

The bus voltages and total loss of the test system after the placement of shunt capacitor at buses 18, 33, and at both weakest buses are compared with the base case values. In all the cases, there is a reduction in total system loss and improvement in the voltage profile. By comparing the results, it is observed that placement of shunt capacitors at both weakest buses shows much improvement in the voltage profile of the test system along with total system loss minimization. The candidate buses and optimal size of STATCOM are given in Table 6. Table 8 gives the voltage profile improvement after the placement of STATCOM. By comparing the voltage profile

Table 6 Sizes and candidate buses for STATCOM

Candidate buses	STATCOM size (kVar)
18	520
33	910

Table 7 Loss before and after placement of STATCOM at both weakest buses

Parameter	Base case	With STATCOM
Active power loss (kW)	203	47
Reactive power loss (kVar)	135	38

and total losses of the radial distribution system before and after the placement of shunt capacitor and STATCOM one at a time, results show that there is improvement in voltage profile of the radial distribution system and total loss minimization compared to base case. But STATCOM shows better performance than shunt capacitor. The improvement in voltage profile and loss reduction is more when STATCOM is placed at the weakest buses than the shunt capacitor (Table 7).

Table 8 Voltage profile of the test system before and after STATCOM placement

Bus No	Before STATCOM placement	After STATCOM placement at buses 18 and 33
1	1	1
2	0.99703	0.99836
3	0.98294	0.99137
4	0.97545	0.98914
5	0.96806	0.9872
6	0.94965	0.98314
7	0.94617	0.98223
8	0.94132	0.98064
9	0.93506	0.98021
10	0.92924	0.98027
11	0.92838	0.98029
12	0.92687	0.98047
13	0.92076	0.98284
14	0.91849	0.98452
15	0.91708	0.98663
16	0.91571	0.98934
17	0.91368	0.99656
18	**0.91308**	**1**

(continued)

Table 8 (continued)

Bus No	Before STATCOM placement	After STATCOM placement at buses 18 and 33
19	0.9965	0.99783
20	0.99293	0.99426
21	0.99222	0.99356
22	0.99158	0.99292
23	0.97935	0.98782
24	0.97268	0.98121
25	0.96935	0.9779
26	0.94773	0.98307
27	0.94516	0.98309
28	0.93372	0.98362
29	0.9255	0.98442
30	0.92195	0.98543
31	0.91778	0.99246
32	0.91687	0.99539
33	**0.91659**	**1**

8   Conclusion

Voltage stability is major concern in power system operation. Voltage stability analysis and its improvement are necessary to operate the system under stable state. In the work reported in this paper, the indicator is formulated and tested on standard IEEE 33 bus RDS. Line stability index is used to find the critical lines of the test system. At the weakest buses, shunt capacitor and STATCOM are placed one at a time. This has resulted in improvement of voltage profile and reduction of total real and reactive power losses.

The work presented an application of cuckoo search optimization technique for sizing the capacitor and STATCOM. It provides good results with a minimum computational effort. The major contribution of this work is application of an algorithm for optimal allocation of FACTS controller in a radial distribution system for improvement of tail end node voltages and power loss reduction. The proposed approach for STATCOM placement in distribution system shows effective performance for the test system.

Appendix

Standard IEEE 33 Bus Radial Distribution System

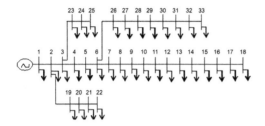

Branch number	Sending bus	Receiving bus	Resistance Ω	Resistance Ω	Nominal load at receiving bus	
					P (kW)	Q (kVAR)
1	1	2	0.0922	0.047	100	60
2	2	3	0.493	0.2511	90	40
3	3	4	0.366	0.1864	120	80
4	4	5	0.3811	0.1941	60	30
5	5	6	0.819	0.707	60	20
6	6	7	0.1872	0.6188	200	100
7	7	8	0.7114	0.2351	200	100
8	8	9	1.03	0.74	60	20
9	9	10	1.044	0.74	60	20
10	10	11	0.1966	0.065	45	30
11	11	12	0.3744	0.1298	60	35
12	12	13	1.463	1.155	60	35
13	13	14	0.5416	0.7192	120	80
14	14	15	0.591	0.526	60	10
15	15	16	0.7463	0.545	60	20
16	16	17	1.289	1.721	60	20
17	17	18	0.732	0.574	90	40
18	2	19	0.164	0.1565	90	40
19	19	20	1.5042	1.3554	90	40
20	20	21	0.4095	0.4734	90	40
21	21	22	0.7059	0.9373	90	40
22	3	23	0.4512	0.3053	90	50
23	23	24	0.898	0.7091	420	200
24	24	25	0.896	0.7011	420	200
25	6	26	0.203	0.1034	60	25

(continued)

(continued)

Branch number	Sending bus	Receiving bus	Resistance Ω	Resistance Ω	Nominal load at receiving bus	
					P (kW)	Q (kVAR)
26	26	27	0.2842	0.1447	60	25
27	27	2S	1.059	0.9337	60	20
28	28	29	0.5042	0.7006	120	70
29	29	30	0.5075	0.2535	200	100
30	30	31	0.9744	0.963	150	70
31	31	32	0.3105	0.3619	210	100
32	32	33	0.341	0.5362	60	40

References

1. Sadat H (2002) Power system analysis. McGraw Hill Series Publications
2. Al Abri RS, El Saadany EF, Atwa YM (2013) Optimal placement and sizing method to improve the voltage stability margin in a distribution system using distributed generation. IEEE Trans Power Syst 28(1):326–334
3. Chakraborty K, Deb G, Deb S (2016) Voltage stability assessment in radial distribution system by line stability indicator (LSI) and its improvement using SVC. In: First IEEE international conference on power electronics, intelligent control and energy systems, vol 16, pp 1–5
4. Majumder Ritwik (2014) Aspect of voltage stability and reactive power support in active distribution. IET Gener Transm Distrib 8(3):442–450
5. Arcanjo DN, Luiz J, Pereira R, Oliveira EJ, Peres W, de Oliveira LW, da Silva Junior IC (2013) Cuckoo search optimization technique applied to capacitor placement on distribution system problem. IET Gener Transm Distrib 7(8):898–904
6. Idris RM, Zaid NM (2016) Optimal shunt capacitor placement in radial distribution system. IEEE Trans Power Deliv 3:18–22
7. Pavan Kumar Y, Phani Raju HB (2014) Static voltage stability margin enhancement using shunt compensating devices. Electr Power Syst Res 7:1–6
8. Reis C, Maciel Barbosa FP (2009) Line indices for voltage stability assessment. In: IEEE Bucharest power tech conference, vol 25, no 3, pp 1–7
9. Nagesh HB, Puttaswamy PS (2012) Power flow model of static VAR compensator and enhancement of voltage stability. Int J Adv Eng Technol 3(2):499–507
10. Yang X-S, Deb S (2009) Cuckoo search via Levy flights. In: IEEE conference on nature and biologically inspired computing, vol 28, no 4, pp 210–214
11. Nguyen KP, Fujita G, Dieu VN (2016) Cuckoo search algorithm for optimal placement and sizing of static VAR compensator in large-scale power systems. J Artif Intell Soft Comput Res 6(2):59–68

Optimal Siting and Sizing of DG Employing Multi-objective Particle Swarm Optimization for Network Loss Reduction and Voltage Profile Improvement

Rudrayya Math and N. Kumar

Abstract Day by day employing Distributed Generation (DG) is increasing and it is becoming an indispensable small capacity generation in the distribution system. It is cost effective, eco-friendly and it can enhance the reliability of the distribution network. This paper proposes a technique for optimal sizing and siting of DG, using modified Particle Swarm Optimization technique. It is proposed for optimal placement and sizing of DG. Since the objective is both reduction of losses and voltage profile improvement the multi objective function is chosen and by choosing appropriately desired level of emphasis is given to both the objectives. Also, by using an index Multi Objective Ranking Index (MORI) the best combination of loss reduction and voltage profile improvement is obtained. The effectiveness of the methodology is tested on standard IEEE-33 bus system and results are presented.

Keywords Distributed generation · Optimal size · Multi-objective optimization · Particle swarm optimization · Voltage deviation index · Power loss reduction index · Multi objective ranking index

1 Introduction

Large scale conventional power plants are located far away from load centers. Conventional large power plants such as thermal power stations, nuclear power plants, and hydro power plants are located far away from the load centers. As the load demand is increasing day by day on distribution system, there is a need for electrical energy near load center itself. This is achieved by placing the energy source near load centers, that energy source is known as distributed generation (DG).

R. Math (✉)
NIE Mysuru, Mysuru, India
e-mail: math.rudrayya@gmail.com

N. Kumar
Department of EEE, NIE Mysuru, Mysuru, India
e-mail: nkmysore@gmail.com

© Springer Nature Singapore Pte Ltd. 2019
V. Sridhar et al. (eds.), *Emerging Research in Electronics, Computer Science and Technology*, Lecture Notes in Electrical Engineering 545,
https://doi.org/10.1007/978-981-13-5802-9_120

According Institute of Electrical and Electronic Engineers (IEEE), DG is defined as distributed resources of electrical power that are not directly connected to a bulk power transmission system. After deregulation of the vertically integrated system DG penetration has become more. In recent years, due to rapid growth in population and industries there is a deficit of power to the consumers, even in such scenario quite a significant amount of power generated is wasted as I^2R loss in distribution network [1].

By locating the DG at optimal size at optimal location network performance improves significantly by the way of improvement in the voltage profile and reduction in the network losses. Further it improves the power quality and reliability of the system. In this work for optimal siting and sizing of DG, Particle Swarm Optimization technique been proposed [2]. DG's are located near the load centers and generally they are not connected to high voltage transmission network directly [3].

2 Present Study of the Work in This Area

Sufficient work has been carried out in the area of optimal siting and sizing of DG. Optimal placement of DG for network loss reduction using analytical approach has been discussed in [5]. In a deregulated environment of the power sector multi objective optimization approach for maximizing voltage profile is discussed in [6]. A technique using Tabu search algorithm is demonstrated for optimal siting and sizing of DG in [7]. For optimal deployment of DG units to reduce system losses using genetic algorithm (GA) has been discussed in [8, 9]. In this paper, the problem of optimum size of a DG source and its optimum location has been determined using particle swarm optimization (PSO). This is tested on standard IEEE-33 bus radial distribution network.

3 Problem Formulation

The problem of optimum optimal siting and sizing of DG is formulated in the form of swarm optimization [10]. The multi objective function of voltage profile improvement and network loss reduction is given below,

a. Minimize

$$f(x) = \sum_{i=1}^{N} W_1 * loss + \sum_{i=1}^{N} W_2 * (1 - V_i)^2 \tag{1}$$

$$W_1 + W_2 = 1 \tag{2}$$

where,

loss   Network real power loss.

W_1 is the weighting factor giving priority to reduction of real power losses and W_2 is weighting factor giving priority to voltage profile improvement. Different weighting factors are assigned in such a way that it should satisfy Eq. (1) and ranging from 0 to 1 in the interval 0.1.

The problem is being tested on standard IEEE-33 bus system. This methodology first runs Newton Raphson load flow method to find the losses and voltage profile improvement secondly it runs PSO algorithm to run to determine the optimum size and location of DG.

And also find the Voltage Deviation Index (VDI) and Power Loss Reduction Index (PLRI) and Multi Objective Ranking Index (MORI).

$$VDI = \sum_{i=1}^{N_{bus}} \frac{(V_i - V_n)^2}{V_n^2} \tag{3}$$

where,

V_n is the nominal voltage in pu. In this it is taken as 1 pu.
V_i is the voltage at the ith bus in pu.

$$PLRI = \frac{PL_{(DG)}}{PL} \tag{4}$$

where,

$PL_{(DG)}$ is the distribution system real loss when DG is connected to the ith bus.
PL is the distribution system power loss without DG connection.

$$MORI = VDI \times PLRI \tag{5}$$

3.1 Constraints

a. Bus Voltage Constraints: The voltage at each bus should be within the specified limits.

$$V_{min} \le V_i \le V_{max}$$
$$i = 1, 2, \ldots, no. \, of \, buses \tag{6}$$

V_{min} is the minimum acceptable voltage at any bus;
V_{max} is the maximum allowable voltage at any bus;

V_i is the voltage of any bus i.

b. Line Load ability Limit: Power flow in the line should not exceed the permissible value.

$$P_{line(i,j)} < P_{line(i,j)max} \tag{7}$$

$P_{line\ (i,\ j)}$ is the line flow between nodes i and j;
$P_{line\ (i,j)max}$ is the maximum line flow capacity of line between nodes i and j.

c. DG Capacity constraint: The total DG power injected should be less than total load and total real power loss.

$$\sum_{i=1}^{Nbus} P_{DGi} = \sum_{i=1}^{Nbus} (P_i + P_L) \tag{8}$$

N_{bus} Total no. of buses.

3.2 Equations

a. Optimal Location of DG:

$$\alpha_i = \frac{\partial P_L}{\partial P_i} = 2\alpha_{ii}P_i + 2\sum_{\substack{j=1 \\ j \neq i}}^{N} \left(\alpha_{ij}P_j - \beta_{ij}Q_j\right) \tag{9}$$

b. Optimal sizing of DG:

$$P_{DGi} = P_{Di} + \frac{1}{\alpha_{ii}} \left[\beta_{ii}Q_i - \sum_{\substack{j=1 \\ j \neq i}}^{N} \left(\alpha_{ij}P_j - \beta_{ij}Q_j\right) \right] \tag{10}$$

P_{DGi} Real power injection from DG
P_{Di} Demand at node i.

4 Particle Swarm Optimization

PSO is an algorithm based on population called swarm and it is first introduced by Eberhart and Kennedy [11]. Swarm consists a group of individuals called particles and each particle moves in N-dimensional search space randomly generated velocity. Each particles velocity and position and is updated by using below Eqs. (1) and (2).

$$V_j(i) = V_j(i-1) + r_1\left(P_{best,j} - x_j(i)\right) + r_2\left(G_{best} - x_j(i)\right)$$
$$j = 1, 2, \ldots, n \tag{11}$$

$$x_j(i) = x_j(i-1) + v_j(i)$$
$$j = 1, 2, \ldots n \tag{12}$$

where, i = iteration, j = Particle Number.
   Modification to Algorithm

$$V_j(i) = \theta V_j(i-1) + r_1\left(P_{best,j} - x_j(i)\right) + r_2\left(G_{best} - x_j(i)\right)$$
$$j = 1, 2, \ldots, n \tag{13}$$

where,

$$\theta(i) = \theta_{max} - \left(\frac{\theta_{max} - \theta_{min}}{i_{max}}\right)i \tag{14}$$

where, θ_{max} is initial value and θ_{min} is the final values of the inertia weight, and i_{max} is the maximum number of iterations used in PSO. The values of $\theta_{max} = 0.9$ and $\theta_{min} = 0.4$ are usually used.
   The PSO-based approach for solving the optimal placement of DG problem to minimize the loss and improving voltage profile takes the following steps:

[i]   Calculate the loss using NR load flow method
[ii] Randomly generates an initial population (array) of particles with random positions and velocities on dimensions in the solution space. Set the iteration counter k = 0.
[iii] For each particle (bus) bus voltage is within limits, evaluate the total system losses using the Newton Raphson Load flow.
[iv] For each particle, if the objective value is lower than Pbest, set this value as current Pbest.
[v]   Choose the particle associated with minimum individual best Pbest of all particles, and set the value of this as the current overall best Gbest.
[vi] If iteration number reaches the maximum limit, print the results.

5 Results and Discussion

The solution methodology has been tested on IEEE-33 bus radial distribution test system. It is a radial distribution system with total active load of 3.715 MW and reactive load of 2.3 Mvar. A Newton Raphson load flow method is used to solve the load flow problem for radial distribution system. PSO technique is used to find the optimum size of DG and optimum location. Simulation is done in MATLAB software of version R2016b and this work is done on standard IEEE-33 bus system.

a. Results for base case
The Newton Raphson load flow is run on standard IEEE-33 bus system and the results are tabulated in Table 1. Figure 1 gives the voltage profile of the base case.

b. Optimal allocation of DG
The algorithm is run for different values of weighting factors W_1 and W_2. W_1 is the weighting factor associated with the system losses and W_2 is the weighting factor associated with the voltage profile. The sum of W_1 and W_2 is 1.0 and the algorithm is run starting from $W_1 = 1$ and $W_2 = 0$. The value of W_1 is reduced in steps and at each step its value is reduced by 0.1 until W_1 becomes equal to zero. For different combinations of weighting factors W_1 and W_2 Table 2 gives the resulting system loss, Table 3 voltage deviation index (VDI) and Table 4 gives multi objective ranking index (MORI) values (Figs. 2 and 3).

   The best case is that combination of W_1 and W_2 which gives minimum value of MORI. It is seen from the Table 4 and Fig. 4 that best combination of W_1 and W_2 is

Table 1 Base case load flow result		
Total active power generation	3.925 MW
Total reactive power generation	2.442 Mvar
Total active load	3.715 MW
Total reactive load	2.3 Mvar
Total active power loss	0.211 MW
Total reactive power loss	0.143 Mvar

Fig. 1 Base case voltage profile

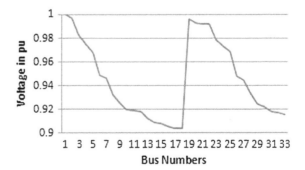

Table 2 Power losses for various weighting factors

W_1 and W_2	Losses (kW)
1 and 0	111.39
0.9 and 0.1	136.33
0.8 and 0.2	187.83
0.7 and 0.3	184.87
0.6 and 0.4	221.8
0.5 and 0.5	232.09
0.4 and 0.6	237.61
0.3 and 0.7	249.76
0.2 and 0.8	286.95
0.1 and 0.9	256.8
0 and 1	279.12

Table 3 VDI values for various weighting factors

W_1 and W_2	VDI
1 and 0	0.033501
0.9 and 0.1	0.00944
0.8 and 0.2	0.004724
0.7 and 0.3	0.01119
0.6 and 0.4	0.024345
0.5 and 0.5	0.026258
0.4 and 0.6	0.27633
0.3 and 0.7	0.028429
0.2 and 0.8	0.31801
0.1 and 0.9	0.2897
0 and 1	0.030997

Table 4 MORI values for various weighting factors

W_1 and W_2	MORI
1 and 0	0.017686
0.9 and 0.1	0.006099
0.8 and 0.2	**0.0042052**
0.7 and 0.3	0.0.0098041
0.6 and 0.4	0.025591
0.5 and 0.5	0.028882
0.4 and 0.6	0.031118
0.3 and 0.7	0.033651
0.2 and 0.8	0.043248
0.1 and 0.9	0.035258
0 and 1	0.041004

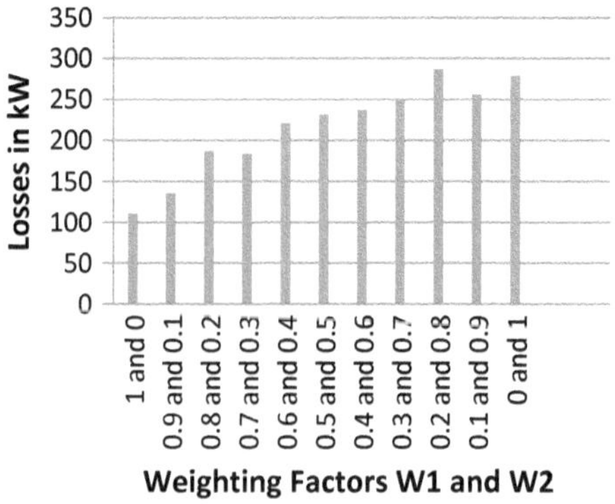

Fig. 2 Losses for various
weighting factor

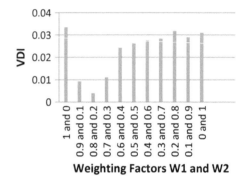

Fig. 3 VDI values for
various weighting factors

Fig. 4 MORI values for
various weighting factors

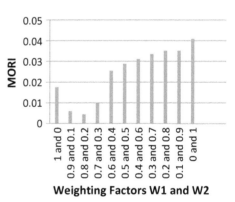

0.8 and 0.2 respectively. Correspondingly the optimal location and size of the DG is given in the following Table 5. The base case losses are also given in the table.

Figure 5 pictorially represents comparison of the system losses of base case and the best case and Fig. 6 pictorially represents the best case voltage profile compared with base case voltage profile.

Table 5 Optimal location and size of DG

Weighting factors		Optimal bus	Optimal size	System real losses for best case	System real losses for base case
W1	W2	8	4 MW	187.83 kW	211 kW
0.8	0.2				

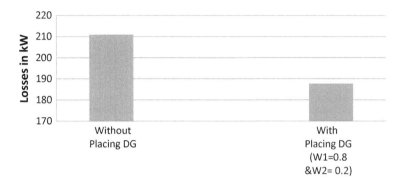

Fig. 5 Comparison of system real losses of base case and best case

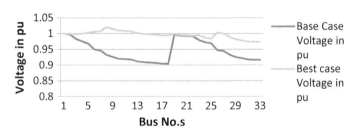

Fig. 6 Comparison of voltage profile of base case and best case

Table 6 Optimal location and size of DG exclusive for maximum loss reduction

Weighting factors		Optimal bus	Optimal size	System real losses
W1	W2	6	2.6006 MW	111.1 kW
1	0			

c. Exclusive for maximum reduction in system losses

For maximum loss reduction the values of W1 and W2 is 1 and 0 respectively, correspondingly the optimal location and size of the DG is given in the following Table 6.

References

1. Prakash DB, Lakshminarayana C (2016) MPSO based DG and capacitor placement for loss reduction. J Electr Eng
2. Mahajan S, Vadhera S (2016) Optimal sizing and deploying of distributed generation unit using a modified multi objective particle swarm optimisation. In: IEEE 6th International conference on power systems (ICPS)
3. Prakash DB, Lakshminarayana C (2016) MPSO based DG and capacitor placement for loss reduction. J Electr Eng
4. El-Khattam W, Salama MMA (2004) Distribution generation technologies, definitions and benefits. Electr Power Syst Res 71:119–128
5. Acharya N, Mahat P, Mithulananthan N (2006) An analytical approach for DG allocation in primary distribution network. Electr Power Syst Res 28:657–678
6. Kumar A, Gao W (2008) Voltage profile improvement and line loss reduction with distributed generation in deregulated electricity markets. In: IEEE Region 10 conference TENCON
7. Nara K, Hayashi Y, Ikeda K, Ashizawa T (2001) Application of tabu search to optimal placement of distributed generators. IEEE PES winter meeting, vol 2, pp 918–923
8. Celli G, Ghiani E, Mocci S, Pilo F (2005) A multiobjective evolutionary algorithm for the sizing and siting of distributed generation. IEEE Trans Power Syst 20:750–757
9. Abou El-Ela AA, Allam SM, Shatla MM (2010) Maximal optimal benefits of distributed generation using genetic algorithms. Electr Power Syst Res 80:857–877
10. Mahajan S, Vadhera S (2016) Optimal sizing and deploying of distributed generation unit using a modified multi objective particle swarm optimization. In: 6th IEEE conference on power systems, New Delhi, India
11. Kennedy J, Eberhart RC (1995) Particle swarm optimization. In: Proceedings of IEEE conference on neural networks, IV, Piscataway, New Jersey, pp 1942–1948

Author Index

Printed by Printforce, the Netherlands